Paediatric Handbook

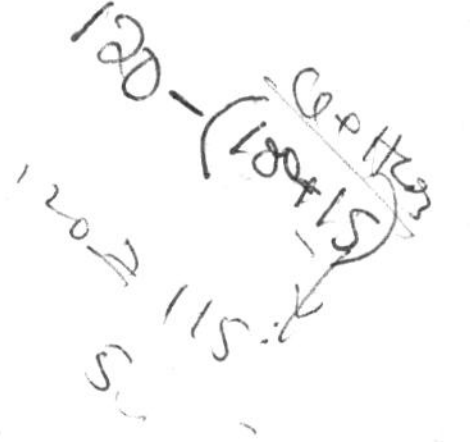

Paediatric Handbook

Seventh Edition

Editors
GEORGIA PAXTON
JANE MUNRO

Associate editor
MICHAEL MARKS

b
Blackwell
Science

Editorial Offices:

9600 Garsington Road,
Oxford OX4 2DQ, UK
23 Ainslie Place, Edinburgh
EH3 6AJ, UK
350 Main Street, Malden,
MA 02148, USA
550 Swanston Street, Carlton
Victoria 3053, Australia
10, rue Casimir Delavigne
Paris 75006, France

Other Editorial Offices:

Blackwell Publishing KK
NK Building, 3F
2-8-12 Iwamotocho, Chiyoda-ku
Tokyo 101-0032, Japan

Iowa State Press
A Blackwell Publishing Company
2121 State Avenue
Ames, Iowa 50014-8300, USA

Set by Graphicraft Ltd, Hong Kong
Production by Blackwell Publishing
Asia Pty

DISTRIBUTORS

Australia

Blackwell Publishing Asia Pty Ltd
550 Swanston Street
Carlton, Victoria 3053, Australia

Orders Tel: +61 3 8359 1011
Fax: +61 3 8359 1120

The Americas

Blackwell Publishing
c/o AIDC
P.O. Box 20
Williston, VT 05495-0020, USA

Orders Tel: +1 800 216 2522
Fax: +1 802 864 7626

Outside Australia and the Americas

Marston Book Services Ltd
P.O. Box 269
Abingdon, Oxon, OX14 4YN, UK

Orders Tel: +44 1235 465 500
Fax: +44 1235 465 555

Cataloguing-in-Publication Data
Paediatric handbook.

7th ed.
Includes index.
ISBN 0 86793 431 X.

1. Pediatrics-Handbooks,manuals, etc.. 2. Children-Hospital care-Handbooks, manuals, etc. I. Marks, Michael, 1961–. II. Munro, Jane, 1973–. III Paxton, Georgia, 1972–.

618.92

For further information on
Blackwell Publishing, visit our website:
www.blackwellpublishing.com

CONTENTS

CONTENTS

DEVELOPMENT

PSYCHOSOCIAL PROBLEMS

MEDICINE AND SURGERY

CONTRIBUTORS

All authors are staff or associates of the Royal Children's Hospital (RCH) unless otherwise indicated.

Roger Allen	Paediatric Rheumatologist Department of General Paediatrics
Peter Barnett	Deputy Director, Department of Emergency Medicine Honorary Senior Lecturer, Department of Paediatrics, University of Melbourne
Robert Berkowitz	Director, Department of Otolaryngology Associate Professor, Department of Paediatrics, University of Melbourne
Julie Bines	Paediatric Gastroenterologist, Head of Clinical Nutrition, Department of Gastroenterology and Clinical Nutrition Associate Professor, Department of Paediatrics, University of Melbourne
Avihu Boneh	Director, Metabolic Service
Fergus Cameron	Deputy Director, Department of Endocrinology and Diabetes Senior Lecturer, Department of Paediatrics, University of Melbourne
Jonathan Carapetis	Consultant in Paediatric Infectious Diseases, Department of General Paediatrics Senior Lecturer, Department of Paediatrics, University of Melbourne Research Fellow, Murdoch Children's Research Institute
George Chalkiadis	Paediatric Anaesthetist, Pain Medicine Specialist Department of Anaesthesia and Pain Management

Noel Cranswick	Director, Clinical Pharmacology Director, Australian Paediatric Pharmacology Research Unit Associate Professor, University of Melbourne
Andrew Court	Paediatric Psychiatrist Mental Health Service
Nigel Curtis	Paediatrician and Head of Paediatric Infectious Diseases Unit, Department of General Medicine Senior Lecturer, Department of Paediatrics, University of Melbourne
Margot Davey	Paediatrician, Centre for Community Child Health and Melbourne Children's Sleep Unit
Lex Doyle	Neonatal Paediatrician Royal Women's Hospital Associate Professor, Department of Paediatrics, University of Melbourne
Daryl Efron	Paediatrician Department of General Paediatrics
James Elder	Director, Department of Ophthalmology
Kay Gibbons	Manager, Nutrition Services Hon. Senior Lecturer, Department of Medicine, Monash University
H Kerr Graham	Orthopaedic Surgeon Professor, Department of Paediatrics, University of Melbourne
Sonia Grover	Gynaecologist, Department of Paediatric and Adolescent Gynaecology Clinical Fellow, Department of Paediatrics, University of Melbourne
Michael Harari	Paediatrician, Department of General Paediatrics
Simon Harvey	Epileptologist, Director, Children's Epilepsy Program, Department of Neurology

CONTRIBUTORS

Marina Hughes	Cardiologist, Department of Cardiology
John Hutson	Director, Department of General Surgery Professor of Paediatric Surgery, Department of Paediatrics, University of Melbourne Associate Director, Clinical Research, MCRI
Jenny Hynson	Paediatrician, Victorian Paediatric Palliative Care Program
David James	Paediatrician, Department of General Paediatrics
Colin Jones	Nephrologist and Director, Department of Nephrology Associate Professor, Department of Paediatrics, University of Melbourne
Steven Kahler	Clinical Geneticist
Andrew Kemp	Director Immunology Paediatrician, Department General Paediatrics Consultant Department Allergy Professor, Department of Paediatrics, University of Melbourne
Nicky Kilpatrick	Paediatric Dentist, Department of Dentistry, Royal Children's Hospital Associate Professor, Department of Paediatrics, University of Melbourne
Chris Kimber	Surgeon, Department of General Surgery Burn Surgeon, Victorian Paediatric Burn Centre
Andrew Kornberg	Neurologist, Department of Neurology Associate Professor, Department of Paediatrics, University of Melbourne
Lionel Lubitz	Paediatrician, Department of Paediatrics, University of Melbourne
James Lucas	Paediatric Dentist, Department of Dentistry, Royal Children's Hospital

Maria McCarthy	Family Therapist, Mental Health Service
Peter McDougall	Director, Division of Medicine Director, Department of Neonatology
Wirginia Maixner	Director Department of Neurosurgery
Catherine Marraffa	Deputy Director, Department of Child Development and Rehabilitation
Michael Marks	Paediatrician, Department of General Paediatrics Senior Lecturer, Department of Paediatrics, University of Melbourne
John Massie	Respiratory Physician, Department of Respiratory Medicine
Michele Meehan	Maternal and Child Health Nurse Consultant
Paul Monagle	Paediatric Haematologist, Director, Division Laboratory Services Associate Professor, Principle Fellow, Department of Paediatrics, University of Melbourne
Colin Morley	Director of Neonatal Medicine Royal Women's Hospital Professor, Department of Paediatrics, University of Melbourne
Annie Moulden	Director Clinical Support Services Paediatrician
Jane Munro	Rheumatology Fellow Department of General Paediatrics
Margot Nash	Paediatrician, Department of General Paediatrics
Mark Oliver	Paediatric Gastroenterologist
Ed Oakley	Consultant Department of Emergency Medicine

George Patton	Director of Adolescent Health Professor, Department of Paediatrics, University of Melbourne
Campbell Paul	Acting Clinical Director Mental Health Service Consultant Child & Adolescent Psychiatrist Associate Professor, Department of Paediatrics, University of Melbourne Honorary Principal Fellow, Infant Mental Health Program, Department Psychiatry, University of Melbourne
Georgia Paxton	Paediatric Fellow, Department of General Paediatrics
Dan Penny	Director of Cardiology Professorial Fellow, Department of Paediatrics, University of Melbourne
Rod Phillips	Paediatrician, Department of General Paediatrics and Centre for Adolescent Health Senior Lecturer, Department of Paediatrics, University of Melbourne
Glynis Price	Endocrinologist Department of Endocrinology and Diabetes
Dinah Reddihough	Director, Department of Child Development and Rehabilitation
Sheena Reilly	Professor of Paediatric Speech Pathology, Speech Pathology Department, School of Human Communication Sciences, La Trobe University
James Rice	Paediatrician Department of General Paediatrics
John Rogers	Senior Clinical Geneticist Genetic Health Services Victoria
Jenny Royle	Paediatrician, Immunisation Service, Department of General Paediatrics

Christine Sanderson Paediatrician, Barwon Health, Geelong Hospital
Senior Lecturer, University of Melbourne

Susan Sawyer Deputy Director, Centre for Adolescent Health
Associate Professor, Department of Paediatrics, The University of Melbourne

Frank Shann Director of Intensive Care
Professor of Critical Care Medicine, University of Melbourne

Yashwant Sinha Paediatric Fellow
Clinical Pharmacology

Sue Skull Deputy Director, Clinical Epidemiology and Biostatistics Unit
Senior Lecturer, Department of Paediatrics, University of Melbourne

Anne Smith Paediatrician, Department of General Paediatrics
Senior Paediatrician, Gatehouse Centre for the Assessment and Treatment of Child Abuse

Mike Starr Consultant in Paediatric Infectious Diseases, Department of General Paediatrics

Mike South Director, Department of General Medicine
Associate Professor & Deputy Head, University of Melbourne

John Su Dermatologist
Department of Dermatology

Mimi Tang Allergist Immunologist, Department of Immunology
Group Leader, Asthma Allergy Immunology Research, MCRI

Russell Taylor Surgeon, Department of General Surgery
Burn Surgeon, Victorian Paediatric Burn Centre

James Tibballs Intensive Care
Associate Professor and Principal Fellow,
Departments of Pharmacology and Paediatrics,
University of Melbourne

Karen Tiedemann Paediatrician, Department of Haematology and Oncology

George Varigos Head of Unit,
Department of Dermatology

Garry Warne Senior Endocrinologist
Director, RCH International
Associate Professor, Department of Paediatrics,
University of Melbourne

George Werther Director, Department of Endocrinology and Diabetes and Centre for Hormone Research
Professorial Fellow, Department of Paediatrics,
University of Melbourne

Dominic Wilkinson Fellow in Paediatrics and Information Technology
Department of General Paediatrics

Margaret Zacharin Paediatric and Adolescent Endocrinologist,
Department of Endocrinology and Diabetes
Endocrinologist, Peter McCallum hospital

EDITORIAL COMMITTEE

EDITORIAL ADVISORY COMMITTEE

FOREWORD

The Royal Children's Hospital, Melbourne, has a long standing commitment to advancing the health and well-being of children, young people and their families not only through the provision of clinical services, but also with respect to research and education. For over three decades, the Paediatric Handbook has represented the endeavours of the staff of the Royal Children's Hospital to make available accessible, up-to-date and practical clinical information relevant to the treatment and care of children and adolescents. This 7th edition of the Handbook continues the tradition, containing much new content that reflects the changing nature of child health and paediatric practice.

All chapters in this new edition have been fully up-dated with new sections on pain management, international child health and failure to thrive. The immunisation section has been comprehensively revised and expanded and there has been the addition of a concise and practical guide to safe prescribing in children. Furthermore, an online supplement has been developed that contains links to clinical guidelines, information tables and visual images.

In an age where there at times seems to be an over-abundance of information, it is of paramount importance for there to be available to practicing clinicians an authoritative source of quality advice and genuine practice wisdom. The Handbook provides just such a source and in an extremely user-friendly format. The Royal Children's Hospital and its staff are rightly proud on this 7th Edition and hope it will continue to make a positive contribution to the work of all those committed to improving the health of children and adolescents.

Glenn Bowes MBBS PhD FRACP
Stevenson Professor and Head
Department of Paediatrics
The University of Melbourne
Royal Children's Hospital Melbourne
Flemington Road, Parkville, 3052
Victoria, Australia

Director, Postgraduate Education and Training
Royal Children's Hospital Melbourne

PREFACE

Welcome to the 7th edition of the Paediatric handbook of the Royal Children's Hospital. The handbook is intended as a practical management guide to the health problems of infants, children and adolescents and is aimed at primary health care providers, junior medical hospital staff and medical students. The handbook draws on the best available evidence and the expertise of the staff of the Royal Children's Hospital. The handbook is not a textbook; it provides a brief synopsis of relevant background information and then a guide to managing common paediatric problems. Additional information is provided on variations from normal in child health and development and conditions that are more uncommon but important to detect.

This edition has been comprehensively revised and updated. The structure of the previous edition has been retained, starting with medical emergencies and practical procedural chapters, followed by development, child public health and psychosocial health, then medical and surgical problems. Large parts of the book have been reformatted, with the intention of making the management guidelines clearer and easier to follow. Many chapters have been extensively rewritten and several new sections have been added. The Antimicrobial guidelines have been updated and the new edition of the pharmacopoeia included. The inside of the front and back covers now contain fold-out charts summarising paediatric resuscitation (front) and the current immunisation schedule (back). Drug doses are included in the text and although every effort has been made to check doses and to ensure consistency between sections, it is possible errors have been missed. We strongly advise that drug doses and product information be checked before administering drugs to patients (see Prescribing guidelines!).

For the first time the handbook is associated with an online supplement with links to sites for each chapter. This will allow access to images and additional sources of information that significantly enhance the text and for additional local information to be provided. It is also a means of updating information about current practice that is bound to change during the lifespan of this edition.

There are many people to thank in putting together this edition of the Paediatric handbook. Firstly, we acknowledge the input of all the people who were involved in previous editions, but not directly in the current edition; their contributions have provided the base upon which the 7th edition is built. Many thanks to all the staff who have been involved with writing the current edition, to the editorial committee and our expert advisory panel. Thanks to Professor Frank Shann for permission to use his drug doses booklet and to the Infectious diseases physicians for reviewing the antibiotics from all the chapters. We are grateful to Bill Reid for use of his illustrations, many of which were included in the 7th edition, and to Alma Ross and Caitlin Matthews at Blackwell Publishing Asia for their help and support. Finally, thanks to Michael Leunig for allowing us to use the image that appears on the front cover. We hope this edition is useful and as well used as the previous editions. Editing it has been a lot of fun.

Georgia Paxton, Jane Munro and Michael Marks

CHAPTER 1
MEDICAL EMERGENCIES

James Tibballs
Ed Oakley

CARDIORESPIRATORY ARREST

Cardiorespiratory arrest may occur in a wide variety of conditions that cause hypoxaemia or hypotension, or both. Examples include trauma, drowning, septicaemia, sudden infant death syndrome, asthma and congenital anomalies of the heart and lung.

The initial cardiac rhythm discovered during early resuscitation is usually severe bradycardia or asystole. The spontaneous onset of ventricular fibrillation in children is uncommon, but it may occur with congenital heart conditions or secondary to poisoning with cardioactive drugs. Respiratory arrest alone is more common.

Diagnosis and initial management

- Cardiorespiratory arrest may be suspected when consciousness is lost, or the patient appears pale or cyanosed. Call for help.
- Assess airway and respiration by observing movement of the chest, as well as listening and feeling for expired breath while positioning the head and neck to open and maintain an airway. Movement of the chest without expiration indicates a blocked airway.
- Assess circulation by palpation of the carotid, brachial or femoral pulse and by other signs of circulation (breathing, movement, consciousness).
- Whenever possible, treat in a treatment room. Carry the patient there if necessary. If this is not possible, fetch the resuscitation trolley from a treatment room.
- Cardiopulmonary resuscitation (CPR) must commence with basic techniques and be continued using advanced techniques (Figure 1.1).

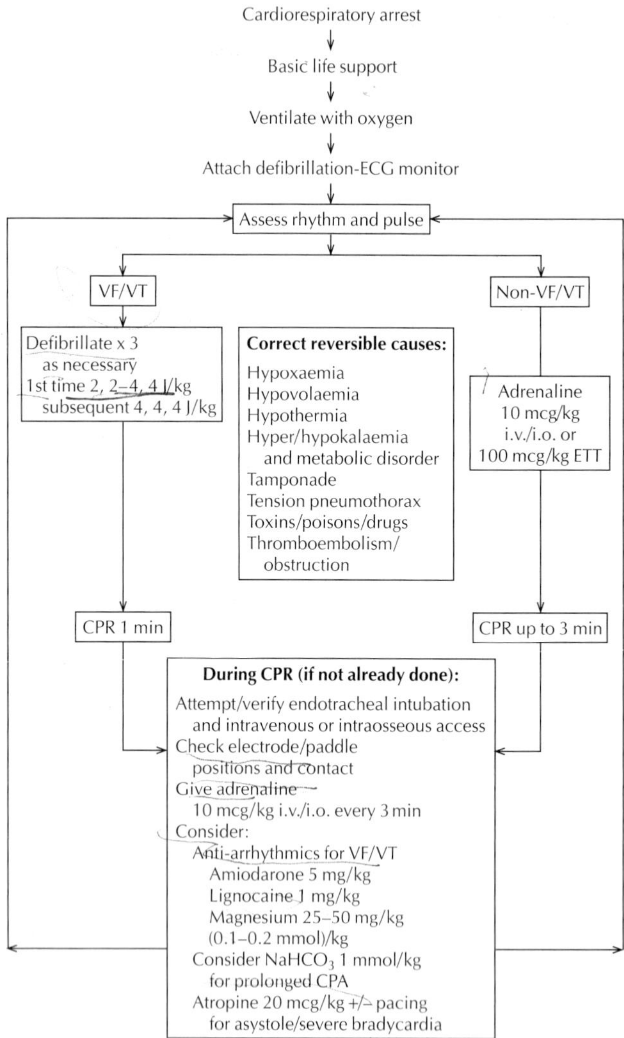

Fig. 1.1 Management of cardiorespiratory arrest. Key: CPA; cardiopulmonary arrest: ECG; eletrocardiograph: ETT; endotracheal tube: i.o.; intraosseus: i.v.; intravenous: J; Joules: kg; kilogram: mg; milligram: mcg; microgram: VF; ventricular fibrillation: VT; ventricular tachycardia.

Airway maintenance and ventilation

- If an airway obstruction is present, quickly inspect the pharynx. Clear secretions or vomitus by brief suction using a Yankauer sucker.
- Maintain the airway with backward head tilt, chin lift or forward jaw thrust.
- If adequate respiration does not resume, ventilate the lungs with a self-inflating resuscitator (e.g. Laerdal, Ambu, Air-viva) with added oxygen 8–10 L/min. If ventilation cannot be achieved with the resuscitator, use a mouth-to-mask technique. Give 5 initial breaths.
- **Whatever technique is used, ensure that ventilation expands the chest adequately.**
- Intubate the trachea via the mouth if able to do so, but do not cause hypoxaemia by prolonged unsuccessful attempts. Select the tube and insert it a depth appropriate to the patient's age in years.

ETT Size and position

- Tube size (internal diameter) = (age/4) + 4 mm (for patients over 1 year of age)
- Depth of insertion is approximately (age/2) + 12 cm from the lower lip

Secure the tube with cotton tape around the neck or affix it firmly to the face with adhesive tape to avoid endobronchial intubation or accidental extubation.

External cardiac compression

Start external cardiac compression (ECC) over the lower sternum if:

- A pulse is not palpable within 10 seconds.
- A pulse is less than 60 beats per minute (all ages).
- Other signs of circulation (respiration, movement, consciousness) are absent.

Place the patient on a firm surface and depress the lower sternum one-third the depth of the chest:

- Newborn infant or an infant (<1 year); two-thumb technique in which the hands encircle the chest.
- Small child (1–8 yrs); the heel of one hand.
- Larger child (>8 yrs) and adult; the two-handed technique.

Avoid pressure over the ribs and abdominal viscera.

- **Whatever technique is used ensure that compression generates a pulse.**

Compression-ventilation rates and ratios

The Australian Resuscitation Council recommends these rates and ratios. Give 5 initial breaths. Then with one or two rescuers give:

- Newborn infants (within hours of birth); give cycles of 3 compressions, followed by one breath.
- Infants and small children (up to 8 yrs); give cycles of 5 cardiac compressions followed by 1 breath. Give *at least* 60 compressions and 12 breaths per minute.
- Larger child (>8 yrs) or adult; give cycles of 15 compressions followed by 2 breaths. Give *at least* 60 compressions and 8 breaths per minute.

If bag-to-mask ventilation or mouth-to-mask ventilation is used, the rescuer giving compressions should count aloud to allow the rescuer giving ventilation to deliver efficient breaths between compressions so that a minimal pause, if any, is required. Compression may be commenced at the end of inspiration. These measures will enable near-continuous ECC and result in an optimum number of compressions and additional breaths each minute.

The *rate* of compression per minute is 100, that is one compression every 0.6 seconds, aiming to give approximately 80–100 compressions each minute.

If ventilation is given by bag and endotracheal tube, ECC may be continued during ventilation (in the recommended ratios) provided lung expansion can be achieved.

Management of cardiac dysrhythmias

- Determine the cardiac rhythm with defibrillator paddles or chest leads.
- Give DC shock if ventricular fibrillation or pulseless ventricular tachycardia is present. See Table 1.1 and Figure 1.1 for monophasic energy doses in DC shock.
- Give adrenaline if any other pulseless rhythm is present (see Figure 1.1).

Table 1.1 Table of drugs, fluid volume, endotracheal tubes and direct current shock for paediatric resuscitation

Age	*0*	*2 months*	*5 months*	*1 year*	*2 years*	*3 years*	*4 years*	*5 years*	*6 years*	*7 years*	*8 years*	*9 years*	*10 years*	*11 years*	*12 years*	*13 years*	*14 years*
*Bodyweight (kg)**	*3.5*	*5*	*7*	*10*	*12*	*14*	*16*	*18*	*20*	*22*	*25*	*28*	*32*	*36*	*40*	*46*	*50*
*Height (cm)**	*50*	*58*	*65*	*75*	*85*	*94*	*102*	*109*	*115*	*121*	*127*	*132*	*138*	*144*	*151*	*157*	*162*
	mL	*mL*	*mL*	*mL*	*mL*	*mL*	*mL*	*mL*	*mL*	*mL*	*mL*	*mL*	*mL*	*mL*	*mL*	*mL*	*mL*
Adrenaline 1 : 1000																	
10 mcg/kg	0.035	0.05	0.07	0.10	0.12	0.14	0.16	0.18	0.2	0.22	0.25	0.28	0.32	0.36	0.4	0.46	0.5
100 mcg/kg	0.35	0.5	0.7	1	1.2	1.4	1.6	1.8	2	2.2	2.5	2.8	3.2	3.6	4	4.6	5
Adrenaline 1 : 10 000																	
10 mcg/kg	0.35	0.5	0.7	1	1.2	1.4	1.6	1.8	2	2.2	2.5	2.8	3.2	3.6	4	4.6	5
100 mcg/kg	3.5	5.0	7.0	10	12	14	16	18	20	22	25	28	32	36	40	46	50
Lignocaine 1% mL																	
1 mg/kg	0.3	0.5	0.7	1.0	1.2	1.4	1.6	1.8	2.0	2.2	2.5	2.8	3.2	3.6	4.0	4.6	5.0
Sodium bicarb. 8.4% mL																	
1 mmol/kg	3.5	5	7	10	12	14	16	18	20	22	25	28	32	36	40	46	50
Fluid volume mL																	
20 mL/kg	70	100	140	200	240	280	320	360	400	440	500	560	640	720	800	920	1000
Endotracheal tube																	
Size (mm) age/4 + 4	3	3.5	3.5	4	4.5	4.5	5	5	5.5	5.5	6	6	6.5	6.5	7	7	7.5
Oral length (cm) age/2 + 12	9.5	11	11.5	12	13	13.5	14	14.5	15	15.5	16	16.5	17	17.5	18	18.5	19
Direct current shock																	
VF, VT 2 J/kg	7	10	20	20	20	30	30	30	50	50	50	50	70	70	70	100	100
VF, VT 4 J/kg	10	20	30	50	50	50	70	70	70	100	100	100	150	150	150	200	200
Unsynchronised																	
SVT 1 J/kg	3	5	7	10	10	10	20	30	20	20	30	30	30	30	50	50	50
Synchronised																	

* 50th percentiles

Source: Oakley, P., Phillips, B., Molyneaux, E. & Mackway–Jones, K. (1993) Updated standard reference chart. *BMJ* 1993; **306**, 1613.

- Insert an intravenous cannula. Although this is the preferred access to the circulation, do not waste time (>90 secs) with repeated unsuccessful attempts, because access can be achieved with the alternative techniques of bone marrow (intraosseous) infusion, (see Procedures, chapter 4) or endotracheal administration (ETT).
- All intravenous drugs and resuscitation fluids can be given via the bone marrow.
- Only adrenaline, atropine and lignocaine can be given via the endotracheal route.
- A quick reference guide to drug doses and fluid volume is provided in Table 1.1 and Figure 1.1.

Other drugs

Calcium

This is a useful inotropic and vasopressor agent but it has no place in the management of a dysrhythmia, unless it is caused by hypocalcaemia, hyperkalaemia or calcium channel blocker toxicity. It is not useful and probably harmful for asystole, ventricular fibrillation or electromechanical dissociation. The intravenous dose is 10% calcium chloride (0.2 mL/kg) or 10% calcium gluconate (0.7 mL/kg). Do not administer calcium by endotracheal tube and do not mix it with bicarbonate.

Adenosine

This is the preferred drug treatment for supraventricular tachycardia (SVT). See management of SVT in Cardiovascular conditions, chapter 18.

ANAPHYLAXIS

See also Allergy and immunology, chapter 16.

The life-threatening clinical manifestations are:

- Hypotension due to vasodilatation and loss of plasma volume due to increased capillary permeability.
- Bronchospasm.
- Upper airways obstruction due to laryngeal or pharyngeal oedema.

Immediate treatment

- Vasopressor and bronchodilator therapy. Give adrenaline 0.01 mg/kg (i.e. 0.1 mL/kg of 1:10,000 solution) by slow intravenous (i.v.) injection (over 10 min) or 0.01 mL/kg of 1:1,000 solution by intramuscular (i.m.) injection. A continuous infusion (0.1–1.0 mcg/kg per min) may be required if manifestations are prolonged.

- Oxygen by mask. Mechanical ventilation may be required.
- Intravenous volume expander. Give or 0.9% saline at 20 mL/kg. Give repeat boluses of 10–20 mL/kg until the blood pressure is restored.
- Bronchodilator therapy with salbutamol – continuous nebulised (0.5%) or i.v. 5 mcg/kg per min for 1 h, then 1 mcg/kg per min thereafter. Secondary therapy with a steroid, aminophylline and an antihistamine may be helpful for prolonged bronchospasm and capillary leak.
- Relief of upper airway obstruction: mild to moderate oedema may respond to an inhalation of nebulised 1% adrenaline (1 mL per dose diluted to 4 mL) or 5 mL of nebulised 1:1,000 solution, but intubation of the trachea may be required.
- Anaphylaxis can be biphasic and the patient may deteriorate again over the next few hours.
- All patients with anaphylaxis should be observed carefully for at least 12 h, followed up for allergen testing and provided with self-injectable adrenaline and a Medi-alert warning.

Allergic oedema causing acute larygeal obstruction

Treat with nebulised 1% adrenaline 1 mL per dose diluted to 4 mL or 5 mL of 1:1,000 solution. Refer to an intensive care specialist or anaesthetist for endotracheal intubation, or an ENT surgeon for tracheostomy.

HAEMORRHAGIC SHOCK

The normal blood volume is 70–80 mL/kg. A child may lose a substantial volume of blood without developing hypotension. Cardiac output and blood pressure are preserved by tachycardia and vasoconstriction, so hypotension is a late sign of blood loss.

- Control external haemorrhage by direct wound pressure, arterial vessel pressure or a tourniquet and elevation of the injured area.
- Administer oxygen by mask.
- Insert a large bore intravenous cannula, preferably in the upper limb. Two cannulae may be required.
- Withdraw blood for group and cross-match.

- Infuse rapidly by pressure 20 mL/kg of 0.9% saline solution. This may also be administered rapidly by syringing with the aid of a three-way tap. Titrate additional volume to the blood pressure and other indices of perfusion. Further boluses of 10–20 mL/kg 0.9% saline solution may be given.
- **If exsanguinating, transfuse urgently** with (in order of preference): (i) cross-matched blood or; (ii) uncross-matched blood of the same group as the patient or; (iii) uncross-matched O-negative blood. Warm the blood.
- Monitor blood pressure, heart rate, oxygenation and urine output.
- Measure the central venous pressure, serum calcium, serum potassium, coagulation and acid-base status if a massive transfusion is required. Calcium (10% calcium chloride 0.2 mL/kg) and fresh frozen plasma are usually needed after 1–2 blood volumes have been transfused.
- Investigate and surgically explore internal haemorrhage if necessary.

SEPTICAEMIC SHOCK

Hypotension is due to leakage of fluid from capillary beds and depression of myocardial contractility.

- Collect blood for culture, but do not delay administration of an antibiotic if a blood sample cannot be collected. If no information is available regarding the source of pathogen, give flucloxacillin 50 mg/kg (max 2 g) i.v. 4-hourly and cefotaxime 50 mg/kg (max 2 g) i.v. 6-hourly. For particular circumstances consult the Antimicrobial Guidelines. For shock due to meningococcaemia, which is usually accompanied by a purpuric rash, give cefotaxime 50 mg/kg (max 2 g) i.v. 6-hourly. Give benzylpenicillin 60 mg/kg (max 3 g) i.v. or i.m. 4-hourly if cefotaxime not available.
- Treat shock with 0.9% saline solution, 20 mL/kg initially – further boluses of 10–20 mL/kg may be needed.
- Commence infusion of an inotropic agent. Dopamine (5–20 mcg/kg per min) is preferred. Administration via a central vein is preferred but it may be given via a peripheral vein as a dilute solution (e.g. 15 mg/kg in 500 mL at 10–40 mL/h = 5–20 mcg/kg per min). Dobutamine (5–20 mcg/kg per min) may be administered into a peripheral vein.

- Give oxygen and monitor blood gases. Mechanical ventilation may be required.
- Defer lumbar puncture, if indicated, until the child has been stabilised.

NEAR DROWNING

There is a global hypoxic-ischaemic injury often associated with lung damage from aspiration of water and gastric contents.

- Adequate oxygenation and ventilation are of paramount importance. Mechanical ventilation is required for severe lung involvement, circulatory arrest or loss of consciousness. Lung hypoxic-ischaemic injury is compounded by pulmonary oedema or aspiration of water or gastric contents.
- Decompress the stomach, which is usually distended with air and water.
- Support the circulation with intravenous infusion of colloid (e.g. 4% albumin) or 0.9% saline solution and infusion of an inotropic agent (e.g. dopamine 5–20 mcg/kg per min into a central vein).
- If signs of cerebral oedema are present (i.e. a depressed conscious state) administer mannitol 0.25–0.5 g/kg i.v. once.
- Correct electrolyte disturbances; hypokalaemia is common. The differences between fresh-water and salt-water drowning are not usually clinically important.
- Administer benzylpenicillin 60 mg/kg (max 3 g) i.v. 6-hourly (to prevent the complication of pneumococcal pneumonia).
- If CPR is required, prevent hyperthermia and induce controlled hypothermia (33–34°C) for 72 h for cerebral protection.

ACUTE LARYNGEAL OBSTRUCTION

The most common cause is laryngotracheobronchitis (croup) and occasional causes are epiglottitis, an inhaled foreign body, allergic oedema and trauma. The hallmark of obstruction is stridor, which when accompanied by a barking cough, suggests croup, or when accompanied by dysphagia/drooling suggests epiglottitis. Severe obstruction stimulates forceful diaphragmatic contraction that results in a retraction of the rib cage, tracheal tug and abdominal protrusion on inspiration. Cyanosis and irregular respiratory effort are terminal signs.

Epiglottitis

See also Respiratory conditions, chapter 33.

- Complete obstruction may occur in just a few hours. In general, tracheal intubation under anaesthesia is required. Arrange promptly.
- Keep the child as calm as possible in a seated position and administer oxygen by mask.
- If complete obstruction is imminent, summon immediate help from an intensivist or anaesthetist. If inexperienced, do not attempt intubation unless the child becomes comatose. Intubate orally initially with a relatively small endotracheal tube. It may be hard to see the larynx because of secretions in the pharynx and the swollen epiglottis. Be prepared to aspirate the pharynx with a Yankauer sucker. Cricoid pressure is very helpful to visualise the vocal cords.
- If intubation proves to be impossible, attempt to ventilate with bag-valve-mask; a good technique may achieve adequate oxygenation and ventilation. If ventilation is impossible, perform cricothyrotomy or tracheostomy (see below).
- Antibiotic therapy: Ceftriaxone 100 mg/kg (max 2 g) i.v. followed by 50 mg/kg (max 2 g) 24 h later.

Croup

See also Respiratory conditions, chapter 33.

- In severe obstruction, give an inhalation of nebulised 1% adrena line 1 mL per dose diluted to 4 mL, or 5 mL of 1:1,000 solution to obtain temporary relief.
- Give corticosteroid i.m./i.v. (e.g. dexamethasone 0.6 mg/kg).
- Obtain intensive care or anaesthetic help with a view to endotracheal intubation. If this is not available, intubate when the child is going into respiratory failure. Use an introducing stylet in an endotracheal tube of size 0.5 or 1 mm smaller than usually calculated by age in years; i.e. (age/4 + 4 mm).

Aspirated foreign body

See also Respiratory conditions, chapter 33.

- Give first-aid (back slaps, lateral chest compressions or Heimlich manoeuvre) if obstruction occurs, otherwise allow the child to cough. Do not instrument the airways if the child is coping, but summon an anaesthetist and ENT surgeon. Give oxygen.
- If complete obstruction occurs, attempt removal of an impacted laryngeal foreign body with forceps – if this is unsuccessful, perform a cricothyrotomy or tracheostomy (see below).
- If respiratory failure is due to a foreign body in the lower trachea or bronchi, attempt ventilation via an endotracheal tube while organising endoscopic removal.

Emergency relief of a totally obstructed upper airway

- Adequate oxygenation (but not normal ventilation) can be obtained by inserting a 14-gauge intravenous cannula percutaneously into the trachea via the cricothyroid membrane (which lies immediately inferior to the thyroid cartilage); the patient should be lying straight, with the cannula in the midline and angled towards the feet. Remove the needle of the intravenous cannula; connect the cannula to a resuscitator or a bagging circuit using a connector from a 3.0 mm endotracheal tube. Oxygenate with sustained 100% oxygen inspirations. Alternatively, connect the cannula to the compressed wall oxygen supply via a three-way intravenous tap (to allow expiration) and a length of plastic tubing. A length of plastic tubing that has a side hole cut may also be used to allow expiration. Aid intermittent expiration by lateral chest compression.
- Alternatively, perform cricothyrotomy. Identify and maintain stabilisation of the thyroid-cricoid region with one hand. Incise the skin over the cricothyroid membrane (between the thyroid and cricoid cartilages). Bluntly dissect into the trachea with forceps in the midline or incise vertically with scalpel. Insert a small tracheostomy or endotracheal tube.
- Alternatively, perform percutaneous mini-tracheostomy.

STATUS ASTHMATICUS

See also Respiratory conditions, chapter 33.

Critical asthma

Children unresponsive to intermittent inhalation of salbutamol should receive:

- Continuous inhalation of undiluted 0.5% salbutamol solution nebulised with oxygen.
- Methylprednisolone 1 mg/kg i.v. (max 50 mg) 6-hourly.
- Nebulised ipratropium may be added as 250 mcg/dose diluted to 2–3 mL every 20 min × 3 and then 4–6-hourly (beware anticholinergic effects).
- Intravenous salbutamol load 5 mcg/kg/min for 60 min followed by infusion 1–2 mcg/kg per min (beware hypokalaemia).
- Aminophylline (subject to prior theophylline use and serum level) 10 mg/kg (max 500 mg) i.v. over 1 h followed by infusion of 1.1 mg/kg per h (age 1–9 years) or 0.7 mg/kg per h (10 years to adult). Check level following loading dose.
- Refractory critical asthma – manage in ICU.

STATUS EPILEPTICUS

See also Neurologic conditions, chapter 30.

A convulsion involving the respiratory musculature and upper airways that does not cease within a few minutes may cause hypoventilation with hypoxaemia and hypercarbia.

- Administer oxygen.
- Be prepared to give mechanical ventilation, particularly if the child has meningitis.
- Check blood glucose, electrolytes, blood gas and septic screen.
- Some initial intravenous anticonvulsant choices include:
  - Diazepam 0.2–0.4 mg/kg (max 10–20 mg) i.v. May be given per rectum if there is no intravenous access. Midazolam 0.1–0.15 mg/kg i.v. or 0.2 mg/kg (i.m.) effective i.m. within 5–10 min.
  - Clonazepam 0.25 mg (<1 year); 0.5 mg (1–5 years); 1 mg (>5 years) i.v.
  - Phenobarbitone 20 mg/kg over 30 min; repeat doses 10–15 mg/kg every 15–30 min up to 100 mg/kg in 24 h (beware of hypotension) if required (adults – max. 600 mg/d).

- Phenytoin 15 mg/kg (max 1.5 g) i.v. over 1 h to avoid negative inotropic effect. Slow onset.
- Thiopentone: titrate dose slowly to effect (usually 2–5 mg/kg). Beware of hypotension.

Prolonged convulsions may require large and repeated doses of anticonvulsant drugs or infusions and, consequently, mechanical ventilation. Repeated doses of a single anticonvulsant such as phenobarbitone (where the serum level correlates with the effects) are preferable to using multiple anticonvulsants. Suspect hyponatraemia as the cause of convulsions in meningitis.

RAISED INTRACRANIAL PRESSURE

Acute intracranial hypertension threatens the blood supply and may cause herniation of the brain. It is recognised by (in approximate sequence):

- Headache, vomiting, papilloedema, deterioration in the conscious state with diminution of spontaneous limb movements.
- Ipsilateral pupillary dilatation and contralateral hemiparesis, limb hypertonicity and spasm if there is uncal herniation into tentorial hiatus with supratentorial lesion. These can be bilateral with an extensive lesion.
- Alteration in pattern of respiration (hyperventilation; irregular respiration), bradycardia and hypertension are near-terminal events due to medullary herniation into the foramen magnum.

Common causes of intracranial hypertension are:

- Acute brain swelling due to cerebral oedema caused by trauma, infection, ischaemia or hypoxaemia.
- Space-occupying lesion, such as an intracerebral haemorrhage, tumour or abscess.
- Obstruction of cerebrospinal fluid circulation.

A neurosurgeon should be contacted immediately where indicated; e.g. in cases of trauma.

- If it is impossible to treat the cause immediately, reduce the intracranial blood volume by using mechanical hyperventilation to lower the $P_{a}CO_2$ and cause cerebral vasoconstriction. (*Note*: prolonged or excessive hyperventilation to $P_{a}CO_2$ of $<25–35$ mmHg may be harmful.)

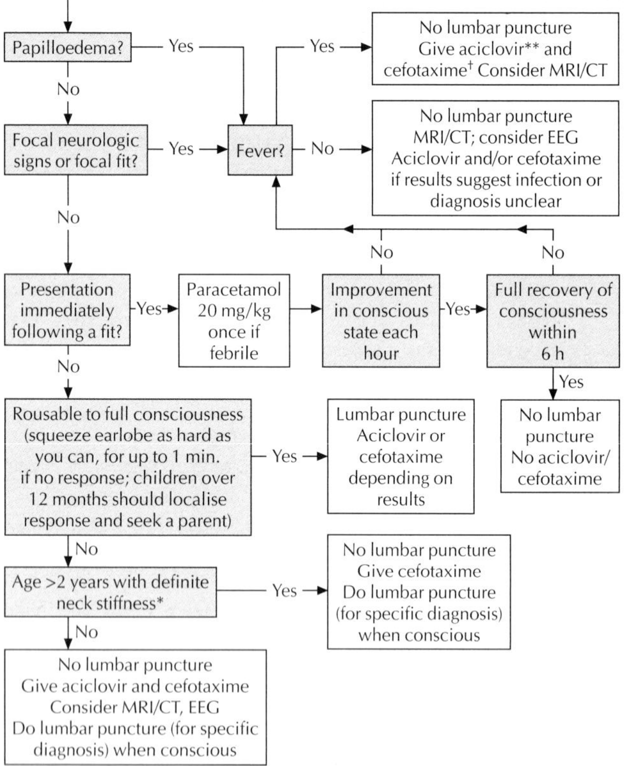

* Neck stiffness is not a reliable sign of meningism in children <2 years

** Aciclovir10 mg/kg i.v. 8 hourly (age 2 weeks–2 years)
500 mg/m^2 i.v. 8 hourly (age 2–12 years)

† Cefotaxime 50 mg/kg (max 2 g) i.v. 6 hourly

Fig. 1.2 A guide to the role of lumbar puncture and the use of chemotherapeutic agents in the child unconscious due to unknown cause.

- Mannitol may be used to reduce cerebral oedema (0.25–0.5 g/kg, i.v.). Fluids should be restricted to avoid cerebral oedema, but not at the expense of causing hypotension. Blood pressure may be maintained with a vasopressor (e.g. dopamine up to 10 mcg/kg per min).
- Hypoxaemia and hypotension must be avoided.

A lumbar puncture should not be performed in the presence of intracranial hypertension because of risk of brain stem coning. A guide to the role of lumbar puncture and chemotherapeutic agents in the undiagnosed unconscious patient is given in Figure 1.2.

CHAPTER 2
POISONING AND ENVENOMATION

James Tibballs

POISONING

Background

Poisoning during childhood occurs mainly among 1–3 year-olds and tends to follow the ingestion of a wide variety of improperly stored agents in the home.

Other circumstances of poisoning are iatrogenic (particularly in infants), the deliberate self-administration of substances by older children for their recreational use or to manipulate their psychosocial environments. Increasingly, the intention is suicidal.

While poisoning in childhood is frequently minor in severity and mortality is low, serious illness may be caused by prescription and 'over-the-counter' drugs and non-pharmaceutical products, including complementary medications.

General management

See Figure 2.1. The principles of management for all poisonings are:

- Resuscitate the patient and remove the poison if indicated.
- Administer an antidote if one exists (see Table 2.1).

Recovery is expected in the vast majority of cases if vital functions are preserved and the complications of poisoning and its management are avoided.

A decision to remove the poison from the body should be dependent on the severity of the poisoning and the likelihood of success in removing the poison without further endangering the patient. Most poisonings in childhood are minor and observation alone or non-invasive treatment is indicated.

The severity of poisoning may be assessed by the:

- Established and expected effects.
- Quantity of the poison(s)

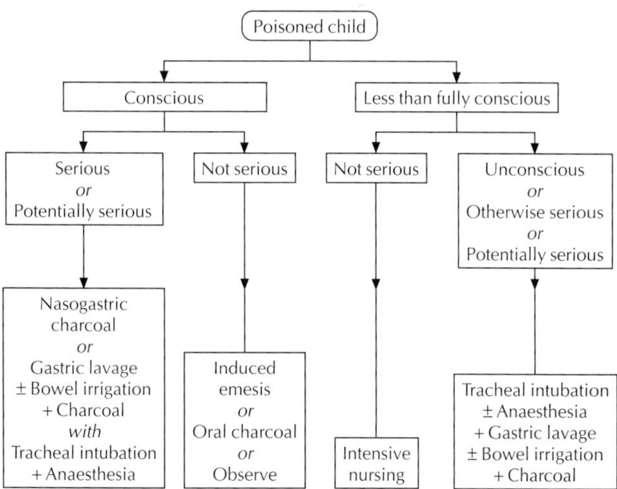

Fig. 2.1 General management of the poisoned child

- Preparation of the poison
- Interval since exposure

Removal from the body usually involves a technique of gastrointestinal decontamination but occasionally other methods, such as dialysis, exchange transfusion, charcoal haemoperfusion, plasmapheresis or haemofiltration are required.

Gastrointestinal decontamination

If the conscious state is depressed, all methods of gastrointestinal decontamination carry a substantial risk of aspiration pneumonitis. These techniques include induced emesis with syrup of ipecacuanha, gastric lavage, activated charcoal and whole bowel washout. Aspiration pneumonitis is not entirely prevented by endotracheal intubation. The most important factor determining the choice of technique is the conscious state. A guideline for the general management of poisoning using these techniques according to severity of poisoning is shown in Figure 2.1.

Table 2.1 Antidotes to poisons

Poison	*Antidotes and doses*	*Comments*
Amphetamines	Esmolol 0.5 mg/kg i.v. over 1 min, then 25–200 mcg/kg per min i.v.	Treatment for tachyarrhythmia.
	Labetalol 0.15–0.3 mg/kg i.v. or phentolamine 0.05–0.1 mg/kg i.v. every 10 min.	Treatments for hypertension.
Benzodiazepines	Flumazenil 5 mcg/kg i.v. repeated at 1 min then 2–10 mcg/kg per h by i.v. infusion.	Specific antagonist at receptor. Titrate to effect. Caution: may precipitate convulsions or arrhythmia in multi-drug ingestion, especially with tricyclics.
Beta blocker	Glucagon 7 mcg/kg i.v. then 2–7 mcg/kg per min i.v. infusion.	Stimulates non-catecholamine cAMP production. Preferred antidote.
	Isoprenaline 0.05–2 mcg/kg per min i.v. Beware β_2 hypotension.	
	Noradrenaline 0.05–0.5 mcg/kg per min i.v.	
Calcium blocker	Calcium chloride 20 mg (0.2 mL of 10%)/kg .v.	
Carbon monoxide	Oxygen 100%	Hyperbaric oxygen may be required.
Cyanide	Dicobalt edetate 7.5 mg/kg (max 300 mg i.v.) over 1 min, then repeat at 5 min if no effect.	Chelates. Give 50 mL 50% glucose after each dose.
	Sodium nitrite 3% i.v. (0.33 mL/kg over 4 min), *then* sodium thiosulphate 25% i.v. 1.65 mL/kg (max 50 mL) at 3–5 mL/min.	Nitrites form methaemoglobin-cyanide complex (beware excess methaemoglobinaemia – restrict to <20%). Thiosulphate forms non-toxic thiocyanate from methaemoglobin-cyanide.

Digoxin	Digoxin F_{ab}. Dose: acute ingestion 1 vial/2.5 tablet (0.25 mg); in steady state vials = serum digoxin (ng/mL) × BW (kg)/100.	
Ergotamine	Sodium nitroprusside infusion 0.5–5 mcg/kg per min.	Treats vasoconstriction. Monitor BP continuously.
	Heparin 100 units/kg i.v. then 10–30 units/kg i.v. per h according to clotting.	Treatment of coagulopathy.
Lead	If symptomatic or blood lead >2.9 μmol/L dimercaprol (BAL) 75 mg/m^2 i.m. 4-hourly 6 doses then calcium disodium edetate (EDTA) 1500 mg/m^2 i.v. over 5 days. If asymptomatic and blood lead 2.18–2.9 μmol/L infuse calcium disodium edetate 1000 mg/m^2 per day for 5 days.	
Heparin	Protamine 1 mg/100 units heparin i.v.	Heparin half-life 1–2 h.
Iron	Desferrioxamine 15 mg/kg per h 12–24 h if serum iron >90 μmol/L or >63 μmol/L and symptomatic.	Beware anaphylaxis.
Methanol, ethylene glycol, glycol ethers	Ethanol, infuse loading dose 10 mL/kg 10% diluted in glucose 5% i.v. and then 0.15 mL/kg per h to maintain blood level at 0.1% (100 mg/dL).	
Methaemoglobin e.g. 2° to drug treatment	Methylene blue 1–2 mg/kg i.v. over several min.	
Opiates	Naloxone 0.01–0.1 mg/kg i.v., then 0.01 mg/kg per h as needed.	
Organophosphates and carbamates	Atropine 20–50 mcg/kg i.v. every 15 min until secretions dry. Pralidoxime 25 mg/kg i.v. over 15–30 min, then 10–20 mg/kg per h for 18 h or more. Not for carbamates.	Restores cholinesterase.
Paracetamol	*N*-acetylcysteine. i.v.; 150 mg/kg over 60 min, then 10 mg/kg per h for 20–72 h. Oral; 140 mg/kg then 17 doses of 70 mg/kg 4 hourly (total 1330 mg/kg over 68 h).	Give for >72 h if still encephalopathic.
Tricyclic antidepressants	Sodium bicarbonate i.v. 1 mmol/kg to maintain blood pH >7.45.	

Activated charcoal

Activated charcoal is more efficacious than induced emesis or gastric lavage and is currently regarded as a 'universal antidote'. It adsorbs most poisons but not metals, corrosives or pesticides. Like other techniques, however, it is contraindicated in the less than fully conscious patient or if ileus is present. If aspirated, charcoal may cause fatal bronchiolitis obliterans. Constipation is relatively common. Addition of a laxative decreases transit time through the gut but does not improve efficacy in preventing drug absorption. It may also upset fluid and electrolyte balance. The initial dose is 1–2 g/kg. Repeated doses of activated charcoal enhance elimination of many drugs, particularly slow-release preparations. A suitable regimen is 0.25 g/kg per h for 12–24 h.

Induced vomiting

Syrup of ipecacuanha is useful as a first aid measure in the home, however, its usefulness in the hospital setting is extremely limited – perhaps only to a case of serious poisoning presenting very early after ingestion when no other effective treatment is possible.

Although it induces vomiting in most children within 30 min of administration, it does not reliably empty the stomach of solids. Moreover, it must be given within 1 h of ingestion to significantly reduce drug absorption. It may cause prolonged vomiting, diarrhoea and drowsiness. The onset of vomiting may be delayed and may mimic the toxic effects of an ingested poison. Contraindications include:

- Impaired conscious state (risk of aspiration pneumonitis).
- Ingestion of a corrosive, hydrocarbon or petrochemical (risks of additional respiratory tract and pulmonary damage).

Gastric lavage

Although gastric lavage appears to be a logical therapy for ingested poisons, it has a limited place in management.

Problems include:

- Poor efficacy in preventing absorption when performed more than 60 min after ingestion.
- Risk of aspiration pneumonitis in the less than fully conscious patient and to a lesser extent in the conscious child.

Gastric lavage is contraindicated after ingestion of corrosives, hydrocarbons or petrochemicals.

In the conscious young child, it is psychologically traumatic and difficult to perform, thus predisposing to minor physical trauma.

If undertaken, care should be taken to avoid water intoxication and intrabronchial instillation of lavage fluid.

Gastric lavage is indicated in serious poisoning when a child is already intubated for airway protection and ventilation. The child should be in the lateral position during lavage. If potentially serious effects are expected, gastric lavage should only be performed after rapid sequence induction of anaesthesia and tracheal intubation.

Whole bowel irrigation

Whole bowel irrigation is performed with a solution of polyethylene glycol (30 mL/kg per h for 4–8 h) and electrolytes administered by nasogastric tube.

It is useful in delayed presentations and for the management of poisoning by slow-release drug preparations, substances not adsorbed by activated charcoal (e.g. iron) or substances which are irretrievable by gastric lavage.

Prevention

Action should be taken according to the circumstance of poisoning to prevent recurrence. Parents should be encouraged to store all medicines in childproof cabinets and to store toxic substances in places inaccessible to young children.

Urgent psychosocial help should be organised for children who have poisoned themselves intentionally.

Steps should be taken to ensure that iatrogenic poisoning is not repeated.

Poisoning with unknown or multiple agents

- Suspect poisoning on presentation with convulsions, depression of the conscious state, hypoventilation, hypotension or an illness that is not readily otherwise explained. A urine drug screen may be useful in diagnosis.

- Multiple poisons may have been ingested. Determine blood levels if there is any possibility of ingestion of paracetamol, iron, salicylate, theophylline, methanol, digoxin or lithium. Blood levels may influence clinical management.
- Contact the Poisons Information hotline for advice.

INDIVIDUAL POISONS

Thousands of poisons exist. The most common poisons in young children presenting to the Royal Children's Hospital, have been paracetamol, rodenticides, eucalyptus oil, benzodiazepines, tricyclic antidepressants and theophylline.

Only the most common serious poisonings, or poisonings peculiar to children are considered here briefly. Some have antidotes (see Table 2.1). **The general principles of management apply to all individual poisons** (see Figure 2.1).

Details of management of specific poisons should be obtained from a Poisons Information Centre, or from appropriate and up-to-date references.

Paracetamol (acetaminophen)

Paracetamol is the most common pharmaceutical poisoning.

Effects

The liver metabolises it to a toxic product, *N*-acetyl-*p*-benzoquinoneimine, which causes hepatic necrosis unless neutralised by the hepatic antioxidant, glutathione. Multi-organ failure and death may occur after 3–4 days if the ingested quantity exceeds 150 mg/kg or with smaller amounts with prior hepatic dysfunction, alcohol or anticonvulsants. Early symptoms are anorexia, nausea and vomiting.

Specific management

N-acetylcysteine (NAC) is an effective antidote if given before hepatic necrosis occurs. Its use is associated with adverse reactions (e.g. rash, bronchospasm and hypotension) that occur more frequently when administered intravenously. If reactions occur, cease NAC temporarily and give promethazine 0.2–0.5 mg/kg i.v. (max 10–25 mg) and recommence the NAC infusion at a reduced rate.

Since the outcome is related to serum levels of paracetamol measured 4–20 h after ingestion, a decision to administer NAC after a single overdose may be made according to time-related plasma levels. Administer if the level exceeds 1000 μmol/L at 4 h, 500 at 8 h, 200 at 12 h, 80 at 16 h, or 40 at 20 h (μmol/L × 0.15 = μg/mL).

- Intravenous NAC: 150 mg/kg in 5 mL/kg of glucose 5% over 60 min, then 10 mg/kg per hour for 20 h or longer if the child is encephalopathic, or presentation is 10–36 h after ingestion.
- Oral NAC: 140 mg/kg, then 17 doses of 70 mg/kg (4-hourly).

Note:

- Serum levels more than 18 h after a single ingestion are unreliable predictors of risk.
- These recommendations do not apply to multiple smaller ingestions (seek expert advice).
- Presentation within 1 h after significant ingestion may be treated with gastric lavage (see previously).
- Monitor liver function tests and serum potassium.

Theophylline

Toxicity is related to serum levels and may be delayed with slow-release preparations.

Effects

- Gastrointestinal – nausea, vomiting (protracted), abdominal pain.
- Metabolic – (i) hypokalaemia due to migration into cells, diuresis and vomiting; (ii) metabolic acidosis; (iii) hyperglycaemia, hyperinsulinaemia and hypomagnesaemia.
- Central nervous system – seizures, agitation, coma (uncommon).
- Cardiovascular – atrial and ventricular ectopy, hypotension.

Specific management

- Prolonged observation if a slow-release preparation is ingested.
- Serum level (anticipate seizures at approximately 300 μmol/L and the need for charcoal haemoperfusion or plasmapheresis at approximately 550 μmol/L or less if there is protracted vomiting).
- Anti-emetic therapy with metoclopramide 0.15 mg/kg (max 10–15 mg) i.v. 6-hourly.
- ECG monitoring. Beware of early hypokalaemia and late hyperkalaemia when potassium re-enters the blood.

Eucalyptus and essential oils

Effects

- Initial coughing, choking.
- Rapid onset (30 min, occasionally delayed) central nervous system depression (convulsions and meiosis are rare).
- Vomiting and subsequent aspiration pneumonitis.

Specific management

- Exclude pneumonitis (perform chest X-ray and measure oxygenation).

Iron

Small quantities (<20 mg/kg) of elemental iron may be toxic. Ingested usually as iron tablets/capsules, mixtures or multi-vitamin preparations.

The principal effects are:

- Immediate nausea, vomiting, abdominal pain and possible gastric erosion.
- Hypotension, hypovolaemia and metabolic acidosis at 6–24 h.
- Multi-organ failure – gastrointestinal (ileus, gastric erosion), central nervous system, cardiovascular, hepatic and renal at 12–24 h.
- Pyloric stenosis at 4–6 weeks.

Specific management

- Serum iron level (mcg/dL × 0.1791 = μmol/L). *Note*: absorption may be slow.
- Abdominal X-ray, which may reveal the quantity ingested.
- Whole bowel irrigation (not if ileus, obstruction or erosion are present). Activated charcoal is useless.
- Infusion of desferrioxamine no faster than 15 mg/kg/h for 12–24 h if patient has ingested >60 mg/kg elemental iron or is hypotensive or has depressed consciousness or in whom iron level is >90 μmol/L or >63 μmol/L and symptomatic.

Tricyclic antidepressants

Sudden death may occur.

Effects

The life-threatening effects are:

- Central nervous system (CNS) depression – coma, convulsions.
- Non-cardiogenic pulmonary oedema.

- Cardiac depression – hypocontractility and hypotension, and sudden dysrhythmias (conduction blocks and ventricular ectopy, including tachycardia/fibrillation).

Specific management

- ECG monitoring – assess heart rate, QRS duration and QT interval.
- Alkalisation of blood to pH 7.45–7.50 with sodium bicarbonate infusion or hyperventilation, or both.
- Anticonvulsant therapy with diazepam 0.1–0.4 mg/kg (max 10–20 mg).
- Antidysrrhythmia therapy – give phenytoin slowly (over 30 min). Beware of hypotension.
- Treatment of hypotension with an α-agonist (noradrenaline 0.01–1 mcg/kg per min). Avoid β-agonists and drugs with mixed α and β actions.
- Treatment of ventricular tachycardia/fibrillation with DC shock, lignocaine (1 mg/kg, then 10–50 mcg/kg per min) and a β-blocker.
- Treatment of torsade de pointes with DC shock, magnesium sulphate (0.1–0.2 mmol/kg i.v.) or lignocaine as above.

Salicylates

Toxicity is expected if >150 mg/kg is ingested.

Effects

- Coma, hyperpyrexia and respiratory alkalosis followed by metabolic acidosis.
- Cardiac depression, pulmonary oedema and hypotension.
- Hepatic encephalopathy (Reye syndrome) with chronic use.

Specific management

- Serum salicylate level, blood glucose, serum potassium and blood pH.
- Correction of dehydration.
- Correction of acidosis and maintenance of urine pH >7.5 (with sodium bicarbonate) and correction of hypokalaemia.
- Haemodialysis / haemoperfusion if the serum level is >25 mmol/L (mcg/mL × 0.0724 = μmol/L).

Petroleum distillates

- Petrol, kerosene, lighter fluid, lamp oils and mineral spirits cause CNS obtundation, convulsions, vomiting or hepato-renal toxicity.
- Pneumonitis must be excluded by chest X-ray and a measure of oxygenation.

Button or disc batteries

- Ingestion may cause electrolysis, corrosion, the release of toxins or pressure effects.
- Impaction in the oesophagus is an emergency – it may cause perforation or an oesophagotracheal fistula and must be removed endoscopically as soon as possible. Surgical follow-up is essential.

Caustic substances

- Automatic machine dishwashing detergents, caustic soda, drain cleaners are strong alkalis and cause burns to the gastrointestinal tract when ingested.
- Significant oesophageal damage may occur in absence of proximal injury.
- Arrange surgical oesophagoscopy and follow-up.

SNAKE BITE

This section applies to bites by Australian snakes of the family *Elapidae*. Snake bites by species in other countries cause different effects not outlined in this handbook. Refer to local publications. Expert advice on envenomation may be obtained from the Australian Venom Research Unit 24-hr advisory service (03 8344 7753).

Of the many species of snakes in Australia, the principal dangerous species are from the genera of:

- Brown Snakes.
- Tiger snakes.
- Taipans.
- Death Adders.
- Black snakes.
- Copperheads.
- Several marine genera.

Venom from these species contains:

- Neurotoxins which cause neuromuscular paralysis with respiratory failure.
- Procoagulants that cause disseminated intravascular coagulation with subsequent haemorrhage due to depletion of clotting factors (Death Adders do not contain significant procoagulant).

Other less important components are haemolysins, anticoagulants and rhabdomyolysins.

Although not all snakes are venomous and envenomation does not always accompany a bite by a venomous snake, every snake bite should be regarded as potentially lethal.

In young children a history of snake bite is often uncertain.

Symptoms and signs of envenomation

The bite site may be identifiable by fang or scratch marks surrounded by bruising or oedema. It is important to note, however, that a bite site may be undetectable and occasionally unnoticed by a victim.

- Headache, nausea, vomiting and abdominal pain may occur within an hour of envenomation
- Early neurotoxic signs are ptosis, diplopia, blurred vision, facial muscle weakness, dysphonia and dysphagia.
- Advanced neurotoxic signs are weakness of limb, trunk and respiratory muscles.
- Spontaneous haemorrhage may occur from mucous membranes, occasionally into solid organs, and from needle puncture sites.
- Hypotension secondary to haemorrhage and respiratory failure
- Renal failure may occur, secondary to hypotension, haemolysis and rhabdomyolysis, particularly if treatment with antivenom is delayed.

The syndrome culminates in respiratory and cardiovascular failure within several hours after envenomation, but may be accelerated in a small child or after multiple bites.

Suspected envenomation

If there is a history of snake bite but no symptoms or signs, the patient should be observed closely for approximately 12 h.

- Test blood coagulation, as it is both a sensitive and reliable indicator of envenomation by major species (in Victoria).

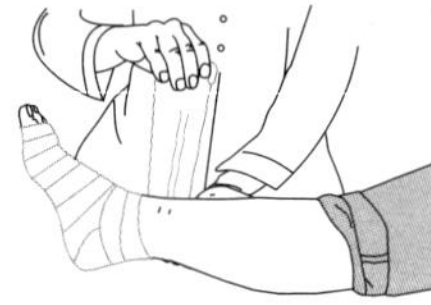

Apply a broad pressure bandage over the bite site as soon as possible. Do not remove clothing, as the movement in doing so will promote the entry of venom into the blood stream. Keep the bitten limb still.

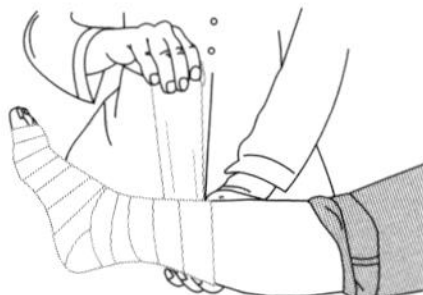

The bandage should be as tight as you would apply to a sprained ankle.

Note: Bandage upwards from the toes or fingers of the bitten limb to help immobilisation. Even though a little venom may be squeezed upwards, the bandage will be far more comfortable than if applied from above downwards; and may be left in place longer.

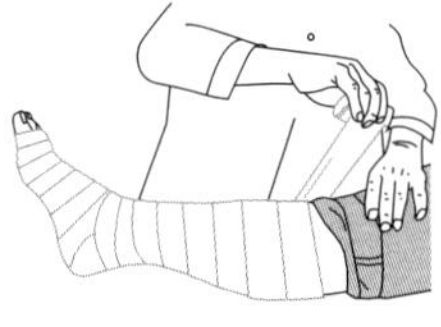

Extend the bandages as far up the limb as possible.

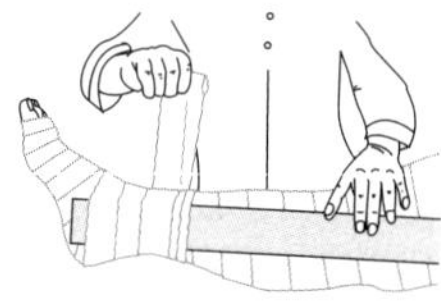

Apply a splint to the leg to immobilise joints on either side of the bite.

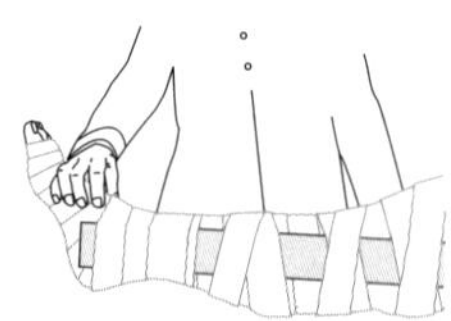

Bind it firmly to as much of the leg as possible. Bring transport to the patients.

Hospital Staff:
Please note that first aid measures are usually removed soon after the patient is seen in hospital. Do not leave on for hours.

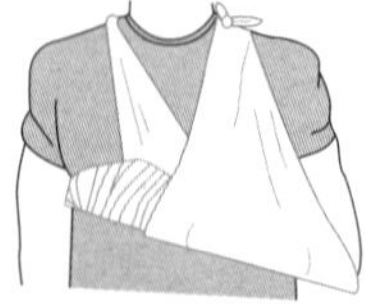

Bites on the hand or forearm
1. Bind to elbow with bandages.
2. Use splint to elbow.
3. Use sling.

Fig. 2.2 Pressure-immobilisation first-aid bandage

- Apply a pressure-immobilisation first aid bandage (Figure 2.2) if not already applied. It can be removed after ensuring that antivenom is available.
- Perform a venom-detection test (see below). A positive test of a swab from the bite site or of a biological sample (urine or blood) indicates which antivenom to administer, if clinically indicated.

Definite envenomation

A number of measures may be required, depending on the severity of envenomation (see Figure 2.3):

- Resuscitation with mechanical ventilation, oxygen therapy and fluid volume restoration.
- Apply a pressure-immobilisation first aid bandage (Figure 2.2) if not already in place. Do not remove an existing first aid bandage until antivenom has been administered. Cut a hole in the existing bandage to obtain a bite site swab if needed and then reinforce.
- Perform a venom test of urine (preferred), blood or bite site swab (or all).
- Administer antivenom (i.v.).
- Coagulation factors (fresh frozen plasma). Occasionally blood transfusion is needed.

Antivenom therapy

Specific antivenoms are available against the Brown snake, Tiger snake, Black snake, Taipan, Death Adder and Beaked Sea snake. A polyvalent preparation contains all the above-named antivenoms except the Beaked Sea Snake. All are given i.v.

- Antivenom is required for clinical signs of envenomation, or for symptomless significant coagulopathy that may cause a serious (e.g. intracranial) haemorrhage. A mild coagulopathy may resolve but requires repeat testing.
- Monovalent preparations are preferred because of a lower incidence of adverse reaction compared with polyvalent antivenom.
- Always premedicate the patient with adrenaline 0.005 mg/kg; (i.e. 0.05 mL/kg of 1:10000 s.c. or 0.005 mL/kg of 1:1,000 for larger patients) before the first dose (only) of antivenom to prevent anaphylaxis or to ameliorate the severity. A course of prednisolone 1 mg/kg orally, daily for 2–5 days may prevent serum sickness, which may occur after polyvalent antivenom or after multiple doses of monovalent antivenom.

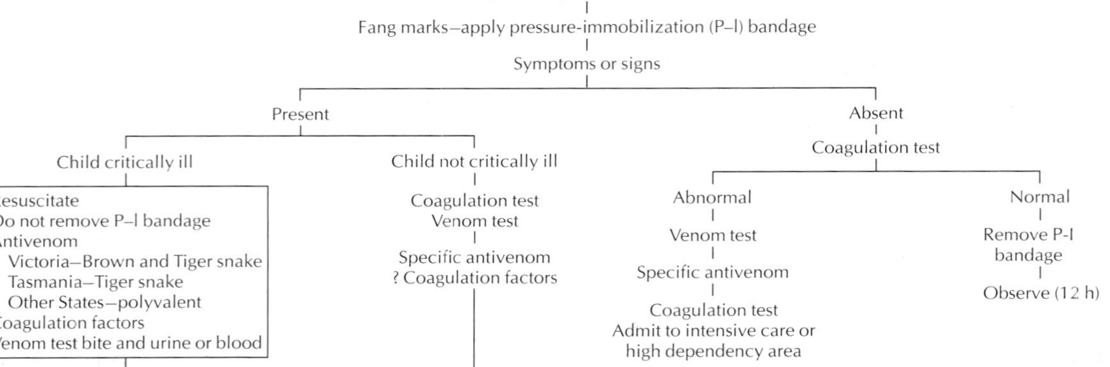

Titrate specific antivenom and coagulation factors against clinical state and coagulation
Admit to intensive care or high dependency area

Dangers and mistakes in management:

- Fang marks may not be visible
- Premature removal of P–I bandage may allow sudden systemic envenomation
- Erroneous identification may cause wrong antivenom to be administered. If in doubt give polyvalent
- Delayed onset of paralysis may be missed
- Insufficient antivenom
- Antivenom without premedication
- Antivenom without clinical or laboratory evidence of envenomation

Fig. 2.3 Management of snake bite

- Selection of antivenom should be based on the result of a venom-detection test or on reliable identification of the snake, as there is little cross-reactivity between antivenoms. Do not rely upon the victim's or witness's identification unless expert.
- If antivenom therapy is required urgently before species identification, administer antivenom according to location. In Victoria give both Brown and Tiger snake antivenom, in Tasmania give Tiger snake antivenom, and elsewhere give polyvalent antivenom. All bites by marine species can be treated with Beaked Sea snake or Tiger snake antivenom. Brown snake, Taipan, Death Adder and Black snake antivenoms are only effective against those species, whereas Tiger snake antivenom is effective against Tiger snakes, Copperheads, Red-bellied Black snake and many minor species.
- Dilute with crystalloid and infuse intravenously over 30 min (faster in life-threatening envenomation).
- The dose of antivenom cannot be predetermined because the amount of venom injected and the patient's susceptibility to it are unknown. Initially administer at least 3 ampoules of Brown snake antivenom or 1 ampoule of other types and titrate additional doses against the clinical and coagulation status. In the treatment of moderate envenomation of children, several ampoules are usually required, while in severe envenomation many ampoules may be required.
- Administer antivenom before giving blood or coagulation factors to forestall further disseminated intravascular coagulation.

Venom Detection Kit

The Venom Detection Kit (VDK) is a bedside or laboratory 3 step enzyme immunoassay, able to detect venom in urine or blood or from a swab of a bite site in very low concentration. It takes about 25 minutes to perform. If positive, it indicates which antivenom to administer (if clinically indicated) but not necessarily the species of snake.

SPIDER BITES

Red-back spider

The venom of this spider contains a neurotoxin that causes release of neurotransmitters. Although potentially lethal, the syndrome of envenomation (latrodectism) develops slowly over many hours, and no deaths have been recorded since an antivenom has been available. A similar syndrome is caused by many species of the genus *Latrodectus* worldwide (Australia, *L. hasselti*; New Zealand, *L. katipo, L. hasselti*).

Symptoms and signs

- Severe local pain.
- Local erythema, persistent pain, oedema, pruritus, sweating and regional lymphadenopathy.
- Systemic effects may include distal limb and abdominal pain, hypertension, sweating, vomiting, fever and headache.
- Myalgia, muscle spasms, arthralgia, paraesthesia and weakness may last many weeks.

Management

- Do not use a pressure-immobilisation bandage.
- If the effects remain mild and localised up to 24 h after a bite, treatment may be symptomatic only.
- Severe local and systemic effects or prolonged mild effects warrant administration of antivenom i.m. (occasionally i.v.). Sometimes several ampoules are needed. Antivenom has been effective even when administered months after envenomation. Although the rate of adverse reactions is low (<0.5%), a premedication with promethazine may be used. In all cases, adrenaline should be at hand to treat anaphylaxis (see Medical emergencies, chapter 1).

White-tailed spider

Bites by this spider are not fatal nor always troublesome, but delayed severe local and extended painful skin necrosis may develop over several days and require excision, grafting and parenteral analgesia.

Funnel-web spiders

Several large aggressive species can threaten life by injecting a venom that releases neurotransmitters and catecholamines. Several dangerous species exist in NSW and Queensland. In some other states (including Victoria) Funnel-web species exist but are not known to be dangerous. Envenomation does not always accompany a bite.

Symptoms and signs

Envenomation is indicated by (in approximate sequence):

- Local muscle fasciculation, piloerection, vomiting, abdominal pain, profuse sweating, salivation and lacrimation.

- Hypertension, tachyarrhythmias and vasoconstriction develop.
- The syndrome culminates in coma, respiratory failure and terminal hypotension.

Management

- Apply a pressure-immobilisation bandage.
- Administer Funnel-web spider antivenom i.v.
- Provide mechanical ventilation, airway protection, atropine and cardiovascular therapy as required.

JELLYFISH STINGS

Chironex Box Jellyfish

This is the world's most venomous animal. It has a cuboid body, approximately 30 cm in diameter and numerous trailing tentacles, and inhabits shallow northern Australian coastal waters. Stings are most common from October to May, but have been recorded throughout the year. Contact with the tentacles leads to the discharge of millions of nematocysts that fire barbs through the epidermis and blood vessels, releasing venom that contains myotoxins, haemolysin and dermatonecrotic toxins, and possibly a neurotoxin. Severity of envenomation is related to the length of tentacles contacting the skin.

Symptoms and signs

- Severe pain and possible cardiorespiratory arrest due to direct cardiotoxicity and possible neurological effects causing apnoea.

Management

- Rescue the victim from water to prevent drowning.
- Cardiopulmonary resuscitation may be required on the beach.
- Dowsing of adherent tentacles with vinegar/acetic acid to inactivate undischarged nematocysts (supplies of vinegar are stocked at popular beaches).
- Analgesia: parenteral for extensive stings, cold packs for minor stings.
- Antivenom i.v. (3 ampoules for life-threatening signs, 1–2 ampoules for analgesia or to prevent skin scarring).

Prevention is most important. Envenomation is prevented by light clothing. Unguarded waters must not be entered when jellyfish are in-shore. Beach warning signs should not be ignored.

Irukandji Jellyfish

This small tropical jellyfish has a bell, measuring 2 × 2.5 cm and 4 tentacles – one from each corner trailing a few to 35 cm. It is almost transparent and difficult to see.

Symptoms and signs

Although the sting is only moderately painful, it is followed after a variable period by a syndrome of:

- Nausea, vomiting, profuse sweating, agitation and muscle cramps
- Vasoconstriction and severe systemic and pulmonary hypertension (due to release of catecholamines). This may cause acute heart failure.

Management

- Mechanical ventilation and vasodilators may be required.

CHAPTER 3
PAIN MANAGEMENT

George Chalkiadis

GENERAL PRINCIPLES OF PAEDIATRIC ANALGESIA

Premature and term neonates, infants and children do experience and suffer pain. There is no evidence that they experience less pain than adults. If unrelieved or inadequately treated, pain has negative consequences.

Consequences of Pain
Physiological

- *Central nervous system*: increase in intracranial pressure, increased risk of intraventricular haemorrhage in premature neonates and spinal cord wind-up (augmented response to subsequent non-noxious afferent input possibly predisposing to persistent pain syndromes).
- *Cardiovascular*: increased heart rate and blood pressure and increased oxygen consumption.
- *Respiratory*: hypoxaemia, impaired ventilation, decreased cough and cooperation with physiotherapy, increased secretion retention and atelectasis.
- *Endocrine*: increase in stress response to surgery and illness.

Psychological

- Anxiety and fear.
- Nightmares and sleep disturbance.
- Behavioural and personality disturbance.

Emotional

- Pain behaviour (distress).

Numerous misconceptions contribute to undertreatment of paediatric pain, including:

- All children are 'sensitive' to analgesics.
- Neonates and children do not experience pain or remember painful events.

- Opioids are addictive or otherwise too dangerous to use in children.
- Pain is character building for children.

ASSESSMENT OF ACUTE PAIN

- Pain scores are important! They are the 5th vital sign on patient's observation charts.
- Pain assessment involves more than simply recording a pain score. In the setting of acute pain, pain assessment involves eliciting a careful history (site, onset, duration, character and radiation) and examining the child before making a decision as to the adequacy of analgesia. Pain-rating scales, behavioural observation and physiological parameters are often helpful.
- In neonates, infants and children who are preverbal, have a cognitive impairment or communication difficulties, pain scores are based (by necessity) on physiological (e.g. heart rate, respiratory rate, blood pressure, muscle spasm) and behavioural parameters (e.g. vocalisation, facial grimacing, posturing, movement). The ability to move (e.g. sitting up after laparotomy) and touch the painful area usually signifies adequate analgesia, whereas a child lying still and withdrawn may be in severe pain.
- Special scoring tools are available for children whose behavioural responses may be difficult to interpret (e.g. those with severe spasticity or self injurious behaviour) but are cumbersome to use. Parents and regular caregivers of these children are often best equipped to interpret what is likely to be pain.
- In children with normal cognition and communication abilities, the child's perception of pain intensity, their ability to use various self-reporting tools and their pain behaviour is influenced by many factors including:
  - Environment.
  - Literacy and numeracy.
  - Sociocultural factors.
  - Affective factors.
  - Coping strategies.
  - Age and development.

- Self-report scores (e.g. Wong Baker Faces Pain Rating Scale, visual analogue scale, verbal numerical rating scale) are subjective and take the above factors into account. Trends of change in an individual's pain score or function (e.g. ability to turn in bed comfortably, ability to walk to the toilet) are more important than the 'raw' score. Children over 4 years can usually use simple Faces Pain Rating Scales.

ANALGESICS FOR ACUTE PAIN

Multimodal analgesia

Using different classes of analgesics in combination after surgery may be beneficial in:

- Optimising analgesia.
- Reducing the dose of each drug.
- Reducing side effects.

Non-steroidal anti-inflammatory drugs (NSAIDs), local anaesthetics, paracetamol, ketamine and opioids administered via any route may be employed in combination.

Paracetamol

- Effective for mild to moderate pain, also antipyretic.
- Thought to act by inhibiting cyclo-oxygenase in the CNS, while sparing peripheral prostaglandin production.
- Opioid sparing effect may be significant.
- May be administered orally or rectally. The oral route is preferable; the time to peak concentration is sooner (30–60 min *vs.* 2–3 h) and absorption is more reliable.
- Hepatotoxicity has been reported in children. Use with caution in patients with severe liver disease, jaundice, malnutrition, glutathione depletion and long-term ingestion.

Codeine

- Weak opioid – ceiling effect to analgesia and increase in opioid side effects with increasing dose.
- Effective for moderate pain in combination with paracetamol and/or NSAIDs.
- After oral administration, peak plasma concentration 60 min.

- Thought to be a prodrug: analgesic effect due to a proportion of codeine being metabolised to morphine.
- The cytochrome P450 enzyme responsible (CYP2D6) shows genetic polymorphism and age dependent activity. The implications are:
  - Codeine is likely to be ineffective in poor metabolisers (9% of English, 1% of Swedish, German and mainland Chinese populations, 30% of Ethiopians and Hong Kong Chinese).
  - Reduced analgesic efficacy in neonates and infants, although enzyme activity increases immediately after birth.
  - Adverse effects of codeine may occur in the absence of analgesia in poor metabolizers.
- Codeine may be regarded as a complicated and unreliable method of giving a low dose of morphine.
- Available in Australia as proprietary mixtures (e.g. Painstop, Liquigesic) and tablets (e.g. Panadeine, Panadeine Forte). All except Panadeine Forte are available as over the counter medications. Painstop and Liquigesic both contain alcohol – a burning pain may result on ingestion after tonsillectomy.

Tramadol

- Acts on mu (μ) opioid receptors peripherally and centrally and by reducing serotonin and noradrenaline reuptake centrally, thus enhancing the function of descending inhibitory pain pathways. Effects only partially reversed by naloxone (30%). Dose-related analgesia.
- May be useful in opioid insensitive pain and patients who can't metabolise codeine, although there are implications regarding poor drug metabolism in this population.
- Less opioid side effects e.g. constipation, respiratory depression and pruritis.
- Nausea and vomiting are common and may be more likely with rapid i.v. administration.
- Less potential for tolerance than opioids and minimal cross-tolerance with morphine are favourable properties for long-term use.
- Oral (immediate and sustained-release) and parenteral (i.m. and i.v.) forms available.

- Risk of inducing seizures in those with a history of epilepsy or those receiving concomitant antidepressants.

Non-steroidal anti-inflammatory drugs

- Analgesic, antipyretic and anti-inflammatory.
- Effective as analgesics in the postoperative period although not powerful enough to be used alone for severe pain.
- Opioid sparing effect significant (reduced likelihood of vomiting, sedation, constipation and respiratory depression).
- Act by inhibiting cyclo-oxygenase (COX) and prostaglandin (PG) production. Old generation NSAIDs inhibit both COX-1 and COX-2 isoenzymes, whereas new generation more selectively inhibit COX-2. COX-1 inhibition is thought to account for the majority of NSAID side effects. COX-2 is induced by surgical trauma and tissue damage and contributes to inflammation and hyperalgesia. Selective COX-2 inhibition is desirable and may account for the therapeutic analgesic and anti-inflammatory actions of NSAIDs.
- COX-1 undesirable side effects:
  - Platelet dysfunction (increased surgical bleeding).
  - Renal dysfunction (maintain hydration).
  - Gastro-intestinal side effects e.g. gastritis, peptic ulceration (administer with food).
  - Possible reduction in osteoblast formation (relevant to use of NSAID after orthopaedic surgery where bone graft used).
  - Bronchospasm in susceptible individuals (i.e. triad of nasal polyps, asthma and aspirin sensitivity).
  - Severe asthma alone is a relative contraindication.
- COX-2 inhibitors:
  - Celecoxib, rofecoxib and meloxicam are available as oral preparations and parecoxib is available for i.v. use.
  - Studies of long-term use in adults show less gastro-intestinal side effects in first 6 months but then similar incidence later.
  - Little evidence to support their use over non-selective NSAIDs for relief of paediatric acute pain.
- Aspirin has been implicated in Reye syndrome and it should not be used as an analgesic in infants and children.

Ketamine

- NMDA (*N*-methyl-D-aspartate) receptor antagonist.
- Potent analgesic in low dose (0.1–0.4 mg/kg/h) i.v. or s.c. continuous infusion. Indications include:
  - In conjunction with opioids:
    - When moderate to severe pain persists despite 'maximal' opioid infusion rate.
    - When opioid tolerance has developed (e.g. cancer pain).
  - Neuropathic pain.
- Restlessness, nightmares, hallucinations and delirium are rarely seen with low dose infusion but may occur after bolus administration.
- Ketamine is a phencyclidine derivative and in higher doses (e.g. 1–2 mg/kg i.v.) results in dissociative anaesthesia (a trance-like state in which the eyes remain open with a slow nystagmic gaze). EEG shows dissociation between the thalamocortical and limbic systems. The patient is non-communicative although wakefulness may appear to be present. Varying degrees of hypertonus and purposeful movement may occur.
- Ketamine may be administered orally/i.v./i.m. for procedural pain management in a monitored environment. In these situations, higher doses are used and problems with CNS side effects, hypersalivation, nausea and vomiting, tachycardia, systemic and pulmonary hypertension and raised intracranial pressure may occur. Airway reflexes may be obtunded; patients should be fasted as for general anaesthesia.

Local anaesthetics

- Local anaesthetics exert their action by blocking sodium channels.
- With increasing concentration of solution, nerve block is denser, with increasing likelihood of motor block in addition to sensory blockade.

Established local anaesthetics:

- *Lignocaine* – safe, rapid onset, relatively short acting. Maximum safe dose 3 mg/kg for plain solution, 7 mg/kg with adrenaline.
- *Bupivacaine* – safe (provided guidelines for use adhered to). Long duration of action. Systemic absorption or intravascular injection may result in toxicity. Bupivacaine-induced cardiotoxicity is difficult to treat. Maximum safe dose 2 mg/kg.

New local anaesthetics

- *Ropivacaine* and *levobupivacaine* are less cardiotoxic than bupivacaine.

Routes of adminstration

Infiltration of subcutaneous tissues

- Provides analgesia for 1–3 h. Useful for suprapubic catheterisation, intercostal chest drain insertion, suturing of lacerations and postoperative analgesia. Longer lasting analgesia may result from continuous infusion into wound via surgically placed catheter.

Topical

- Eye drops for removal of corneal foreign body in cooperative patients, lignocaine gel applied to urethra for urethral catheterisation, cophenylcaine spray to nostrils and nasopharynx for nasogastric tube insertion. (See Procedures, chapter 4).

Peripheral nerve block

- Excellent analgesia for suturing extensive lacerations or fractures (e.g. femoral nerve block for femur fracture), repair of nail bed injuries (digital nerve blocks). The most peripheral nerve to anaesthetize the operative field should be blocked:
  - Lower limb: digital, sural, saphenous, common peroneal, femoral and lateral cutaneous nerve of thigh nerves.
  - Upper limb: digital, median, ulnar, radial nerves.
  - Chest wall and abdomen: intercostal nerves.
  - Face and lip: supraorbital, infraorbital, mental nerves.

Intravenous regional anaesthesia

- Prilocaine or lignocaine is used via this route to provide limb anaesthesia. (See Procedures, chapter 4).

Central nerve block

- Central nerve blocks such as caudal epidurals, lumbar epidurals and spinals are the domain of anaesthetists in operating theatres.
  - Spinals in the paediatric population are performed mainly in neonates undergoing inguinal hernia repair to reduce the risk of postoperative apnoea. Spinal anaesthesia with bupivacaine is short acting (60 min) in this age group.

- Epidurals provide intra-operative analgesia that extends into the postoperative period. Single shot caudal epidural analgesia administered in the operating theatre may be effective for up to 12 h. Inserting an epidural catheter with the tip placed in the region of the dermatomes that need to be blocked allows for the continuous infusion of analgesia.

Local anaesthetic toxicity

- Inadvertent intravascular injection of local anaesthetic drugs may result in death. Quoted 'safe' ranges are only a guide and toxicity can result even when these are adhered to.
- Always aspirate prior to injection.
- As plasma concentration of local anaesthetic increases, toxicity is manifest by (in order):
  - Tongue and peri-oral numbness.
  - Lightheadedness.
  - Blurred vision.
  - Tinnitus.
  - Muscular twitching.
  - Unconsciousness.
  - Convulsions.
  - Coma.
  - Respiratory arrest.
  - Cardiovascular depression and arrhythmias.
- In order to detect toxicity early, it is important to maintain verbal communication with the child as local anaesthetic is injected. In the case of non-verbal children, recognising the early signs of toxicity may be difficult. Observe for increasing irritability or behavioural changes while injecting the local anaesthetic.
- If a sufficiently large dose of local anaesthetic is administered systemically, the initial signs of CNS excitation are rapidly followed by CNS depression (i.e. seizure activity ceases) or CNS depression may occur without a preceding excitatory phase (especially if CNS depressants have already been administered).
- Arrhythmias (especially those induced by bupivacaine) may be refractory to treatment. Cardiopulmonary bypass may be necessary.

Clonidine

- An α_2 adrenergic receptor agonist.
- Epidurally thought to stimulate descending noradrenergic medullospinal pathways that inhibit the release of nociceptive neurotransmitters in the dorsal horn of the spinal cord.
- Prolongs the duration of local anaesthetic block administered as a single shot caudal epidural injection.
- Improves the quality of the local anaesthetic block administered via continuous epidural infusion.
- Provides excellent analgesia (in combination with bupivacaine) after intra-articular administration following knee arthroscopy.
- Used intravenously for analgesia and sedation in some paediatric ICU.
- Useful in patients susceptible to, or experiencing opioid withdrawal.
- Side effects include sedation, hypotension and bradycardia.

Strong opioid analgesics

General principles

- Opioids act principally by binding to mu (μ) opioid receptors as full agonists, resulting in dose dependent analgesia.
- Opioids remain the most powerful parenteral analgesics for children in severe pain.
- Published dosage guidelines are appropriate for opioid naïve patients. Ultimately the dose should be titrated to effect.
- Patients already on regular opioids may require higher doses to achieve adequate analgesia.
- Tolerance to opioids occurs over time. The dose may need to be increased if tolerance develops. This is not usually an acute phenomenon e.g. in the acute postoperative period.
- Consider the co-administration of non-opioid analgesics and adjuvant agents (anticonvulsants or tricyclic antidepressants) where appropriate.
- Patients who have been on opioids for an extended period of time may develop signs and symptoms of opioid withdrawal if they are rapidly weaned or ceased. Slow weaning may be necessary.

Table 3.1 Opioid side effects

Common	*Dose dependent*	*Histamine release*
Nausea	Respiratory depression	Hypotension
Vomiting	Miosis	Rash
Pruritis	Euphoria	Bronchospasm
Constipation	Sedation	
	Bradycardia	

Routes of administration

Oral

- Low oral bioavailability.
- Morphine, oxycodone, methadone and hydromorphone are available as oral and immediate release liquid preparations.
- Morphine and oxycodone are available as slow release preparations. They are indicated where the need for opioid analgesia is likely to be prolonged and continuous e.g. cancer pain. Plasma concentrations remain stable and plateau within 24 h after dose alteration. These preparations are generally not suitable for the management of acute exacerbations of pain.
- Available as tablets which must be swallowed whole to preserve the integrity of the slow release coating. Morphine is available as granules, which allow easier administration via gastrostomy tube and administration of small doses more suitable for small children.
- Morphine's oral bioavailability is 30% – to convert 24 h intravenous morphine consumption (mg) to oral equivalent dose (mg/24 h), multiply by 3. If slow release preparations are to be used, divide this new total by 2 and administer 12 h apart.
- Immediate release preparations are indicated when treating acute exacerbations of pain.
- The dose consumed over 24 h can be totalled and used to estimate the total daily dose required for conversion to slow release preparations. This can be done using the immediate release preparation for breakthrough pain when the patient is already receiving a slow release opioid. If breakthrough is required, mainly during the day or night, it may be appropriate to increase the dose of the slow release preparation for the corresponding

time. This can also be achieved by totalling intravenous opioid usage administered by a patient-controlled analgesia or nurse-initiated boluses and calculating the equianalgesic opioid dose for oral administration.

Intravenous

- Parenteral opioids should not be administered without the availability of oxygen, resuscitation equipment and naloxone to reverse the opioid effect.
- Morphine or fentanyl are the preferred opioids for intravenous use in children. Pethidine is no longer recommended due to the risk of convulsions (secondary to accumulation of its metabolite norpethidine).

Intermittent bolus of morphine:

- Indications include rapid attainment of analgesia.
- Infants under 6 months may be more sensitive to opioids. To ensure safe administration in this age group, morphine should be titrated to effect in smaller increments than in older children. Caution should also be exercised in situations where the child may be at added risk e.g. head injury, cardiorespiratory compromise (underlying disease, trauma, infection) and severe developmental delay.

Recommended initial boluses of morphine are:

- Children <12 months: 20 mcg/kg
- Children >12 months and <50 kg: 40 mcg/kg
- Children >50 kg: 2 mg

- Titrate to effect. Wait 5 min before administering repeat bolus.
- Before administering initial or repeat bolus, check that the patient is:
  - In moderate or severe pain.
  - Awake or easily roused to voice.
  - Respiratory rate is:
    >20/min if <12 months
    >15/min if <50 kg
    >12/min if >50 kg
  - In addition to the observations above, monitoring of heart rate and pulse oximetry should be performed while titrating intravenous opioid analgesia.

Continuous Infusion

- Nurse controlled infusion
  - Continuous opioid infusion indicated for ongoing pain relief.
  - Maintains stable plasma concentration.
  - Nurses may administer opioid bolus for breakthrough pain or procedures (and usually increase the continuous infusion rate).
  - Suitable for all ages.
- Patient controlled analgesia (PCA)
  - Suitable for children older than 6 years of age who have the ability to understand the concept of pressing a button to relieve pain and the willingness to use it.
  - It is safe, as children will fall asleep and stop bolusing when plasma levels rise.
  - Indications include postoperative pain, oncology, burns and frequent painful procedures.
  - It offers several advantages:
    - Immediate on-demand analgesia.
    - No opioid administered unless the patient demands it.
    - The ability to program a continuous background infusion if required.
    - Saves nursing time.
    - Enables rapid estimation of a patient's opioid requirements (e.g. cancer pain)

Subcutaneous

- Very effective.
- Suitable for intermittent bolus or continuous infusion of morphine.
- Convenient in the child with difficult intravenous access or where the child is to be treated at home by palliative care services.
- A cannula can be safely placed under the skin without risk of trauma.
- The dose (mg) is the same as for intravenous administration. The solutions are more concentrated than intravenous infusions to minimize the volume infused.

Other

Rectal – problems with reliability of absorption.

Intramuscular – discouraged for paediatric use.

Transdermal – Fentanyl patches suitable for use in children (smallest patch delivers 25 mcg/h). Appropriate for long-term use. Indicated in oncology and other palliative conditions.

Oral Transmucosal – Fentanyl lollypops (not available in Australia).

Management of excessive sedation or respiratory depression

- Cease administration of opioid immediately.
- Administer 100% oxygen by mask.
- Commence bag and mask ventilation if necessary.
- Administer naloxone 0.01 mg/kg i.v. stat (up to 0.1 mg/kg (max 2 mg) for severe respiratory depression/coma).

PROCEDURAL PAIN

Everyday events such as blood collection, cannula insertion, port cannulation, lumbar puncture and suturing are a source of major fear and anxiety for children. Children with illnesses that necessitate undergoing multiple painful procedures must be treated with care and sensitivity from the outset to avoid psychological trauma and unnecessary distress. Physical restraint should be used only where absolutely necessary.

Consideration must be given to the type of procedure, its urgency, its duration, the age of the patient and the emotional and physical condition of the child when any procedure is planned.

There is no substitute for adequate preparation of the child and their parents. Parents may be as anxious as their child!

- Parents should be informed about the procedure, what to expect and what they are expected to say and do. A strong and encouraging parent may help instil confidence in their child while comforting them physically and providing emotional support.
- An explanatory video/CD ROM may be helpful in preparing the child and their parent for the procedure.

A combination of pharmacological and non-pharmacological techniques is often indicated.

Non-pharmacological techniques

- Non-pharmacological strategies can be used alone for less painful procedures, or as adjuncts to drugs.

- Intervention needs to be tailored to the child and family. Parental presence should be encouraged except where the parent themselves have poor coping strategies and where their behaviour further increases their child's fear and anxiety. Some suggested techniques are listed below.

Neonates and Infants

Sensorimotor aids such as pacifiers with or without sucrose, feeding, warm blankets, holding and rocking. Magnetic resonance imaging scans are performed in neonates without sedation using a wrap-around inflatable foam cuddly, which serves as a restraint.

Older children

Guided imagery and cognitive techniques such as hypnosis, relaxation, distraction, music, art, play, virtual reality devices, positive encouragement and rehearsal may be useful. The use of calico dolls to simulate the procedure has been shown to be effective.

Physical techniques

Application of heat or cold, massage, exercise, rest or immobilisation.

Occasionally the distress of a child may warrant the presence of an anaesthetist to provide intravenous sedation or general anaesthesia.

Pharmacological techniques

Topical local anaesthetic (EMLA or amethocaine)

- The insertion of intravenous drips, lumbar punctures and blood sampling are all potentially distressing for children.
- Application of local anaesthetic cream 1 h before these procedures ensures an area of analgesia of the skin several millimetres deep.
- Iontophoresis of lignocaine results in good skin anaesthesia within 10 min. Delivery device and disposable electrodes are costly.
- EMLA is a mixture of prilocaine 5% and lignocaine 5%, and often vasoconstricts the area under application (onset 60 min).
- Amethocaine 1% is a topical local anaesthetic with a more rapid onset than EMLA (onset 40–60 min). It has vasodilator properties and may cause a painless erythema of the skin that resolves within a few hours. Erythema is common if amethocaine is left on longer than 1 h.

Local anaesthetic infiltration (lignocaine, ropivacaine, bupivacaine or levobupivacaine)

- The skin and subcutaneous tissues can be effectively infiltrated with local anaesthetic solutions.
- Lignocaine stings as it is injected. Adding 1 mL 8.4% sodium bicarbonate to 9 mL of Lignocaine solution will eliminate the stinging sensation.
- The addition of adrenaline 1 in 200,000 or 1 in 400,000 (or 5–10 mcg/mL) may increase the duration of action, slow systemic absorption by up to 50% and reduce bleeding.

Adrenaline should not be used in end organs such as fingers, toes, penis, nose or ears due to the risk of ischaemia.

Anxiolytics and sedatives

- Midazolam oral 0.5 mg/kg (max 15 mg) or intranasal 0.4 mg/kg (max 10g) 20–30 min prior to treatment.
- Sedation is not analgesia!
- Sedation alone is useful for non-painful procedures e.g. diagnostic ultrasound.
- For painful procedures, analgesia is also necessary.

Midazolam should not be given to children with respiratory insufficiency or neuromuscular problems.

Nitrous oxide

Increasing use is being made in burns and oncology units of nitrous oxide, which is a very useful inhalational analgesic.

- Provides potent short-term analgesia for painful procedures such as wound dressings and the removal of catheters.
- Rapid onset and offset.
- Side effects may include sedation, nausea and vomiting and bone marrow depression with prolonged exposure (>12 h). The latter is unlikely to pose a problem for a single procedure but should be considered in the child requiring daily repeat procedures.
- It should not be used in patients with head injuries, pneumothorax, obtunded patients or cardiac patients.
- The person administering nitrous oxide should have adequate airway management skills.
- Patients should be fasted prior to its administration.

- Methods of delivery include:
  - Entonox (a mixture of 50% nitrous oxide and 50% oxygen).
  - Quantiflex (variable demand delivery system of nitrous oxide and oxygen).

CHRONIC OR PERSISTENT PAIN MANAGEMENT

Acute and chronic pain are distinct entities that require vastly different diagnostic and management skills.

Acute pain

- Tangible and understandable by the patient, family, friends and the treating doctor.
- Usually brief, evoked by a recognised noxious stimulus and associated with an adaptive biological significance (e.g. protection of injured part to encourage healing).
- Usually improves rapidly and is associated with functional improvement and pain score reduction on a daily basis.
- Usually related to the nature and extent of tissue damage.
- Responds to pharmacological intervention.

Chronic or persistent pain

- Often nothing to see or minimal evidence of tissue damage.
- Often presents for prolonged duration.
- May be evoked by minor trauma.
- Improves slowly over time with an undulating course. Improvement and deterioration may be linked to life stresses.
- Not necessarily related simply or directly to the nature and extent of tissue damage.
- Does not always respond to pharmacological intervention.
- Often associated with secondary gains (e.g. school, sport or chore avoidance).

Patient assessment

It is important to assess the physical and psychosocial causes for the child's presentation. Integrated multidisciplinary assessment is ideal and facilitates the co-ordinated implementation of treatment. The factors contributing to and maintaining persistent pain vary and will determine treatment. Treatment may involve all or part of the multidisciplinary team.

Team members should include a pain medicine specialist, physiotherapist, clinical psychologist, occupational therapist and a child psychiatrist. The team should have access to an orthopaedic surgeon, neurosurgeon, paediatrician, paediatric rheumatologist and a rehabilitation specialist.

Evaluate the contribution of:

- Nociception – is the pain:
  - Nociceptive (arising from peripheral or visceral nociceptors)?
  - Neurogenic (arising at any point from the primary afferent neurone to higher centres in the brain)?
  - Psychogenic (occurs in the absence of any identifiable noxious stimulus or injurious process)?
- Fixed factors (age, cognitive level, previous pain experience, witnessed examples of how other family members react to pain).
- Situational factors (school, learned pain triggers, independent pain reducing strategies).
- Suffering (fear, anxiety, anger, frustration, depression).
- Pain behaviour (overt distress, secondary gain, visiting multiple health professionals because of pain, moaning, splinting, complaining of pain).

Assess for:

- Unhelpful belief systems of child and/or family (e.g. if pain were cured the other problems would not exist).
- Unrealistic expectations (e.g. it is others responsibility to fix the problem).
- Functional disability (e.g. inability to play sport, socialise with peers, school absenteeism).

Examine the painful site:

- What is causing the pain?
- Are there signs of complex regional pain syndrome? (See page 56)
- Is there any evidence of secondary deconditioning (muscle wasting, joint stiffening, tendon shortening)?

Treatment goals

- Eliminate pain.
- Restore function.
- Reduce pain behaviour.

Ideally it would be possible to identify the cause of pain, treat it and eliminate it. This is not always possible; therefore resuming a more active and fulfilling lifestyle less constrained by pain and reducing pain behaviour become the treatment goals. Coordination of outpatient appointments facilitates achieving these goals by minimising school absenteeism, time off work for parents and discouraging adoption of the sick role.

Rationale for cognitive behavioural therapy

Unhelpful thoughts or beliefs associated with chronic or persistent pain may relate to:

- Self-efficacy.
  - Refers to the belief about one's ability to change one's life.
  - Often low in children and adolescents with persistent pain.
  - A factor of depression and fear.
  - Due to experience of treatments over which control is taken by powerful others.
- Attribution of causality.
  - Need to make sense of the experience.
  - 'Face-saving' resolution may be necessary in some cases.
- Attribution of blame.
  - Need to attribute blame or responsibility for the pain.
  - Anger directed at those who caused pain.
  - May be accompanied by threats of litigation.
- Catastrophising.
  - Consequences of events quickly and anxiously blown out of proportion.

Pain behaviour is exacerbated where the following reinforcements are present:

- Where pain is central to communication (e.g. to receive a diagnosis or treatment).
- Where the child is fearful of increased pain (e.g. with movement).
- Where the meaning of pain is fear inducing.
- Where there is an absence of reinforcement for non-pain communication.

The child and their parents may hold unhelpful beliefs and inadvertently maintain suffering, disability and dependency. The parent(s) or child may obtain significant secondary gain from the child's maintained pain.

Non-pharmacological techniques

Cognitive behavioural techniques address the (often unhelpful) thoughts that accompany and maintain pain and disability:

- Pain coping strategies:
  - Relaxation: muscle relaxation via body awareness techniques, meditation, self-hypnosis or biofeedback.
  - Distraction: art, play or music therapy.
- Pain education
  - An understanding that stress, anxiety and anger may contribute to pain. Addressing what is contributing to these feelings (often school or family stressors) or managing the feelings more effectively, may reduce or eliminate pain.
  - Pain does not always mean damage: understanding that pain is not a hindrance to return to function.
- Illness information (if one has been identified) outlining implications for the future.
- Pacing activity with reasonable goals:
  - Return to school.
  - Physiotherapy reconditioning programs involve gradual return to function utilizing:
    - Muscle stretches.
    - Postural exercises.
    - Reconditioning programs (secondary deconditioning occurs rapidly, especially when fear of touch or movement exists).
    - Stress loading (e.g. 'scrub and carry' techniques for the upper limbs, weight bearing for lower limbs).
- Thought stopping or challenging.
- Behaviour modification: based on modifying the consequences of the child's pain experience and pain behaviour by rewarding positive behaviour.
- Management of setbacks.
- Sleep management.

Other non-pharmacological techniques

- Family therapy: how family dynamics may maintain pain; how pain affects the rest of the family (e.g. lack of attention for well siblings).
- Parental counselling: to address helplessness and loss of control. Parents may inadvertently support illness and ignore non-pain activities. Equip parents with strategies to manage pain behaviour.

- Vocational counselling.
- Assertiveness training.
- School liaison.
  - Address bullying.
  - Modifications to allow return to school despite disability.
  - Equip teachers with strategies to deal with pain behaviour.
  - Graded return to school programs with involvement and education of teachers.
- Physiotherapy:
  - Ultrasound treatment.
  - Heat/cold treatment.
  - Transcutaneous electrical nerve stimulation (TENS) – activates large myelinated primary afferent fibres (A-fibres) that act through inhibitory circuits within the dorsal horn to reduce nociceptive transmission through small unmyelinated fibres (C-fibres). This is more likely to be effective if pain responds to heat or cold.
- Hydrotherapy.
- Acupuncture.

Pharmacological techniques

Paracetamol

- Limit the dose for long-term administration to 90 mg/kg per day.

Steroids

- Triamcinolone used for joint injections, trigger point injections, tendon sheaths and neuralgias.
- Dexamethasone administered by iontophoresis for soft tissue injuries.
- Methylprednisolone via epidural administration for localised nerve root irritation due to disc herniation without motor weakness.

NSAIDs

- Topical gels (diclofenac, piroxicam, ibuprofen).
- Oral and rectal preparations (described above).

Capsaicin

- Acts by releasing substance P at nerve endings. Applied topically and useful in rheumatic and neuropathic pain.

Tricyclic antidepressants

- Indications include severe unremitting pain, especially if neuropathic, complex regional pain syndrome (CRPS), associated depression or poor sleep. Noradrenergic and serotonergic reuptake inhibitors provide more effective analgesia.
- Improve pain even if depression is not present; tricyclic antidepressants suppress pathological neural discharges.
- Effective within days, once appropriate dose reached.
- Amitriptyline 0.2 mg/kg increasing over 2 weeks to 2 mg/kg/day. Administer as a single dose before bed to take advantage of sedative properties. Increase dosage until the side effects become unacceptable; e.g. dry mouth and morning somnolence.

Anticonvulsants

- Indicated in neuropathic pain and CRPS.
- Dosage should be in the therapeutic anticonvulsant range, although there is no evidence of any relationship between analgesic effect and the plasma level. Some recommend increasing the dosage to the point of side effects or analgesia.

Opioids

- Only partially modulate central sensitisation. Usually ineffective in controlling neuropathic pain or pain secondary to CRPS.
- Indicated in cancer pain and nociceptive pain.
- Tramadol may be useful

Ketamine

- Reduces primary and secondary hyperalgesia. It is a more potent modulator of central sensitisation than opioids.
- Useful in chronic pain syndromes, especially where pain is neuropathic.

Sympathetic nerve blocks

- These may be useful where sympathetically maintained pain is present (e.g. CRPS Type I or II, see page 56).
- Their main function is to facilitate physiotherapy by reducing allodynia (pain elicited by a stimulus that is usually not painful) and pain on movement.
- Intravenous regional upper or lower limb block – guanethidine/phentolamine.

Peripheral nerve block

- Bupivacaine +/– steroid.
- Diagnostic: used to identify where the pain is originating (e.g. rectus sheath block for abdominal pain).
- Therapeutic (e.g. in occipital neuralgia and meralgia paraesthetica).

Baclofen

- GABA-B agonist acting on spinal cord reflex mechanisms.
- Used to treat spasticity in patients with spinal cord injury or upper motor neuron conditions; e.g. cerebral palsy and post-cerebrovascular accidents.
- May produce hypotonia, sedation and gastric upset.
- May be used orally or intrathecally via continuous infusion.

Clonidine

- Useful in neuropathic or sympathetically maintained pain.
- May be used orally, transdermally or via epidural.

Anti-arrhythmics

- Lignocaine i.v.: in neuropathic pain (diagnostic) followed by oral mexiletine (for maintenance).

Surgical techniques

These measures are reserved for intractable pain not responsive to conventional methods; e.g. neurectomy, sympathectomy, rhizotomy and cordotomy.

COMPLEX REGIONAL PAIN SYNDROME (TYPES I AND II)

This condition of unknown aetiology is more common in paediatrics than is generally realised. It is essentially a clinical diagnosis. Early recognition is important because the earlier they are identified the easier they are to treat:

- Type I was formerly known as reflex sympathetic dystrophy (RSD). It often occurs after a noxious stimulus to the affected limb (e.g. minor trauma or surgery). Symptoms are disproportionate to the inciting event.
- Type II was formerly referred to as causalgia. It differs from Type I because it occurs after peripheral nerve injury.

The affected area, usually a limb, manifests autonomic, sensory and motor symptoms consisting of:

- Pain:
  - Regional non-dermatomal distribution.
  - Diffuse pain exacerbated by touch (hyperaesthesia).
  - Allodynia (pain elicited by a stimuli that is not usually painful).
- Temperature change (affected limb often colder).
- Changes in skin blood flow – often red/purple colour change.
- Abnormal sweating.
- Oedema.
- Loss of function.
- Abnormal hair growth, skin and/or nail atrophy.

Investigations

- Bone scan often abnormal – increased or decreased uptake.
- Plain X-ray – osteopenia in prolonged cases.
- Acute phase markers normal.
- MRI – diffuse marrow infiltration is sometimes present.

Management

- Management requires early identification, skilful physical therapy, avoidance of immobilisation and multidisciplinary pain management (consider psychiatric assessment, pharmacological and interventional techniques).

NEUROPATHIC PAIN

- Typified by continuous burning with an intermittent electric shock, stabbing or shooting-type discomfort.
- May be paroxysmal or spontaneous.
- Pain in an area of sensory loss.
- Pain in the absence of ongoing tissue damage
- Is associated with dysaesthesia (unpleasant abnormal sensation e.g. ants crawling on skin), allodynia and hyperalgesia (increased pain in response to noxious stimuli)
- Increased sympathetic activity may be present.
- Usually poor response to opioid medication.
- Causes include: CRPS type II, tumour, spinal cord injury, nerve damage (e.g. neuropraxia or avulsion, neuroma).

PAIN IN CHILDREN AND ADOLESCENTS WITH DISABILITIES

Pain assessment in individuals with cerebral palsy, cognitive impairment and/or communication difficulties can prove challenging. No simple pain assessment tools exist. Caregivers are best placed to distinguish pain from 'normal' behaviour in the individual. Pain may manifest as crying, screaming, frequent waking, grimacing, arching, muscle spasm or self-injurious behaviour but some individuals with cerebral palsy may exhibit these behaviours without experiencing pain.

Differential diagnosis includes seizures, anxiety, depression and anger.

Common causes of pain (and possible treatments) include:

- Gastro-oesophageal reflux: (antacids, proton pump inhibitors, H2 antagonists, fundoplication).
- Muscle spasms: look for the underlying cause of pain (e.g. hip subluxation / dental problems). Baclofen (oral or intrathecal), botox and obturator phenol nerve blocks may attenuate adductor scissoring.
- Orthopaedic deformities and inflammation secondary to spasticity and contractures, (mainly affecting limbs and back).
  - Capsulitis.
  - Osteoarthritis.
  - Joint stiffening.
  - Tendon shortening.
  - Joint subluxation.
  - Joint dislocation.

Night waking is frequent with implications for the productivity of siblings and parent. Most settle with re-positioning. Tricyclic antidepressants, via their analgesic and sedative effects, may be useful in reducing the frequency of waking.

WHEN TO REFER TO A MULTIDISCIPLINARY PAIN CLINIC

Refer when:

- Pain persists longer than anticipated (e.g. after an injury).
- Pain is more intense than anticipated.
- Character of pain different to that expected.
- Pain behaviour manifests (e.g. suffering, disability and dependency).
- Loss of function resulting in secondary deconditioning (e.g. muscle wasting).
- Pain interferes with sleep, socialising with peers, school attendance and leisure activities.
- Poor response to medication.
- Complex regional pain syndrome.
- Neuropathic pain.

CHAPTER 4
PROCEDURES

Peter Barnett
Georgia Paxton

Procedures are painful and a source of fear for children. Appropriate analgesia is required and non-pharmacological techniques such as distraction and the presence of a parent can help alleviate distress. Suggested analgesia is included for procedures in this chapter, further details are included in Chapter 3, Pain management. Universal precautions should be taken during any procedure. Gloves and protective eyewear should be worn and a hard plastic container should be within easy reach for the disposal of sharps. When performed, procedures should be documented.

VENEPUNCTURE

Sites

- Cubital fossa.
- Dorsum of the hand.
- Others, as dictated by availability or necessity.

Suggested analgesia

- Topical local anaesthetic (e.g. amethocaine or EMLA [lignocaine, prilocaine]).
- Consider nitrous oxide.

Technique

- In adolescents and older children, blood can be collected with a needle and syringe, as in adults. In infants and small children, a 23–gauge butterfly offers more stability.
- Some visible veins are too small to be used to take blood. A palpable vein is more likely to be successful than a visible but non-palpable vein.

- With small children, an assistant can act as both a restraint and tourniquet.
- An alternative technique is to snap the hub off a 21 or 23–gauge needle, or cut off the tubing of a butterfly then insert the needle into a vein and allow the blood to drip out directly into collection tubes. Several millilitres can be collected this way.

INTRAVENOUS CANNULA INSERTION

Sites

- Dorsum of the hand is preferred, on the non-dominant hand if possible.
- Alternative sites include the anatomical snuffbox, volar aspect of the forearm, dorsum of the foot, great saphenous vein or cubital fossa.
- The site of the cannula usually requires splinting and this needs to be considered (e.g. elbow, foot in a mobile child).
- Scalp veins should only be used when there are no other possibilities (shaved scalp hair regrows very slowly).

Suggested analgesia

- Topical local anaesthetic.
- Consider injectable local anaesthetic in older children (e.g. lignocaine 1%).
- Consider nitrous oxide or sedation (e.g. midazolam 0.5 mg/kg oral, max = 15 mg).

Technique

- Be patient and look carefully for the best option.
- Ensure that the child is warm and there is adequate light.
- Wrapping small patients in a sheet is often helpful to minimise kicking and wriggling.
- If using the back of the hand in infants, grasp the wrist between the index and middle fingers with the thumb over the patient's fingers, flexing the wrist. This achieves both immobilisation and tourniquet (see Fig. 4.1).
- Insert the cannula just distal to and along the line of the vein at an angle of 10–15°. When a large vein is entered, a 'flash' of blood

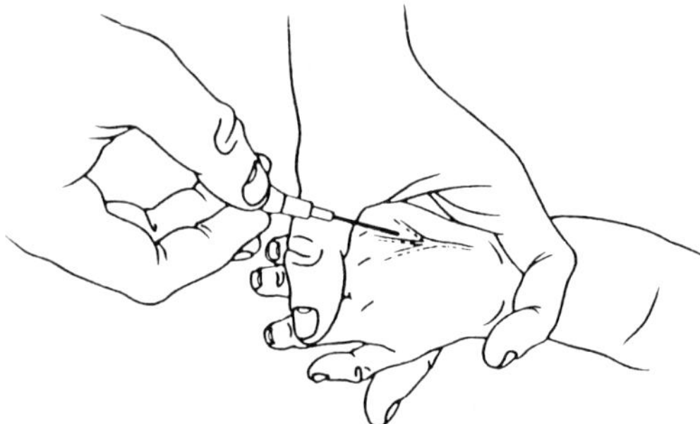

Fig. 4.1 Intravenous cannula insertion

will enter the hub of the needle. Advance the cannula a further 1–2 mm along the line of the vein, then remove the needle while advancing the cannula along the vein. If the cannula is in the vein, blood will flow out along the cannula and continue to fill the chamber. When trying to cannulate a small vein, there may not be a flashback of blood. Insert the cannula and when it is likely to be in the vein, remove the needle and watch for blood moving slowly down the cannula. Advance the cannula along the vein gently.

- Take blood samples at this stage then securely strap the cannula in place. In younger children use two inverted cross-over straps and another tape over the top. In older children an adhesive clear plastic dressing may be used.
- Flush the cannula with saline to confirm intravenous placement. Connect the intravenous tubing and splint the arm to an appropriately sized board (keeping the thumb free). Wrap the whole distal extremity in a crepe bandage.

LONG LINE INSERTION

Indications

- Prolonged venous access.
- Central venous placement for parenteral nutrition.

Sites

- Basilic and cephalic veins in older children.
- Basilic, cephalic, axillary and saphenous veins in neonates and infants.

Suggested analgesia

- See intravenous cannula insertion.

Technique

- Strict asepsis is required.
- Silastic catheters are used in neonates and adolescents and can be inserted via a butterfly or intravenous cannula.
- Semi-rigid long lines are an alternative in children and are inserted into an intravenous cannula, which is left in place.
- Measure the distance from the site of insertion to the desired location of the catheter tip (e.g. right atrium for central venous placement or axilla for midline placement). If necessary cut the catheter to the required length.
- Prime catheter with sterile saline. Insert the introducer needle or cannula into the vein until free-flowing blood return is obtained. Release the tourniquet.
- Using smooth forceps, grasp the catheter very close to the tip and feed the catheter through the introducer needle/cannula to the desired length (see Fig. 4.2a).
- If using a silastic line, slowly withdraw the needle/cannula keeping it parallel to the skin and leave the catheter in position. When the needle clears the skin, secure the catheter by trapping it with a gloved finger at the skin exit site (see Fig. 4.2b). Attach the catheter to the appropriate intravenous line.
- If using a semi rigid line, the cannula is left in place and the wire stylet is removed before attaching intravenous tubing.
- Flush the catheter.
- Secure catheter in place with steristrips then a sterile transparent dressing.
- If the line is for central access, confirm catheter tip placement radiologically. This may be aided by the injection of 0.3 mL of a contrast agent.

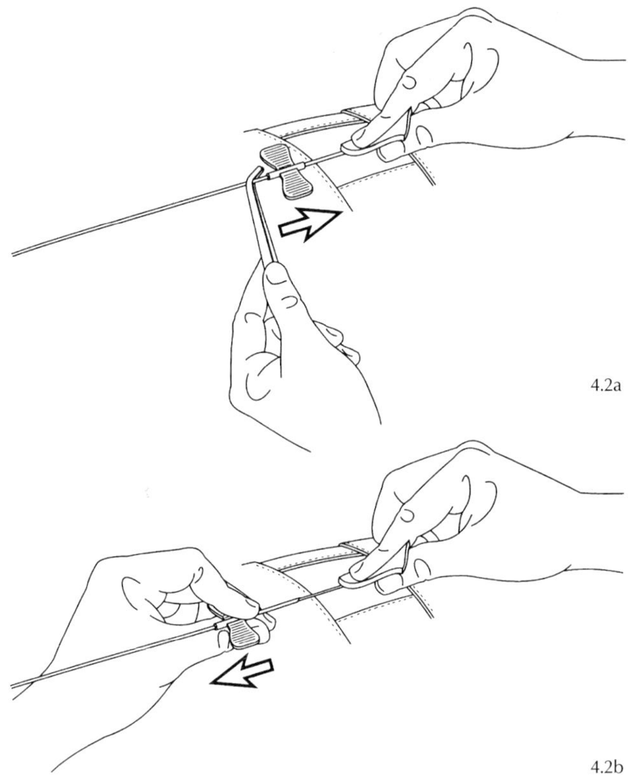

Fig. 4.2a and b Long line insertion

UMBILICAL VEIN CATHETERISATION

Indications

Used in neonates up to 7 days of age for:

- Emergency vascular access for resuscitation.
- Intravenous access for exchange transfusion.
- Central venous pressure monitoring.
- Venous access in low birth weight infants.

Technique

- Measure the distance of a line drawn from the tip of the shoulder to the level of the umbilicus.
- Using Fig. 4.3 determine the catheter length needed to place the tip between the diaphragm and the left atrium. Add length for the height of the umbilical stump.
- Strict asepsis is required.
- Flush the catheter with sterile saline.
- Loosely tie a sterile umbilical tape around base of the cord. Cut through the cord horizontally 1.5–2 cm from the skin; tighten the umbilical tape to prevent bleeding if necessary.
- Identify the large thin-walled vein and smaller thick-walled arteries. Clear any thrombi with forceps, gently dilate the vein with curved iris forceps and insert the catheter. Aim the tip at the right shoulder.
- Gently advance the catheter to the desired distance. Do not force.
- Secure the catheter with both a purse string suture around the cord and a tape bridge. Confirm the position of the catheter tip radiologically.

UMBILICAL ARTERY CATHETERISATION

Indications

Used in low birth weight neonates for:

- Monitoring blood pressure and arterial blood gases.
- Access and infusion site.

Technique

- Measure the distance of a line drawn from the tip of the shoulder to the level of the umbilicus. Use Fig. 4.3 to determine the catheter length needed for:
  - Low line position: between L3–L5 (below renal and mesenteric arteries); tip just above aortic bifurcation.
  - High line position: between T6–T9; tip above the diaphragm.
- Strict asepsis is required.
- Flush the catheter with sterile saline.
- Stabilise and cut the umbilical stump (see above).

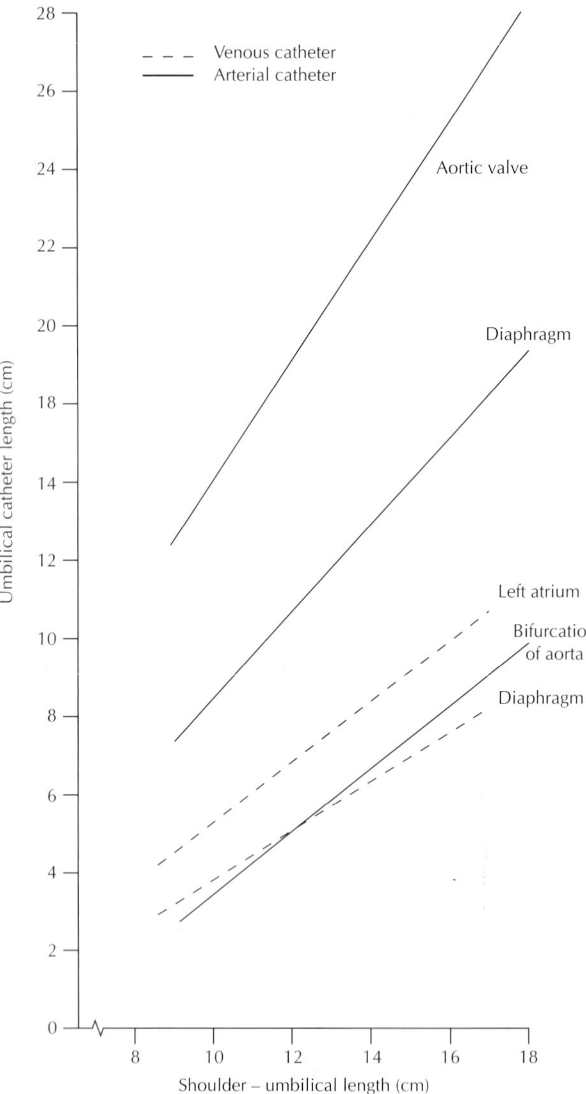

Fig. 4.3 Determining umbilical vein and artery catheter length

- Identify the artery, clear any thrombi and dilate with curved iris forceps. Insert catheter and advance gently. Aim the tip towards the feet.
- Secure the catheter and confirm tip position (as above).
- Check for any complications caused by catheter placement, especially blanching or cyanosis of lower extremities.

ARTERIAL PUNCTURE

Indications

- Suspected hypoxaemia, hypercapnia or severe acidosis with poor peripheral perfusion

Note: Acid-base status can also be assessed by a capillary or venous collection.

Sites

- Radial or brachial artery

Note: The femoral artery is used only in emergencies when no other arteries are palpable. Never use the ulnar artery.

Suggested analgesia

- Injectable local anaesthetic (lignocaine 1%) can be used however this does not prevent pain caused by puncturing the artery.

Technique

- Clean the skin with an alcohol swab.
- Use a pre-heparinised 2 mL syringe and a 23– or 25–gauge needle.
- Pierce the skin at a 15–30° angle directly over the artery. On entering the artery, blood will fill the hub; however, gentle aspiration is usually required to fill the syringe.
- If there is no flashback at full depth or when the bone is contacted, withdraw the needle very slowly while aspirating. Blood will often be obtained at this point if the artery has been transfixed.
- Only 0.5 mL of blood is required for arterial blood gas, sodium, potassium and haemoglobin measurements.
- After obtaining a specimen, remove the needle quickly and apply firm pressure to the puncture site for 3–5 min.

INTRAOSSEOUS CANNULA INSERTION

Indications

- For emergency vascular access when efforts to cannulate a vein are unsuccessful.

Sites

- Preferred sites of insertion are:
- Up to 3 years of age:
  - Proximal tibia (1–2 cm inferomedial to tibial tuberosity).
  - Distal femur in the midline (approximately 3 cm above the condyles) (see Fig. 4.4).
- Any age:
  - Medial malleolus of the tibia (just above the ankle).

Suggested analgesia

- Performed in emergency situations. Injectable local anaesthetic (lignocaine 1%) if the patient is conscious.

Technique

- Prepare the insertion site. If an intraosseous needle is not available, a short lumbar puncture needle or bone marrow aspiration needle may be used (intravenous cannulae or venepuncture needles are not appropriate).

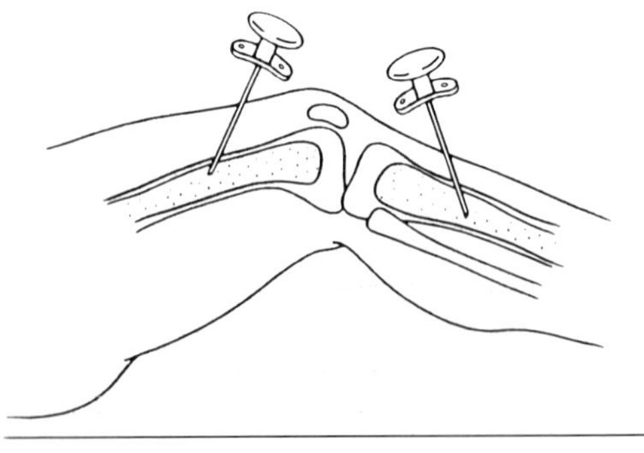

Fig. 4.4 Intraosseous needle insertion sites

- Penetrate the skin and then angle the needle at 10–15° from vertical – caudad for proximal tibial insertion and cephalad for femoral or medial malleolus insertion (see Fig. 4.4). Apply downward pressure with a rotary motion to advance the needle. When the needle passes through the cortex of the bone into the marrow cavity, resistance suddenly decreases. The needle should stand without support (except in a very young infant).
- Remove the stylet and attach a 5 mL syringe; aspirate to confirm that the needle is in the bone marrow (this is not always possible). Flush the needle with saline to confirm correct placement and connect intravenous tubing. Often fluids will not flow by gravity into the marrow – a three-way tap and syringe or pressure infusion may be needed.
- Watch the infusion site for fluid extravasation, or the calf becoming tense. The needle should be removed once intravenous access has been obtained.
- Any fluid or drug that can be given intravenously can be administered through the intraosseous route.

SUPRAPUBIC ASPIRATION

Indications

- Suspected urinary tract infection (UTI)/clean urine collection as part of septic workup.

Note: Not recommended in age >12 months (unless the bladder is palpable or percussible).

Technique

- Wait at least 30 min after the last void. If performing a septic work-up, do the suprapubic aspiration (SPA) first. If available, bladder ultrasound is helpful.
- Position the patient with legs either straight or bent in the frog-leg position. In males, hold the tip of the penis to prevent voiding. Have a sterile bottle handy for a clean catch in case the child voids.
- The site of entry is the skin crease above the symphysis pubis, in the midline.
- Prepare the skin with an alcohol swab. Insert a 23-gauge needle attached to a 2 or 5 mL syringe perpendicular to the abdominal

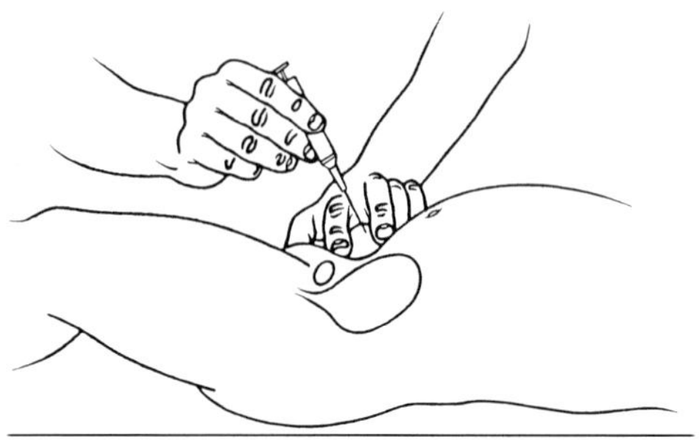

Fig. 4.5 Suprapubic aspiration

wall (see Fig. 4.5). Pass almost to the depth of the needle and then aspirate while withdrawing. If urine is not obtained, do not remove the needle completely. Change the angle of the needle and insert it again, first angling superiorly and then inferiorly.

- In the event of obtaining no urine, either: (i) perform urethral catheterisation; or (ii) wait 30 min, giving the child a drink during this time. Repeat the suprapubic aspiration (SPA). It is a good idea to place a urine bag on to determine if the child has voided before proceeding with a further SPA.

URETHRAL CATHETERISATION

Indications

- Suspected UTI where midstream specimen is not possible.
- Acute urinary retention.

Suggested analgesia

- Local anaesthetic topical gel (e.g. lignocaine 2% gel).
- Consider nitrous oxide

Technique

- An assistant is required to hold the child's legs apart, in the frog-leg position. Prepare the area with a water-based disinfectant solution and drape with sterile towels.

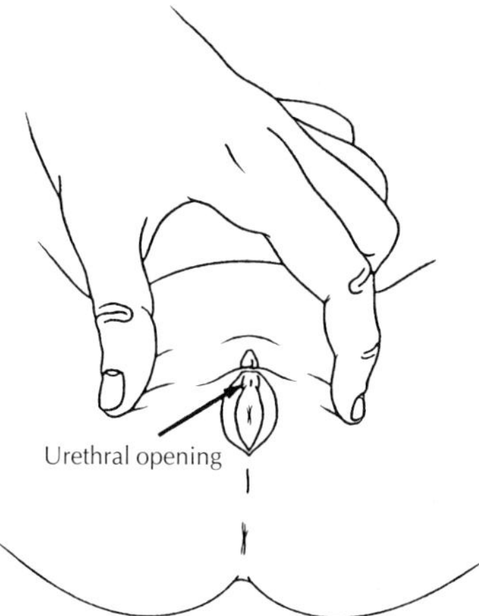

Fig. 4.6 Urethral orifice in girls

- For diagnostic catheterisation, use a size 5 or 8 feeding tube (depending on age). For in-dwelling catheters, use a silastic catheter with an inflatable balloon. Lubricants will aid insertion.
- Using a sterile technique, locate the urethral orifice (see Fig. 4.6). In males the foreskin need not be retracted fully for successful catheterisation. Advance the catheter posteriorly with care until urine is obtained.
- For indwelling catheters: only inflate balloon when urine has been obtained, attach catheter to collection device and tape catheter securely to leg.

LUMBAR PUNCTURE

Indications

- A febrile, sick infant or child with no focus of infection.
- Fever with meningism.
- Prolonged seizure with fever.

See also Fig. 1.2, page 14.

Contraindications

- Coma.
- Focal neurological signs.
- Focal or tonic seizures, recent seizures (within 30 min) or prolonged seizures (over 30 min).
- Signs of raised intracranial pressure: papilloedema, altered papillary responses, absent doll's eye reflex, decerebrate or decorticate posturing, abnormal respiratory pattern, hypertension or bradycardia.
- Cardiovascular compromise/shock.
- Thrombocytopenia/coagulopathy.
- Local superficial infection.
- Strong suspicion of meningococcal infection (typical purpuric rash in ill child).

Note: Coma – rapid deterioration in conscious state or absent or non-purposeful responses to painful stimuli (squeeze earlobe hard for up to one minute. Children should localise response and seek a parent). If in doubt, do not proceed to a lumbar puncture.

Note: Drowsiness, irritability, vomiting and isolated tonic-clonic, myoclonic, absence or atonic seizures are not contraindications in themselves.

Suggested Analgesia

- Topical local anaesthetic plus:
- Injectable local anaesthetic (lignocaine 1%) in age >6/12 plus:
- Consider nitrous oxide or sedatives (e.g. midazolam). Sedatives may complicate assessment of conscious state.

Technique

- A lumbar puncture needle with introducing stylet should be used. A 22- or 25–gauge needle is usually appropriate. The correct needle size is:
  - 30 mm for neonates and infants.
  - 40 mm for 1–4 year olds.
  - 50 mm for 4–10 year olds.
  - 60 mm for older children.

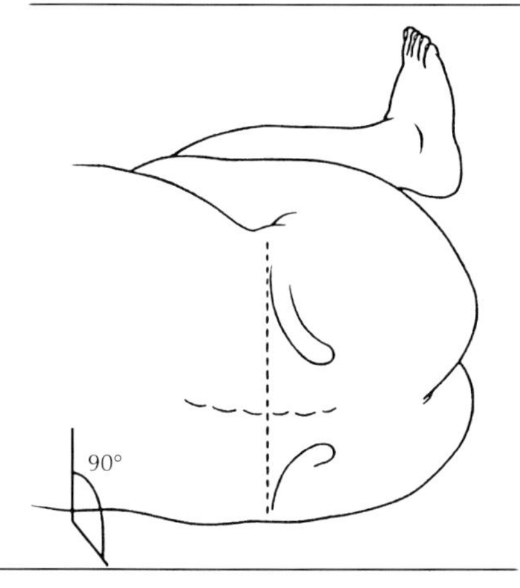

Fig. 4.7 Position for lumbar puncture

- Positioning of the patient is crucial and an assistant is needed. Restrain the patient in the lateral position on the edge of a flat surface. A line drawn between the iliac crests should be perpendicular to the table surface. Maximally flex the spine without compromising the airway. In small babies flex from the shoulders only; neck flexion can cause airway obstruction.
- The iliac crests are at the level of L3–4. Use this space or the space below (see Fig. 4.7). Using a strict aseptic technique, cleanse the skin and drape the patient.
- Anaesthetise the area to near the dura (i.e. about two-thirds the length of the appropriate lumbar puncture needle).
- Grasp the spinal needle with the bevel facing upwards. With the needle perpendicular to the back, insert it through the skin between the spinous processes slowly, aiming towards the umbilicus (i.e. slightly cephalad). Continue advancing the needle until there is decreased resistance (having traversed ligamentum flavum), or the needle has been inserted half its length. Remove the stylet and advance the needle about 1 mm.

- Wait at least 30 s for CSF to appear in the hub. Rotation of the needle 90–180° may allow CSF to flow. Advance 1 mm at a time if no CSF has appeared. If no CSF is obtained when bone is contacted or the needle is fully inserted, withdraw the needle very slowly until CSF flows, or the needle is almost removed. Reinsert the stylet, recheck the patient's position and needle orientation, and repeat the procedure.
- Collect 0.5–1 mL of CSF in each of two tubes, for microbiological and biochemical analysis. Remove the lumbar puncture needle with one quick motion. Press on the puncture site with a cotton ball for about 30 s. Cover with a light dressing.

NASOGASTRIC TUBE INSERTION

Indications

- Oral rehydration.
- Administration of medications (e.g. charcoal, golytely).
- Decompression of stomach (e.g. bowel obstruction, abdominal trauma).

Suggested analgesia

- Topical anaesthetic spray (e.g. cophenylcaine) and lubrication with lignocaine-containing lubricant.

Technique

- Select the correct tube size (these sizes may vary depending on the use of the nasogastric):
  - 8 Fr for newborns
  - 12 Fr for 1–2 year olds
  - 16 Fr for adolescents
- Measure the correct length of insertion by placing the distal end of the tube at the nostril and running it to the ear and to the xiphisternum. Add a few centimetres. Mark the tube with permanent marker at this point so the position can be checked.
- If the tube is too pliable, stiffen it by immersing in cold water or freezing briefly.
- Grasp the tube 5–6 cm from the distal end and insert it posteriorly. Advance it slowly along the floor of the nasal passage (see Fig. 4.8).

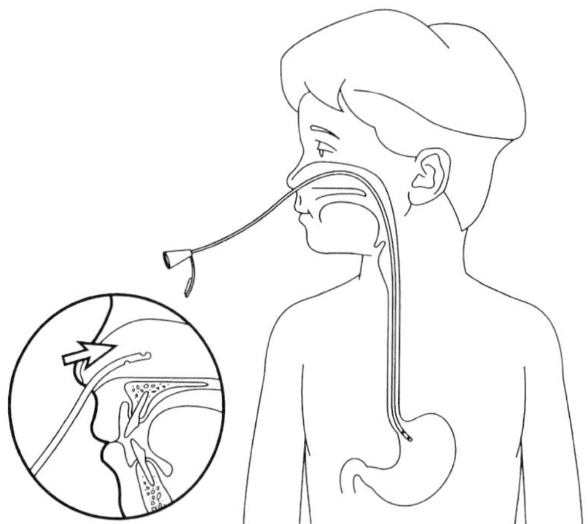

Fig. 4.8 Nasogastric tube insertion

- Firm pressure is needed to pass the posterior nasal opening; this may cause some minor bleeding.
- If the child is cooperative, once the tube is in the naso/oropharynx, ask the child to flex their neck and swallow.
- If the child coughs and gags, their voice becomes hoarse or the tube emerges from the mouth, pull the tube back into the nasopharynx and start again.
- Once the tube has been passed to the measured length, check its position by aspirating fluid and testing for an acid pH. Confirm position with X-ray if necessary.
- Secure the tube to the side of the face using adhesive tape.

GASTROSTOMY TUBE REPLACEMENT

Indications

- Burst balloon/malfunctioning parts.
- Displacement/extrusion of tube.

Suggested analgesia

- Nitrous oxide or sedation (e.g.: midazolam).

Technique

- Check the balloon of the new tube by injecting 3–5 mL of air into the side port. Deflate the balloon fully.
- Slide the skin flange on the new tube to the 8–10 cm mark. Close off the feeding ports and apply a small amount of lubricant to the tube.
- If the old tube is still *in situ*, attach an empty syringe to the side port and deflate the balloon by removing the water (*Note:* there is usually less than the expected 4 or 15 mL of water left in the balloon).
- Gently pull on the tube and rotate it slowly until it is removed.
- Place the tip of the new tube at the opening of the stoma. Hold the distal end of the tube and slowly put pressure on the tube to push it into the hole.
- The new tube should insert easily. Insert it to 6–8 cm.
- Inflate the new tube to either 4 or 15 mL (i.e. not to its capacity) with water. Slowly pull back on the tube until resistance is felt.
- Slide the skin flange down until there is a snug fit, but not too tight. This is usually at the 2–4 cm mark.
- In the case of a MIC key, the correct tube for that patient should be inserted to its full depth before inflating the balloon.
- Gastrostomy buttons or Malecot catheters need introducers and should only be replaced by experienced staff.

Note: if there is any difficulty inserting the tube, then a radiographic study (i.e. contrast through the tube) should be performed to check correct positioning.

WOUND MANAGEMENT

Assessment

Lacerations are common in childhood. Most are superficial and tend to occur on the face, scalp and extremities. When assessing a wound consider:

- Is the wound contaminated?
- Are there likely to be other associated injuries?
- Is there injury to deeper structures?

- Is blood supply impaired or is this an area of end-arteriolar supply? Do not use local anaesthetic with adrenaline on such wounds.

Cleaning Wounds

- Superficial wounds can be cleansed with normal saline or aqueous chlorhexidine.
- Adequate analgesia is required for complete examination, cleaning and repair of all but the most superficial wounds.
- Consider an X-ray if there is a possibility of a foreign body (particularly glass).

Suggested analgesia

Topical local anaesthetic

- LAT (lignocaine 4%, adrenalin 1:2000 and tetracaine 2%) or ALA (adrenalin/lignocaine/amethocaine). Dose = 0.1 mL/kg bodyweight.
- Apply on a piece of gauze or cotton wool placed inside the wound and held in place with an adhesive clear plastic dressing.
- Leave for 20–30 min. An area of blanching (~1 cm wide) will appear around the wound. Anaesthesia lasts about 1 hour.
- Test the adequacy of anaesthesia by washing and squeezing the wound, if pain free, suturing will usually be painless.
- The sensations of pulling and light touch are preserved. This should be explained to the child and parent.

Injectable local anaesthetic (lignocaine 1%)

Injectable lignocaine 1% can be used:

- When LAT/ALA are contraindicated (e.g. areas of end arteriolar supply).
- In adolescents.
- To supplement topical local anaesthetic if adequate anaesthesia has not been achieved.

There are several ways to decrease the pain from injecting local anaesthetic:

- Use topical anaesthesia first.
- Use 27–32-gauge needles.
- Inject slowly.
- Place the needle into the wound through the lacerated surface, not through intact skin.

- Pass the needle through an anaesthetised area into an unanaesthetised area.
- Use 1% lignocaine rather than 2%.
- Buffer lignocaine with sodium bicarbonate (10:1 dilution).

Sedation/Other

- Nitrous oxide or sedation (e.g. midazolam).
- Ketamine may be used in children over 12 months by staff experienced in its use.

Regional blocks

- See end of chapter.

Wound closure

Tissue glues

- Tissue glue (e.g. histacryl glue) is an alternative to suturing in wounds that are small (<3 cm), straight, easily approximated and under no tension. It must not be used on mucosal surfaces.
- Topical anaesthesia will reduce bleeding from the wound and the discomfort of gluing.
- Clean the wound with normal saline or aqueous chlorhexidine and let dry. Hold the edges firmly together and apply a small amount of glue (approximately 0.05 mL) to the line of the laceration. Do not allow glue to enter the wound itself.
- Hold the wound edges together for 30 s. Steristrips should be applied (using tincture of benzoin) to prevent the child picking the glue off.
- The wound should be kept dry for 3–4 days. It then can be washed. The scab will come off in 1–2 weeks.

Suturing

- Absorbable sutures (e.g. catgut) are appropriate for use on areas where the cosmetic advantages of non-absorbable sutures are not required (e.g. scalp and hand). Using absorbable sutures avoids the stress and potential pain of suture removal.
- Non-absorbable sutures (e.g. nylon and polypropylene) are used in areas where cosmetic appearance is important.
- Deep sutures (absorbable) should be used to close deep tissues; this reduces cavitation and dead space, which increase the risk of infection.

- The size of suture and timing of suture removal depends on the area affected:
  - Scalp 4/0–5/0 5 days.
  - Face 5/0–6/0 5 days.
  - Arm/hand 4/0–5/0 7 days .
  - Trunk/legs 4/0–5/0 10–14 days.

Note: Areas of stress (e.g. over joints) need longer.

- Splint any sutured wound that is under tension (e.g. across joints or on the hand), for at least 1 week. This decreases pain and promotes healing.

Special circumstances

Lips

- Accurate approximation of vermilion border and skin is essential.
- May need general anaesthetic and plastic surgical repair in small/ uncooperative child.
- Sutures: mucosa/muscle – 4/0 gut, skin – 6/0 nylon.
- Lacerations of the inner lip rarely need intervention however degloving to the gum margin requires specialist referral.

Palate

- Rarely requires suturing unless laceration is wide, extends through posterior free margin or is actively bleeding.
- Beware retropharyngeal injury (needs specialist opinion. See Ear, nose and throat conditions, chapter 21).

Tongue

- Small lacerations do not require suturing.
- Plastic surgical opinion is required if the laceration is large, bleeding actively, extends through the free edge or is full thickness.

Finger tips

- Areas of skin loss up to 1 cm^2 are treated with dressings and heal with good return of sensation. Greater areas require specialist referral.
- Involvement of the nail bed requires plastic surgical consultation.

Other

- Lacerations involving cartilage (e.g. nose, ear) require specialist opinion.

Tetanus prophylaxis

See: The Australian Immunisation Handbook, current Edition.

For clean minor wounds, if the patient has had a:

- Tetanus course (≥3 doses), last dose within the past 10 years: no requirement.
- Tetanus course (≥3 doses), last dose more than 10 years ago: give tetanus toxoid.
- Unimmunised/incomplete/unknown treatment: give tetanus toxoid.

For tetanus-prone wounds, if the patient has had a:

- Tetanus course (≥3 doses), last dose within the past 5 years: no requirement.
- Tetanus course (≥3 doses), last dose more than 5 years ago: give tetanus toxoid.
- Unimmunised/incomplete/unknown treatment: full three-dose course and tetanus immunoglobulin.

Note: Tetanus toxoid: give DTPa/DT/Td as appropriate.

Dose of tetanus immunoglobulin is 250 IU <24 h, 500 IU >24 h.

Antibiotics

Antibiotics are not indicated for simple lacerations. They are usually given for bites and wounds with extensive tissue damage, but are of secondary importance to the initial decontamination of the wound.

Recommended antibiotics are amoxicillin clavulanate (400/57 mg per 5 mL), 12.5–22.5 mg/kg/dose, 12-hourly for 5 days.

FEMORAL NERVE BLOCK

Indication

- Pain relief for proximal femur fractures.

Technique

- After skin preparation, palpate the femoral artery below the inguinal ligament. Raise a wheal with local anaesthetic just lateral to the artery.

- Introduce a short bevelled needle (such as a lumbar puncture needle or a 23–gauge needle) through this wheal and advance downwards perpendicular to the skin. A characteristic 'pop' or loss of resistance is felt as the needle goes through the fascia lata and again as it penetrates the fascia iliaca (if using a lumbar puncture needle).
- Aspirate to ensure that the needle is not in a blood vessel. Inject local anaesthetic solution (usually bupivacaine in a dose of 2 mg/kg). The anaesthetic should inject smoothly without subcutaneous swelling. Paraesthesia need not be elicited.

BIER'S BLOCK

Indication

- Children over 5 years with forearm fractures requiring manipulation.

Technique

- Keep child nil orally and give adequate pain relief.
- Two trained staff must be present and full resuscitation equipment available. Radiology should be notified.
- Insert an intravenous cannula into a distal vein on each hand.
- Elevate the affected arm above the level of the heart while compressing the brachial artery for 1 min.
- Inflate the tourniquet cuff to 200 mmHg. This reading should be maintained throughout the procedure.
- Infuse lignocaine 0.5% 0.6 mL/kg (3 mg/kg) max = 40 mL. Full anaesthesia takes 5–10 min.
- Release tourniquet cuff **at least** 20 min after lignocaine infusion, after procedure is complete and position confirmed radiologically.

DIGITAL NERVE BLOCK

Indication

- Anaesthesia of finger for minor surgical procedures (e.g. suturing, drainage of paronychia).

Use local anaesthetic (e.g. lignocaine 1%). Do **not** use adrenaline.

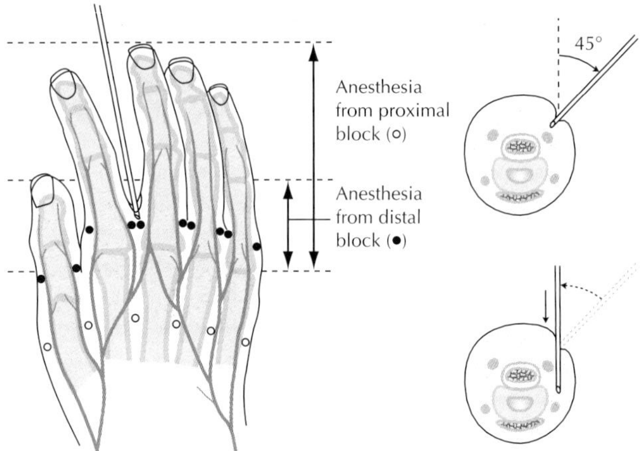

Fig. 4.9 Digital nerve block

Technique

Digital nerve block

- With the palm facing up, insert a 25-gauge needle at the base of the finger on either medial/lateral side at a 45° angle to the vertical (see Fig. 4.9).
- Inject when needle hits periosteum.
- Rotate needle to vertical and inject along the side of the finger to at least $^3/_4$ of the depth of the finger.
- Remove needle and repeat on the other side.

Proximal nerve block

- Insert a 25-gauge needle between the fingers at the interdigital fold in line with the web space (see Fig. 4.9).
- Insert until needle tip is level with the head of the metacarpal bone.
- Inject 1–2 mL at this level.
- Repeat on the other side, or for index/5th finger; inject half ring wheal around the outer side of the finger.

CHAPTER 5
FLUID AND ELECTROLYTE THERAPY

Frank Shann

There are marked differences between children and adults in fluid and electrolyte composition and maintenance requirements. Maintenance fluid requirements are the daily water needs per kg of bodyweight in a disease-free state. They are high in infancy and gradually decrease throughout childhood.

Table 5.1 Fluid distribution

	Total body water (mL/kg)	*Intracellular fluid (mL/kg)*	*Extracellular fluid (mL/kg)*	*Blood volume (mL/kg)*
Neonate	800	350	450	85
Infant	700	400	300	80
Child	650	400	250	70
Adult	600	400	200	60

Table 5.2 Daily maintenance intravenous fluid requirements

Bodyweight	*Requirements*
3–10 kg	100 mL/kg per day
10–20 kg	1000 mL + (50 mL/kg per day for each kg over 10 kg)
20 kg and over	1500 mL + (20 mL/kg per day for each kg over 20 kg)

Table 5.3 Hourly maintenance intravenous fluid requirements

Weight (kg)	4	6	8	10	12	14	16	20	30	40	50	60	70
mL/h	16	24	32	40	45	50	55	65	70	80	90	95	100

Table 5.4 Adjustments to maintenance intravenous fluid requirements

Condition	*Adjustment to fluid intake*
Renal failure	× 0.2 + urine output
Basal state	× 0.7
High ADH (e.g. brain injury, meningitis)	× 0.7
High room humidity	× 0.7
Breathing humidified gas	× 0.75
Fever/hypothermia	± 12% per °C from 37 °C
Burns	
Day 1	+ 4% per 1% burn
Subsequent days	+ 2% per 1% burn

HYPOVOLAEMIC SHOCK

Dehydration without shock can usually be managed with oral rehydration fluid plus food.

Children with shock (hypotension and acidosis) caused by hypovolaemia should be given parenteral fluid immediately: administer 20 mL/kg repeatedly until the plasma volume is restored (they may need 20–100 mL/kg). The fluid can be given intravenously or into the bone marrow (see Procedures, chapter 4). Nasogastric or intraperitoneal fluid is not effective in shock.

Use 0.9% saline to restore intravascular volume in hypovolaemic shock. Do not use albumin or Haemaccel (polygeline). Dextrose solutions may cause hyperglycaemia if infused rapidly, and hyponatraemia if they contain less than 0.9% saline.

In states of hyponatraemia or hypernatraemia, the correction of serum sodium towards normal should not occur at more than 0.5 mmol/L per hour.

REPLACEMENT THERAPY

Three basic aspects are considered:

- Existing deficit.
- Continuing losses during therapy.
- Maintenance requirements.

Existing fluid deficit

The fluid deficit is most reliably estimated from the loss of body weight if a recent weight is available. Otherwise the degree of dehydration can be estimated using the following clinical features:

- Decreased peripheral perfusion (pallor or reduced capillary return).
- Deep (acidotic) breathing – not useful in diabetic ketoacidosis.
- Decreased skin turgor.
- Increased thirst.

A history of oliguria, restlessness, lethargy, sunken eyes, dry mouth, sunken fontanelle and the absence of tears have poor sensitivity as signs of mild to moderate dehydration in children. For:

- <3–4% bodyweight loss there are no clinical signs
- 4–6% bodyweight loss there are clinical signs present and the severity of the signs is a guide to the degree of dehydration
- ≥7% bodyweight loss there may be hypotension and acidosis

In general, fluids to replace the existing deficit are given over the first 24 h. For hypernatraemic or hyponatraemic dehydration, at least 48–72 h should be taken for replacement.

Electrolyte deficit

The type and amount of electrolyte deficit depends on the diagnosis (e.g. in gastroenteritis, the loss of base leads to acidosis; in pyloric stenosis, the loss of acid and chloride leads to hypochloraemic alkalosis).

Potassium should rarely be infused intravenously faster than 0.2 mmol/kg/hour and never faster than 0.4 mmol/kg/hour. Concentrations of potassium greater than 40 mmol/L should be used only with extreme caution.

Electrocardiographic monitoring should be considered in massive potassium replacement. Infusions of concentrated solutions should be controlled with the use of a pump.

Continuing losses

It is essential to have an accurate recording on a fluid balance chart of the volumes of vomitus or gastric aspirates, drainage from fistulae, diarrhoea, urine output and other fluid losses. These will determine both the volume and type of fluid and electrolyte replacement required

Table 5.5 Composition of some body fluids in children

Fluid	*Na^+ mmol/L*	*K^+ mmol/L*	*Cl^- mmol/L*	*HCO_3^- mmol/L*	*Other*
Gastric fluid	20–80	10–20	100–150	0	H^+ 30–120
Bile	140–160	3–15	80–120	15–30	
Pancreatic fluid	120–160	5–15	75–135	10–45	Basal state
Jejunal fluid	130–150	5–10	100–130	10–20	
Ileal fluid	50–150	3–15	20–120	30–50	
Diarrhoeal fluid	10–90	10–80	10–110	20–70	
Sweat					
Normal	10–30	3–10	10–35	0	
Cystic fibrosis	50–130	5–25	50–110	0	
Burn exudate	140	5	110	20	Protein 30–50 g/L
Saliva	10–25	20–35	10–30	2–10	Unstimulated

(see Table 5.5). It is also important to monitor weight and clinical features during rehydration: weigh every 6 h for the first 24–48 h.

Maintenance requirements

These are given in addition to the replacement of the existing deficit and continuing losses. See Tables 5.1–5.5.

ACID-BASE PROBLEMS

The maintenance of pH within narrow limits is a result of two mechanisms:

- Buffer systems – the bicarbonate system is quantitatively the most important in plasma (70% of the total).
- Excretory mechanisms – via the kidneys and lungs.

Acidosis (low pH) and alkalosis (high pH) may be respiratory or non-respiratory (metabolic) in origin. Respiratory disorders result from changes in the excretion of volatile carbon dioxide and, consequently, in the levels of carbonic acid. Metabolic disorders occur with changes in concentrations of non-volatile acids and, consequently, in the concentration of buffer base – mainly bicarbonate.

The four primary disorders are:

- *Metabolic acidosis.* This arises from increased production of non-volatile acid (e.g. ketoacids and lactic acid), failure of the kidney to excrete non-volatile acid or conserve base, or excess loss of buffer base (e.g. gastroenteritis or intestinal fistula).
- *Metabolic alkalosis.* This arises from excess loss of non-volatile acid (e.g. pyloric stenosis), excess intake of buffer (e.g. bicarbonate infusion), or potassium depletion where an extracellular alkalosis occurs as hydrogen ions are lost in the urine (e.g. renal tubular syndromes, pyloric stenosis or diuretic therapy).
- *Respiratory acidosis.* Hypercapnia is the result of alveolar hypoventilation from any cause (e.g. central, neuromuscular or pulmonary).
- *Respiratory alkalosis.* This is caused by hyperventilation.

Indicators of acid-base status

pH

This reflects the actual hydrogen ion concentration and alters in response to both respiratory and metabolic changes.

$P\text{CO}_2$ (Partial pressure of carbon dioxide)

In arterial and capillary blood samples, this represents the $P\text{CO}_2$ in blood leaving the lungs. Alterations reflect the disturbance in the respiratory component of the acid-base state (and not the metabolic component).

Base excess

This is an estimate of the change in total buffer base that would be present if the $P\text{CO}_2$ were normal (40 mmHg). Changes in the base excess reflect a disturbance in the metabolic component of the acid-base status (and not the respiratory component). In metabolic alkalosis, the total buffer base is increased and thus the base excess is positive. Other calculated measures of the metabolic component are the standard bicarbonate and the total buffer base.

Actual bicarbonate

This is the plasma concentration of bicarbonate; it is influenced by both metabolic and respiratory components.

In practice, isolated metabolic and respiratory disorders are uncommon. Most disorders have both a metabolic and a respiratory component. Usually one is the primary disorder and the other occurs secondarily to correct the change in pH. Sometimes, however, primary metabolic and respiratory disturbances occur together; for example, in respiratory distress syndrome, when hypoxia leading to lactic acid accumulation produces metabolic acidosis and carbon dioxide retention produces a respiratory acidosis (see Tables 5.6 and 5.7).

Table 5.6 Changes in arterial capillary blood (before compensation)

	pH (mmol/L)	*Pco_2 (mmHg)*	*Base excess (mmol/L)*	*Actual bicarbonate (mmol/L)*
Normal range	7.36–7.44	36–44	–5 to +3	18–25
Metabolic acidosis	Decrease	Normal	Decrease	Decrease
Metabolic alkalosis	Increase	Normal	Increase	Increase
Respiratory acidosis	Decrease	Increase	Normal	Increase
Respiratory alkalosis	Increase	Decrease	Normal	Decrease

Table 5.7 Changes in indicators of acid–base status seen in combined disorders

	pH (mmol/L)	*Pco_2 (mmHg)*	*Base excess (mmol/L)*	*Actual bicarbonate (mmol/L)*
Normal	7.36–7.44	36–44	–5 to +3	18–25
Primary metabolic acidosis + compensatory respiratory alkalosis (e.g. gastroenteritis, diabetic ketosis)	Decrease or normal	Decrease	Decrease	Decrease
Primary metabolic alkalosis + compensatory respiratory acidosis (e.g. pyloric stenosis)	Increase or normal	Increase	Increase	Increase
Combined primary respiratory and metabolic acidosis (e.g. respiratory distress syndrome)	Decrease	Increase	Decrease	Normal

The interpretation of changes in base excess and $P\text{CO}_2$ as primary or secondary changes must be made clinically.

Correction of metabolic acidosis

Metabolic acidosis will often resolve rapidly once the cause has been corrected and administration of bicarbonate is usually not required. Consider giving bicarbonate if there is a marked metabolic acidosis (large base deficit, normal $P\text{CO}_2$) with a pH less than 7.10. Give bicarbonate for metabolic acidosis with a pH less than 7.15 caused by bicarbonate loss, as shown by a normal anion gap of less than 12 mmol/L

Anion gap = Na – bicarbonate – Cl

A guide to the amount of bicarbonate required is given by:

mmol of HCO_3 required = basic deficit (mmol/L) × weight (kg) × 0.3

The factor (weight × 0.3) represents the volume of extracellular fluid through which the base deficit (negative base excess) is distributed. In babies less than 5 kg, the factor is (weight × 0.5) due to the greater percentage of extracellular fluid. It is usual to give only half the amount of bicarbonate suggested by these formulae and to repeat the blood gas measurement before giving any more.

The rate of administration of bicarbonate will be determined by the cause of the metabolic acidosis and the clinical state of the patient; for example, in cardiac arrest, infuse bicarbonate rapidly. If acidosis has been present for more than 6 h, the correction should usually be undertaken over at least 6 h (and mild to moderate acidosis will resolve with rehydration alone). Rapid correction of metabolic acidosis will cause a fall in extracellular potassium.

The principles of correction of metabolic alkalosis are discussed in the section on pyloric stenosis (see below).

MANAGEMENT OF SOME SPECIAL CONDITIONS

Pyloric stenosis

All infants with pyloric stenosis should have their acid-base and electrolytes measured. Hydrogen ion and chloride loss predominate, with consequent hypochloraemic alkalosis. Losses of potassium in vomitus and urine can lead to significant hypokalaemia. In severe cases, hypokalaemia will lead to a renal compensatory mechanism, in which hydrogen ions are lost in an attempt to conserve potassium. This leads to paradoxical aciduria.

The duration and severity of vomiting will determine the degree of fluid and electrolyte imbalance.

Assessment

All patients require biochemical assessment, but not all will require intravenous therapy pre-operatively. Any child who is clinically dehydrated or has significant biochemical derangement requires intravenous therapy.

Intravenous therapy

- In severe dehydration (≥7%), commence with 0.9% saline until adequate circulation has been established and continue with 0.45% saline and 5% dextrose.
- In moderate dehydration (4–6%), commence with 0.45% saline and 5% dextrose.
- In mild dehydration await electrolyte results before commencing therapy if only mildly dehydrated.
- Adequate potassium and chloride replacement is necessary for the correction of the acid-base abnormality. As soon as urine flow is established, potassium chloride is given up to a maximum of 0.2 mmol/kg per h. Usually 20–40 mmol/L is adequate.

Acute oliguria and anuria

The definition of severe oliguria is a urine output of less than 0.5 mL/kg per h.

Initial management

Three clinical situations occur:

- Sudden and complete anuria should arouse suspicion of urinary obstruction, provided the catheter is correctly placed and not blocked.
- Renal hypoperfusion causing oliguria should be suspected in the presence of clinical dehydration or septicaemia leading to hypotension; the urinary sodium is usually less than 20 mmol/L. Blood volume expansion is necessary.
- Renal tissue injury (e.g. acute post-streptococcal glomerulonephritis or secondary to hypoperfusion or nephrotoxin). The urinary sodium is usually more than 40 mmol/L. Frusemide (1–2 mg/kg) should be given i.v. and, if there is no response, treatment for continuing anuria should be instituted.

Continuing anuria

Fluid intake is restricted to the previous 24 h urine output and any abnormal losses; approximately 20% of normal maintenance requirements must also be given to replace insensible water loss.

At least 20% of full calorie requirements are given as carbohydrate to spare tissue protein from catabolism for energy, which accentuates the rise in blood urea. Intravenous 10–20% glucose, or oral high caloric supplements (e.g. Caloreen or Polyjoule) are suitable.

Peritoneal dialysis or haemofiltration will be required for hyperkalaemia, severe uraemia (blood urea >50 mmol/L), acidosis or water overload leading to hyponatraemia, oedema or hypertension, and should always be considered if anuria persists for more than 24 h.

Hyperkalaemia

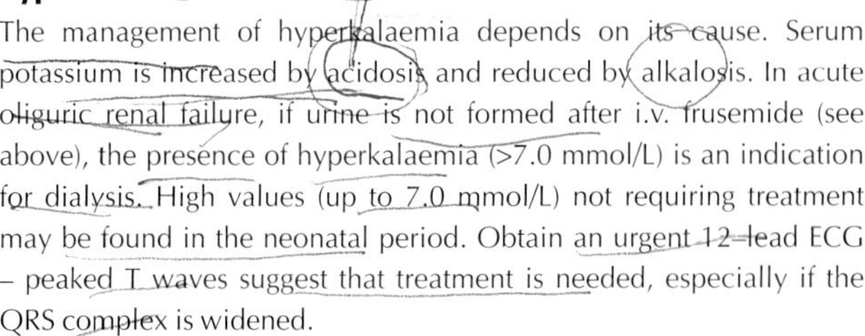

The management of hyperkalaemia depends on its cause. Serum potassium is increased by acidosis and reduced by alkalosis. In acute oliguric renal failure, if urine is not formed after i.v. frusemide (see above), the presence of hyperkalaemia (>7.0 mmol/L) is an indication for dialysis. High values (up to 7.0 mmol/L) not requiring treatment may be found in the neonatal period. Obtain an urgent 12-lead ECG – peaked T waves suggest that treatment is needed, especially if the QRS complex is widened.

If cardiac arrhythmias are present, rapid but temporary benefit may be achieved by giving:

- Sodium bicarbonate 1 mmol/kg, i.v.
- Short-acting (regular) insulin 0.1 unit/kg given with 2 mL/kg of 50% dextrose, i.v.
- Calcium gluconate 10% 0.5 mL/kg, i.v. given slowly.
- Sodium polystyrene sulphonate (Resonium) 1 g/kg rectal or nasogastric.

Hypokalaemia

Metabolic alkalosis may cause hypokalaemia, but this will resolve if the alkalosis is treated. Severe hypokalaemia causes a long QT interval, often with prominent U waves. Treatment involves giving potassium orally, or by adding it to maintenance fluid. Potassium should rarely be given faster than 0.2 mmol/kg/h and **never** faster than 0.4 mmol/kg/h.

Hypernatraemia

If hypernatraemia is due to water deficit (hypernatraemic dehydration), the sodium should fall no faster than 0.5 mmol/L/h with treatment. This should be done by giving water slowly; the composition of the solution used is less important than the rate of administration.

If hypernatraemia is due to salt poisoning and has been present for less than 12 h, it should be corrected rapidly by haemofiltration or dialysis. If hypernatraemia has been present for more than 24 h, the sodium should fall no faster than 0.5 mmol/L/h.

Hyponatraemia

Low serum sodium should be corrected slowly, especially if the abnormality is long-standing. It should never be increased faster than 0.5 mmol/L/h, and usually at 0.25 mmol/L/h or less. To increase the sodium by 0.25 mmol/L/h, infuse saline at a rate (mL/h) = Wt (kg) / (% saline infused).

Other conditions

See acute infectious diarrhoea (p. 370), haemorrhagic shock (p. 7), burns (p. 264), diabetes mellitus (p. 328) and Meningococcal septicaemia (p. 8, 433).

THE NEWBORN

Babies are different from older age groups because they have:

- Proportionately more body water in all compartments.
- Greater insensible water losses.
- Reduced renal capacity to compensate for abnormalities.
- Less integrated and responsive endocrine controls (see Table 5.8).

These differences are of practical importance only in very sick babies – those requiring in-patient care in Level 2 or Level 3 nurseries.

This section highlights major practical differences between the sick newborn and older age groups. However, any baby needing intravenous therapy should be in a Level 2 or Level 3 nursery.

Insensible water losses can vary from around 30 mL/kg per 24 h at term, to greater than 200 mL/kg per 24 h below 27 weeks gestation.

The newborn kidney is less able to concentrate or dilute urine, retain Na^+ and K^+ or shed excess loads or to excrete H^+ to shed acid loads.

Water requirements

There is often confusion between babies' water and milk requirements. For normal nutrition, babies need 150–200 mL/kg of milk per 24 h. For most babies this is 2–3 times their water requirements. This difference is only of practical importance in babies suffering illnesses that are made worse by excess water administration; for example acute and chronic lung disease, heart failure or renal impairment.

Water requirements depend on:

- Gestational age – the earlier the gestation the greater the skin losses and the poorer the renal concentration.

Table 5.8 Neonatal body water distribution

	<28 weeks	*Term*
Total body water	85% (of bodyweight)	75%
Extracellular water	55%	45%
Circulating blood volume	90–100 mL/kg	85 mL/kg

Intermediate gestations lie between these figures.

Table 5.9 Water requirements in newborn babies

	Days 1–2	*Days 6–7*
Mature 35 weeks +	40–50 mL/kg per day	60
Immature 27 weeks	80–120	60–80

Intermediate gestations lie between these figures. Lower figures are for babies on ventilators.

- Postnatal age – skin losses decrease and renal function improves steadily from day 1.
- Conditions of nursing – dressed babies lose least; naked babies under radiant heaters lose most. Humidified respiratory circuits (e.g. ventilators) reduce respiratory losses.

Water requirements are summarised in Table 5.9.

Before 27 weeks' gestation, requirements are too variable to tabulate: start at 120 mL/kg and modify 6–12 hourly according to the clinical state, serum Na^+ and urine osmolality.

Sodium

Babies are less able to conserve sodium or excrete excess loads. Daily requirements are 2–4 mmol/kg per 24 h; the earlier the gestation, the higher the need.

Hyponatraemia (Na^+ <132 mmol/L)

This may be due to excess water administration, inadequate sodium administration, excess sodium loss or inappropriate ADH secretion. The cause should always be defined; do not just treat blindly.

It is easy to overload sick babies with water in the first days after birth. This is a common cause of hyponatraemia. In general, intravenous rates greater than 60 mL/kg per 24 h in sick mature babies will provide excessive water in the first 48 h.

When the cause is water overload, serum Na^+ correction by water restriction alone is very slow in the newborn. As serum Na^+ <125 mmol/L can result in fits and may be injurious to the CNS, it should be treated with Na^+ administration, even when the primary cause is water overload. The dose required can be calculated as follows:

Dose of Na^+ (mmol) = bodyweight × 0.8 × (140 − current serum Na^+)

The aim is to correct this condition slowly over 36 h, once the level of 125 mmol is reached. Using this regimen, serum Na^+ should be checked every 6 h: if correction is occurring rapidly, Na^+ administration can be ceased once the serum levels are safe.

Hypernatraemia (Serum Na^+ >154 mmol/L)

This may be due to excess Na^+ administration, inadequate water administration or excess loss of water in relation to sodium. The cause should always be defined.

It is easy to overload sick babies with sodium-containing intravenous fluids (e.g. 1 mL/h of normal saline = 4 mmol Na^+ per 24 h, the entire Na^+ requirements of a 1000 g baby and more than half the daily requirements of a 2000 g baby). The use of sodium bicarbonate for correction of acidosis also often leads to sodium overload.

Hypernatraemia may be injurious to the CNS and should be avoided if possible.

Na^+ should be added to intravenous maintenance fluids from the beginning of day 2, taking into account separate sodium administration as sodium bicarbonate or heparinised saline.

Potassium

Potassium requirements are 2–4 mmol/kg per 24 h. Serum K^+ does not reflect body K^+. With high or low levels, the cause should be defined.

Except with anuria, K^+ should be added to maintenance intravenous fluids from the beginning of day 2.

With diuretic therapy, Na^+ and K^+ losses are much greater in babies than in older age groups.

Glucose

Blood glucose levels are unstable in sick babies. Fasting babies require intravenous solutions containing at least 10% dextrose. Average glucose requirements are 4–7 mg glucose/kg per min (6–10 g/kg per day), but some sick babies require more and others less.

Acid–base problems

Metabolic acidosis is the commonest acid–base disturbance in sick babies. The cause should always be defined. Correction with sodium bicarbonate is controversial, but it is reasonable to begin correcting pH <7.10 fairly quickly, i.e. over 30–60 min and pH 7.10–7.20 slowly, that is, over 2–4 h.

$$\text{mmol of } HCO_3 \text{ required} = \text{base deficit (mmol/L)} \times \text{weight (kg)} \times 0.5$$

Acid–base status should be re-evaluated once half the dose of bicarbonate has been given and the dose adjusted if necessary. When given at the rates recommended there is no need to dilute 8.4% sodium bicarbonate before administration. Other measures to control the acidosis (e.g. volume expansion) should be instituted at the same time.

SPECIFIC INTRAVENOUS SOLUTIONS

4% Albumin

This solution contains human albumin 40 g/L, sodium 140 mmol/L, chloride 128 mmol/L and octanoate 6.4 mmol/L. It has an osmolality of 260 mOsm/kg and a pH of 6.7–7.3. It should not be used for rapid correction of hypovolaemia (use 0.9% saline).

20% Albumin

This solution contains albumin 200 g/L, sodium 46–58 mmol/L and octanoate 32 mmol/L. It has an osmolality of 80 mmol/kg and a pH of 7.0. Dose (mL/kg) = 0.25 × (desired increase in serum albumin in g/L).

Additives

- Molar potassium chloride (0.75 g in 10 mL) = 1 mmol/mL of K^+ and Cl^-.
- Sodium chloride (20%) = 3.4 mmol/mL of Na^+ and Cl^-.
- Molar sodium bicarbonate (8.4%) = 1 mmol/mL of Na^+ and HCO_3.
- Calcium gluconate 10% = 0.22 mmol/mL of Ca^{2+}, which is 8.9 mg/mL of Ca^{2+}.
- Magnesium chloride for injection (0.48 g anhydrous in 5 mL) = 1 mmol/mL of Mg^{2+}.

Table 5.10 Commonly used intravenous solutions

	Na^+ (mmol/L)	Cl^- (mmol/L)	K^+ (mmol/L)	Lactate (mmol/L)	Ca^{2+} (mmol/L)	Glucose (g/L)
0.9% NaCl (Isotonic or normal saline)	150	150	–	–	–	–
0.45% NaCl with 5% glucose	75	75	–	–	–	50
0.18% NaCl with 4% glucose	30	30	–	–	–	40
0.18% NaCl with 4% glucose and KCl 20 mmol/L	30	30	20	–	–	40
Hartmann's solution	130	110	5	30	2	–
Hartmann's solution with 5% glucose	130	110	5	30	2	50

FORMULAE AND DEFINITIONS

Conversion factors

- Sodium chloride 1 g contains 17 mmol Na and 17 mmol Cl.
- Potassium chloride 1 g contains 13 mmol K and 13 mmol Cl.
- Sodium bicarbonate 1 g contains 12 mmol Na and 12 mmol HCO_3.

Molarity

Osmolality is the number of osmotically active molecules in a solution per kg of solute (usually mmol/kg of water).

Osmolarity is the number of osmotically active molecules in a solution per litre of solute (usually mmol/L of water).

Useful formulae

- Anion gap = Na – (bicarbonate + Cl); normal ≤12.
- Number mmol = mEq/valence = mass (mg)/mol. weight.
- Sodium deficit: mL 20% NaCl = wt × 0.2 × (140 – serum Na).
- Water deficit (mL) = 600 × weight (kg) × [1 – (140/Na)] (if body Na normal).
- Non-catabolic anuria: urea rises of 3–5 mmol/L per day.
- Bicarbonate dose (mmol) = base excess × weight ÷ 3 (give 1/2 this. *Note:* this is different in neonates).
- Osmolality serum = 2Na + glucose + urea (normal 270–295 mmol/L).

CHAPTER 6
NUTRITION

Julie Bines
Kay Gibbons
Michelle Meehan

BREAST-FEEDING

Breast milk alone is adequate nutrition for infants for the first 6 months of life. Breast-feeding is the best means of feeding babies and all efforts should be made to promote, encourage and maintain breast-feeding for as long as possible (see Table 6.1).

Normal variations of breast-feeding

Frequency of feeds

Breast-fed infants usually feed every 2–5 h on both sides each feed. Young babies feed frequently but demand feeding (i.e. feeding when hungry) will usually have the baby settle into a fairly predictable pattern of feeds. The frequency of the feeds is determined by the baby's appetite and gastric capacity, as well as the amount of mother's milk available.

Length of feeds

The duration of the feed is determined by the rate of transfer of milk from the breast to the baby, which, in turn, depends on the baby's suck and the mother's 'let down'. This may vary from 5–30 min. Young infants tend to feed for longer. It is the cessation of strong drawing sucks and the appearance of shorter duration bursts of sucking that indicate the 'end' of the feed – not the time.

If the mother feels the baby is on the breast 'all the time' it is better to look at the point where the pauses between bursts of sucking are longer than the sucking and take the baby off or swap sides at this time (rather than timing it).

Appetite spurts

Babies seem to experience appetite spurts at 2 weeks, 6 weeks and 3 months. It is crucial that parents are aware of this or the baby's natural increase in frequency of feeds may be mistaken for diminution of milk

Table 6.1 How to assess good breast-feeding

	Good	*Problem*
Baby's body position	On side-chest to chest	On back angled away from mother
Mouth	Open wide	Lips close together
Chin	Touching or pressing into the breast	Space between chin and breast
Lips	Flanged out	Tucked in, inverted
Cheeks	Well rounded	Dimpled or sucked in
Nose	Free of or just touching the breast	Buried in breast, baby pulls back
Breast in mouth	Good mouthful, more of bottom part of breast in mouth	Central, little breast tissue in mouth or only nipple in mouth
Jaw movement	Rhythmic deep jaw movement	Jerky or irregular shallow movement
Sounds	Muffled sound of swallowing milk	No swallowing, clicking sounds
Body language of the baby	Peaceful, concentrated	Restless, anxious
Body language of the mother	Comfortable, relaxed	Tense, hunched, awkward
Awareness of feelings during feed	Pain free, may feel a drawing feeling deep in breast or 'let down'	Nipple or breast pain
Nipple, post-feed	Nipple elongated, well shaped	Not elongated, compressed 'stripe' or blanched

Source: Murray S., *Breast Feeding Information and Guidelines for Paediatric Units*, Royal Children's Hospital, Melbourne, 1992.

supply. This is especially true at 6 weeks when breasts are no longer carrying extra fluid and the supply is settling to the demands of the baby. Unfortunately, many women wean at this time through poor advice. Let the baby feed on demand, even 2-hourly, and this should settle in 48 h.

Qualities of breast milk

Breast milk is naturally thinner in consistency than an artificial formula and may have a bluish tinge – this is normal, healthy and nutritious. The composition of breast milk varies during the feed. The fat content of milk varies diurnally: it is lowest about 6 am and gradually increases to its highest point about 2 pm. At any one feed, the highest concentration of fat is at the end of the feed in the 'hind milk'. The change in the concentration is a gradual merging over the feed and is part of the process of the feed. Hind milk is not 'better' than the early 'fore milk'. Fore milk is higher in water and lactose and provides liquid to quench the baby's thirst and a quick surge of energy.

The presence of blood in the milk may cause a red or pinkish brown discoloration. If this is present when the mother first starts expressing colostrum it may be due to duct hyperplasia. This gradually disappears and is of no significance. The most common cause of blood-stained milk (usually first noticed when the baby possets) is trauma to the nipple.

Bowel actions

The motions of breast-fed infants are normally bright yellow and soft to loose. The baby may have a bowel action with every feed (strong gastro-colic reflex) or once every 5–8 days.

Mastitis is a common reason for early weaning. Any reports of pain by the mother should be actively addressed (see Neonatal conditions, chapter 29).

Temporary cessation of breast-feeding

If the feeding pattern is interrupted due to illness, a planned fast for a procedure or the mother's absence, the mother will need to express to maintain the milk supply.

- Milk can be expressed by hand or by pump.
- Express as often as the baby would normally feed (i.e. 6–8 times a day). Several volumes of expressed milk can be added to the same bottle or storage bag (bags are available from commercial pharmacies), but a new container should be used every 24 h.

- Milk may be kept in the freezer section of the refrigerator for 2 weeks or in the deep freeze for 3 months.
- To thaw frozen milk, place a bag/bottle in a container of cool water and run hot water in until it is standing in hot water. When the milk is thawed it will be cold; continue to heat in hot water or place in the fridge until required for a feed.
- Thawed milk should be used within 24 h.

How much milk to express?

If the mother wants to express to give a feed by bottle or to substitute a feed as she is weaning, how much will the baby need?

Daily requirements of milk are:

- From 0–6 months: 150 mL/kg/day.
- Over 6 months: 120 mL/kg/day.

Divide this amount by the usual number of feeds to calculate the amount required per feed.

Growth in breast-fed infants

Growth patterns differ between breast-fed and artificially fed infants. Average weights of breast-fed babies are similar to or higher than formula-fed until 4–6 months, after which breast-fed babies slow significantly in their weight gains. Length and head circumference remain similar.

There are as yet no standard weight charts for breast-fed infants. It is not appropriate to interpret their naturally slower weight gain, taken in isolation, as abnormal.

Maternal illness

When the mother is unwell, breast-feeding should continue. In the case of maternal infection, antibodies will be passed on in the breast milk to protect the baby.

Maternal drugs

If the mother has to take medication, the risk-benefit ratio should be weighed carefully by the prescriber. The mother should continue to breast-feed unless the use of the drug is absolutely contraindicated during lactation and there is no safe alternative. There are very few drugs that are absolutely contraindicated and almost all have a safe alternative. If the mother is concerned about continuing breast-feeding, even if the drug is safe, suggest that she takes the drug after a feed to minimise the concentration, or to divide the dose if possible.

FORMULA FEEDING

If breast milk is not available, either from the breast or as expressed milk, a commercially prepared iron-fortified formula should be chosen. These are based on cow milk, modified to lower the protein, calcium and electrolytes to levels better suited to the human infant and contain added amino acids, vitamins and trace minerals. See tables of formula composition on the website associated with this chapter.

The introduction of some formula (e.g. returning to work, low milk supply) need not mean the end of breastfeeding. A combination of breast and formula may be quite manageable and suitable for the infant.

Cow milk-based formulas

- Formulas may be classified as whey dominant or casein-dominant, describing the main protein type in the formula. Most standard formulas are whey dominant.
- Changes between types of formula are made for a variety of reasons. In the normal thriving infant there is little indication to change the type of formula.

Children over 6 months – follow-on formulas

For infants over 6 months, follow-on formulas may be used. They have a higher protein and renal solute load and are not suitable for infants under 6 months of age.

Soy formulas

If a soy-based feed is chosen, a soy infant formula should be chosen. These are nutritionally adequate for infants. Follow-on soy formulas are available.

Formulas with long chain polyunsaturated fatty acids

Formulas with long chain polyunsaturated fatty acids (LCPUFA) are a suitable (and more expensive) alternative to standard cow milk formulas. There is little evidence of benefit for long-term development when used in full-term infants.

Antiregurgitation formulas

Thickened formulas are aimed at reducing regurgitation. Their use should be limited to the stepwise treatment of gastro-oesophageal reflux (see Gastrointestinal Conditions, chapter 24). They are not recommended in healthy infants without regurgitation.

Low-lactose formulas

Infant formulas with a low lactose content are recommended only in cases of proven lactose intolerance (see Gastrointestinal Conditions, chapter 24).

NUMBER OF FEEDS

Babies less than 6 weeks of age usually feed every 3 h; however, they may take more each time and feed 4-hourly. Babies rarely sleep through the night before 6–8 weeks. When they miss a night feed (usually sleeping 5–6 h straight) they will have 5 feeds. They will consequently have more milk each feed. Babies who sleep longer in the day (e.g. 5 h between feeds) often need to feed overnight to maintain adequate intake. Parents may need to wake the baby after 4 h in the daytime. There is no need to wake a baby overnight if the intake and weight gain are adequate.

INTRODUCTION OF WHOLE COW MILK

The introduction of cow milk products as part of an expanding diet is appropriate, but the main milk intake should be breast milk or formula until 12 months of age because of the risks of iron deficiency and allergy. Small amounts can be used on cereal, in custard and yoghurt from about 7–8 months.

Full cream dairy products should be used for children up to 2 years; skim milk should not be used for children under 5 years.

INTRODUCTION OF SOLIDS

Breast milk or formulas will meet all nutrient needs for the first 4–6 months. At this stage the development of head control and oropharyngeal function are sufficient to allow introduction of solids in most children. From this time solids can be introduced, to increase the intake of nutrients such as iron and as part of the educational process of learning to eat.

Solids can be iron-fortified baby cereal, smooth vegetables or fruits. Foods should be introduced one at a time to allow observation of tolerance. Meat can be introduced at about 6–7 months. Texture should be increased so that by about 8–9 months the infant is managing lumps and varying textures, and is starting to manage finger foods.

By about 12 months, most family foods can be offered. Increasing intake of solids should result in a reduction of milk intake to about 600 mL/day by 12 months. Much higher intakes of cow milk will limit the intake of other foods; continued high intake of cow milk, (with its low iron content), is associated with the development of iron deficiency.

Iron deficiency and associated anaemia is the commonest nutrient deficiency in children in Australia. It is associated with the early introduction of cow milk, high intake of cow milk in the second year and low intake of iron-rich foods, such as meat and pulses.

WEANING

There is no set rule for weaning time. Solids should be introduced by 6 months and cup-drinking started as a skill by 7–9 months. There is no need for the baby to be weaned to a bottle – if they are old enough they can go straight to a cup.

Sudden cessation of breast-feeding leaves the mother at risk of developing mastitis. Ideally, weaning is achieved by reducing the feeds by one a week. Start by offering a drink in a cup or bottle instead of a breast feed at midday, and gradually increase these other drinks.

Many mothers retain the early morning feed or the last feed at night for a little longer.

Persistent difficulty in weaning usually requires someone to support the mother, giving the baby a feed and allowing the baby some time away from the mother to help with mutual separation. Both need to be ready to let go. Specialist lactation advice may be needed.

TODDLERS WHO WILL NOT EAT

An assessment of the toddler who refuses food includes the following steps:

- Plotting weight and height to assure the parents of the child's normal growth.
- Using the growth chart to demonstrate that the growth rate normally slows in the second year.
- Linking this to a lessened need for food and subsequent drop in appetite.
- Emphasising developmental progress.

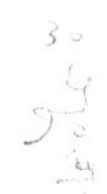

Advise parents that:

- A healthy child will eat when hungry – *quit the fight!*
- Showing independence is an important part of toddler development – choosing and refusing food is an expression of independence.
- Serve small portions – lower expectations.
- Serve some food that they like. Cereal is okay for lunch! A lack of variety is not a major worry at this age.
- Try to avoid arguments over food. Remember: 'It's my job to offer food, it's the child's job to eat it!'
- Avoid filling up on milk and juice – large volumes of milk (over 600 mL a day) can make the child feel full. Juice is not necessary in the child's diet.
- Give the child time to enjoy the meal without comment. Remove the food after 1/2 h or if they dawdle or lose interest.
- Learning to eat is fun. Switch to finger food if they refuse to be fed.
- Try not to use food as a punishment or reward. It only increases its potential power.

FOOD NEEDS OF PRESCHOOLERS

The following is a guide to the quantities suitable for 2–5 year olds. Many parents are surprised at how little children of this age need. However, because total needs are small there is relatively little place for high-fat, high-sugar extras such as savoury snack foods and soft drinks.

Daily

Milk group

Three serves (1 serve = 250 mL of milk, 200 g of yoghurt or 35 g of cheese).

Full cream products are recommended.

Bread and cereal group

Four to five serves (1 serve = 1 slice of bread, 1/2 cup of pasta or 2 cereal wheat biscuits).

Vegetable and fruit group

Four or more serves (1 serve = 1 piece of fruit or 2 tablespoons of vegetables).

Meat or protein group

Two serves (1 serve = 30 g of lean meat, fish or chicken, 1/2 cup of beans or 1 egg).

ENTERAL FEEDING

Enteral nutrition is the provision of nutrients to the alimentary tract through a feeding tube. It can be used to provide the total nutritional needs of a patient (either short or long term), or to provide additional nutrients when voluntary oral intake is inadequate.

Enteral feeding has certain advantages over total parenteral nutrition:

- Less risk of infection.
- Less risk of metabolic abnormalities.
- The nutrients provided to the alimentary tract enhance intestinal growth and function.
- It is cheaper.

Indications

Enteral feeding is used for patients who:

- Cannot feed orally (e.g. neurological damage or prematurity).
- Have increased metabolic requirements for nutrients (e.g. burns or congenital heart disease).
- Fail to achieve their nutritional requirements (e.g. failure to thrive or cystic fibrosis).
- Require unpalatable specialised feeds to treat their medical condition (e.g. metabolic disorders or liver disease).

Contraindication

Enteral feeding is contraindicated in patients with a non-functioning gastrointestinal (GI) tract.

Administration

The most commonly used route is nasogastric, its main benefit being ease of insertion. When long-term feeding is required, a gastrostomy tube may be indicated. Most gastrostomy tubes are now placed endoscopically rather than surgically.

When gastric motility is poor or when gastric residues are persistently high, a nasojejunal tube may be of benefit. However, feeding directly into the jejunum limits the choice of formula and may increase the risk of bacterial overgrowth.

Implementing feeds

When choosing a method consider the feeding route, the expected length of time the feed will be required and the type of feeding regime to be used (see Table 6.2). The introduction of hyperosmolar feeds should be done gradually.

Selection of feed

A full nutritional assessment (current nutritional status, current intake, requirements and the consideration of medical condition/fluid restrictions) should be carried out by a dietician to establish which feed will be optimal.

In general, infants can be managed using breast milk (if available) or an infant formula, or both. The formula will usually require additional fortification with both energy and other nutrients at around 6 months of age; this is suitable for up to about 2 years of age.

Table 6.2 Types of enteral feeding regimens

	Advantages	*Disadvantages*
Bolus feedings	Most closely mimics physiological feeding Increases patient mobility Little equipment is needed Volume given can be precisely measured	Can be time consuming for caregiver May decrease voluntary oral intake
Gravity drip	Little equipment needed	Rate of delivery cannot be closely monitored
Pump-assisted continuous	Feeding most likely to be tolerated Feeding can be delivered while patient sleeps Larger volumes can be tolerated than if given by bolus method	Requires feeding pump

Children over 2 years can be managed adequately using a proprietary product (see Table 6.3).

It is inappropriate to put pureed foods down feeding tubes as the amount of fluid required to achieve a suitable consistency dilutes the energy and nutrient content, while increasing the risk of microbial contamination and tube blockage.

Monitoring enteral nutrition

When monitoring patients on enteral feeds, mechanical, metabolic, gastrointestinal, nutritional and growth parameters must be assessed routinely. In the early stages of feeding, the patient's tolerance of the feeding regimen is critical to the success of feeding.

Once the feeding plan has been fully implemented, a regular assessment of the patient's nutrient requirements is needed to ensure that the adequacy of nutritional support is maintained and to indicate when enteral feeding can be ceased.

From total parenteral nutrition to enteral feeding

Initiating enteral feeds in critically ill patients (even in small amounts) helps to preserve gut function and structure, and to minimise the hypermetabolic response to stress. When initiating enteral feeds in patients

Table 6.3 Commonly used enteral feeds

Type	*Example*	*Notes*
Polymeric foods	Pediasure	Contains fibre
1 kcal/mL (4.2 kJ/mL)	Osmolite	
	Nutrini	
	Ensure	
	Jevity	
High energy polymeric	Resource plus	
1.5 kcal/mL (6.3 kJ/mL)	Ensure Plus	Hypertonic
2.0 kcal/mL (8.4 kJ/mL)	Twocal HN	Hypertonic
Specialised formula (elemental)	Vital HN Elemental 028 Vivonex paediatric	Contains short chain peptides; not suitable for infants under 1 year
	Neocate*	Suitable for infants
Modular feeds		
Protein source	Promod, Maxipro HBV	Nutritionally incomplete; requires vitamin and mineral supplement
CHO source	Polyjoule, Polycal, Maxijul	
Fat source	Calogen	
LCT	Liquigen, MCT Oil*	
MCT	Duocal	
Fat and CHO source		

All feeds are lactose free. CHO = carbohydrate
* Australian Pharmaceutical Benefits Schedule listed.

maintained on total parenteral nutrition (TPN), an isotonic, lactose-free formula perfused at a low constant rate is usually best tolerated. The transition from parenteral to enteral nutrition should be gradual with a tapering of TPN and advancing enteral feeds. This helps to prevent hypoglycaemia and fluid overload. Total parenteral nutrition should be ceased when enteral feeds provide approximately 75% of nutritional requirements.

From enteral to oral feeding

The goals for enteral feeding should be set at the outset. Once the patient is able and willing to eat by mouth the enteral feed can be reduced in proportion to the amount consumed orally. Transition from continuous feeds to overnight feeds may help establish oral intake while ensuring the patient is not nutritionally compromised.

Home enteral feeding

The decision to provide home enteral feeding should take into consideration the patient's medical needs and the social, psychological and financial factors that influence the family's ability to cope with a home feeding program.

Children on home enteral feeding, especially those who have minimal or no voluntary oral intake, require close monitoring of their growth and need their feeding regimens altered appropriately.

Common problems

- *Gastrointestinal disturbance*: is the most common problem (diarrhoea, cramping, nausea and vomiting). These problems can be minimised with the correct formula selection and administration in conjunction with a review of medications. High gastric residues should be treated by reducing the rate of feed given, or feeding small volumes, continuously reassessing the concentration of feed and assessing GI function. Directing feed into the jejunum alleviates the problems caused by slow gastric emptying.
- *Other problems*: include overhydration, dehydration, electrolyte imbalance, hyperglycaemia, hypoglycaemia and constipation. These need to be assessed and managed appropriately.
- Malnutrition is associated with major changes in electrolyte balance. Enteral feeding should be initiated with caution in patients with significant and long-standing under-nutrition. Serum phosphate, potassium, magnesium and glucose levels should be assessed regularly (see Refeeding syndrome, p. 120).
- *Food aversion*: young children who have been fed enterally during infancy or for long periods of time may miss important developmental steps in self-feeding. Non-nutritive sucking and mouth contact or taking small amounts of appropriate food/fluid orally will help establish or maintain eating and feeding skills, or both. A speech pathologist may be of assistance in this area.

FEEDING THE SICK NEWBORN

Feed type

Options available for feeding:

- Breast milk, including expressed breast milk (EBM).
- Artificial formulas, including specialised 'low birthweight' formulas.
- Specialised feeds for pathological states.

Breast milk

Breast milk feeding should be the primary aim for very sick babies. When babies are too ill or too premature to suckle at the breast, most mothers can establish lactation by expression. Expressed breast milk can be fed by gavage (nasogastric or orogastric) tube or other artificial means until the baby is well enough to be put to the breast. In this way breast milk feeding can be achieved in extremely premature babies and for those with the most major malformations, birth defects and other serious illnesses. The only situations in which breast milk feeding is not possible are:

- When an informed mother chooses not to express.
- Specific inborn errors of metabolism, which require exclusion formulas.
- Some complex malabsorption syndromes.

Evidence is accumulating that EBM feeding of sick babies reduces morbidity and mortality, and improves the developmental outcome compared with artificial feeding.

Lactation by expression

Every mother planning to express breast milk for her baby needs ready access to lactation specialists.

Expression by hand or pump should be started within 24 h of delivery preferably by 4–8 h. Episodes should be every 3–4 h, lasting about 30 min with a break for sleep. Hand expression is best until lactation is established. Expressed breast milk, if used with clean and straightforward techniques, does not have to be sterilised or pasteurised. In general EBM for sick babies should not be frozen; the freshest EBM available at the time should be used first.

Supplements and fortifiers

'Fortifiers', derived from cow milk, are available to add to EBM to increase its content of protein, energy and other nutrients. Babies who may benefit from fortifiers are those with greatly increased nutritional requirements (e.g. very low birthweight babies, (VLBW)) and those requiring fluid restriction (i.e. babies with heart failure or chronic lung disease).

Very low birthweight babies may need folate and iron (in addition to a fortifier); extra sodium; and vitamins C, D and E. The addition of fortifier should be delayed until feeds are fully established (i.e. 150–200 mL/kg per 24 h).

Iron should not be started until 12 weeks of age. VLBW babies who receive multiple blood transfusions may not need supplemental iron.

Phototherapy

Phototherapy for jaundice can impede breast-feeding by placing physical and psychological barriers between mother and baby and by causing diarrhoea. Breast-feeding can be assisted by interrupting the phototherapy frequently. Breast-feeding should be continued despite diarrhoea or sugar in bowel fluid. Although insensible water loss is increased by some phototherapy devices, the increase is only 10–20 mL/kg per 24 h. Thus, as long as usual amounts of breast milk are available by suckling or expression, supplements of water or formula are not necessary.

Artificial formulas

These are used when breast milk is not available.

Low birthweight (LBW) formulas are designed for very premature (<32 weeks) babies. In general, these contain more protein than standard formula (and may provide this as protein hydrolysate), more easily assimilated additional calories and increased calcium, phosphorus, trace elements and some (but not all) additional vitamins. Low birthweight formulas include LCPUFA as part of their fat content, based on evidence of better developmental outcomes in premature infants given a source of LCPUFA.

Standard cow milk formula may require fortification where nutritional requirements are high, or fluid is restricted (see previous section).

Strengthening formula feeds

Standard formulas provide 270–290 kJ/100 mL (65–70 kcal/100 mL or 20 kcal/30 mL). To increase energy to 350 kJ/100 mL (25 kcal/30 mL):

- Use *additional* formula powder (i.e. for formulas where the standard dilution is 1 scoop to 30 mL of water use 1 scoop to 25 mL of water, or for formulas where the standard dilution is 1 scoop to 60 mL of water use 1 scoop to 50 mL of water). This will also increase protein and other nutrient intakes. Care should be taken in infants with renal or liver impairment.
- Add glucose polymer (polyjoule, polycose) using 2 level teaspoons to 100 mL formula, or 5 mL fat emulsion (calogen, liquigen) to 100 mL formula. These additions will increase energy value only.

To increase energy to 420 kJ/100 mL (30 kcal/30 mL), use additional formula powder as above with the addition of either glucose polymer or fat emulsion (as above).

Specialised feeds

Specialised feeds are available for the treatment of complex malabsorption, allergy, inborn errors of metabolism and liver and renal disease.

Feed volumes, frequency and delivery

For sick babies who cannot be fed to appetite or 'demand', schedules specifying volume, frequency and delivery method are required.

Factors determining schedules include:

- Intestinal motility, gut enzyme and hormonal activity, which are low at birth and take time to switch on. This process is depressed by hypoxia, acidosis, sepsis and drugs, especially narcotics. This limits the volumes tolerated.
- A full stomach and bowel, which can press on the diaphragm, impairing breathing.
- Frequent reflux or vomiting which makes milk aspiration a risk.
- Aggressive schedules increase the risk of necrotising enterocolitis.

Mature babies need 150 mL milk/kg per 24 h. This is usually reached over 5–7 days, starting at 30–40 mL/kg per 24 h and increasing by 30 mL/kg per 24 h as tolerated. Expressed breast milk should never be diluted for use. Feed frequency should be 3–4-hourly, although with reflux or abdominal distension, smaller volume and more frequent feeds may help.

By using LBW formulas or concentrated standard formulas, adequate nutrition may be achieved with 120–150 mL/kg per 24 h. Very low birthweight (VLBW) babies require 180–200 mL/kg per 24 h of EBM or standard formula, or 150–180 mL/kg per 24 h of fortified EBM or LBW formula, starting at 20–30 mL/kg per 24 h and increasing by 30 mL/kg per day as tolerated. Regimes should be modified according to condition and stability in VLBW infants. Initial feed frequency should be 1–2-hourly. Hourly feeds may be necessary in babies less than 1000 g.

Intragastric feeding tubes are necessary for babies who cannot suck: use No. 5–6 French tube for babies less than 2000 g and No. 6–8 French tube for larger babies. Orogastric tubes should be used in babies less than 1250 g, as nasogastric tubes cause significant airways obstruction. Continuous intragastric infusion of feed rather than intermittent boluses may help if reflux, gastric distension or apnoea are persistent. Transpyloric duodenal or jejunal feeding provide no advantages and present additional risks.

THE NUTRITIONAL MANAGEMENT OF THE UNWELL CHILD

In order to define specific nutritional requirements and the optimal method of delivery, an evaluation of the medical history and nutritional status is required. Dietary manipulation or enteral feeding, or both, are always preferred over parenteral nutrition (PN) in any patient with a functioning gastrointestinal tract. Children with severely delayed gastric emptying or who are at risk of aspiration may still be successfully fed enterally through a transpyloric tube.

General indications for parenteral nutrition

- Recent weight loss of greater than 10% of usual bodyweight and a non-functional GI tract.
- No oral intake for more than 3–5 days in a patient with sub-optimal nutritional status and a non-functional GI tract.
- Anticipated need for PN for a minimum of 3–5 days.

Medical/surgical conditions that may require parenteral nutrition

- Patients unable to tolerate enteral feeding because of gastro-intestinal dysfunction; i.e. postoperative neonates, extensive short bowel syndrome or severe malabsorption.

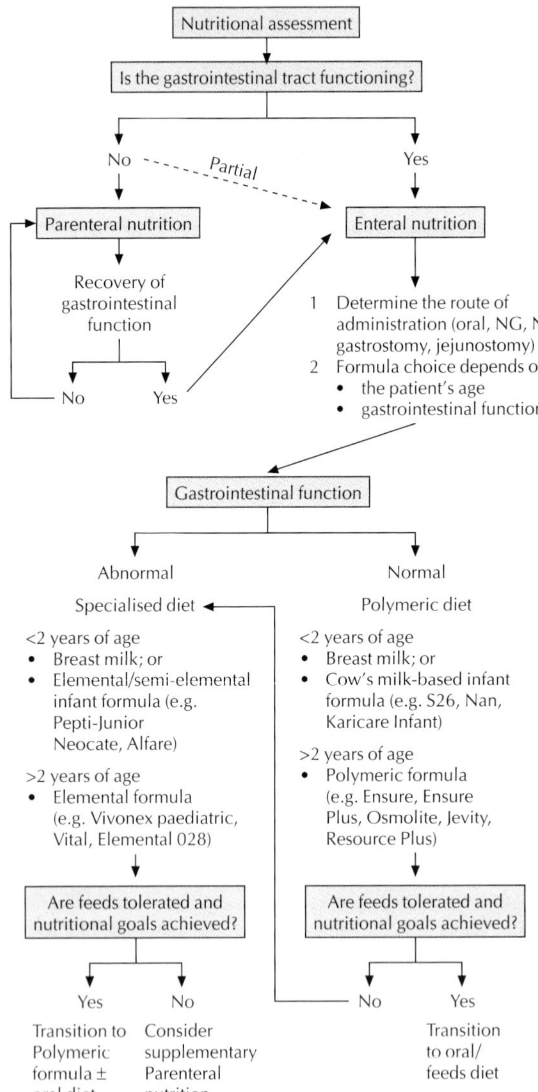

Fig. 6.1 Nutrition support algorithm

- Patients with increased metabolic requirements that may not be adequately treated with enteral therapy; i.e. severe burns, cystic fibrosis or renal failure.

DETERMINING NUTRITIONAL STATUS

Medical history

- Type and duration of illness.
- Degree of metabolic stress.
- Treatment (medications or surgery, or both).

Dietary assessment

- Twenty-four hour dietary recall.
- Three-day food record.

Physical examination

- General impression of wellbeing: wasting, oedema, lethargy and muscular strength.
- Specific micronutrient deficiency: pallor, bruising, skin, hair and neurological or ophthalmological complications.
- Anthropometry:
  - Weight for age.
  - Length/height for age.
  - Weight for length/height.
  - Head circumference.
  - Growth velocity.
  - Skinfold thickness, mid-arm circumference.
- Laboratory assessment
  - Protein status: albumin, total protein, pre-albumin, urea, 24 h urinary nitrogen, carnitine.
  - Fluid, electrolyte and acid-base status: serum electrolytes and acid-base urinalysis.
  - Iron status: serum ferritin and full blood examination.
  - Mineral status: calcium, magnesium, phosphorus, alkaline phosphatase, bone age and bone density.
  - Vitamin status: vitamins A, C, B_{12}, D, E/lipid ratio, folate and INR.
  - Trace elements: zinc, selenium, copper, chromium and manganese.

- Lipid status: serum cholesterol, HDL cholesterol and triglycerides.
- Glucose tolerance: serum glucose, HbA1c.

ESTABLISHING A NUTRITION TREATMENT PLAN

Calculating fluid requirement

See Fluid and electrolyte therapy, chapter 5.

Calculating nutritional requirements

(1) Energy

Estimated energy requirements for the sick child are usually calculated by using either:

- The requirements of a normal well child of the same sex and age.
- An estimate of basal requirements with additional activity.
- Measurement of energy expenditure using indirect calorimetry.

Energy requirements can be expressed as kilocalories (kcal) or as kilojoules/megajoules. The conversion equation is:

$$\text{kcal} = \frac{\text{mJ} \times 1000}{4.2}$$

Recommended energy requirements for infants

The recommendations for infants are based on studies in formula-fed infants. Recent data suggest that the energy expenditure and energy intake of breast-fed infants in the first months of life are significantly less (17 and 27% respectively) than that of formula-fed infants. These differences in energy metabolism are lost after weaning.

Breast-fed infants

- 0–5 months – 100–110 kcal/kg per day
- 6–12 months – 70–80 kcal/kg per day

Preterm infants – parenteral energy recommendation

In acute metabolic stress requirements, 110–120% of basal energy expenditure (~55–65 kcal/kg per day) is required.

Low birthweight infants who receive an energy intake of 80 kcal/kg per day with 3 g/kg per day amino acid intake gain weight at approximately the rate achieved *in utero*. However, this amino acid intake may be difficult to achieve by PN alone using some amino acid solutions such as Vamin-N®, due to the potential risk of excessive serum concentrations of some amino acids at doses greater than 2 g/kg per day in preterm infants.

(2) Protein

Optimal protein utilisation depends on a balanced energy and protein intake. If energy intake is less than the maintenance energy requirement then protein is shunted through gluconeogenesis to produce glucose. Optimal protein utilisation requires a non-protein energy intake of 60 kcal/kg per day to utilise 2.5 g/kg per day protein (or 0.4 g/kg per day nitrogen), which is a ratio of 150:1. This ratio may be altered in metabolic stress.

Amino acid recommendations are usually higher in parenteral nutrition as the patients who require this type of therapy generally have higher protein requirements due to their primary disease or treatment.

Increased protein intake is recommended in:

- Protein-losing states; i.e. enteropathy and nephrotic syndrome.
- Chronic malnutrition.
- Burns.
- Renal dialysis.
- HIV.
- Haemofiltration (~2 g/kg per day).

Reduced protein intake is recommended in patients with:

- Hepatic encephalopathy (0.3 g/kg per day)
- Severe renal dysfunction (not dialysed).

(3) Fat

Fat is a concentrated source of energy and an integral component of all cell membranes for the transport of fat-soluble vitamins and hormones. Essential fatty acid (EFA) deficiency can occur in neonates within days of initiating fat-free parenteral nutrition. Clinical signs of deficiency include reduced growth rate, poor hair growth, thrombocytopenia, increased susceptibility to infections and impaired wound healing.

Essential fatty acid deficiency is prevented by intravenous lipid (0.2–1 g/kg per day) or an enteral supplement with corn oil, sunflower oil or safflower oil.

(4) Micronutrients

Special consideration is needed when estimating the micronutrient requirements of sick children (see Table 6.4).

For ordering and monitoring parenteral nutrition, refer to the guidelines on the web page for this chapter.

Table 6.4 Diseases that increase micronutrient requirements

Disease	*Increased requirement*
Burns	Vitamins C, B complex, folate, zinc
HIV/AIDS	Zinc, selenium, iron
Renal failure: dialysis	Vitamins C, B complex, folate (reduce or omit copper, chromium, molybdenum)
Haemofiltration	Vitamins C, B complex, trace elements
Protein energy malnutrition	Zinc, selenium, iron
Refeeding syndrome	Phosphate, magnesium, potassium
Short bowel syndrome, chronic malabsorption states	Vitamins A, B_{12}, D, E, K, folate, zinc, magnesium, selenium
Liver disease	Vitamins A, B_{12}, D, E, K, zinc, iron (reduce or omit manganese, copper)
High fistula output, chronic diarrhoea	Zinc, magnesium, selenium, folate, B complex, B_{12}
Pancreatic insufficiency	Vitamins A, D, E, K
Inflammatory bowel disease	Folate, B_{12}, zinc, iron

REFEEDING SYNDROME

After a period of prolonged starvation, aggressive nutritional therapy may precipitate a cascade of potentially fatal metabolic complications. These include:

- Hypokalaemia.
- Hypophosphataemia.
- Hypomagnesaemia.
- Glucose intolerance.
- Cardiac failure.
- Seizures.
- Myocardial infarction/arrhythmias.

At particular risk are patients with:

- Anorexia nervosa.
- Classical marasmus.
- Kwashiorkor.
- No nutrition for 7–10 days in adolescents (much less in infants and children) with significant metabolic stress.
- Acute weight loss of ≥10–20% of usual bodyweight, and possibly metabolic stress, or >20% of usual bodyweight.
- Morbid obesity with massive weight loss (i.e. postoperative).

Management

- Identify risk and chronicity.
- Identify and treat metabolic stress if present (e.g. infection).
- Establish baseline status: weight, height/length, head circumference, fluid status, electrolytes, urea, creatinine, calcium, phosphate, magnesium, phosphate and magnesium, prior to commencing nutritional rehabilitation.
- Establish modest nutritional goals initially (e.g. basal requirements until stability is assured), then aim to provide for catch-up growth. During the first week of nutritional therapy, weight gain may not be seen or, if present, may reflect fluid gain rather than muscle or fat gain.
- Monitor closely over the first week until a nutritional plan is established with: pulse rate, fluid balance, weight, caloric intake, glucose, electrolytes, urea, creatinine, phosphate and magnesium. Bloods are required daily for the first 3 days.
- Administer vitamin and mineral supplement.

CHAPTER 7
WEIGHT RELATED PROBLEMS

Michael Harari
David James
Kay Gibbons

FAILURE TO THRIVE

Failure to thrive (FTT) is arbitrarily defined as being <3rd percentile for weight or dropping two or more percentile tracks. It implies failure to gain weight, with height and head circumference being initially well preserved. Short stature is discussed elsewhere (see Endocrine conditions, chapter 22). The majority of cases do not have an organic cause. Clues to the cause usually lie in history and examination of the child, along with assessment of growth patterns of other family members. Investigations should be limited and focused.

Is this weight normal or is it failure to thrive?

- Birth weight percentile does not necessarily predict future weight. In the first 6 months of life, deceleration of growth may be normal, until infants equilibrate to their 'true' growth channels.
- Later in childhood, some children will be <3rd percentile for weight because of genetic or constitutional factors. These children will appear healthy, with good muscle bulk, adequate subcutaneous fat and normal activity and development. Reference to the family's growth parameters may be helpful.
- Further evidence of adequate growth can be sought in anthropometric measurements such as skinfold thickness.

Categories of failure to thrive

- Poor caloric intake – nutritional, chronic illness.
- Increased caloric losses – vomiting, malabsorption.
- Poor utilisation.
- Increased metabolic requirements.

Causes

Non-organic failure to thrive

Non-organic FTT accounts for >50% of FTT in Australia.

- Normal variant (see above)
- Not enough food – careful dietary history
- Psychosocial factors in parent or child. This includes maternal depression, deprivation and neglect of the child
- Rumination

Organic failure to thrive

Organic FTT may also have non-organic component.

- Poor intake – numerous causes.
- Renal disease – UTI, renal tubular acidosis, chronic renal insufficiency.
- Cardiorespiratory – chronic upper airway obstruction, congenital heart disease, cardiomyopathy, bronchopulmonary dysplasia, cystic fibrosis (CF).
- Gastrointestinal – cleft lip and palate, Pierre Robin syndrome, gastro-oesophageal reflux, pyloric stenosis, coeliac disease, pancreatic insufficiency (CF, Shwachman syndrome), inflammatory bowel disease (IBD), Hirschprung disease.
- Endocrine – hyper and hypothyroidism, adrenal insufficiency, diabetes insipidus.
- Central nervous system – congenital and acquired CNS or muscle disease may cause inadequate feeding. Tumours – diencephalic syndrome.
- Chronic infection – immune deficiency, tuberculosis.
- Genetic, chromosomal or intrauterine causes – intrauterine growth retardation, trisomy syndromes.
- Metabolic – galactosaemia, phenylketonuria, acrodermatitis enteropathica, amino and organic acidopathies, hypercalcaemia.

History

History should focus on intake, any excessive losses that may be present and the previous and familial patterns of weight gain and growth. It should also cover psychological and developmental issues. Consider:

- Intake – what is consumed, how it is made up, when were solids added.

- Output – amount and colour of vomit, stool frequency and consistency.
- Birth – weight, gestation, complications.
- Past history – chronic illness, recurrent infections.
- Family history – possible maternal depression, growth pattern of other family members, illnesses and consanguinity.

Examination

Examination is focussed on growth parameters and nutritional status (see Nutrition, chapter 6). Look for signs of macro/micronutrient deficiency and evidence of system-based disease.

Investigations

Avoid random tests. The history and examination should guide the direction and tempo of investigation. If the cause of failure to thrive is not readily apparent after history, examination and limited investigations (e.g. FBE, urine M/C/S) further investigations and management should be in consultation with a specialist. Second line investigations might include: liver function, renal function, inflammatory markers, faecal microscopy, screening for coeliac disease, rickets, occult infection or immune dysfunction and a sweat test.

Management

The underlying cause will determine the treatment. Admit to hospital for:

- Severe undernutrition.
- Failed outpatient management.
- Child abuse or neglect.
- Extreme parental anxiety or depression that requires time to allow a constructive patient-doctor relationship to develop.

Admission may facilitate further assessment of feeding technique, the parent-child interaction and will allow the involvement of a multidisciplinary team.

OBESITY

Obesity is an increasingly prevalent problem among children in Australia. Up to 25% of Australian children and young people can be defined as overweight or obese.

Childhood obesity increases the risk of adult obesity and is associated with substantial psychosocial morbidity in childhood and adolescence. Childhood onset obesity that persists into adulthood accounts for a disproportionate share of severe adult obesity. A history of childhood obesity is associated with increased mortality and morbidity independent of adult weight. Parental obesity is the strongest risk factor for the persistence of obesity in children.

Definition

- Greater than 120% of the expected weight for height, estimated from the growth chart see Appendix.
- A clinically useful definition that reflects excess body fat and is simple to use is the body mass index (BMI).

BMI = bodyweight in kg divided by the square of height in metres (kg/m^2). Standard growth charts now include BMI centile charts.

- Overweight = BMI between 85–95th centile for age and sex.
- Obesity = BMI greater than 95th centile for age and sex.

International data sets have been used to develop BMI centiles showing equivalence to the adult BMI cut-offs for overweight and obesity of 25 and 30 respectively.

Causes

Children become obese because their energy intake exceeds their energy requirement. The understanding of factors that influence this energy balance equation is incomplete: genetic, hormonal, metabolic and environmental factors interact to contribute to the development and maintenance of obesity. Genetic factors may account for 25–40% of obesity. The gene pool changes slowly and so lifestyle changes are more likely to be responsible for the increase in the prevalence of obesity. Lifestyle factors include increased sedentary activities such as television and computer games, less time partaking in physical activities, and increased access to a dietary intake high in fat.

Endocrine causes of obesity are rare and are usually associated with growth retardation, which distinguishes them from the accelerated linear growth accompanying exogenous obesity (see Endocrine conditions, chapter 22). Syndromic causes of obesity are often recognised by the presence of a significant developmental disability and less frequently by dysmorphic features.

Clues to syndromatic or endocrime causes of obesity

- Height <50th centile (or less than genetic potential).
- Dysmorphic features.
- Developmental disabilities.

Complications of obesity

- Psychosocial – depression, teasing, school avoidance and low self-esteem.
- Cardiovascular – hyperlipidaemia, hypertension, increased heart rate and cardiac output, and exercise intolerance.
- Endocrine – glucose intolerance, insulin resistance, non-insulin-dependent diabetes mellitus (NIDDM), accelerated linear growth and bone age, early onset of puberty, polycystic ovary syndrome and menstrual dysfunction.
- Orthopaedic – Blount's disease, slipped capital femoral epiphysis and coxa vara.
- Respiratory – obstructive sleep apnoea.
- Gastrointesinal – gall-bladder disease and hepatic steatosis.
- Dermatological – intertrigo, furunculosis and acanthosis nigricans (a marker of insulin resistance).
- Neurological – benign intracranial hypertension.

Assessment

The aim is to identify:

- Individuals at high risk of associated disease.
- Underlying syndromes.
- Complications.

History

A detailed personal, family, developmental and past history complemented by a thorough dietary and activity history, and a detailed physical examination will be sufficient in most cases.

For high-risk factors, check the family history of obesity, heart disease, diabetes, hypertension, dyslipidaemias and other complications of obesity.

Examination

- The physical examination should include an assessment of body build, posture, distribution of adiposity, pigmentation of neck and axilla (acanthosis nigricans), striae, pubertal and developmental status.
- Blood pressure should be measured with an appropriate cuff.
- Height and weight should be plotted on percentile charts. Calculate and plot BMI.
- Waist circumference measured at umbilicus is useful for monitoring.

Investigations

- Screening for hyperlipidaemia, diabetes and hepatic steatosis should be considered in the child with obesity and is advisable when complications or a strong family history of adiposity-related morbidities are present.
- When obesity is suspected to be secondary, further investigation is required (see Endocrine conditions, chapter 22).

Management

The goals are to diminish morbidity and morbidity risk, rather than to achieve a normal bodyweight. The weight goal is generally to maintain weight over time as the height increases, or to slow weight gain compared to normal weight gain for age.

The highest success in the achievement of sustained weight loss is found in long-term family-based intervention, including behavioural change. The aim is a shift in energy balance achieved by:

- Lowering energy intake through targeted changes in the family eating pattern and a reduction in energy density. This includes regular meals and snacks, with an emphasis on cereals, fruit and vegetables, lean protein foods and low-fat dairy products, and a reduction in high-fat items.
- Increasing energy expenditure through an increase in age-appropriate physical activities and a reduction in sedentary activities. Endurance walking (>20 min per session) is useful for older children. Organised sport is useful for social activity, but often provides little sustained activity, especially for the overweight child.

Useful approaches include:

- Intervention, which can begin at any age, after identifying the problem.
- Identifying the family's readiness to change (consider deferring treatment or referring for family assessment).
- Providing families with information about:
  - Medical complications of obesity.
  - The concept of energy balance.
  - Healthy eating.
  - Appropriate physical activities.
  - Behavioural strategies.
- Involving all family members and caregivers.
- Permanent lifestyle changes as opposed to short-term diets or exercise programs aimed at rapid weight loss. Medications are not indicated.
- Monitoring diet and physical activities to help maintain changes.
- Professional input that encourages support and understanding.

Referral to a specialist is indicated when there is:

- Suspicion of pathological causes.
- The presence of complications.
- A lack of progress.
- Massive obesity.
- Parental or patient request.

CHAPTER 8
IMMUNISATION

Jenny Royle
Sue Skull

Immunisation is one of the most cost-effective public health measures available. Modern vaccines are safe and effective. They prevent clinical manifestations of disease altogether or substantially reduce severity. Health professionals have a responsibility to offer vaccination to those under their care at every available opportunity.

In Australia, vaccinations are not compulsory; they are recommended. Childcare payments and school entry are linked to reporting of vaccination status. All parents must feel comfortable about immunising their children. As a disease becomes less common through a successful immunisation program, the occurrence of side effects takes on greater relative importance. Health care providers may need to emphasise the risks of the diseases themselves and inform parents clearly that disease complications far outweigh the potential vaccine side effects.

Use every health care visit as an opportunity to update the vaccination status of an infant, child or adolescent. The Australian Childhood Immunisation Register (ACIR) can be used to check vaccination status (1800 653 809). For each dose of scheduled vaccine – notify ACIR and up-date the Child Health Record.

Further information

Please refer to the current edition of the Australian Immunisation Handbook (National Health and Medical Research Council), the Commonwealth Government immunisation website (http://www.immunise.health.gov.au) or for parent fact sheets: http://immunise.health.gov.au/publications.htm.

VACCINATION TECHNIQUE

- Clean the site; antisepsis is unnecessary.
- Use a new syringe and needle for each injection (take extra care with multidose vials).
- Use needles of 23–gauge and 25 mm in length. Smaller gauge needles may be used for premature babies, subcutaneous injections into the upper arm or intradermal (e.g. BCG) vaccinations.
- All intramuscular vaccines should be injected deep into a muscle. Insert needle at an angle of 60° into the anterolateral thigh and pointing towards the knee (<12 months of age) and into the deltoid pointing towards the shoulder (≥12 months of age). Never use the buttock for vaccination as the sciatic nerve is vulnerable and vaccine absorption at this site may be suboptimal.
- Multiple vaccines: two injectable vaccines can be given into the same limb – separated by at least 25 mm.
- Cold chain: never use a vaccine if there is any doubt about its safe cold chain storage. Vaccines should be kept in a refrigerator reserved for vaccine/medicine storage at 2–8°C and never frozen.

COMMON MISCONCEPTIONS FOR MISSING VACCINATIONS

Anti-vaccination issues

Only about 1–2% of parents refuse vaccination for their children because they oppose vaccination. Health professionals missing opportunities to vaccinate contributes to children being under immunised for their age. Some common misconceptions about vaccination are: natural infection is the best way to achieve immunity, vaccination weakens the immune system and homeopathic 'immunisation' is safer and more effective. Parents require their concerns to be addressed, but it is very important to emphasise the well-established risks associated with not vaccinating their child, as well as providing reassurance about vaccine safety. In Australia and elsewhere, authoritative booklets are now available to help parents and practitioners understand why these anti-vaccination concerns are ill-founded.

Table 8.1 False contraindications to vaccination

Children *should* still be vaccinated, even if they:

- Have a cold, or low grade fever (<38.5°C)
- Have a family history of any reactions following vaccination.
- Have a family history of convulsions.
- Have had a pertussis-like illness, measles, rubella or mumps infection.
- Are premature (vaccination should not be postponed).
- Have a stable neurological condition such as cerebral palsy or Down syndrome.
- Have been in contact with an infectious disease.
- Have asthma, eczema, hay fever or 'snuffles'.
- Are on treatment with antibiotics.
- Are on treatment with locally-acting (inhaled or low-dose topical) steroids.
- Have a pregnant mother.
- Are being breast-fed.
- Were jaundiced after birth.
- Are over the age recommended in the standard vaccination schedule.
- Have had recent or imminent surgery.
- Are of low weight but otherwise healthy.
- Have been treated with replacement corticosteroids.

Table 8.1 adapted from The Australian Immunisation Handbook, 7th Edition (National Health and Medical Research Council, March 2000).

Table 8.2 Contraindications to vaccination

All vaccines	• Acute febrile illness (if fever >38.5°C, postpone vaccine) • Previous anaphylaxis contraindicates further dosage of the same vaccine
DTPw or DTPa	• Encephalopathy within 7 days of previous DTP vaccination*
Live vaccines (e.g. MMR, OPV, varicella)	• Usually contraindicated in immune-suppressed children e.g. chemotherapy or high dose corticosteroids (2 mg/kg/day for >1 week). • OPV is contraindicated in household contacts of immunosuppressed people. • MMR and varicella vaccines should be deferred if <3 months after injection of a blood product (immunogenic response may be diminished). • MMR and varicella should be given on the same day or separated by 1 month (this does not apply to OPV or any killed vaccines).
Other vaccines	• Severe adverse reactions (extremely rare)

* defined as severe acute neurological illness with prolonged seizures and/or unconsciousness and/or focal signs due to another identified cause.

Table 8.3 Current vaccines, their abbreviations and available forms with tradenames

Disease	*Vaccine*	*Available Products*
Hepatitis B	hepB	Engerix-B; H-B VaxII
Diphtheria, tetanus, pertussis	DTPa	Infanrix; Tripacel
Diphtheria, tetanus, pertussis	DTPa (adult)	Boostrix
Diphtheria, tetanus, pertussis, hepatitis B	DTPa-hepB	Infanrix-HepB
Diphtheria, tetanus	dT	ADT Vaccine
Haemophilus Influenzae type B	Hib (PRP-OMP)	PedvaxHIB
Haemophilus Influenzae type B, hepatitis B	Hib (PRP-OMP)-hepB	Comvax
Poliomyelitis	OPV	Polio Sabin
	IPV	IPOL (also available in combination with DTPa)
Measles, mumps, rubella	MMR	MMR II; Priorix
Influenza	Influenza vaccine	Fluarix; Fluvax; Vaxigrip; Fluvirin
Pneumococcal disease	23 valent Polysaccharide Pneumococcal vaccine, 23vPSV	Pneumovax23
	7 valent Pneumococcal conjugate vaccine, 7vPCV	Prevenar
Meningococcal C disease	Meningococcal C Conjugate vaccine, MCCV	Meningitec; Neis-Vac; Menjugate
Meningococcal disease	Polysaccharide Meningococcal vaccine	Mensevax; Menomune
Varicella	VZV	Varilrix; Varivax

THE AUSTRALIAN STANDARD VACCINATION SCHEDULE 2000–2002

Table 8.3 indicates current vaccines, their abbreviations and available forms with tradenames. The NHMRC recommends the vaccination schedule in Figure 8.1. The latest changes to the schedule involve

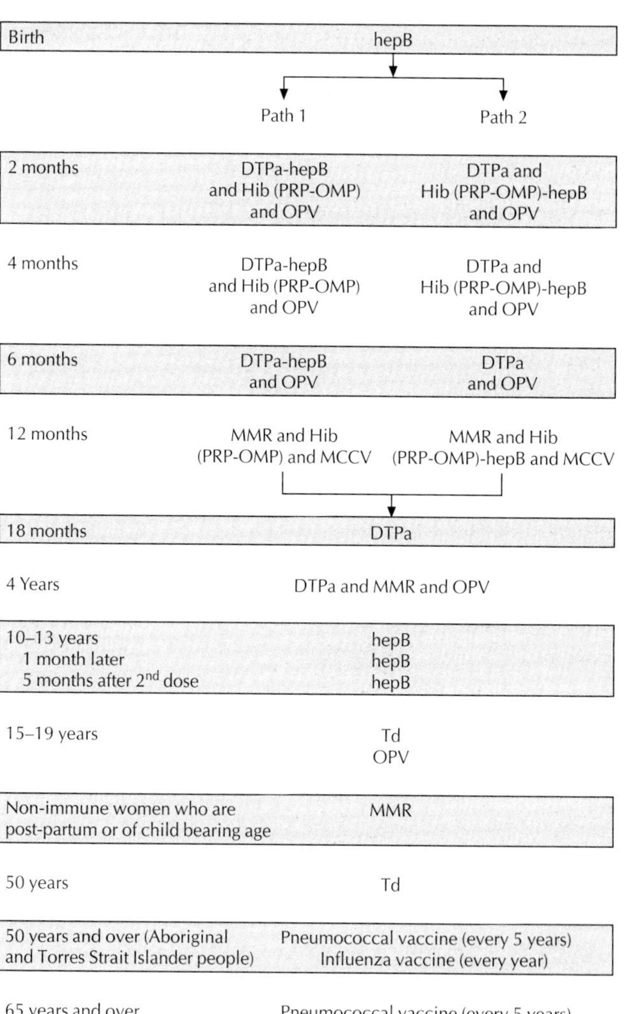

	Path 1	Path 2
Birth	hepB	
2 months	DTPa-hepB and Hib (PRP-OMP) and OPV	DTPa and Hib (PRP-OMP)-hepB and OPV
4 months	DTPa-hepB and Hib (PRP-OMP) and OPV	DTPa and Hib (PRP-OMP)-hepB and OPV
6 months	DTPa-hepB and OPV	DTPa and OPV
12 months	MMR and Hib (PRP-OMP) and MCCV	MMR and Hib (PRP-OMP)-hepB and MCCV
18 months	DTPa	
4 Years	DTPa and MMR and OPV	
10–13 years 1 month later 5 months after 2nd dose	hepB hepB hepB	
15–19 years	Td OPV	
Non-immune women who are post-partum or of child bearing age	MMR	
50 years	Td	
50 years and over (Aboriginal and Torres Strait Islander people)	Pneumococcal vaccine (every 5 years) Influenza vaccine (every year)	
65 years and over	Pneumococcal vaccine (every 5 years) Influenza vaccine (every year)	

When infants and children have missed scheduled vaccine doses, a 'catch up' schedule should be commenced. Details can be found in the Australian Immunisation Handbook, current edition.

Fig. 8.1 The Australian Standard Vaccination Schedule

the introduction of universal meningococcal C vaccine for 1 year olds, hepatitis B vaccine for neonates and the introduction of further infant combination vaccines. The schedule differs slightly in different states of Australia. For vaccinations at 2, 4, 6 and 12 months, two options for the use of combination vaccines are presented. Victoria uses path 2.

VACCINES IN THE AUSTRALIAN SCHEDULE – FURTHER INFORMATION

DTPa

Importance of completing the first 3 doses on time

Protection for pertussis following the first DTPa dose at 2 months is minimal. This vaccine is highly effective once the primary course is completed. If there has been a delay in the first DTPa dose, the second dose can be given 1 month after the first dose.

Previous proven pertussis

Children who have had culture-positive pertussis after the age of 3 months do not need to receive pertussis vaccine. However, vaccination of children who have been previously infected is not dangerous. If there is any doubt, vaccinate.

Does DTP vaccine cause encephalopathy?

There is no evidence to support claims that pertussis containing vaccines cause an encephalopathy. However, infants having had the timely association of encephalopathy within 7 days after a pertussis containing vaccine should not receive further such vaccines.

Targeting adolescents and adults to protect young children: pertussis booster vaccine

Young babies are at risk of pertussis infection from their parents and other adults, who have been shown to be the major source of the disease in the community. Target immunisation of adults in contact with young babies can reduce the chance of serious pertussis infection in infants. A booster pertussis vaccine (Boostrix®) is now registered in Australia for use in children and adults over the age of 8 years and should be considered for health care workers, parents etc. Further data are needed to determine whether repeat boosters may be required in adults to maintain adequate immunity.

MMR

Two doses

Two doses of MMR vaccine are now given (12 months and 4 years) to improve seroconversion.

Egg allergy

The MMR vaccine is safe for children with egg allergy, even anaphylactic egg allergy, as it is produced in chicken fibroblasts (not eggs). Give under supervision. Skin testing with small doses of vaccine is of no value.

Does MMR vaccine cause Inflammatory Bowel Disease or Autism?

There is no link between MMR vaccination and inflammatory bowel disease or autism. Families with further concerns about this topic should discuss them with a specialist.

Co-administration with other vaccines

The MMR vaccine can be given on the same day as the varicella vaccine at a separate site. If the dose is not given on the same day as the varicella vaccine, it should be spaced by 4 weeks (or more). The MMR vaccine can be given at any time, before, after or with OPV.

Post-exposure prophylaxis

The MMR vaccine can be administered to susceptible contacts >9 months of age within 72 h, of exposure to measles as post-exposure prophylaxis, **or** immunoglobulin given within 7 days of contact. Immunoglobulin can also be used for subjects with contraindications to MMR such as immunocompromise.

Previous proven measles, mumps or rubella

Children require protection from all components of MMR. As vaccination of children who have been previously infected is not dangerous, MMR should be given to all children.

Religious objection to pork products

The MMR II vaccine contains a small amount of porcine gelatin as a stabiliser. Families with a religious objection to pork products can be given a different brand of MMR vaccine (Priorix®), which is free of pork products and is now funded by the government for this particular use.

Hepatitis B

Neonatal schedule

The first dose should be given within 7 days of birth. Passive protection with 100 IU hepatitis B immunoglobulin (0.5 mL) on the day of birth is also required for infants born to hepatitis B surface antigen positive mothers, (preferably within 12 h). Active vaccination against hepatitis B should be commenced at the same time.

Infant schedule

Three further doses of hepatitis B vaccine are required for all infants in the first year. The dosage schedule differs slightly in different states. In Victoria, the 3 further doses of hepatitis B vaccine are given in combination with Hib vaccine at 2, 4 and 12 months.

Adolescent schedule

Immunisation for all pre-adolescents aged 10 to 13 years either at the end of primary school or at the beginning of secondary school commenced in Australia in 1998 as part of the routine schedule. This dosage regimen is 3 doses, the 2nd dose is given 1 month after the first dose and the 3rd dose is 5 months after the second dose. The adolescent program will continue until the neonatal schedule has vaccinated all children up to 13 years. Families can choose to have children younger than 10 years vaccinated with the same spaced 3 doses in early childhood. A 2-dose schedule may be introduced as an alternative to the standard 3-dose schedule for adolescents aged 11–15 years of age.

OPV

Polio eradication

Polio eradication is now a possibility, as was achieved for smallpox. Many countries are now polio-free, including Australia. However, these countries remain susceptible to imported cases and until the disease is eradicated worldwide, high levels of immunisation coverage need to be maintained.

Oral versus injectable polio vaccine

Discussions are underway about whether the scheduled oral live-attenuated polio vaccine will be changed to the killed injectable formulation (IPV) because of vaccine-associated polio. Vaccine-associated polio can occur at a rate of 1 per 2.4 million doses with OPV and is not an adverse event associated with the use of IPV. Polio vaccine can be excreted in the bowel for up to 6 weeks following vaccination. Household contacts of immunosuppressed people should receive IPV. The OPV vaccine should not be given to patients while in hospital because of bowel excretion.

Meningococcal group C conjugate vaccine

Meningococcus causes septicaemia and meningitis. There are at least 13 serogroups, of which groups B and C are the most common. A vaccine against serogroup B is not yet available. The incidence of meningococcal disease in Australia is increasing, it is highest in infants and young people aged 15–19 years. Group C disease is now more common than B in adolescents and young adults.

The conjugate vaccine

There are 3 brands of protein-conjugated group C meningococcal vaccine in Australia. Each brand is safe and effective at preventing group C meningococcal disease at all ages, including young infants. The vaccine is given intramuscularly and can be given at the same time as the routine childhood vaccinations. The conjugate vaccine provides long-term immunity. Ongoing research will provide information on whether a booster dose is needed later in life.

Who should be vaccinated?

Conjugate meningococcal C vaccine is recommended for all children >6 weeks, adolescents and adults. It is particularly important for children with medical conditions which predispose them to meningococcal disease (e.g. asplenia and complement component deficiency). In 2003, the government introduced funded vaccination for 1–20 year olds.

Schedule

- 2–4 months — 3 doses at least 1 month apart (e.g. 2, 4 and 6 months of age).
- 4–12 months — 2 doses 1 month apart.
- All persons >12 months: 1 dose.

ADDITIONAL VACCINES

There are an increasing number of vaccines available in addition to those in the current schedule. Some of these are particularly important for certain risk groups; others are simply not currently part of the routine schedule and hence are only available in the private sector.

Influenza vaccine

- Recommended for children who are at increased risk of influenza-related complications (including children with chronic lung diseases, and congenital heart disease, around those receiving immunosuppressive therapy). Also recommended for people who may transmit the virus to at-risk individuals (e.g. health care workers and family members of those at increased risk of severe influenza disease).
- Annual vaccination is recommended.
- Children >9 years and adults are given a single annual dose. Children <9 years are given 2 doses (at least 1 month apart) in the first year they receive the vaccine. Subsequent single annual doses are then given. The dose depends on age:
  - 6 months–2 years = 0.125 mL.
  - 2–6 years = 0.25 mL.
  - >6 years = 0.5 mL.
- Influenza vaccine can be administered concurrently with other vaccines including pneumococcal vaccine and all the scheduled childhood vaccinations.
- Individuals with anaphylactic hypersensitivity to eggs should not be given the influenza vaccine. It is contraindicated because the current influenza vaccines are grown in the allantoic cavity of embryonated eggs.
- Symptoms post-vaccination may mimic influenza infection but current influenza vaccines do not contain live virus and cannot cause influenza disease.

Conjugate pneumococcal vaccine

- *Streptococcus pneumoniae* is an important cause of infections in children, particularly in those <2 years of age. Infections include meningitis, pneumonia, septicaemia and otitis media. A 7–valent conjugate pneumococcal vaccine (7vPCV) was licensed for use in Australia in December 2000. This vaccine is almost 100% effective against invasive pneumococcal disease due to the 7 vaccine serotypes (responsible for approximately 60–80% of cases in Australia). The vaccine is also safe and effective over the age of 2 years, though the risk of invasive pneumococcal disease declines in this age group.

- Conjugate pneumococcal vaccine is recommended for all children under 2 years of age. This vaccine is not currently part of the routine funded schedule in Australia.
- The National Childhood Pneumococcal Vaccination Program offers funded vaccination to particular high-risk groups who have a significantly higher rate of invasive pneumococcal disease than the rest of the community.
- *High-risk groups:*
  - All Aboriginal and Torres Strait Islander children <2 years of age.
  - All Aboriginal children 24–59 months of age in Central Australia and regions of similar very high incidence of pneumococcal disease.
  - Non-Aboriginal children in Central Australia <2 years of age.
  - Children <5 years of age with medical risk factors which predispose them to high rates or high severity of pneumococcal infection. This includes children who have a compromised immune response to pneumococcal infection (e.g. congenital immunodeficiencies, children receiving immunosuppressive therapy, asplenia, HIV, renal failure or nephrotic syndrome) and children with certain anatomical abnormalities associated with higher rates or severity of pneumococcal disease (e.g. cyanotic cardiac disease and CSF leaks).

Number of doses varies with age and risk group

Primary Vaccination

- 3 doses: 2, 4 and 6 months
- Vaccination dosage of infants commenced after 6 months of age for children not in high-risk categories.
  - 7–17 months: 2 doses, 2 months apart.
  - 18 months and older: single dose.

Booster doses

The following children should have booster doses (not required by other children).

- Children with impaired immunity: a booster dose of 7vPCV at 12 months of age.
- Aboriginal and Torres Strait Islander children in Northern Territory and Central Australia: a booster of the 23-valent-polysaccharide pneumococcal vaccine (23vPSV) between 18 and 24 months.

Meningococcal polysaccharide vaccine

A short acting polysaccharide meningococcal vaccine has been available for many years, which is particularly useful for travel. This offers protection for up to 3–5 years against serotypes A, C, Y and W135. This unconjugated vaccine is ineffective in infants <2 years. It is used in patients with poor immunity against polysaccharide antigens (e.g. asplenia) and as a travel vaccine.

Varicella vaccine

Varicella vaccine is highly effective against severe varicella disease. Mild breakthrough cases occur in vaccinated subjects at around 1–2% per year.

Recommended for all persons over 1 year of age without a definite history of chickenpox except those who are immunocompromised. Highly recommended for non-immune subjects who are in contact with immunosuppressed subjects (e.g. family members and health care workers). If vaccinees develop a rash (approximately 2–4% chance of rash), they should avoid contact with immunocompromised persons for the duration of the rash.

Varicella vaccine is safe to administer at the same time as any of the routine childhood vaccinations. In infants, it is convenient to administer the vaccine at the same time as the 12-month MMR dose or the 18-month DTPa dose (at a separate site). Varicella vaccine should be spaced 4 weeks (or more) after MMR vaccination if it is not given on the same day.

Schedule

- 1–13 years without a definite history of chicken pox: single dose, no serology beforehand.
- ≥14 years without a definite history of chicken pox: 2 doses, at least 4 weeks apart for those with proven lack of immunity on serology.

- Approximately 40% of adults who do not think they have had chicken pox are found to be immune on serology and do not need vaccination. However, there is no known harm giving the vaccine to immune subjects.
- Health care workers (HCW) with a negative or uncertain history of varicella should be serotested and vaccinated if negative. If a HCW develops a vesicular rash following the vaccine, they should be reassigned to duties that do not require patient contact or placed on sick leave for the duration of the rash (not for 4–6 weeks as per product information). The duration of the rash is likely to be less than 1 week.
- Serotesting after vaccination is not necessary.

Post-exposure prophylaxis

Varicella vaccine is effective in preventing varicella in those already exposed if used within 3–5 days, with earlier administration being preferable. It is not 100% effective following exposure, however, as with pre-exposure vaccination, if varicella occurs it is usually milder.

ADVERSE EVENTS ASSOCIATED WITH VACCINATIONS

The vast majority of adverse events that may be experienced after the scheduled vaccinations are minor (e.g. fever, local redness, swelling or tenderness) and do not contraindicate further doses of the vaccine. Parents who have questions regarding potential adverse events should discuss these with their vaccine provider. A summary of potential vaccine side-effects compared with the effects of diseases is tabled on the back cover of the current Australian Immunisation Handbook. The Immunisation handbook has a comprehensive section on adverse events following immunisation and also discusses adverse events separately with each vaccine throughout the book.

Anaphylaxis

Anaphylaxis is a rare but potentially fatal reaction that can follow administration of almost any drug or vaccine. Overall, it occurs approximately/ 1/1–4 million vaccine doses. Because of this small risk, recipients of any vaccine should remain in the vicinity of the vaccination area for approximately 15 min. For treatment of anaphylaxis, refer to Medical emergencies, chapter 1.

IMMUNISATION GUIDELINES FOR SPECIAL GROUPS

Immunosuppressed or immunodeficient children

Inactivated vaccines (such as pertussis and hepatitis A vaccines), modified toxins (such as diphtheria and tetanus vaccines) and sub-unit vaccines (such as Hib and hepatitis B vaccines) can be given safely to children receiving immunosuppressive therapy, but may be less effective. Live vaccines (e.g. OPV, varicella vaccine, MMR, BCG) should not, as a general principle, be given to immunosuppressed individuals. The OPV vaccine should never be given to an immunosuppressed child. The MMR vaccine can be given to some children with HIV. Children who have received bone marrow transplants may require booster doses or revaccination, depending on their serological and clinical status. Children who have received i.m. immunoglobulin are recommended a 3-month delay in receiving MMR and varicella vaccines to avoid reduced effectiveness of the vaccine (delay 9 months following i.v. immunoglobulin). Children who have received high dose oral steroid therapy (prednisolone 2 mg/kg/day for more than 1 week, or 1 mg/kg/day for more than 1 month) should delay live vaccine administration until at least 3 months after therapy has stopped. The use of inhaled steroids is not a contraindication to vaccination with either live or inactivated vaccines. For further details of immunisation in immunosuppressed children refer to the current Australian Immunisation Handbook.

Household contacts of children with immune deficiency

Siblings and close contacts of immunosuppressed children should be given MMR, varicella and IPV (but not OPV). Immunisation will ensure that they have less chance of infecting their immunosuppressed siblings.

Premature infants

Preterm babies should be immunised with the recommended schedule according to their actual (not corrected) age, provided they are well and that there are no other contraindications. Some preterm babies do not respond as well to the hepatitis B and Hib vaccines and may require an extra dose of each. For details see the current Australian Immunisation Handbook.

Functional or anatomical asplenia

All splenectomised individuals should receive pneumococcal and meningococcal vaccinations in addition to the vaccinations of the standard schedule. In cases of elective splenectomy, the vaccinations should be given 2 weeks before the operation. There is a detailed immunisation protocol for children with asplenia available from the RCH immunisation service.

Vaccination of Immigrants to Australia

See Immigrant child health, chapter 9.

CHAPTER 9
IMMIGRANT CHILD HEALTH

James Rice
Susan Skull
Jonathan Carapetis

Newly arrived immigrants to Australia come from many parts of the world under a variety of entry programs. Some come from countries where health facilities and programs have been disrupted or may be minimal.

Pre-departure health screening for children is limited and includes a chest X-ray to exclude pulmonary tuberculosis if there is clinical suspicion or a known contact, urinalysis if aged over 5 years and hepatitis B serology if the child is unaccompanied. In some states of Australia (including Victoria) routine post arrival health checks are not performed. Although it is known that immigrants and refugees have high rates of physical and mental health problems, access to health services upon arrival may be limited, particularly by language and cultural differences.

Immigrant and refugee children may:

- Come from situations of conflict and persecution.
- Have experienced torture or severe human rights violations.
- Have experienced loss of, or separation from family members.
- Have spent long periods in refugee camps inside or outside their home country.
- Not speak English as their first language.
- Experience anxiety about the medical consultation.
- Distrust authority figures.

The health care visit needs to be handled sensitively, taking into account the above factors, and ideally a qualified interpreter should assist.

At the initial visit

- Rule out acute illness.
- Focus on medical issues – including growth, development, pre-existing illness, hearing or visual difficulties and dental problems.

- Examine the child fully with a special focus on infection, parasitic infestation, previous trauma, dental health and evidence of micronutrient deficiency.
- Perform baseline screening investigations, tailored to the health issues in their region of origin.
- Determine immunisation history and perform initial immunisations as required.

At subsequent visit

- Follow-up on results from initial visit.
- Explore less acute and chronic illnesses.
- Begin exploring psychosocial issues.
- Arrange referrals to specialists and other agencies as appropriate (including dental services).
- Plan follow-up with existing local general practitioner and immunisation services or liaise with interested local providers to whom the family can be referred.

Investigations

The following investigations are suggested for all immigrant children from settings of poverty or deprivation (e.g. refugees, asylum seekers, or immigrants from developing countries):

- Full blood count (anaemia and eosinophilia).
- Ferritin (iron deficiency anaemia).
- Mantoux test.
- Stool sample (intestinal parasites).
- Hepatitis B serology.
- Strongyloides and Schistosomiasis serology (according to region of origin).
- Vitamin A levels.
- Vitamin D levels.

Note that pre and post-test counselling must accompany hepatitis B serology and Mantoux testing. Tuberculosis carries great stigma in some countries and issues around testing must be handled sensitively.

Investigations in febrile immigrant children

- Full blood count and blood culture.
- Baseline markers of inflammation.
- Exclude malaria in children from endemic areas (thick and thin films × 3, 8–12 h apart).

Immunisation

If the family of a child has no written documentation to verify previous immunisation, a 'catch-up' course of immunisation should be commenced (refer to 'Catch-Up' Vaccination section, The Australian Immunisation Handbook, current edition).

Vitamin D deficiency

- Common and poorly recognised among child immigrants with dark pigmentation in Australia.
- Most are asymptomatic but will have diagnostic features on laboratory testing and radiographic examination.
- If serum 25 OH Vitamin D level <25 nmol/L, further investigations are required:
  - Parathyroid hormone, alkaline phosphatase, calcium, phosphate, urea and creatinine.
  - X-ray wrist and knee if the child is still growing.

Treatment of Vitamin D deficiency

- Symptomatic rickets (including tetany, severe hypocalcaemia and stridor) requires inpatient management.
- Non-symptomatic Vitamin D deficiency – treat with Ergocalciferol 1,000 to 4,000 units/day for a minimum of 4 weeks then reassess. Alternative regimens such as megadoses of (minimum) 100,000 units every 6–8 weeks are presently being investigated. Specialist consultation is essential.
- Screen other family members, including children born in Australia and pregnant women. Infants (breast or bottle fed) may be particularly affected due to maternal deficiency and routine supplementation of Vitamin D 400 units daily (e.g. Pentavite) is recommended. Check serum Vitamin D level before cessation.

Intestinal parasites

- Commonly found in the stool of children particularly from Africa and South-East Asia.
- Most organisms do not produce a clinical illness and many are considered non-pathogenic and do not require treatment. The following generally require treatment and specialist advice may be helpful.
  - Ascaris.

- Giardia intestinalis (lamblia).
- Ancylostoma (Hookworm).
- Strongyloides.
- Schistosoma.
- Taenia (Tapeworm).
- Trichuris (Whipworm).
- Hymenolepis.
- Entamoeba histolytica (may or may not require treatment – discuss with specialist).

Tuberculosis

Tuberculosis (TB) is common in developing countries. Immigrants to Australia aged over 16 years are screened only for pulmonary TB by chest X-ray. One of the highest risk periods for reactivation for TB is during the 5 years immediately following immigration. Children are more likely to have extrapulmonary TB than adults and 15% of children exposed to TB will develop signs of primary or disseminated disease.

All children who come from countries where TB is prevalent should have a Mantoux test. The test is positive if:

- Reaction >10 mm diameter in a child without a BCG scar.
- Reaction >15 mm in a child with a BCG scar.

Discuss positive results with a specialist.

Human immunodeficiency virus

Many children come from regions with high prevalence of HIV infection (e.g. Sub-Saharan Africa, South-East Asia). There is no requirement for routine pre-arrival HIV screening, except in adults. It is unusual for children and non-sexually active adolescents to have asymptomatic HIV infection after the age of 1 or 2 years, as most cases are acquired perinatally and will manifest in the first 2 years of life.

Human immunodeficiency virus testing should be considered in:

- Children with symptoms of possible HIV infection (e.g. failure to thrive, chronic respiratory infections, persistent thrush).
- Infants from high-risk areas.
- Where parents are known or suspected to be HIV positive.

Pre-test counselling for HIV is complex and detailed. Specialist advice is usually needed.

Hepatitis B

Hepatitis B infection is a major public health concern in immigrants, particularly those from Asia, Africa and Oceania where prevalence rates are between 12 and 22%. Chronic infection results in chronic hepatitis, cirrhosis and/or hepatocellular carcinoma in up to 1/3 of affected individuals and is most likely to result after exposure at birth or in the first 5 years of life. Universal immunisation of all infants against hepatitis B is recommended.

Dental disease

Assessment of dental health is particularly important in refugee patients, as the patient may have had limited access to dental care services, poor diet, or sustained injuries. A dental review should be recommended for all recent immigrants.

Mental health

Refugees entering under the Humanitarian Program are likely to have had traumatic experiences in, or during their flight from their countries of origin and may be experiencing physical and/or psychological sequelae. In children this can result in withdrawal, fear, aggression, behavioural or somatic complaints. Many children have witnessed violence to family members or have themselves been victims of violence. Health professionals seeing refugees may need to orient their consultation and management to accommodate the negative effects of reaction to past trauma, their prior experience of health care, cultural differences and the stresses of resettlement. Referral to appropriate mental health services or community support groups may be necessary. Establishing trust is the key to successful interactions.

Parents

Recently arrived immigrant parents are also likely to have unmet health needs. They should be advised to see their family doctor to discuss the above issues.

CHAPTER 10
BEHAVIOURAL, DEVELOPMENTAL AND SLEEP PROBLEMS

Daryl Efron
Margot Davey
Sheena Reilly

Concerns regarding children's behaviour are common and need to be assessed within a developmental framework. Many presentations are in fact normal behaviour (e.g. toddler tantrums), however, parents need empathic support and practical management advice.

Child behaviour is the result of interaction between innate biological or temperamental characteristics and environmental influences including family constitution, socioeconomic status and available resources, parental mental health, ethnic and cultural factors and educational setting.

Developmental status must always be evaluated in a child who presents with behaviour disturbance. Developmental delays or disabilities may present in this way. Physical causes for behaviour disturbance must be excluded (e.g. iron deficiency causing irritability, nocturnal seizures causing sleep disturbance). Behaviour modification strategies must be pitched at a developmentally appropriate level.

INFANT DISTRESS ('COLIC')

A common research definition of colic is crying for more than 3 h per day for 3 or more days per week for more than 3 weeks. However, parental tolerance of infant crying varies and it is more useful clinically to define the problem in terms of the parent's concerns.

The typical clinical scenario is an extended period of distressed behaviour. The infant cries vigorously and the parents may interpret this as pain, often using the term 'screaming'. There are usually repeated bouts with sudden onset. The legs are often drawn up and the face red.

The worst period is typically in the late afternoon and early evening, however some infants seem to be irritable at any time of day.

It occurs equally in both sexes and in both breast-fed and formula-fed infants. It begins in the early weeks of life and abates by 3 months of age in 60% and by 4 months in more than 90% of infants. There are no predictable long-term associations.

Assessment

A detailed history should be taken, noting:

- Temporal associations with feeds.
- Variation with contextual or environmental factors.
- Parental response (both affective and practical).
- Level of support for the parents should be assessed.

A detailed physical examination is important; particularly to reassure the parents that identifiable organic causes have been excluded. If the infant is thriving and developing normally, then physical causes are rare.

History and examination should rule out conditions such as otitis media, UTI, reflux oesophagitis (rare in the absence of vomiting) and raised intracranial pressure.

Associations with foods are difficult to prove and random changes of maternal diet (in breast fed infants) or formula in the absence of specific indicators are not usually helpful. Cow milk protein intolerance or allergy will usually have some associated features including vomiting, diarrhoea or skin rash. Lactose intolerance causes frothy stools with perianal excoriation and abdominal distension.

Management

- Reassurance that the infant is healthy is important and often extremely helpful. Explain that some infants appear excessively sensitive to both internal and environmental stimuli in the early months of life, but that it will settle with maturation.
- Minimise environmental stimulation – low level background noise, soft lighting and comfortable ambient temperature and avoid excessive handling.
- Maintain predictable routines.

- Carrying the infant in a sling (snuggly) is often helpful and allows the parents to free their hands. Patting, rocking, gentle massage, a dummy and swing may be tried.
- Medications such as antispasmodics and sedatives should *not* be used and over the counter anticolic preparations are rarely helpful. Antacids or ranitidine may be tried if the history suggests gastro-oesophageal reflux (see Gastrointestinal conditions, chapter 24).
- Encourage contact and support from extended family, friends, maternal and child health nurse, etc.

TEMPER TANTRUMS

It is developmentally normal for toddlers to express frustration as they strive for autonomy and some control over their world. From the second year of life most children will have temper tantrums, often persisting through to the preschool years. These are often more prominent in children with delayed speech development and associated frustration.

Management

- Assess contextual factors and the parent's response. Behaviour modification techniques are more likely to be successful if applied as consistently as possible. This involves the same consequence being applied each time a particular behaviour occurs, across different environmental settings and caregivers.
- Toddlers and preschool aged children generally respond to Pavlovian style conditioning, that is, positive reinforcement of socially acceptable behaviour and negative reinforcement of undesirable or unacceptable behaviour. Consequences should be decided upon in advance (with all carers agreeing) and explained to the child. They should be applied immediately when the behaviour occurs, as calmly as possible with minimal discussion and no negotiation or bargaining.
- Avoid over stimulation or excessive fatigue.
- Apply rules consistently.
- Ignoring. This involves the parents withdrawing any feedback that may be a positive reinforcer of the tantrum behaviour. The parent needs to stand some distance from the child, withdraw

eye contact and not speak to the child at all. The parent should continue doing what they were doing. Sometimes the parent may need to walk away from the situation. Following the tantrum, acceptable behaviour should be praised. Some children may need reassurance that they are okay after a period of prolonged or severe loss of control.

- When an ignoring program commences the behaviour may escalate initially. However, if the parents can persist through this period, the frequency of tantrums will decrease.

BREATH HOLDING SPELLS

Breath holding spells are extremely frightening for parents, particularly initially. The peak incidence is between 1–3 years of age, although they generally begin in infancy, sometimes in the newborn period.

The most common type is a cyanotic spell. In response to relatively minor frustration or a painful stimulus (e.g. knock to the head), the child cries briefly before involuntarily holding the breath in expiration and becoming rapidly cyanosed. In some cases loss of consciousness or even a brief hypoxic seizure results.

Pallid breath holding spells are less common. The precipitating event is similarly minor and the child holds the breath and becomes markedly pale and limp. This is due to an excessive vagal response resulting in bradycardia or transient asystole.

Management

- Breath holding spells need to be distinguished from seizures. This is usually possible on history, as the cyanosis occurs before the loss of consciousness in breath holding spells, whereas if cyanosis occurs in a seizure it follows loss of consciousness and the onset of seizure activity.
- Place the child on their side until spontaneous recovery, which is usually rapid.
- Do not provide the child with excessive attention, which may promote secondary gain.
- Minimise unnecessary struggles with firm consistent behaviour management. Ensure the child is not iron deficient (dietary history) as this is associated with breath holding spells.

HEAD BANGING

Head banging is a behaviour manifested by young children that usually begins in the first year of life. There are a broad range of repetitive movements, with head banging being the most common, but head rolling and body rocking may also occur. Sometimes these movements are accompanied by vocalisations and humming, which can be disruptive to other family members.

Head banging occurs in 5–15% of normal children and tends to decrease with increasing age, the majority having settled by 5 years. Rarely these movements persist into adolescence. The child almost never sustains significant injuries although bruising and abrasions can occur. In children with severe developmental disabilities head banging can occur for many years and may result in more marked injury to the head and eyes (corneal abrasions and cataracts).

Management

- Reassurance of the parents that head banging is a normal self-limiting condition and will not cause brain damage.
- Strategies to reduce the noise disruption at night such as putting the cot/bed in the middle of the room away from a wall or placing the mattress directly on the ground.
- If the rocking behaviour seems attention seeking, avoid reinforcing the behaviour.
- Sometimes head banging can occur during prolonged periods of wakefulness in bed so restricting the time in bed may be useful.

AGGRESSION/OPPOSITIONAL-DEFIANT BEHAVIOUR

Most children will exhibit some defiant and non-compliant behaviours as they negotiate progressive developmental stages. Parents may seek help when relationships within the family are strained or the child's behaviour is extreme, antisocial, or impairs learning and social development.

Symptoms vary with age and sex. Young children particularly display verbal and physical aggression when unhappy or frustrated. Underlying contributing factors such as developmental and learning difficulties, family and parenting problems and the influence of violent video games need to be considered, along with factors discussed in the introduction, in a biopsychosocial model.

Management

Positively reinforce acceptable behaviour

Parents should be encouraged to 'catch the child being good', noticing and rewarding acceptable behaviour. Encourage abundant use of praise.

Structured reward systems are often extremely helpful in children from about 2½ to 5 years of age. An example of this is for the child to make a colourful 'Big Boy' or 'Good Boy' chart. The child is rewarded with stickers (0–2/day) and once they accumulate 5 stickers they earn a special surprise in the form of a lucky dip selected from a box. Healthy competition can be set up with the model sibling to increase motivation. Stickers should not be removed from the chart as punishment (rewards and punishments should be separate).

Ignore minor irritating behaviours

In many families a great deal of energy is spent arguing about relatively inconsequential behaviours such as whingeing, nagging or not tidying up. This is not sustainable as the parents usually become exhausted. It is preferable to save energy for serious indiscretions.

Consequences for serious oppositional behaviour

This generally involves hitting or kicking somebody, or damaging property. Toddlers and preschool age children generally respond very well to time out when used consistently. This involves calmly and immediately placing the child in a chair or in their room for a timed period of 1 minute per year of age for certain predetermined defined behaviours. If they are calm at the end of the time they can come out, otherwise the clock starts again. Most children learn to abide by time out rules if used consistently, as they recognise they need containment.

For school aged children withdrawal of privileges (e.g. television, video games) is generally the best strategy. Again this should be introduced immediately after the behaviour occurs and applied for a brief period only (e.g. 1–2 days).

Smacking should be discouraged as it models violence and is usually not effective.

Serious antisocial or delinquent behaviours such as frequent high level violence, cruelty to animals, arson or repeated stealing are indicators of a significant conduct disorder and warrant referral to a child and adolescent mental health service. It is important, however, to recognise that isolated incidents are common and not necessarily indicative of severe psychopathology.

ATTENTION DEFICIT HYPERACTIVITY DISORDER

Attention Deficit Hyperactivity Disorder (ADHD) is the somewhat unsatisfactory umbrella term currently applied to a variety of children who share certain core features, principally poor impulse control and limited sustained attention to task, often with motor hyperactivity. Common associated features include oppositional defiant behaviour, anxiety, perceptual and motor coordination difficulties and learning difficulties. The DSM-IV diagnostic criteria for ADHD are provided in the Table 10.1. The majority of children diagnosed with ADHD have the combined type. The predominantly inattentive subgroup often present later with academic difficulties, as they do not generally display disruptive behaviour.

Assessment

- History – A detailed history is critical, focusing on attachment, early development, social skills and academic progress. The timing and nature of initial concerns along with secondary effects such as depression, low self-esteem and social ostracism should be noted. It is important to identify the child's strengths as well as their weaknesses. Standardised behaviour rating scales – completed by parents and teachers (e.g. Connors, Achenbach) are helpful.
- Past and present school reports.
- Psychoeducational assessment in children with significant learning difficulties.
- Physical examination should focus on neuro-development assessment including fine and gross motor coordination, visual-motor integration, auditory and visual sequencing etc.
- Audiology including auditory processing assessment is often helpful. Other investigations are not usually required.

Management

Children with ADHD have multiple special needs and difficulties and the emphasis often shifts over time. The child, family and often school need sustained and skilled support over many years, including the doctor

Table 10.1 DSM IV diagnostic criteria for ADHD

A. Either 1 or 2

1. *Inattention*

At least six of the following nine symptoms have persisted for at least 6 months to a degree that is maladaptive and inconsistent with developmental level

- Often fails to give close attention to details or makes careless mistakes in school work, work or other activities
- Often has difficulty sustaining attention in tasks or play activities
- Often does not seem to listen to when spoken to directly
- Often does not follow through on instructions and fails to finish schoolwork chores or duties in the workplace (not due to oppositional behaviour or failure to understand instructions)
- Often avoids or dislikes tasks (such as schoolwork or homework) that require sustained mental effort
- Often has difficulty organising tasks or activities
- Often loses things necessary for tasks or activities (e.g. school assignments, pencils, books, tools or toys)
- Often easily distracted by extraneous stimuli
- Often forgetful in daily activities

2. *Hyperactivity/Impulsivity*

At least six of the following nine symptoms of hyperactivity/impulsivity have persisted for at least 6 months to a degree that is maladaptive and inconsistent with developmental level

Hyperactivity

- Often fidgets with hands or feet and squirms in seat
- Often leaves seat in classroom or in other situations in which remaining seated is expected
- Often runs about or climbs excessively in situations where it is inappropriate (in adolescents or adults may be limited to feelings of restlessness)
- Often has difficulty playing or engaging in leisure activities quietly
- Is often on the go and acts as if driven by a motor
- Often talks excessively

Impulsivity

- Often blurts out answers to questions before the questions have been completed
- Often has difficulty awaiting turn
- Often interrupts or intrudes on others (e.g. butts into conversation or games)

B. Onset no later than 7 years of age

C. Symptoms must be present in two or more situations (e.g. at school, at home and/or at work)

D. The disturbance causes clinically significant distress or impairment in social, academic, or occupational functioning

E. Does not occur exclusively during the course of a pervasive developmental disorder, schizophrenia, or other psychotic disorder, and is not better accounted for by a mood disorder, anxiety disorder, or dissociative disorder, or a personality disorder

working in collaboration with other health, educational and community professionals. A multimodal strategy is required.

Behaviour modification

The methods described previously under oppositional defiant behaviour are generally helpful.

- Parents and teachers need to apply structured behavioural modification strategies as consistently as possible. Predictable routines are required both at home and at school.

Educational strategies

- An individualised plan should be developed to optimise learning and promote appropriate behaviour.
- Classroom adaptations include seating the child at the front of the classroom near a good role model, using written lists and other visual prompts. Some children need individualised instructions and encouragement to complete tasks, with increased adult one to one supervision such as a teacher's aide. Frequent breaks with the opportunity to move around the classroom help the child remain on task. Tasks such as collecting lunch orders similarly break up the work and are also good for self-esteem.
- Clear rules and predictable routines are important. Positive reinforcement should be provided for acceptable behaviour.

Medication

Psychostimulant medication is the single most effective intervention for children with ADHD (see Table 10.2). It is successful in about 75% of cases, helping children control antisocial verbal and physical impulses and sustain attention to tasks to enable work completion and academic success nearer their potential. Secondary benefits in terms of improved peer status, family functioning and self-esteem often accrue over time.

A number of other medications are useful in some children with ADHD. These include:

- Antidepressants (tricyclics, SSRI, SNRI), particularly if there is associated anxiety.
- Clonidine, which can help smooth out explosive behaviour and assist with sleep onset. If clonidine is used in combination with a stimulant, twice-daily dosing is preferable and the total daily dose should not exceed 100 mcg.

Table 10.2 Stimulant Medication

Generic Name	*Methylphenidate*	*Methylphenidate long-acting*	*Dexamphetamine*
Brand name	Ritalin, Attenta	Ritalin LA	–
Capscale/ Tablet sizes	10 mg	20 mg/30 mg/40 mg	5 mg
Dosage	10–60 mg/day	20–60 mg/day	5–30 mg/day
Onset of action	30–60 min	Biphasic relase – 50% immediate – 50% delayed (4 h later)	30–60 min
Half life	3–4 h	–	4–6 h
Dosing frequency	Breakfast, lunchtime, occasionally after school for homework	Once daily	Breakfast, lunchtime
Common side effects	Appetite suppression	Appetite suppression	Appetite suppression Initial insomnia Irritability & tearfulness (usually abate over several weeks)

Drug holidays – Not for most children. Preferred by some families on weekends and school holidays if the main problem is attentional

Other strategies

The parents of children with ADHD commonly try a variety of unproven complementary therapies. There is no evidence that these interventions are helpful and some are expensive and/or potentially harmful. A small minority of children may benefit from elimination of synthetic food colourings and preservatives.

Prognosis

Most children with ADHD will continue to have some difficulties through adolescence and into adulthood, although many develop good compensating strategies and function very well. A significant minority suffer long-term complications including academic underachievement, school drop-out, delinquency, vocational disadvantage and relationship difficulties. Children with ADHD treated with stimulant medication appear to be less likely to develop substance abuse in adolescence than those left untreated.

TICS AND TOURETTE SYNDROME

Motor tics are stereotypic, involuntary, rapid jerking movements including eye blinking, head jerking and facial grimacing. Transient motor tics are relatively common in school-aged boys. Tourette syndrome is diagnosed when multiple motor tics are associated with vocal tics such as repetitive sniffing, throat clearing or grunting if the symptoms persist for more than a year. More florid vocal tics such as barking sounds or words including obscenities are less common. Tourette syndrome is 10 times as common in boys as in girls.

Associated problems include obsessive-compulsive disorder, ADHD and learning difficulties. Tics may be exacerbated by stress or stimulant medication.

Management

- Most children with a transient tic disorder require no treatment.
- Intervention is indicated if the child is embarrassed by the tics, or there are functional impairments in social or academic functioning.
- Medication treatment may include haloperidol, pimozide and clonidine or an SSRI. These should only be prescribed by a paediatrician or child psychiatrist.
- Behaviour management and educational support is often required to help with associated problems.

LEARNING DIFFICULTIES

There are many reasons why a child may experience learning difficulties and often multiple factors are involved. These include specific learning disabilities (commonly language-literacy based), intellectual disabilities, attentional deficits, sensory impairments (hearing, auditory processing, vision), emotional disturbance, chronic illness, family and social difficulties and suboptimal teaching or educational placement. A specific learning disability is defined as a discrepancy between a child's intellectual ability and their academic achievement.

Management

- Obtain information from both parents and teachers.
- Obtain previous school reports.
- Formal educational psychology assessment.
- Neurodevelopmental assessment undertaken by a developmental paediatrician is important in identifying areas of difficulty such as language receptivity, short-term auditory memory, motor planning and fine motor coordination.
- The doctor has an important advocacy role.
- Liaise closely with the school to ensure that appropriate assessments are undertaken and that an individualised educational plan is devised taking account of the child's special needs and is reviewed periodically.
- In severe cases an application for integration assistance should be made to the education department.
- Some children benefit from remedial tuition either within or outside school hours. It is important for parents not to over burden children, who need normal recreational time.
- Parents need support in understanding their child's potential and the ways in which they can help optimise their child's learning.

SLEEP PROBLEMS

Sleep physiology

- Sleep is divided into 2 states depending on the presence or absence of rapid eye movements (REM) – REM sleep and Non-REM sleep. Non-REM sleep is further divided into 4 stages –NREM1 (light sleep) through to NREM4 (deep sleep).
- Sleep is made up of cycles of REM/NREM sleep that occur at intervals of 60 min in the infant and lengthen to 90 min in the preschooler.
- Newborn infants sleep around 16 h per day, reducing to 14.5 h by 6 months and then 13.5 h by 12 months.
- Around 3 months of age the infant's circadian rhythm is emerging with sleeping patterns becoming more predictable and the majority of sleep occurring at night. By 6 months of age most full-term healthy infants have the capacity to go through the night without a feed.

- Towards the end of the first year of life the child's sleep architecture becomes similar to that of an adult with the majority of deep sleep (NREM3/4) occurring in the first third of the night and REM sleep concentrated in the second half of the night.
- Infants who develop the ability to transition from sleep cycle to sleep cycle without parental assistance appear to sleep through the night.

Assessment

1/3 of families will complain of difficulties with their child's sleeping patterns. To help in the diagnosis and management look at:

- Detailed sleep history over 24 h, looking at how and where the child goes to sleep, frequency and character of wakings, snoring and daytime functioning.
- Sleep patterns during weekends/holidays and with different caregivers.
- A sleep diary may help clarify the situation.
- Family and social history to examine the presence of contributing problems such as maternal depression, marital problems and drug or alcohol abuse.
- Medical history and examination to exclude medical conditions contributing to disrupted sleep patterns, for example; obstructive sleep apnoea, asthma, eczema, nocturnal seizures, gastroesophageal reflux, otitis media with effusion and nasal obstruction.

Bedtime struggles and night-time waking

For infants less than 6 months of age no interventions other than schedule manipulation and anticipatory guidance are used.

Treatment plans must be individualized and adapted for each family.

Aetiology

- Sleep associations occur when a child learns to fall asleep in a particular way, so that every time the child has a normal arousal they wake up fully and are unable to put themselves back to sleep unless those particular conditions are set up again. Examples include rocking, feeding or falling asleep in the pram or car.
- Frequent feeding can cause wakings by both sleep associations and the child developing a 'learned hunger' response. The latter group can develop patterns that lead to large quantities of milk being consumed overnight. Most healthy full-term babies can go without a night-time feed by 6 months.

- Erratic scheduling can contribute by inappropriate timing of naps and lack of a regular bedtime routine.
- Inconsistent limit setting in the toddler and preschooler can exacerbate bedtime struggles and nighttime wakings.

Management

- Detailed explanation about normal sleep and sleep cycles in a non-critical manner.
- Strategies to deal with inappropriate sleep associations all aim to provide the child with the opportunity to learn to fall asleep without parental assistance. Interventions range from extinction (letting the child cry it out), graduated extinction or controlled crying (checking the child at increasing periods of time until they fall asleep by themselves) to a more gradual approach whereby slowly all 'props' are removed.
- If frequent feeding is a problem discuss reducing the amount of fluid over 7–10 days and allowing the child to develop other ways to settle to sleep. Increasing the interval between breast feeds, decreasing the amount of fluid in bottles or substituting water for milk/cordial/juices are all useful strategies that parents can adopt.
- A regular day and night routine needs to be established. An age appropriate enjoyable bedtime routine should be introduced to help the child learn to anticipate going to bed. Sometimes a gate is useful when the child has graduated to a bed and the newfound freedom creates bedtime struggles.
- Medication (Promethazine or Trimeprazine 0.5 mg/kg (max 10 mg) as single night-time dose) may be used in conjunction with behavioural techniques over a 1–2 week period. Medication is not recommended for children less than 2 years.

Night-time fears and anxiety

Aetiology

Night-time fears may present in the preschool and school age child with bedtime struggles and refusal to sleep by themselves. There may be a precipitant (frightening movie, bullying at school) or it may be a manifestation of an anxiety disorder.

Management

- Address separation issues for the child, which may include the introduction of a transitional object.
- Camper bed technique: a camper bed and a parent are moved into the child's room. The parent spends the entire night in the child's bedroom for 2 weeks helping them overcome their fears and gaining confidence in their own bed and room. This is often used in conjunction with a reward/sticker chart. The parent then gradually moves out of the child's bedroom, once the child is sleeping through the night.
- Self control techniques including relaxation, guided imagery and positive self-statements may also be used, again often in conjunction with reward/sticker chart.
- Make sure that the child is not in bed too early, allowing them the opportunity to further fuss and worry, which will interfere with sleep onset.

Night terrors and sleep walking

Aetiology

- These are disorders of arousal, which occur, in the first third of the night during transition from NREM 3/4 sleep to another sleep stage.
- They share common characteristics of the child being confused and unresponsive to the environment, autonomic activation (dilated pupils, sweating, tachycardia) and retrograde amnesia.
- Sleepwalking occurs at least once in 15–30% healthy children and is most common between 6–12 years. It can range from quiet walking, performance of simple tasks such as rearranging furniture or setting tables, to more frenetic and agitated behaviour.
- Night terrors are most common between 4–8 years and have a prevalence of 3–5%. They usually begin with a terrified scream and the child may either thrash around in bed or get up and run around the house. Efforts to calm the child often make the episode worse.
- Night terrors can be distinguished from nightmares by the following characteristics (see Table 10.3).
- The other important differential diagnosis to consider is frontal lobe epilepsy, where attacks present as repetitive stereotypical movements +/– vocalisations. These episodes are brief but occur frequently through the night and are sometimes associated with awareness by the patient.

Table 10.3 Characteristics of night terrors verus nightmares

	Night Terrors	*Nightmares*
Sleep Stage	NREM	REM
Time of night	First third	Last half
Wakefulness	Unrousable	Easily roused
Amnesia	Yes	No
Return to Sleep	Easy	Difficult
Family History	Yes	No

Management

- As these events are generally self-limiting, explanation and reassurance, with discussion of safety issues is all that is usually required.
- Avoid sleep deprivation as this can precipitate events.
- Scheduled awakening (waking the child 30 min before an event) is useful if events occur at predictable times most nights.
- Sleep study may be required if events are very frequent, violent or are atypical. In these situations, low dose clonazepam before bedtime may be useful for 4–6 weeks.

Sleep studies

A sleep study involves the continuous recordings of the following physiological parameters: EEG, EOG, EMG, ECG and respiratory activity; assessing nasal-oral airflow, respiratory effort, O_2 and CO_2.

Sleep studies are indicated for:

- Obstructive sleep apnoea; primary snoring versus sleep disordered breathing.
- Excessive daytime sleepiness (include multiple sleep latency testing in addition if narcolepsy suspected).
- Atypical night-time disruptions including very frequent or violent wakings.
- A full EEG montage is required if seizures are suspected.
- Periodic limb movement disorder.

The majority of sleep disorders can be diagnosed by a careful sleep/wake history and sleep diary, and do not require a sleep study.

SPEECH AND LANGUAGE PROBLEMS

Language delay/impairment can involve receptive skills (ability to understand spoken language), expressive skills (language production) or both. Articulation/phonological problems may also occur, resulting in reduced speech intelligibility.

Background

- Impaired language affects between 5–8% of 4–5 year old children.
- Delay in speech and language may be very specific and occur in the absence of any other developmental problems, or may reflect a general delay in the child's overall development.
- Children with autism may present with concerns regarding speech and language development. These children have distinct early communicative, social and behavioural difficulties that differ from children with primary language impairment (see Developmental delay and disability, chapter 11).
- Children with language delay at 1 and 2 years are at risk of later language impairment, however, not all children identified early with language delay will have language impairment at 4–5 years.
- Some children spontaneously recover or 'grow out' of their early delay. It is not currently possible to differentiate with any certainty those who will recover from those who will go on to have persistent speech and language problems.

Prognosis

Preschool children with persistent speech and language impairment tend to have:

- Learning and social difficulties when starting formal schooling.
- Increased risk for later literacy problems.
- Increased rate of emotional and behavioural disorders.

These problems may persist into adolescence and adulthood and affect employment opportunities.

Factors raising concern about speech and language

- Parental report of concern regarding speech and language development.
- History of hearing loss.

Table 10.4 Speech and language milestones: indicators of concern

Age (years)	*Reason for concern*
6 months	No response to sound, not cooing, laughing or vocalising.
12 months	No localising to sound or vocalising. No babbling or babbling contains a low proportion of consonant vowel babble (e.g. *baba*). Doesn't understand simple words (e.g. '*no*' and '*bye*') or recognise names of common objects or responds to simple requests (e.g. '*clap hands*') with an action.
18 months	No meaningful words except '*mum/dad*' Doesn't understand and hand over objects on request.
2 years	Expressive vocabulary is less than 50 words and no word combinations. Cannot find 2–3 objects on request.
3 years	Speech is not understood within the family. Not using simple grammatical structures (e.g. tense markers). Doesn't understand concepts such as colour and size.
4 years	Speech is not understood outside the family. Not using complex sentences (4–6 words). Not able to construct simple stories.
5 years	Speech is not completely intelligible. Does not understand abstract words and ideas. Cannot reconstruct a story from a book.

- Family history of speech and language difficulties.
- Receptive and expressive language skills both delayed.
- Concern about other aspects of development and lack of developmental progress.
- Autistic features, for example, poor social interactions, limited use of gesture/facial expressions, stereotypic and repetitive behaviours, 'in their own world'.
- Concern regarding general stimulation received.
- Parental report of regression in babbling or language.

Management

- Assess other areas of the child's development, if uncertain or concerned refer to a specialist. Formal cognitive assessment may be needed.
- Exclude hearing loss as a contributing factor by referral to an audiologist.

- Referral to a speech pathologist is recommended as early as possible. Don't delay! The 'watch and wait' approach is no longer considered best practice for all children. Speech pathologists may decide to 'watch and wait' but only after they have considered factors such as the child's speech and language profile, environmental factors, family history, developmental history and progress to date.
- In cases where regression in language is suspected refer, promptly to a paediatrician. In a child under 2 years, a sign of regression may be losing a number of words that had been well established and used spontaneously and frequently for at least 4 weeks.

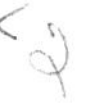

Stuttering

Stuttering is a disorder that affects the fluency of speech production. Stuttering may occasionally appear for the first time in school aged children and even more rarely in adulthood. Stuttering in children is more amenable to treatment than stuttering in adults, however, stuttering beyond 9 years of age usually persists.

- Speech is disrupted by abnormal repeated movements of the speech mechanism, such as *'I w-w-w-w-w-was saying . . .'* and fixed postures of the speech mechanism during which speech stops.
- Many features of stuttering are superfluous behaviours such as body tics and abnormal patterns of speech respiration.
- Stuttering has a strong genetic link with 50–75% of people who stutter having at least one relative who also stutters.
- Stuttering is now considered to be a developmental anomaly rather than a psychological disorder.

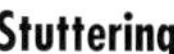

- About 5% of children start to stutter, usually during the third and fourth year.
- Some children recover from stuttering naturally.
  - More girls recover naturally than boys.
  - The period of time that has lapsed since the onset of stuttering is a strong predictor with little chance of natural recovery in children over 9 years old.
  - Family history of recovery may also increase the child's chance of recovering naturally.

Management

- Do not ignore the stutter.
- Refer to a speech pathologist early.

CHAPTER 11
DEVELOPMENTAL DELAY AND DISABILITY

Catherine Marraffa
Dinah Reddihough

Approximately 3–5% of children have developmental delay of at least mild–moderate severity that may remain undiagnosed unless specific assessment is undertaken. In general, problems affecting motor development and speech present early, while problems affecting receptive language, socialisation and cognition present late. The clinician's role is to ascertain whether a child's development is significantly aberrant for his or her age and to determine the underlying reasons for this, realising that most developmental delay does not have a clearly identifiable medical basis.

DEVELOPMENTAL SURVEILLANCE

Developmental surveillance is a flexible continuous process of skilled observation as part of providing routine health care. It should occur opportunistically whenever a child comes into contact with a health professional.

If a parent is concerned about a child's development it is highly likely that evaluation will confirm developmental delay, however, a lack of concern from parents is no guarantee that the child's development is normal.

Informal clinical judgement is unreliable as a method for detecting developmental problems.

The PEDS (Parents Evaluations of Developmental Status) consists of 10 questions based on research of parents concerns. It aims to systematically elicit parents' concerns and guide referral decisions. It is validated from birth to 8 years. It is simple to administer and can be used in primary care settings.

Milestone checklists (see Table 11.1) serve as an aide to memory by recording what is expected of the average child at each age in several domains of developmental function. Because they record average expectations for each age, it is often difficult to distinguish the child with

Table 11.1 Developmental milestones

*Age**	*Gross motor*	*Fine motor adaptive*	*Language*	*Personal–social*
1 m	Lifts head momentarily while prone (0–3 w)	Visual following to mid-line (0–5 w)		Watches face (0–4 w)
2 m	Lifts head momentarily to erect position when sitting	Hands predominantly open	Vocalises (0–7 w)	Smiles responsively (0–7 w)
3 m	Lifts head to 90° while prone (0–10 w)	Visual following past mid-line (0–10 w)	Laughs (6–10 w)	
4 m	Head steady when held erect (6–17 w)	Plays with hands together (6–15 w)	Goos and gurgles	Excited by approach of food
5 m	No head lag when pulled to sitting (3–6 m) Rolls over	Grasps rattle (10–18 w) Reaches for object with palmar grasp (3–5½ m)	Squeals (6–18 w)	Smiles spontaneously (6 w–5 m)
6 m	Lifts head forward when pulled to sit (9–19 w)	Passes block hand to hand (4½–7½ m)	Turns to voice (3½–8½ m)	Friendly to all comers
8 m	Maintains sitting position without support		Repetition of syllables (e.g. baba, Dada)	Feeds self biscuit (5–8 m) Tries to get toy out of reach (5–9 m)
10 m	Stands holding on (5–10 m)	Index finger approach	'Mum', 'Dad' without meaning (6–10 m)	Shy with strangers Plays peek-a-boo
12 m	Walks holding on to furniture (7½–12½ m)	Crude finger–thumb grasp (7–11 m)	Imitates speech sounds (6–11 m)	Gives up a toy

Continued overleaf

Table 11.1 Developmental milestones *cont'd*

*Age**	*Gross motor*	*Fine motor adaptive*	*Language*	*Personal–social*
15 m	Walks alone (11 1/2–15 m)	Neat pincer grasp of pellet (9–15 m)	'Mum', 'Dad' with meaning (9–15 m)	Indicates wants (10 1/2–14 1/2 m)
1 1/2 y	Walks well (11 1/2–18 m)	Builds tower of two blocks (12–20 m)	Three words other than 'Mum', 'Dad' (12–20 m)	Drinks from cup (10–17 m)
2 y	Walks up steps without help (14–22 m)	Scribbles (12–24 m)	Points to one named body part (14–23 m)	Feeds self with spoon (12–24 m)
2 1/2 y	Throws ball (15–32 m)	Builds tower of four blocks (15–26 m)	Combines two words (14–27 m)	Helps in house – simple tasks (15–24 m)
3 y	Pedals tricycle (21 m–3 y)	Imitates vertical line (18 m–3 y) Copies circle (2 1/2–3 1/2 y)	Uses three word sentences	Puts on clothes (2–3 y)
4 y	Balances on one foot (2 3/4–4 1/2 y)	Copies square	Gives first and last name (2–4 y)	Dresses with supervision (2 1/2–3 1/2 y)
5 y	Hops on one foot (3–5 y)	Draws person in three parts (3–5 y)	Knows some colours (3–5 y) Knows age	Dresses without supervision (2 1/2–5 y)

w, weeks; m, months; y, years.

* Age indicates when at least 90% of a normal group of children will achieve the test. Figures in parentheses represent the range from 25th to 90th centiles for achievement.

true developmental delay from the normal child with below-average milestone attainment.

Formal screening tests such as the *Denver II* and the *Australian Developmental Screening Test* allow the objective discrimination of the child who *probably* has a developmental delay from the child who *probably* does not. Results of screening tests are not definitive; a fail on such a test requires referral of the child for formal developmental assessment.

Formal assessment involves a synthesis of the findings from history, physical and neurological examination, and developmental testing using standardised assessment tools such as the *Bayley Scales of Infant Development* and the *Griffith's Developmental Scales.*

The type of testing undertaken depends on the presence or absence of several risk factors for developmental delay (see Table 11.2).

Table 11.2 Children at risk of developmental problems

Risk group	*Risk factors*	*Action*
High	Developmental regression Abnormal neurology Dysmorphism Chromosomal abnormality Hearing or vision problems	Bypass developmental screening. Refer for comprehensive developmental assessment
Moderate	Parents suspect developmental delay History of severe pre- or perinatal insult Very low birthweight (<1500 g) Family history of developmental delay Severe socio-economic or family adversity	Administer a formal screening test *Pass* – reassure that development is within normal range and continue surveillance through a local doctor/maternal and child health nurse. *Questionable* – repeat the test 4 weeks later. *Fail* – refer for comprehensive paediatric consultation and developmental assessment
Low	No parental or professional concerns No other risk factors	Developmental surveillance by a local doctor/maternal and child health nurse is recommended Should there be later parental or professional concerns, a formal screening test is recommended. If there are no further concerns continue surveillance monitoring.

DEVELOPMENTAL DELAY AND DISABILITY

Children with developmental delay or disability, or both, have the same basic needs as non-disabled children. They have the potential for further development and the principles of normal development apply.

Specific disabilities in one area may cause secondary disabilities in other areas (e.g. children who have motor disabilities with reduced opportunity for exploration may suffer delayed development of their comprehension abilities).

Transient developmental delay may be associated with:

- Prematurity.
- Physical illness.
- Prolonged hospitalisation.
- Family stress.
- Lack of opportunities to learn.

Causes of *persistent developmental delay (developmental disability)* include:

- Language disorders.
- Intellectual disability.
- Cerebral palsy.
- Autism.
- Hearing impairment.
- Visual impairment.
- Degenerative disorders.
- Neuromuscular disorders.

Once suspicion regarding a child's development has been raised, a complete paediatric consultation is required. This should include full details of the family, obstetric, neonatal and developmental histories. Liaison with the family doctor and a maternal and child health nurse to obtain background information is often helpful. A history of loss of previously attained developmental skills is suggestive of regression rather than delay and requires more comprehensive investigation to exclude neurodegenerative conditions. Observation of how the child looks, listens, moves, explores, plays, communicates and socialises is essential prior to the formal examination. Understandably, parents will be anxious and a sensitive approach is essential at all times.

Developmental assessment provides the family with an understanding of the child's development and outlines developmental goals and strategies to facilitate development and reduce any handicapping effects of the disability. Assessment and management may include input from physiotherapists, speech pathologists, educationalists, occupational therapists, psychologists and social workers.

Principles of assessment

These include:

- Utilisation of play as a fundamental assessment tool.
- Promotion of optimal performance of the child.
- Gearing of the assessment towards remediation rather than merely producing a profile.
- Involvement of the parents in the assessment process.
- Close linking of the assessment service with services offering help and support.

Early intervention

Early intervention includes prevention and early detection of disabilities, as well as health, educational and community services that assist the child, family and community in adapting to the child's disability and developmental needs. Services are based on the principles of normalisation and the least restrictive alternative.

The aims of early intervention are to minimise the handicapping effects of the child's disability on their development and education and to support the family in understanding and providing for their child's individual needs. Services include individual teaching and therapy (speech and occupational therapy), family support and counselling, providing resources and support to child care, preschools and respite care. Services are usually regionally based and are provided by government and non-government agencies.

Education

There are a range of special educational strategies to optimise learning and development, dependent on the child's abilities and disabilities, with increasing opportunities for integration as resources are moved from special to local schools. A range of special schools is also available.

Family supports

Parents need to be aware of the services that are available to them to assist in the care of their child with a disability. Supports include social security benefits, home help and respite care through foster agencies and community residential units. Consumer organisations can provide parent support, information and advocacy.

INTELLECTUAL DISABILITY

The definition of intellectual disability comprises three elements: (i) a significantly sub-average general intellectual functioning (i.e. 2 standard deviations below the mean of the intelligence quotient) that exists concurrently with; (ii) deficits in adaptive behaviour; and (iii) manifests during the developmental period.

This definition is used by service providers, as well as academics and legislators. The term *developmental disabilities* is used increasingly to reflect the complexity of development.

Up to 2.5% of children have an intellectual disability: approximately 2% mild and 0.5% moderate, severe or profound.

Causes of intellectual disability

Prenatal

- Chromosomal; e.g. trisomy 21 and Fragile X syndrome.
- Genetic; e.g. tuberous sclerosis and metabolic disorders.
- Major structural anomalies of the brain.
- Syndromes; e.g. Williams, Prader-Willi.
- Infections; e.g. cytomegalovirus.
- Drugs; e.g. alcohol.

Perinatal

- Infections.
- Trauma.
- Metabolic abnormalities.

Postnatal

- Head injury.
- Meningitis or encephalitis.
- Poisons.

Presentation

- At birth with a known syndrome or malformation.
- At follow up in high-risk infants.
- Language delay.
- Global developmental delay.
- Learning difficulties.
- Behaviour problems.
- With associated medical complications (e.g. epilepsy).

A biological cause for moderate, severe and profound intellectual disability can be identified more readily than in those with a mild intellectual disability. In disability requiring extensive support, a cause may be identified in up to two-thirds of cases. In people with mild intellectual disability, the cause is identifiable in less than 20% of cases. Where a cause is identified, the majority are caused by problems during the prenatal period with 10% due to perinatal and 5% due to postnatal insults. The two most common identifiable causes of intellectual disability are trisomy 21 and Fragile X syndrome.

Investigations

It is important to establish aetiology where possible in order to understand prognosis, provide genetic counselling and to ensure that associated problems are detected.

The following investigations should be considered:

- Chromosomes, especially for Fragile X, William and Prader–Willi syndromes using DNA probes.
- MRI of the brain.
- Creatinine phosphokinase in boys.
- Plasma amino acids.
- Urinary organic and amino acids.
- Thyroid function tests.
- Mucopolysaccharide screen.

- Investigation for congenital infection: ophthalmological and audiological examination, maternal/infant serology and viral culture (cytomegalovirus).

Despite thorough investigation, the cause is often not identified.

Management

- Support and information for parents.
- Referral to and liaison with other practitioners, early intervention, family support and educational services.
- Child advocacy.
- Regular assessment of vision and hearing.
- Investigation for associated anomalies (e.g. cardiac and thyroid status with trisomy 21).
- Treatment of associated disorders (e.g. epilepsy).
- Monitoring of development.

CEREBRAL PALSY

Cerebral palsy is a persistent, but not unchanging disorder of movement and posture due to a defect or lesion of the developing brain. It occurs in about 2 per 1000 live births.

Aetiology

Cerebral palsy is not a single entity but a term used for a diverse group of disorders, which may relate to events in the prenatal, perinatal or postnatal periods. The cause is unknown in many children. Perinatal asphyxia accounts for less than 10% of cases and postnatal illnesses or injuries for a further 10%. There is a significant association with prematurity. Infants with birth weights less than 1500 g are especially vulnerable to cerebral palsy, with a childhood prevalence of 60 per 1000 compared with an overall prevalence of 2 per 1000.

Classification

This is according to:

- The type of motor disorder (e.g. spasticity or athetosis).
- The distribution (e.g. hemiplegia, diplegia and quadriplegia).
- The severity of the motor disorder.

Associated disorders

- Visual problems.
- Hearing deficits.
- Communication disorders.
- Epilepsy.
- Intellectual disability.
- Learning disabilities.
- Perceptual problems.

Some children have only a motor disorder.

Management

Management of the child with cerebral palsy involves:

- An accurate diagnosis with genetic counselling.
- An assessment of the child's capabilities and referral to the appropriate services for the child and family. Liaising with the kindergarten, school and general practitioner is important.

Management of the commonly associated disabilities and health problems

- All children require a hearing and visual assessment.
- Careful assessment and management of epilepsy is required.
- Children may benefit from formal cognitive assessment.
- *Nutritional problems* – obesity can occur due to an imbalance between intake and physical activity. Conversely, children may be underweight, particularly in the presence of oromotor problems that may result in major feeding difficulties. Dietary advice is important. The presence of severe failure to thrive, major feeding problems or aspiration, or all of these, may be indications for non-oral feeding by a nasogastric or gastrostomy tube.
- *Gastro-oesophageal reflux* occurs commonly in cerebral palsy.
- *Constipation* requires dietary and laxative advice.
- *Aspiration and lung disease* may be associated with impaired oromotor control. Chronic cough with wheeze or repeated lower respiratory infections may indicate the presence of chronic lung disease. Videofluoroscopy is a useful test for the detection of aspiration.
- *Osteoporosis* with pathological fractures may occur in cerebral palsy.
- *Psychological and social difficulties* require careful attention.

Management of the consequences of the motor disorder

- *Saliva control* can be improved with techniques employed by speech therapists, or by the use of anticholinergic medication or surgery in a small group of children.
- *Spasticity management* is aimed at improving function, comfort and care and requires a team approach. Options include:
  - Oral medications, e.g. diazepam, dantrolene sodium and baclofen.
  - Inhibitory casts to increase joint range and facilitate improved quality of movement.
  - Botulinum toxin A for localised spasticity.
  - Intrathecal baclofen is suitable for a small number of children with severe spasticity.
- *Orthopaedic problems.* The orthopaedic management of cerebral palsy requires a team approach. Dynamic spasticity, which interferes with function in young children, is best managed by conservative methods (e.g. orthotics, inhibitory casts or the use of botulinum toxin A). Surgery is mainly undertaken on the lower limb, but is occasionally helpful in the upper limb. Some children also require surgery for scoliosis. Physiotherapy is an essential part of postoperative management. Gait laboratories are useful in planning the surgical program for ambulant children. The critical parts of the body to observe are:
  - *The hip* – non-walkers and those only partially ambulant are prone to hip subluxation and eventual dislocation. Early detection is important and hip X-rays should be performed at yearly intervals or more frequently if there is concern. Dislocation, which may cause pain and difficulty with perineal hygiene, is extremely difficult to treat once it occurs and prevention by early adductor releases is a better strategy. Hip problems may also occur in mobile children; e.g., those with severe hemiplegia, however, this is rare.
  - *The knee* – hamstring surgery may be necessary to improve gait pattern, or the ability to stand for transfers.
  - *The ankle* – there may be a range of problems around the foot and ankle. Conservative treatments are used in young children but surgical correction is frequently required later.

- *Multilevel surgery*
  - Sometimes children require surgery at several different levels, e.g. hip, knee and ankle.

Referrals

Referral to and ongoing liaison with allied health professionals is essential to enable children to achieve their optimal physical potential and independence.

- *Physiotherapists* give practical advice to parents and carers on positioning, handling and play to minimise the effects of abnormal muscle tone and encourage the development of movement skills. They also give advice regarding mobility aids, the use of orthoses or special seating. They may provide individual or group treatments or refer to appropriate community services.
- *Occupational therapists* help parents to develop their child's upper limb and self-care skills, and are also involved in suggesting suitable toys, equipment and house adaptations for home care.
- *Speech pathologists* provide guidance for those with severe eating and drinking difficulties, and communication and augmentative communication systems for children with limited verbal skills.
- *Orthotists* provide advice and design and fabricate various braces. These braces are used to improve function, support, align, prevent or correct deformities to different parts of the child's body – more commonly the lower limbs. As part of the allied health team, orthotists work closely with orthopaedic surgeons and physiotherapists to optimise the child's potential.
- *Other professionals* that may be helpful include medical social workers, nurses, psychologists and special education teachers.
- *General practitioners* play an important role in supporting these children and their families in the community.

SPINA BIFIDA (MYELOMENINGOCELE)

Spina bifida is the commonest severe congenital malformation of the nervous system. The degree of impairment from the spinal cord pathology varies. Most children have some element of lower limb dysfunction, sensory loss and a neurogenic bladder and bowel. Eighty per cent have progressive hydrocephalus requiring surgery. Many children have specific learning problems.

Prevention

Peri-conceptional folic acid supplementation (in the month before and in the first 3 months of pregnancy) has been shown to reduce the risk of recurrence in any at-risk family (by about 75%), as well as reduce occurrence in any family. Recommended doses are:

- Low-risk women (no family history of neural tube defects): 0.5 mg daily.
- Women with a previous child with a neural tube defect (or personal, partner or close family history): 4 mg daily (5 mg if 4 mg not available).
- Women with epilepsy on anticonvulsants should also be advised to take the larger dose.

Note: Multivitamin supplements are not recommended because of the potential risks of vitamin overdose to the developing foetus.

Fortification of staple foods with folate has been recommended in many countries. Fewer children are now being born with neural tube defects, mainly due to antenatal diagnosis and termination of pregnancy. The effect of folate supplementation on incidence is not yet clear.

Management

Management requires collaboration between health, education and welfare professionals and the child and family. Most children attend regular schools. Families require a great deal of support.

An interdisciplinary team of physicians, a neuropsychologist, physiotherapist, orthotist, occupational therapist, social worker and stomal therapist is required to develop an appropriate developmental and rehabilitation program, in collaboration with the family, general practitioners and community agencies (including local primary care service providers).

Initial management

- *Neurosurgical and paediatric assessment* of the newborn infant is undertaken to determine if early surgery to close the spinal defect should be recommended. Clinical and ultra-sound observation to detect and monitor the presence of hydrocephalus is important. Insertion of a ventriculoperitoneal shunt may be necessary.
- *Orthopaedic and urological consultations* and investigations are undertaken in the neonatal period to provide baseline

information for subsequent management. A small number of infants require early management of talipes or a high-pressure neurogenic bladder.

- The families must be fully informed about the diagnosis, natural history and prognosis, and be reassured that assistance is available.

Specific aspects of management

Medical and therapy staff should monitor children regularly.

- *Mobility*
  - Independent mobility is the primary goal of the orthopaedic surgeon, physiotherapist and orthotist.
- *Urinary tract*
  - The primary goal is the maintenance of satisfactory renal function and the establishment of urinary continence (dryness) at a developmentally appropriate age.
  - Clean intermittent catheterisation is now the preferred method of treatment, starting in the neonatal period. Additional support may be necessary in the form of medication (e.g. oxybutynin 8–12 hourly), protective clothing and condom drainage. Bladder augmentation and/or insertion of artificial urinary sphincters may be required.
  - Urinary tract infection is common.
- *Neurological functioning*
  - Children with shunts should have neurosurgical assessment regularly (in infancy every 6–9 months; in childhood and adolescence at least every 1–2 years). See also Neurologic conditions, chapter 30.
  - Tethering of the spinal cord to surrounding structures occurs in most children. In a small number, traction on the cord causes deterioration in neurological functioning. Surgical detethering may be required.
  - Children often have specific cognitive difficulties and a neuropsychological assessment is usually carried out prior to school entry and repeated before transition to secondary school.
- *Miscellaneous medical problems*
  - Constipation is common and dietary advice, laxatives and enemas may be required. For children with severe continence problems anal plugs can be used following careful assessment by the stomal therapist.
  - Scoliosis is a common management problem.

- Pressure sores occur in all children with spina bifida at some time, most commonly on the feet or the buttocks.
- Epilepsy occurs in 15 % of cases.
- Latex allergy is much more common in children with spina bifida and has serious implications. Testing is offered to all children.
- Weight issues can be a problem.

- *Adolescent issues;*
  - Delayed or precocious puberty can occur.
  - Specific adolescent issues including sexuality, relationship difficulties and contraception should be addressed.
  - Mental health should be monitored.
  - Vocational support is important.
  - Transition and transfer to adult services provides a big challenge and needs careful planning and support for the young person.

AUTISM SPECTRUM DISORDER

Autism is now seen as part of a spectrum of disorders. Diagnosis requires the presence of 3 core features by 3 years of age:

- Qualitative impairment of social interaction.
- Qualitative impairment in communication.
- Restricted, repetitive and stereotyped patterns of activities, behaviour and interests.

Prevalence estimates vary with definitions used but autism spectrum disorders may affect up to 60/10 000 children <8 years, with a sex ratio of 3 males: 1 female.

Aetiology

The aetiology of autism is unknown. Factors involved may include:

- Genetic: recurrence rate in families of 2–6%.
- Syndromal: there is an association with tuberous sclerosis, Fragile X syndrome and congenital rubella. Careful medical assessment to exclude these conditions is important.
- Structural: subtle brain abnormalities are described in some cases.

Associated disorders

- Intellectual disability (75%).
- Epilepsy (20%).
- Other: ADHD, affective disorders, Tourette syndrome.

Clinical features

Parents will often identify that something is different about their child before the second birthday. Early features include *lack of*:

- Pretend play.
- Pointing out objects to another person.
- Social interest.
- Joint attention.
- Social play.

Language development is delayed with an unusual use of language. Regression of language may be seen.

Diagnosis

There is no single test for autism spectrum disorders. Diagnosis is best made by a multidisciplinary team of a paediatrician/child psychiatrist, speech pathologist and psychologist.

Management

Management is multidisciplinary. It includes:

- Parent support and education.
- Appropriate screening of vision/hearing, investigation for associated disorders/syndromes if suspected.
- Early intervention programs, including a well structured and predictable environment with:
  - Behavioural modification.
  - Speech therapy.
  - Special education.
  - Sensorimotor programs.
- A combination of educational, developmental and behavioural treatments has been shown to improve a child's rate of progress.
- Drug therapy is sometimes used to treat comorbid psychopathology (e.g.: attentional and behavioural problems, anxiety, self injury). It does not affect the core autistic symptoms.
- Advice regarding educational options.

- Support groups.
- Access to respite care.

Families of children with autism spectrum disorder will often seek alternative health care, sometimes at considerable cost. It is important to be aware and informed of what is available and the evidence supporting/refuting such strategies to help families make an educated choice.

Asperger syndrome

Asperger syndrome is used to describe individuals with:

- Normal intelligence.
- No delay in language development.
- Impaired social and communication skills with a narrow range of obsessional interests.

CHAPTER 12
ADOLESCENT HEALTH

Susan Sawyer
Andrew Court
George Patton

Adolescence is the transitional period of development between relatively dependent childhood and relatively independent adulthood.

Chronological age is not always a good reflection of developmental stage. The term 'adolescent' refers to those aged between 10 and 19 years and 'youth' refers to those aged from 15–24 years. More recently, the term 'young person' has been used in the context of health policies, referring to those between the age of 10 and 24 years.

A social health perspective

The health profile of young people has changed in recent decades with higher rates of psychosocial disorders such as substance abuse, depression and eating disorders now evident. These health problems have arisen as a result of broad social and economic changes in communities. The lifestyles of young people have changed as a result of the longer time required for key social transitions such as completing education, leaving home, commitment to long-term relationships and having children. In addition, unemployment, poverty and increased drug availability have a special impact on young people who are more vulnerable as a consequence of their developmental tasks.

Adolescent developmental tasks

Engaging adolescents in a productive therapeutic relationship requires the clinician to have a good understanding of both the social context of young people's lives and the developmental tasks they confront. The key developmental tasks are around the issues of:

- Autonomy and independence.
- Body self-integrity and personal identity.
- Peer relationships and recreational goals.
- Educational and vocational goals.
- Sexuality.

Developmental outcomes as health outcomes

Clinicians must have clear goals for therapy of young people's health problems. Assisting young people achieve their developmental tasks should be a goal of consultation. Management approaches are more likely to be successful when they are developed in the context of the developmental goals of adolescence and the individual needs of the young person.

A CLINICAL APPROACH TO ADOLESCENTS

Allowing adequate time is essential to the conduct of a successful consultation. Young people often perceive that they are not listened to, not given adequate time to put their views across and that their opinions are dismissed. A clinician who listens respectfully and acknowledges a young person's point of view will make an excellent start in establishing a therapeutic relationship.

Starting the consultation

Greet the young person by name, make eye contact with them and give them your full name. When parents are present, try to greet the young person first and then the parents. The young person is the patient and must be given some time alone with the clinician during the consultation.

Confidentiality

Maintenance of confidentiality enhances trust and honesty, which enables more appropriate health care. Explain the issue of confidentiality at the beginning of the first contact with every adolescent. An example is:

> *'Health consultations are confidential. That means that I cannot talk about anything we discuss today with your parents or anyone else, unless you and I have agreed to do so. However, there are some exceptions. I cannot maintain confidentiality if you are at risk of harm, such as threat of suicide, self harm, or sexual abuse.'*

Young people benefit from reminders about confidentiality when sensitive information is discussed (see Table 12.1).

Table 12.1 Confidentiality

- Define the term at the start of the interview
- Consider all information from an adolescent as confidential until discussed or clarified.
- In most states, confidentiality is a legal requirement over 16 years of age. Negotiation or compromise may be required for adolescents under 16 years.
- Exceptions to confidentiality are when the adolescent is at risk of significant harm, such as risk of suicide or if they are subject to physical or sexual abuse.

Developmental screening

Young people are most likely to present for clinical care as a consequence of a minor complaint, such as a viral illness or injury. Irrespective of the primary reason for presentation, in all adolescents take the opportunity for a developmental assessment and psychosocial screening. Considering risk behaviours, mental health state, health promotion and disease prevention.

One approach to developmental screening is to use the HEADSS framework to take a psychosocial history (see Table 12.2). Questions can be asked in any order, although the first three themes generally involve less sensitive questions in comparison to the latter three themes. Taking a psychosocial history is a powerful way of engaging a young person in the consultation and establishing rapport. It also provides an opportunity for assessment of developmental stage (maturity), assists in identifying the balance of health risk and protective factors, and identifies opportunities for early intervention and health promotion.

Physical examination

A thorough physical examination should be conducted whenever appropriate. Protection of the adolescent's modesty and privacy is very important. Use friendly and reassuring dialogue that explains the reason for the particular examination. Many young people are anxious about many aspects of normal development and benefit from reassurance. Provide feedback on examination findings as much as possible. Plotting growth on a growth chart and explaining it in the context of the normal range can be very reassuring.

Table 12.2 Adolescent developmental screening: HEADSS*

	Area	*Questions*
H	Home	Where do you live and who lives there with you?
E	Education and employment	What are you good at in school? What grades do you get?
A	Activities	What do you do for fun? What things do you do with friends?
D	Drugs	Many young people experiment with drugs, alcohol and cigarettes. Have you ever tried them?
S	Sexuality	Most young people become interested in sex at your age. Have you had a sexual relationship with anyone?
S	Suicide risk/ Depression Screening	See Table 12.3

* Goldenring and Cohen, *Contemporary Pediatrics*, July, 1988, pp. 75–80.

YOUNG PEOPLE WITH CHRONIC ILLNESSES AND DISABILITIES

Young people with chronic illnesses and disabilities are frequently the most experienced consumers of the paediatric health care system. Clinicians are encouraged to acknowledge and respect the experience and views of these young people and their families.

Conflict of priorities

It is not uncommon for a conflict of priorities to occur between the therapeutic goals of the clinician (focused on disease control and management) and the developmental goals that are frequently the main concern of young people. For example, a young person with persistent asthma who goes on a school camp may be too embarrassed to take their preventer medication while on their camp, preferring instead to put up with the unknown consequences (and the unspoken wishful thinking that their asthma will be fine). Negotiating management approaches with the young person is the key to achieving medical goals in ways that the young person is developmentally comfortable with. Providing the young person with a choice of acceptable management options is one useful strategy.

Adherence

Promoting adherence with treatment regimens is a challenge for clinicians irrespective of the age of the patient. It can be especially difficult with adolescents with chronic illness, as they are less influenced by long-term health goals than adults. There may be conflict between the young person's (developmentally appropriate) pursuit of increasing autonomy and independence and the clinician's desire to improve their health. Practical tips include:

- Provide a clear rationale for all treatments.
- Simplify the treatment regimen.
- Discuss the acceptability of treatment in relationship to peers.
- Use simple language. Write down all instructions.
- Don't use threats.
- Work with both parents and young people. Parents may need to be either more involved or encouraged to 'back off' and be less over-protective.

Multidisciplinary teams and mixed messages

The value of a multidisciplinary team is well established, however, there is the potential for individual health professionals within a team to give conflicting messages to young people and their families. Excellent communication within a team is crucial to ensure that a mutually agreed set of messages is delivered to the young person and their family.

Transition to adult health care

Transition is the purposeful and planned movement of adolescents with chronic illness and disability from child-centred to adult-oriented health-care systems. Transfer refers to the physical move from one hospital or health-care setting to another. In contrast, the term 'transition' refers to a process that, ideally, has been anticipated by patient, parents and health-care professionals, with strategies put in place to increase the likelihood of success. Anticipation of transfer to an adult setting from the time of diagnosis is one way of ensuring that the physical move is truly part of a transition process. A planned, coordinated approach is essential. An adult specialist or team that is both interested and capable of providing tertiary care is fundamental. Compilation of a detailed medical and allied health summary by the paediatric team is important, as is good communication between paediatric and adult providers. Community providers, such as general practitioners, are an important source of continuity of care. Starting to see young people alone (for at least part of the health consultation) from the age of 14–15 years is part of the process of transition to adult health care.

Working across the sectors

The emotional health and wellbeing of young people is influenced by many factors, including families, peers and schools. It is valuable to gain information from these other sources provided young people and their parents consent to the sharing of such information. Sources of information may include:

- School and other educational agencies.
- Welfare agencies.
- Recreational programs.
- Peer support groups.

HIGH-RISK YOUNG PEOPLE

High-risk young people include those with significant health risk behaviours (e.g. regular drug use) or mental health problems. A small proportion of young people are considered to be at a very high health risk. This includes adolescents who are socially disadvantaged by homelessness, those engaged in multiple health risk behaviours, those with major mental health problems or those within the juvenile justice setting. These young people commonly do not receive appropriate health care. Close consultation and liaison with existing case-managers in the community is a priority and is more effective than referral to new services. Case managers may be based within a range of community-based facilities, such as general practice, youth mental health services, or protective services. Youth-focussed services are preferred over adult specialist services.

ADOLESCENT MEDICINE REFERRALS

Specialist adolescent medicine units are a resource for general practitioners.

Common reasons for referral include:

- Complex health problems that are relatively unique to the adolescent age group, including eating disorders, deliberate self-harm and suicide attempts, school problems and behaviour disorders.

- Problems occurring at the interface between adolescent general health and adolescent mental health, such as early depression, psychosomatic disorders and chronic fatigue syndrome.
- Complex interactions between young people, diseases and disease treatments.
- Concerns about physical growth, puberty and sexual behaviours.
- Problems requiring access to networks and programs dealing with young people.

ADOLESCENT MENTAL HEALTH

The notion of adolescence as a time of inevitable emotional turmoil, with few implications for future mental health, has given way to a view that the teens and early twenties are critical years for the development of major psychiatric disorders that persist into adulthood (see also Child psychiatry, chapter 13). Major disorders with high rates of first onset in young people include:

- Depression.
- Anxiety disorders.
- Obsessional neurosis.
- Schizophrenia.
- Bipolar affective disorders.
- Substance abuse.
- Personality disorders.
- Anorexia and bulimia nervosa.

The recognition and early diagnosis of adolescent mental health disorders is a clinical challenge. Presenting features may be less well-developed than in an adult population. The mounting evidence that psychological and social treatments are most effective at this early stage of illness underlines the necessity for early diagnosis and referral for treatment.

Adolescent mental health disorders generally arise in a context of interpersonal and social problems. During assessment and treatment, consideration should be given to recent stresses arising from grief (e.g. death or illness in the family or among friends), conflict (e.g. victimisation by peers or arguments with parents), relationship breakdowns and problems with school work. Many young people, have long standing problems with parents, school and a lack of emotional and interpersonal skills, as well as having to deal with the developmental tasks of adolescence (e.g. difficulties in initiating social contact, dealing with new sexual feelings and negotiating greater independence within the family).

DEPRESSION, DELIBERATE SELF-HARM AND SUICIDE

Suicide is the second most common cause of death in 15–25 year olds in Australia, after motor vehicle accidents. Factors most commonly associated with completed suicide are a history of deliberate self-harm, major depression, substance abuse and antisocial behaviour.

About 1 in 200 young people present to emergency departments each year for deliberate acts of self-harm, typically in the form of an overdose. An even greater number do not present for medical care at all. In most instances, deliberate self-harm is not true suicidal behaviour with the intent of causing death. Most self-harm is associated with a degree of psychiatric disturbance. Key features of assessment of the potentially suicidal adolescent are shown in Table 12.3. Assessment of the act of self-harm should include:

- Attention to suicidal intent.
- Perceived lethality of the act.
- Actual harm incurred.
- Degree of planning.
- Actions taken by the patient after the event.

Assessment should also be made of any associated psychiatric disorders, and the level of social and interpersonal difficulties in the young person's life (see Table 12.3).

Depression is the most common major psychiatric disorder of young people. Symptoms are similar to those found in adults and typically include:

- Extended periods of low mood.
- Loss of pleasure in activities.
- Irritability.
- Fatigue.
- Somatic complaints.
- Social withdrawal.

Table 12.3 Assessment of suicide risk following an act of self-harm

Act itself	Impulsive or planned? Suicidal intent? Method and perceived lethality? Does life feel worthless or hopeless? Any acute precipitant? Actions post attempt (e.g. disclosure)?
Background	Stressors (family and peer relationships, school, sexuality) Recent suicidal ideation or attempts
Comorbidity	Depression Drug and alcohol use Anxiety disorders Personality disorders (disturbed past relationships and behaviours)

- Impaired concentration and deteriorating function at school.
- Early and mid insomnia.
- Suicidal ideation.

In most instances a young person will give a better account of these symptoms than parents or other informants. Assessment should include consideration of organic causes (e.g. recent steroid therapy, hypothyroidism, or substance abuse). Fluctuations in mood in response to a significant stressor may respond to short-term problem-solving strategies but evidence of significant lowering of mood lasting longer than 2 weeks requires specific treatment. This may include psychotherapy (cognitive behavioural and interpersonal psychotherapies have been shown to be effective) and/or antidepressant medication. Specific serotonin re-uptake inhibitors (SSRI) are often used as first-line antidepressants as they are usually well tolerated and are safe.

THE VIOLENT YOUNG PERSON AND EMERGENCY RESTRAINT

Physical restraint and emergency sedation should only be used when other reasonable methods of calming the patient down are unsuccessful. **If a patient who is acting out does not need acute medical or psychiatric care, they should be discharged from the hospital rather than restrained**.

When restraint is required a coordinated team approach is essential. Roles should be clearly defined and swift action taken swiftly. Unless contraindicated, sedation should usually accompany physical restraint.

Emergency restraint should be considered in any patient who requires urgent medical or psychiatric care with aggressive and combative behaviour, that is:

- Compromising the provision of urgent medical treatment (physical or psychiatric)
- Placing the patient at risk of self-harm.
- Placing staff at risk.

Alternative means of calming the patient include prevention of a crisis by anticipating and identifying irritable behaviour (consider the patient's past history), early involvement of mental health services, provision of a safe 'containing' environment, listening and talking, and possibly planning 'collaborative' sedation (e.g. oral medication).

Contra indications to physical restraint and emergency sedation

- Safe containment possible via alternative means.
- Inadequate personnel/setting/equipment.
- Situation judged as too dangerous e.g. patient has a weapon (call police if concerned regarding the safety of staff or others).
- Known adverse reaction to drugs usually used (e.g. neuroleptic malignant syndrome).

Procedure

- Establish roles, including defining person in charge (usually attending doctor).
- Assemble team. Person in charge to assemble team of 7 people.
- Draw up drugs. **Drugs of preference are midazolam 5 mg, and haloperidol 5 mg (draw up together).** Ensure benztropine is available.
- Secure the patient quickly and calmly. At least 5 people are required – one for the head and one for each limb (assign roles before approaching the patient). The patient should be prone, with hands and feet held flexed behind back.
- **Administer midazolam 5 mg (onset rapid) and haloperidol 5 mg (onset 15–20 minutes) by intramuscular injection into lateral thigh.** Beware the risk of needle-stick injury. Further titrated doses of 0.1 mg/kg may be required (preferably i.v.).

- Sedated patients must have continuous O_2 saturation monitoring. They must have a nurse present continuously, with close observation of conscious state, respiration, HR, BP and temperature.
- Explain the procedure to the parents/carers if possible.
- Following restraint, the patient must have a complete medical and mental health assessment to guide subsequent management. In some cases certification and transfer to an in-patient mental health facility may be required (Section 9 of the Mental Health Act 1986). Consider the need for on going physical restraint and/or for on going sedation.
- Document fully.

Complications of emergency sedation include anaphylactic reactions, respiratory depression, hypotension, tachycardia and extrapyramidal reactions. Dystonia may occur with major tranquillizers, particularly as the benzodiazepine is wearing off (treat with benztropine (0.02 mg/kg i.v. or i.m.) or repeated small doses of diazepam).

CHRONIC FATIGUE SYNDROME

Chronic Fatigue Syndrome (CFS) is characterised by unexplained, prolonged (>3 months) and disabling fatigue along with constitutional and neuropsychological symptoms. It occurs in children but is more common in adolescents. Most patients have a history of suspected or confirmed viral illness. Diagnosis is clinical. Differential diagnoses include connective tissue diseases, inflammatory bowel disease, coeliac disease and gastrointestinal infection.

History

Symptoms include:

- Prolonged fatigue.
- Increased need for sleep.
- Pain: headaches, myalgias, abdominal pain.
- Nausea.
- Depressive symptoms.
- Loss of concentration
- Difficulty with balance.

Examination

- Usually normal.

Investigations

- Full blood examination, ESR, U & E, creatinine, LFT, TFT and urinalysis.

Management

- Management must be developed with patient, family and local doctor in a team approach.
- An individual management plan should focus on addressing the psychosocial features and impact of the illness.
- Aim for reintegration to normal life. Plan balanced activities and encourage social contact.
- Manage focal problems (e.g. sleep difficulties) symptomatically.

Prognosis

- Most recover with normal function, however, it often takes several (e.g. 2–4) years.
- A small number remain unwell.

EATING DISORDERS

Anorexia nervosa and bulimia nervosa typically arise in the early to mid-teens. The commonest eating disorders to present clinically are subsyndromal forms where the mental state is similar but the clinical features have not developed. Such disorders may pass spontaneously but should be treated seriously. Where symptoms persist beyond 3 months, referral for more specific treatment is warranted.

Adolescent dieting is the usual forerunner of an eating disorder. Although most dieters do not go on to develop an eating disorder, pre-occupation with dieting that leads to the avoidance of other activities (e.g. not going out with friends because of feeling fat) deserves attention.

Anorexia nervosa

Diagnostic criteria of anorexia nervosa are:

- Refusal to maintain body weight over a minimum normal weight for age and height.

- Intense fear of gaining weight or becoming fat, even though underweight.
- Distorted body image.
- Amenorrhoea.

Severity indices of post-pubertal anorexia nervosa include the current weight, rate of weight loss, methods employed (e.g. abstinence, self-induced vomiting, purging and exercise) and any associated depression or other mental health disturbance (e.g. obsessional neuroses). Consideration should be given to the exclusion of other primary psychiatric disorders (e.g. major depression or obsessional neurosis) and physical disorders (e.g. thyrotoxicosis and malabsorption).

Multidisciplinary outpatient care is the basis of most specialist centres where there is commonly input from medical, nutritional and mental health professionals. The earlier the onset of the disorder (e.g. peripubertal) the greater the concern for long term physical complications such as growth retardation and reduced bone mineral density.

Hospital admission is indicated in adolescents where there is evidence of physiological compromise, such as bradycardia and hypotension, rather than by the extent of weight loss per se. Admission is also indicated when outpatient treatment has failed.

Refeeding is the mainstay of most acute admissions. Nasogastric feeding is commonly used in inpatient settings to achieve physiological stability. Refeeding can be associated with significant metabolic and physiological consequences. Refeeding syndrome most commonly occurs with parenteral feeding after prolonged starvation, but it is also seen with NGT feeding and oral refeeding. Refeeding syndrome can be fatal. Close attention must be paid to electrolyte and cardiovascular status, especially in the first week of refeeding (see Nutrition, chapter 6).

Bulimia nervosa

Bulimia nervosa is characterised by frequent loss of control of eating (bingeing), self-induced vomiting and fear of fatness.

Intercurrent depression and difficulties with impulse control in other areas (e.g. alcohol use, sexual behaviour and deliberate risk-taking) are common. The psychosocial context in which bulimia arises is often similar to that found in depression, but an antecedent history of dieting is usually evident.

Treatment is usually on an outpatient basis and focal psychotherapies such as cognitive-behavioural therapy are effective both in individual and group treatment settings. Antidepressant medications, such as SSRI, are indicated when severe depressive symptoms are evident, as well as to prevent relapse.

CHAPTER 13
CHILD PSYCHIATRY

Maria McCarthy
Campbell Paul

Mental health is defined as a state of emotional and social wellbeing in which the individual realises their own abilities, can cope with the normal stresses of life, can work productively or fruitfully, and is able to make a contribution to their community (WHO 1999).

One in five people will experience mental health problems in their lifetime. Approximately 14% of children and adolescents in Australia have a mental health problem. The majority of childhood mental health problems are managed by general practitioners, paediatricians, schools and community services. Only a small percentage of children and young people are treated in specialist mental health services/facilities. It is important that other health professionals working with children and adolescents are able to undertake some mental health and developmental assessment. Medical practitioners are often well placed to identify mental health problems and facilitate appropriate management. It is important to remember that the child's family is the most powerful therapeutic force in the child's life.

Key skills required by medical practitioners

- To be able to listen and engage children and young people and their families around emotional/psychological issues in a comfortable manner.
- To be able to manage more common or 'straightforward' mental health problems either independently or with consultation from appropriate health professionals.
- To be able to identify when mental health issues are more serious, complex and/or chronic and to facilitate referral to appropriate mental health services.

APPROACH TO MENTAL HEALTH PROBLEMS

Interview and assessment

Each interview of a child and family should provide an assessment and evaluation of the child (including their strengths and difficulties) and the family's contribution to these difficulties and capacity to help overcome them. Parents are respectful of the clinician who tries to understand their child directly.

- See the child with their parents and siblings.
- Aim to speak with the child directly and engage other family members. This enables a therapeutic relationship to be established with the child.
- Assess the presenting problem, attending to the language and narrative used by the child and family.
- Observe the verbal and non-verbal interaction between the child and each parent and siblings if present.
- Aim to make a formulation of the problems based on the initial assessment, decide on an initial management plan and whether to refer for specialist mental health assessment.

A clinician needs to be able to answer the following questions:

- What is the problem now?
- How did this problem come about?
- What have been the precipitating, perpetuating, predisposing and protective factors?
- What is this child usually like?
- How does this child's mind work now?

History

- The presenting problem – how long has it been present, severity, exacerbating or relieving factors?
- What is the parent's theory about this problem?
- Family medical and psychiatric history.
- Details of the experience of pregnancy, delivery and the child's early months.
- Ask about:
  - The child's feeding, sleeping and toileting habits where appropriate.
  - Friendships, relationships within the family.

- Possible traumatic events at home, at school, directly experienced or witnessed. Consider physical or sexual abuse and ask sensitive questions directly where appropriate.

The child and family should come to feel the problem is taken seriously and understood by the clinician.

Mental State Examination

Table 13.1 Mental state examination

Observe the child's play and behaviour before, during and after the formal consultation. The young child communicates through play. Access to simple toys, such as a doll, a ball or pencil and paper will allow the clinician access to the child's level of self-organisation as well as their inner world of imagination and thought. Ask the child to draw a person or a house. Interview with the parents.

1. General appearance and behaviour
- Observe the child's appearance, demeanour, gait, motor activity and relationship with examiner.
- What is the child's apparent mood?
- Do they seem sad, happy, fearful, perplexed, angry, agitated?

2. Speech
- How does the child communicate?
- Are the speech quality, rate, articulation and flow appropriate for the developmental level?

3. Affect
- Observe the quality, range, communicability, modulation and appropriateness of affect.

4. Thought
- Stream: Are there major interruptions to flow of thinking?
- Content: What is the child thinking about?
- Do they seem preoccupied by inner thoughts, obsessional ideas, delusions, fears or have suicidal ideation?

5. Perception
- Do they have hallucinations?

6. Cognition
- Conscious state & orientation: Does the child know where they are, what time it is, who they are and who is around them?
- Concentration: Is the child able to concentrate on developmentally appropriate tasks?

Continued overleaf

Table 13.1 Mental state examination *cont'd*

- Memory: How well do they remember things of the recent past and more distant past?
- Do they understand questions posed to them and can they think in a problem solving way?

7. Insight

- Does the child seem aware of their illness?

Much of this information can be obtained from the child in a non-threatening way if the clinician asks them directly in detail about things such as their family, home, school, address, telephone number and their immediate context.

Principles of intervention

At the conclusion of the therapeutic assessment the clinician will have formed a provisional diagnosis and assessed the severity and urgency of the presenting problem.

Further options for intervention:

- Explain and reassure if the problem is transient or minor. Suggest further contact with general practitioner or community counsellor.
- Further mental health intervention through paediatric or primary care service. Offer follow up appointment or telephone contact.
- For further input seek telephone consultation with regional mental health service or colleague.

Available mental health interventions:

- Brief therapies – family or individual.
- Cognitive behavioural therapies.
- Psychodynamic psychotherapy.
- Family therapy.
- Supportive intervention for the child and family (clinic, school or home based).
- Psychopharmacology.

When and how to make a mental health referral

The manner and process in which a referral to mental health is discussed with a child and family can influence their engagement with mental health services, their expectations and understandings and even treatment outcome.

- Avoid coercion (unless the patient is at serious risk to themselves or others).
- Ensure an open and honest discussion about why you believe a mental health referral is indicated/helpful.
- Explain what the child and family should expect from an initial mental health consultation in clear and simple language.
- Examine your own responses/feelings about mental health and ensure you do not impose these views on a child or family, e.g. being sceptical about the usefulness of mental health services but referring anyway, or presenting the mental health clinician as the potential cure to all current and future difficulties!
- Where appropriate, continue your involvement and interest in a child and family.

Some children and/or families will readily accept a mental health referral whereas others will be much more wary or even openly opposed to a referral. In the latter scenario, referral should be considered as a process that may be discussed with a child and or family over a period of weeks or even months before the referral can be made.

Stigma around mental health continues to be a powerful influence. Families may interpret the suggestion of a referral as an indication that you think they are 'mad' or 'crazy'; beliefs that may not necessarily be overt. Families may need reassurance.

Talking to children and families in more everyday language, e.g. talking about the *stress* they are dealing with or the *worries* they seem to have or about how *down* they have been feeling, may facilitate their engagement with the concept of referral. For the hospitalised child or child who has been the subject of significant medical interventions, it may be important to reassure the child that the mental health clinician is a talking person, not someone who gives needles etc. Terms such as *'the talking doctor'* can be useful for the younger hospitalised child. Similarly, talking to parents about your mental health *colleagues* as you would talk about other medical/surgical referrals can help reduce stigma or concerns they may have.

INFANT MENTAL HEALTH

Infant mental health is an area of study and clinical work aimed at understanding the psychological and emotional development of infants from birth to 3 years and the particular difficulties that they and their families might face.

Babies come into the world with a range of capacities and vulnerabilities and, together with their parents, negotiate the next months and years. This process of attachment, growth and development may be challenged by a range of experiences that stress or interrupt this course, e.g. traumatic events, developmental concerns, hospitalisation of the infant or parent, prematurity, illness or disability, an experience of loss, changing family circumstances or postnatal depression.

Referral to an appropriate mental health clinician may be considered for:

- Persistent crying, irritability or 'colic'.
- Gaze avoidance.
- Bonding difficulties.
- Failure to thrive.
- Persistent feeding or sleeping difficulties.
- Persistent behavioural symptoms e.g. tantrums, nightmares, aggression.
- Family relationship problems.
- Infants with chronic ill health.
- Premature babies and their families.

ANXIETY DISORDERS

Anxiety is a normal emotion and children commonly experience anxiety as part of the normal developmental process.

- In infants and toddlers, anxiety often manifests at separation from parents/caregivers.
- Pre-schoolers and school-aged children may be fearful of the dark or specific situations.
- Older children and adolescents may exhibit performance anxiety associated with exams, social situations etc. Anxiety is most

Table 13.2 Common symptoms of anxiety disorders

Symptoms
Distress and agitation when separated from parents and home
School refusal
Pervasive worry and fearfulness
Restlessness and irritability
Timidity, shyness, social withdrawal
Terror of an object (e.g. dog)
Associated headache, stomach pain
Restless sleep and nightmares
Poor concentration, distractibility and learning problems
Reliving stressful event in repetitive play
Family factors
Parental anxiety, overprotection, separation difficulties
Parental (maternal) depression and agoraphobia
Family stress: marital conflict, parental illness, child abuse
Family history of anxiety

Reproduced with permission from Tonge B. Medical Journal of Australia, 2001; 63–70

commonly experienced at times of transition e.g. moving house, starting/changing schools.

Anxiety disorders may be characterised by:

- Persistent fears and/or developmentally inappropriate fears.
- Irrational worries or avoidance of specific situations that trigger anxiety.
- Impaired ability to perform normal activities for example; inability to go to school.

Management

- Obtain a thorough account of the problem including anxiety symptoms, the length of time the anxiety has persisted, and the degree to which the child is impaired in their day-to-day activities and relationships.
- If symptoms are relatively mild, explore behavioural and/or family support interventions with the child and family and review.
- Specific fears (e.g. phobias) and more severe or generalised anxiety disorders will require specialist intervention. In this situation, referral to local mental health services is appropriate.

SCHOOL REFUSAL

School refusal is often an indicator of separation difficulties with the child frightened to leave their parent or home. Children refusing to attend school will often present with somatic complaints such as abdominal pain.

It is important to ascertain the basis of the child's anxiety, which may be related to factors at home such as a parent's physical or mental health, or parent relationship difficulties, or factors at school such as bullying, peer relationship difficulties or anxiety related to academic performance.

Management

- Conduct a physical examination if the child presents with somatic symptoms.
- Assess the source of the anxiety and consider whether further management is required, e.g. family therapy, school based services such as school counsellor etc.
- Return to school is a high priority. If necessary this can be graduated with the child increasing their time at school over a short period of time.

OBSESSIVE COMPULSIVE DISORDER

Obsessive-compulsive disorder is one of the more severe forms of childhood anxiety disorders. Obsessive-compulsive disorder is relatively rare (affecting 1–2% of children and adolescents), although obsessive-compulsive behaviour can be associated with childhood anxiety and depressive disorders and pervasive developmental disorders. Symptoms include intrusive thoughts, rituals, checking and compulsive behaviour.

Management

- Provide support and explanation to the child and family.
- Refer for assessment and management by a specialist.
- Cognitive-behavioural therapy alone or in combination with medication can be very effective treatment.

POST TRAUMATIC STRESS DISORDER

It is now widely recognised that trauma can contribute to the development of mental health difficulties in children and young people and can manifest in the syndrome recognised as Post Traumatic Stress Disorder (PTSD).

In relation to childhood trauma the following is known:

- Children show a variable response to trauma.
- PTSD is not an *expected* outcome of trauma.
- The development of PTSD is not strongly correlated to the severity of the trauma.
- The cluster of symptoms characteristic of PTSD are intrusion, avoidance and arousal.
- PTSD criteria are not particularly sensitive to trauma effects in very young children.

Management

For the diagnosis of PTSD to be met, the traumatic event must *precede* the symptoms and symptoms must be present for at least 1 month. Other mental health disorders can occur co-morbidly with PTSD. Furthermore,

Table 13.3 Common symptoms of post traumatic stress disorder

Symptoms
Intrusive thoughts and 're-experiencing' of the event(s) – this may be evidenced through play, enactment or drawings
Fear of the dark
Nightmares
Difficulty getting to sleep and/or nocturnal waking
Separation anxiety
Generalised anxiety or fears
Developmental regression e.g. toilet training, language skills
Social withdrawal
Irritability
Aggressive behaviour
Attention and concentration difficulties
Memory problems
Heightened sensitivity to other traumatic events

these presenting symptoms may be indicative of a different mental health problem such as anxiety disorder or depressive disorder rather than PTSD. When symptoms have persisted beyond a period for a few days or weeks, refer to mental health services for further assessment, diagnosis and treatment.

DEPRESSION

Depression occurs in childhood although it is probably relatively underdiagnosed. Symptoms can vary according to the age and developmental stage of the child. Infants and younger children may present with irritable mood, failure to gain weight and lack of enjoyment in play and other activities. Depression becomes increasingly common in adolescence (almost a quarter of adolescents will experience a major depressive episode) and is associated with an increased risk of suicide (see Adolescent health, chapter 12). Co-morbidities are common and may include anxiety disorder, conduct disorder or attention deficit hyperactivity disorder.

Table 13.4 Common symptoms of childhood depression

Symptoms
Persistent depressed mood, unhappiness and irritability
Loss of interest in play and friends
Loss of energy and concentration
Deterioration in schoolwork
Loss of appetite and no weight gain
Disturbed sleep
Thoughts of worthlessness and suicide (suicide attempts are rare before age 10 years, then increase)
Somatic complaints (headaches, abdominal pain)
Comorbid anxiety, conduct disorder, attention deficit hyperactivity disorder, eating disorders or substance abuse
Family Factors
Family stress (ill or deceased parent, family conflict, parental separation)
Repeated experience of failure or criticism
Family history of depression

Reproduced with permission from Tonge B. Medical Journal of Australia, 2001; 63–70

Management

- Recognition of depressive symptoms in childhood is very important. Untreated childhood depression increases an individual's risk for depression in adulthood. Additionally, depression in childhood and, particularly in adolescence, increases the risk of suicide and self-harming behaviours.
- Referral to local mental health services for further assessment and treatment is generally required.
- General practitioners can play an important role in providing ongoing support and counselling to the child and/or family.

SUICIDE RISK AND SELF HARM

(See Adolescent health, chapter 12)

PSYCHOSOMATIC PROBLEMS

Somatic responses to stressful situations are a well-known phenomenon (e.g. the experience of sweating during a job interview, or diarrhoea prior to taking an exam). Somatic complaints in children are also believed to be relatively common and appear as physical sensations related to affective distress.

Psychosomatic or somatoform disorders refer to the presence of physical symptoms suggesting an underlying medical condition without such a condition being found, or where a medical problem cannot adequately account for the level of functional impairment.

Common symptoms include:

- Headache.
- Abdominal pain.
- Limb pain.
- Fatigue.
- Pain/soreness.
- Disturbance of vision.
- Symptoms suggestive of neurological disorders.

Conversion disorder may present with dramatic symptoms such as:

- Gait disturbance
- Paraesthesia
- Paralysis
- Pseudoseizures

In this situation the onset of the symptom is closely associated to a psychological stressor. Conversion disorders are generally believed to be relatively short lived and are often alleviated with appropriate identification and management of a stressor(s) and in some instances, symptomatic treatment of the physical problem.

Somatisation disorders may present in children whose families have a history of illnesses or psychosomatic disorders. Such patterns may be evident at a multi-generational level where physical symptoms appear to be the 'currency' by which affective states are communicated and responded to. Possible family relationship difficulties (including sexual abuse) should be considered as part of taking a thorough history.

MENTAL HEALTH PROBLEMS ASSOCIATED WITH CHRONIC ILLNESS

Children and adolescents with chronic illnesses such as asthma and diabetes may present with exacerbations of their physical symptoms that relate to their affective state. Such responses may be related to a precipitating stressor or may reflect the child's changing responses to their illness. Increased cognitive understanding of the illness and its implications and developmental changes will influence a child's responses to their medical condition. Children and adolescents may experience anger, resent the limitations their condition imposes and may be particularly sensitive to being different from their peers. Additionally responses of parents (e.g. over or under protective responses) may contribute to adjustment difficulties. Along with somatisation, other difficulties may emerge such as non-compliance with treatment and family relationship problems.

Management

Management will depend on the nature, severity and duration of the problem. Some general principles are:

- It is important to recognise the child's physical symptoms as genuine and distressing.
- Appropriate medical examination/investigation is required. Hospital admission may be required for appropriate medical and mental health assessment.
- Early introduction of the concept of possible psychological factors and mind-body interactions is useful. This may allow the child and family to begin to think and talk about possible psychological stressors and may reduce resistance to mental health referral.
- Symptomatic treatment e.g. heat packs, relaxation exercises, physiotherapy, mild analgesia etc. may be appropriate along with supportive counselling and/or mental health referral.
- Avoid medical over-investigation based upon the family's coercion or unwillingness to consider psychological factors.
- It is important that the child and family do not feel they have 'wasted your time' if there is no evident medical problem. Maintain an interest in the child and family with a review appointment or follow-up telephone enquiry as appropriate.

FAMILY RELATIONSHIP DIFFICULTIES

Almost invariably, a family sensitive approach is crucial to the assessment and management of childhood mental health issues. Behavioural and/or emotional difficulties in a child can occur in the context of chronic family dysfunction. Conversely, such difficulties can arise in the context of well functioning families where issues relating to the child's temperament, personality or precipitating stressors may lead to behavioural/emotional difficulties for the child and/or parent child relationship difficulties. When a child is presenting with behavioural and/or emotional difficulties, assessment should include gathering an understanding of the family situation including:

- Family constellation.
- Quality of family relationships.
- Early attachment relationships.
- History of significant losses, stressors, precipitating factors.
- Social/family support networks.
- Identifiable 'risk' factors such as poverty, illnesses, absent social supports.

Keep in mind that children can be symptom-bearers for family and/or couple relationship difficulties. In such instances, treatment of the presenting symptom is unlikely to be successful in the long term without appropriate family and/or couple counselling.

When working with families:

- Establish a practice of conducting at least one family interview when dealing with a child with significant behavioural or emotional difficulties.
- Interview all family members (including siblings, who are often insightful commentators on family life) and provide an empathic response to each member's point of view. In the case of young children observing and commenting upon play themes is useful.
- Do not assume that different family members agree on what is the presenting problem. It is often useful to ask family members to rank their concerns such as:
  - *What is the problem you are most worried about today?*
  - *What is the number one worry you have at the moment . . . number 2 . . . number 3?*
  - *Who in the family is most worried about this problem? Who is the least worried?*
- If family members are not present seek further understanding by questions such as:
  - *If your husband were here today what would he say about this problem?*
  - *Who else in the family has noticed the changes you have described today?*
- Encouraging families to find solutions to their difficulties is more likely to provide long-term change. This may involve helping families identify negative or unhelpful patterns of interaction, helping families identify strengths and resilience and noting small changes/improvements.

OPPOSITIONAL BEHAVIOUR

(See Behavioural, developmental and sleep problems, chapter 10)

GRIEF AND LOSS

Experiences of grief and loss are inevitable. Where losses are severe or traumatic or where a child has pre-existing vulnerabilities, these experiences can contribute to mental health difficulties or result in complicated grief reactions. Children may harbour beliefs that they somehow caused a loved one's death or illness. Bereaved children may feel different from other children or have difficulty managing the reactions of their peers.

In most instances, the bereaved child can be supported through available family, school, community and/or religious supports. Family-based counselling/therapy can be a very helpful way in which a child's difficulties can be addressed in the context of other family members' grief and may feel less blaming for the child.

Grief and loss experiences for children occur in situations other than bereavement (e.g. chronic illness, refugees or a parent with a mental illness). A very common and significant loss is experienced by children when parents divorce. Grief associated with this situation can be very complicated and often remains unacknowledged by significant adults. Children may experience feelings of guilt and self blame, harbour fantasies of a parental reunion, struggle with divided loyalties and feel anxious about their own future relationships. Feelings of anger, rejection and sadness may lead to behavioural or emotional manifestations of their grief.

Management

- Acknowledge the child's loss in an empathic and appropriate manner; this can be helpful even when a loss is not recent.
- Where a grieving child presents with behavioural or emotional difficulties, gently probing their beliefs about why the loss occurred can be helpful to understanding the child's predicament. For example:
  - *Sometimes when I see children who have lost their (mum/brother etc.) they feel like it's their fault that they died or got sick. Does it ever feel like that for you?*
  - *How do you imagine your life would be different if your mum and dad were still together?*
  - *Why do you think people get (cancer etc.)?*

- Assist the family in gaining access to appropriate support and counselling.
- Seek further specialist mental health services when a child continues to exhibit extreme distress or prolonged behavioural or emotional difficulties.

EATING DISORDERS

(See Adolescent health, chapter 12)

PSYCHOSIS

Psychosis is a general term for states in which mental function is grossly impaired, so that reality testing and insight are lacking, and delusions, hallucinations, incoherence, thought disorder or disorganised behaviour may be apparent.

In the case of 'organic' psychosis there may also be a clouding of consciousness, confusion and disorientation, as well as perceptual disturbances. Short-term memory impairment is common in organic brain syndromes.

Anticholinergics, anticonvulsants, antidepressants, antimalarials and benzodiazepines have been associated with psychotic reactions in young people, as have substances of abuse (amphetamines, cocaine, marijuana, opiates and hallucinogens). Organic brain syndromes may follow even minor head injury.

Adolescents may occasionally present in an acutely psychotic state with no prior history of drug ingestion or head injury. In this case the possibility of a 'functional' psychosis, schizophrenia or bipolar disorder should be considered. The latter often presents with an elated mood, grandiose ideas, increased energy and reduced sleep requirements.

Management

- In most instances, children presenting with such symptoms require admission for a full psychiatric and medical assessment.

PRINCIPLES OF PSYCHOTROPIC MEDICATIONS

- Limited application in childhood.
- With well-verified attention deficit hyperactivity disorder, methylphenidate or dexamphetamine can enhance concentration and attention and reduce morbidity (see Behavioural, development and sleep problems, chapter 10).
- With severe depression, selective serotonin uptake inhibiters such as fluoxetine may be helpful on a case-by-case basis.
- With severe anxiety disorders, imipramine may be helpful. Benzodiazepines may produce paradoxical inhibition in childhood and have no proven role in anxiety or depressive disorders in children.
- With psychosis in adolescents, recent trials have demonstrated the value of early treatment with newer anti-psychotic medication in collaboration with specialised youth psychiatric service.

CHAPTER 14
CHILD ABUSE

Anne Smith
Chris Sanderson

Health care providers should consider the possibility of child abuse whenever they evaluate and treat an injured child. Doctors are encouraged to access advice and opinion from local medical professionals with expertise in this area. As the body of knowledge related to child abuse increases and as the demand for expert court testimony also increases there is an additional expectation that doctors will provide evidence and opinion that will withstand the rigours of cross examination in court.

DEFINITIONS

Child abuse

Child abuse may be defined as the harming (physically, emotionally or sexually), ill treatment, abuse, neglect, or deprivation of any child or young person.

Child physical abuse

Child physical abuse is physical trauma inflicted on a child. Objective evidence of this violence may include bruising, burns and scalds, head injuries, fractures, intra-abdominal and intrathoracic trauma, suffocation and drowning. Impact, penetration, heat, a caustic substance, a chemical or a drug may cause the injury. The definition also includes physical harm sustained as a result of Munchausen syndrome by proxy.

Child neglect

Child neglect is the failure of caregivers to adequately provide for and safeguard the health, safety and wellbeing of the child. Neglect is defined as any situation in which the basic needs of children are not met with respect to nutrition, hygiene, clothing and shelter. It also comprises failure to provide access to adequate medical care, mental health care and education.

Child sexual abuse

Child sexual abuse is the involvement of dependent, developmentally immature children and adolescents in sexual activities that they do not fully comprehend and to which they are unable to give consent.

Psychological maltreatment

Psychological maltreatment of children and young people consists of acts that are judged on the basis of a combination of community standards and professional expertise to be psychologically damaging. Such acts are committed by individuals, singly or collectively, who by their characteristics (e.g. age, status, knowledge and organisational form) are in a position of differential power that renders a child vulnerable. Such acts damage, immediately or ultimately, the behavioural, cognitive, affective or physical functioning of the child. Examples of psychological maltreatment include acts of spurning (hostility, rejecting or degrading), terrorising, isolating, exploiting or corrupting and denying emotional responsiveness.

Signs of neglect and emotional abuse are often non-specific, but suspicion should be raised when infants, preschoolers or school age children behave in the following ways:

- They are persistently angry, socially avoidant, defiant, disobedient and overactive.
- They are anxiously attached, watchful of their patients, have a limited ability to enjoy things, or are intensely ambivalent to parents.
- They have low self-esteem, are depressed or unresponsive, have developmental and emotional retardation, poor social skills and over-inhibition.

Signs of sexual abuse are also usually non-specific, but may include the above and various behaviour problems (phobias, bad dreams, eating and sleeping disorders, depression, school problems or delinquency). There may be overt manifestations of sexual preoccupation, including precocious and inappropriate sexual activity, promiscuity and aggressive sexual behaviour.

Psychiatric consultation is often useful in conjunction with the involvement of local child protection services.

CHILD PHYSICAL ABUSE

In assessing and treating an injured child, there is a duty to exclude child abuse from the differential diagnosis. Most of the children examined will have injuries as a result of accidental childhood trauma. If the patterns of injury are familiar and the injuries are consistent with the alleged mechanisms of injury, then the child can be investigated and treated without mentioning the possibility of deliberately inflicted trauma.

Table 14.1 identifies aspects of history-taking, which might be alerts to the need for further investigation.

Aims of assessment

- Differentiate accidental from deliberately inflicted trauma.
- State an opinion about the likely cause of the child's injuries.
- Investigate and manage all medical aspects of the case.
- Take action to protect the child from additional harm. This usually involves working in partnership with police, protective workers and support agencies.
- Intervene to prevent re-injury to this child or another child in the family.

History

Professionals dealing with injured children must become familiar with the manifestations of accidental and inflicted trauma and take a thorough and detailed history of the alleged mechanism of injury:

- Determine when, where and how the injury occurred.
- Note who witnessed the injury.
- Note the child's developmental capabilities.

Examination

When an injury appears to be inflicted rather than accidental, it is important to obtain details of the child's past medical, social and family history.

A thorough physical examination must be performed. **A parent or legal guardian must give informed consent prior to the child's physical examination**. Record injuries on a body chart and use diagrams whenever possible. Accurate measurements are essential. Include details of the site, size, colour and shape of all injuries, and skin lesions (including injuries thought to result from accidental trauma).

Table 14.1 Aspects of history taking in the evaluation of an injured child

Alerts on History Taking	*Examples*
1. History of the alleged mechanism of injury seems unlikely given the child's developmental level.	A parental allegation that a 6 week-old baby rolled from a couch onto the carpet.
2. History of the alleged mechanism of injury seems unlikely.	A parental suggestion that a 17 month-old sibling could fracture a newborn baby's ribs, skull and femur. Alternative explanations for the infant's injuries are probable.
3. History is inconsistent.	A parent gives differing versions of the sequence of events prior to the child's presentation to hospital.
4. The history varies between historians.	The child's parents give different versions of their whereabouts for the time prior to the child's presentation to hospital and the disparity in their histories indicates at least one of the parents is offering information that is not factual.
5. The child implicates an adult as the cause of the injuries.	A child alleges '*Mummy's moke burn hot*' when you examine skin lesions suggestive of cigarette burns.
6. The injured child's parent seems to be hinting that they and/or their partner have been extremely stressed during recent days. First time parents with distressed infants are particularly vulnerable. Be sensitive to the needs of a parent with an injured child who might be seeking help to improve their parenting and avoid inflicting additional injuries. Ask specifically about shaking and 'rough handling' when assessing injured infants.	
7. The pattern of injury is not one usually associated with accidental trauma.	Abdominal wall bruising and bruising over the scapula in a toddler with no history of accidental trauma.
8. The pattern of injury is inconsistent with the explanation offered.	A parent suggests that an 18 month-old might have sustained contact burns when he accidentally bumped into a heater but the pattern of injury suggests a contact burn to the palm and dorsum of the hand with sparing of the digits.
9. The pattern of injury suggests deliberately inflicted trauma.	The presence of a large curved bruise on a baby's arm consistent with a bite mark with indentations from an adult's teeth.
10. One parent alleges that someone else injured their child.	

Look for:

- Skin injuries such as bruises, petechiae, lacerations abrasions, and puncture wounds. Note injuries that may be inflicted by a human hand (finger marks from a slap or fingertip bruising from a firm grip) or an instrument.
- Intra-oral injuries such as a torn frenulum, contused gums, dental trauma or petechiae on the soft palate.
- Nasal trauma such as a nasal septal haematoma.
- Ear trauma – remember to inspect behind the pinnae and examine both tympanic membranes.
- Eye trauma – examine for objective evidence of injury from the lids to the retinae.
- Internal injuries – injuries to internal organs in the thorax and abdomen.
- Genital trauma.

Investigations

- Consider clotting studies and a full-blood examination for children with bruising.
- X-ray sites of clinically suspected fracture(s).
- Bone scan if the child is less than 3 years and occult or healing fractures are suspected. (*Note*: a bone scan is not a sensitive tool for the detection of skull fractures, therefore perform a skull X-ray as well if skull fracture is considered.)
- A skeletal survey should be performed if a bone scan is not available for the child less than 3 years and an occult or healing fracture is suspected.
- Photography is a very important means of documenting injuries. Note the need for a colour wheel and a tape measure/ruler. Also note that photography augments a detailed written description of injuries.

Interviewing parents

- A non-judgemental, sensitive approach is essential.
- Ask open, non-directive questions. Use verbatim quotes whenever possible.

CHILD NEGLECT

Detail information related to the child's health, growth, nutrition, physical and emotional wellbeing.

Examination includes the nature and appropriateness of a child's clothing, cleanliness of the skin and nails, nutritional status, growth percentiles, evidence of infections and infestations, as well as evidence of other medical conditions.

Medical opinion should reflect the doctor's assessment of objective signs of physical neglect, as well as historical evidence of environmental neglect (e.g. if an infant is left unattended in the bath) or medical neglect (medical conditions not treated).

CHILD SEXUAL ABUSE

Aim for one examination by a suitably trained medical practitioner who has access to facilities for paediatric genital examination and photo documentation. This doctor should have expertise in the preparation of medical reports and presentation of evidence in court. All other medical practitioners are encouraged to seek advice from regional experts.

These guidelines are for the uncommon situation when the examination cannot be deferred and a clinician with expertise in the assessment of child sexual abuse is not available.

History

A full paediatric assessment is required. The evaluation should include:

- The nature of the sexual contact (digital, penile, vaginal, rectal, oral or a foreign object).
- The time and circumstances of the alleged abuse, whether ejaculation occurred and whether a condom was used.
- The identification of the alleged perpetrator(s).
- Genital complaints (pain, discharge or bleeding).

Examination

An examination should be performed as soon as possible after the alleged assault. Note signs of injury on general examination.

- Ask the child to indicate the exact sites on their body where there was contact with the offender.
- The external genitalia should be carefully examined for debris from the crime-scene and signs of injury.
- Girls may be examined in the frog-leg position using labial traction or labial separation techniques. Adequate visualisation of the posterior hymenal rim may be achieved with the girl in the knee-chest prone position.
- Boys may be examined in the supine position, flexing the boy's knees to visualise the anus.
- An otoscope provides light and magnification when a colposcope is not available. Many medical examination lights provide a source of magnification and are 'cold' to touch. Ensure the child is comfortable with the procedure and understands the equipment being used.
- Semen may fluoresce under ultraviolet light.
- Speculum examination is not usually required in prepubertal girls or adolescent girls who are not sexually active. Examination under anaesthetic should only be considered if the clinician suspects internal injuries that might require surgical repair.
- Collect the child's clothing (including underwear) for forensic evaluation. Collect forensic specimens. Seek advice if uncertain about what specimens to collect. Forensic swabs should be air-dried, labelled and handed to police. Document the chain of transmission of evidence, i.e. record the name of the person to whom the forensic specimens are handed and the time and date this occurs.
- Swabs and slides for microbiological tests should be performed as clinically indicated. Blood tests for hepatitis B and C, as well as screening tests for syphilis (VDRL) and HIV should be considered when the history raises concern about the transfer of body fluids. Note the need for repeat serology after 3 months. Consider urine Polymerase Chain Reaction (PCR) for identification of Chlamydia.

- Consider pregnancy prophylaxis if the child is within 72 h of sexual contact. Arrange for a follow-up pregnancy test (see Gynaecologic conditions, chapter 25).
- Consider STD prophylaxis with azithromycin.
- Arrange for follow-up tests for STD.
- All abused children and their parents should have access to appropriate counselling.

Management

- Multidisciplinary assessment of the child and their family is recommended for all children in whom child abuse is suspected.
- A child with moderate or severe injuries should be admitted to hospital for evaluation.
- Medical staff are expected to attend case conferences with police and protective workers in order to share information and plan intervention.
- Medical reports should be prepared by the senior medical staff responsible for the child's care. The report should use language appropriate for non-medical professionals. The report should be clear, concise and informative, including an opinion as to the possible causes of the injuries.
- Prior to appearing in court, medical staff are advised to consult with senior medical colleagues who are experienced in this field.

Tertiary referral centres

Most major metropolitan paediatric hospitals have established tertiary reference centres for the assessment and treatment of child abuse. Paediatricians and other medical professionals working in these centres provide expert advice in relation to the assessment of injuries and the management of suspected child abuse.

MANDATORY REPORTING

In most states of Australia, medical practitioners are legally required to notify the relevant statutory authorities about children who have experienced, or are likely to experience, child abuse. The wording of legislation varies between states/territories in Australia but the common theme is a legal requirement to notify local child protection agencies when child abuse is considered. Medical practitioners are encouraged to inform themselves of relevant legislation in their own state or territory.

Report writing

Senior medical staff should write (or supervise the preparation of) the medical report. This report will provide information to non-medical agencies. The report can form the basis of a statement, it will need to be signed and witnessed by the police at a later date. The statement can then form part of the evidence in bringing criminal charges to court. Subsequently, doctors may receive a subpoena (sometimes years later) to give evidence as a witness. It is very useful to have a clear report as a reminder of the case details. Doctors are also required to take the original notes (or hospital record) of the consultation to court and can be cross-examined about the details of this record. Ensure the original notes are clear and non-ambiguous. Use simple medical language in the report.

Remember that providing a medical report involves describing what was observed, which draws on the report writer's experience as adoctor with knowledge of anatomy, physiology, growth and development. However, doctors are not expected to be detectives. For example, they can offer a description of bruising and may be able to reach a conclusion about the likely mechanism of injury but should refrain from saying whom they believe did it and when.

Hints on format for report writing

Heading

Do not use any identifying patient details apart from name and date of birth. Do not include address. Confidentiality cannot be ensured of a report which may pass to legal and welfare systems. Even so, all reports should be headed 'confidential'.

Introduction

Document credentials clearly. This may include academic qualifications and year of graduation/conferring of degrees, relevant past experience and current position. State who was examined, when and where it took place and who else was present in the room, part or all of the time.

Consent

Record the name of the person giving consent for the medical evaluation and the preparation and release of the report.

Presenting history

- Circumstances – who referred the child, what information they provided e.g. *Senior Constable Jack Cracklaw requested a medical examination of child A following allegations of attempted digital vaginal penetration by person X, occurring two days prior.*
- History taken from child/adolescent e.g. *I obtained the following history from child B. Child B told me that 'person X touched, etc. Child B told me . . .*
- History taken from accompanying person e.g. *Child B's mother told me that 'I went into child B's bedroom and saw . . .'*

This style of narrative can seem repetitious but provides an unambiguous record and structured report (without winning a literary award). The medical report does not need to contain details of non-relevant medical history (though this should form part of the original history).

Physical examination

- General statement includes whether the child was cooperative, overview of level of function and growth parameters.
- General physical examination should mention relevant positive findings in detail, e.g. the following bruises were noted . . . A numbered list is useful in avoiding any ambiguity and helps divide those injuries for which there is an explanation from those where the mechanism remains unclear.
- Genital examination should be described separately when this is relevant. It is important to note the position of the child and the additional lighting and magnification that was used. It is stressed that experience is required in the interpretation of abnormal genital signs and that this examination should not be undertaken without full consideration of possible management options, including the need for collection of forensic specimens.

Investigations

- Investigations should be noted, with results and interpretation.

Conclusions and opinion

Keep concise. Try to answer the question that is being asked (e.g. the pattern, extent and distribution of bruising observed exceeds that likely to occur as a result of accidental childhood trauma).

Court appearances

Few doctors are familiar with the court system and are therefore uncertain about this foray into foreign territory. Some key points relevant to the process and giving evidence as a witness are as follows:

Process

- Swearing in (the oath).
- Evidence in chief – the prosecutor takes the doctor through their statement – non-leading questions.
- Cross examination – to test the evidence and raise doubts about the validity of the factual basis upon which an opinion has been expressed. To test whether there are alternative explanations and how firmly the doctor holds their view.
- Re-examination – to clarify any remaining points.

Table 14.2 Key points for court appearances

1. Address (and look at) the magistrate or jury rather than the cross-examining counsel.
2. Answer the question asked.
3. Beware of expressions of absolute certainty. Make concessions if and as required.
4. Be dispassionate and not combative or hostile.
5. Never try to be an advocate.
6. Prepare by talking with experienced colleagues.

CHAPTER 15
THE DEATH OF A CHILD

Peter McDougall
Jenny Hynson
John Rogers

The death of a child causes an intense grieving process in surviving family members that may last for years. For the family's future well-being it is very important that the health-care team ensures that the processes surrounding death are carried out in a sensitive and caring manner. The purpose of this chapter is to provide some practical guidelines.

BEFORE DEATH

Often the death of a child can be anticipated. Although hospital admission is frequently necessary, most children and families will wish to spend as much time at home as possible. With appropriate planning and support, the majority of symptoms can be controlled effectively at home. Domiciliary medical care can be provided by the general practitioner in consultation with hospital staff. Palliative care agencies can provide specialised nursing care as well as a range of other services. While home care offers many advantages to the family, it is not without difficulties and parents are subject to physical, emotional and financial stress. Readmission to hospital or hospice should be easily and readily available. A letter detailing the child's condition, plans in case of sudden deterioration and people to contact will facilitate appropriate care in an emergency.

Giving bad news to families: the interview in a hospital setting

The way in which difficult information is communicated sets the stage for the working relationship between staff and family. Staff need to be aware of how their own feelings of anxiety, sadness and impotence may influence this process. Most families appreciate honest information given in an empathic way and tempered with a sense of hope. Realistic hope may be offered in terms of ongoing support, attention to symptoms and help to maximise the child's quality of life.

Personnel

The consistency of the health-care team in a child's final illness is essential. Medical interviews with families, in hospital, should be led by a senior doctor together with a junior doctor, nurse, social worker or member of the clergy. The presence of more than two of these people at an interview may be difficult for the family. Other health-care team members, especially the family doctor, community nurse and others outside the hospital, must be closely informed.

Comfort

Choose a physically comfortable location where interruptions can be avoided. The open ward or corridor are not the places for interviews. Whenever possible divert phones and have someone answer pagers. Try and allow plenty of time for the discussion.

Giving clear and simple information

- Begin by asking the family to give their understanding of the situation.
- The prognosis is usually best given first.
- Give an explanation of the disease process.
- Try and determine what it is the family wish to know.
- Avoid the use of unexplained medical jargon.
- Avoid information overload. There is time to deal with complex medical issues at later interviews.
- Avoid ambiguous phrases such as 'we might lose the battle' or 'he's passed away'. The words death, die or dying should be used.
- Allow expression of emotion.
- Offer to help the parents tell important others such as grand-parents and siblings.
- Initial shock may render parents unable to process detailed information so multiple opportunities for discussion should be provided.

Respect silences

When bad news is delivered it is best to remain silent until the parent responds. This sometimes takes minutes and can be very uncomfortable. These are important moments; they should not be interrupted.

Responsibilities of the accompanying members of the health-care team

At a medical interview, the accompanying members of the health-care team need to be sensitive to the parents' needs and to watch for misunderstandings. If they do not understand the medical message, it is unlikely that the parents will. At an appropriate time, the accompanying team member may ask the doctor to clarify some of the explanations given, but it is important not to interrupt a train of conversation or the silences that occur.

The senior doctor will, when appropriate, inform the family that all possible reasonable measures were taken to preserve their child's life. It is not necessary to repeat this message.

Interpreters

The availability of trained interpreters for people with a language other than English is essential. Do not use other family members or friends as interpreters.

Adequate relief of pain and distress of the child

It is important to actively ask about symptoms and consider potential contributing factors. Fatigue, for example, may be an expected part of terminal illness but it may also be due to factors such as anaemia and depression, which may be amenable to treatment.

Many parenteral medications (e.g. morphine, midazolam, haloperidol) may be successfully administered subcutaneously rather than intravenously and this offers many advantages to children needing palliative care. Community palliative care teams are able to help establish and monitor subcutaneous infusions if the family wish to be at home. Planning for symptom development and escalation is essential in this situation such that appropriate medications are available in the home for use in a crisis.

Communicating with children about death and dying

Parents may feel compelled to protect their children from 'bad news'. Children very often know a great deal about their disease and prognosis even when they have not been 'told'. They may not reveal what they know for fear of upsetting their parents who may falsely assume the child knows very little. Attempts to protect the child from accurate information may leave them feeling anxious and isolated as they sense distress in those around them and generate incorrect explanations for this such as '*I have been bad*' or '*Mummy and Daddy are angry with me*'. In general, it is best to encourage parents to be honest with children but information needs to be provided in a manner appropriate to their cognitive ability and developmental level. It may be helpful to anticipate questions and work with the family in planning responses.

It is important to listen to what the child is asking. The child who asks '*Am I going to die*' may actually not be concerned about dying as such but more about who will look after their parents, what their friends will think, or whether they will be in pain. A response such as '*What makes you ask me that*?' will provide further information upon which to base an answer.

Children may not wish to express themselves verbally or directly. Stories, artwork, music and play allow expression, build trust and facilitate communication.

Concepts of death

The child's concept of death becomes more complete with development and life experience. A number of variables influence this process so statistical averages serve as a guide only. Preschoolers typically view death as a reversible phenomenon (e.g. Snow White) and do not yet appreciate that people die as a consequence of age, illness or trauma. Magical thinking may lead them to believe they have caused death through bad behaviour or thoughts. By 7 years of age most children understand the concepts of irreversibility, causality, universality and cessation of bodily functions. Eight year olds also understand that dead people cannot feel pain or fear.

Siblings

Siblings of children with life-threatening conditions suffer not only the distress of having a brother or sister who is sick and dying but the isolation of having parents who are frequently either physically or psychologically unavailable to them. They may feel guilty that they do not have the condition, or may fear for their own health. They may resent the attention given to the sick child. They may feel they have somehow caused the illness. Siblings often wish not to burden their parents with their concerns and may express distress through developmental regression, school failure and physical symptoms.

Siblings benefit from inclusion in visits to the hospital and where possible, the care of the child. Staff can help by dedicating special time to children in which they may be given information and allowed to ask questions. Specific reassurance that the illness is not their fault may be needed, especially for siblings who have donated organs.

Preparations for death

Time and space

The health-care team must not overwhelm families. Parents need to spend time alone together and with their child, either in the hospital ward, a quiet room, at home, or at a children's hospice.

Arrangements

These may need to be made for baptism, religious advice, photographs, videos and other memories of the child.

Permission

Many families have specific needs and sometimes they are unsure whether these are permissible. If these issues can be anticipated and discussed, the family's wishes may be facilitated.

The child

The preparation for death is largely dependent on the age and particular illness of the child. The older child with a chronic illness is often aware of impending death, and the health-care team needs to be sensitive to the family's and child's wishes in the delivery of information.

The place of death

Decisions need to be made about where the child will die. This largely depends on the family, but it may be at home, in a hospice or the hospital. When appropriate, the child may be included in this planning.

Taking the body home

Some families wish to take their child home after death. This may be for a brief period or several days. This allows family and friends to say goodbye and can be very helpful in facilitating the grieving process. Funerals may then commence from home, or the family may be happy to allow an undertaker to remove the body earlier.

SUDDEN UNEXPECTED DEATH

The sudden death of a child from a wide variety of causes may occur in the community, the emergency department, or the ward of a hospital. Sudden infant death syndrome (SIDS – see p. 237) is particularly traumatic because it is the unexpected and unexplained death of a previously well infant. Although most of the preceding guidelines are applicable, there are some additional considerations regarding sudden death.

Resuscitation

This is frequently attempted either at home or in hospital. Some parents may wish to be present and they should not be excluded, but an experienced health professional needs to be available to provide them with support.

When it becomes clear that further resuscitative attempts are futile, it is the responsibility of the senior hospital doctor, general practitioner or senior ambulance officer to:

- Introduce themselves and explain their role in the child's care.
- Explain to the family what happened and what treatments were attempted (this may need to be repeated).
- Listen to the family's account of the events.
- Allow the family to express their emotions.
- Provide a non-judgemental understanding for any pre-existing difficult family relationships.
- Provide access to telephones for the notification of relatives.
- Facilitate the attendance of siblings and other important family members at the hospital.
- Encourage the family to see the child's body, say their farewells and take as much time as required.
- Ensure the family can reach home safely.

The family response

The immediate responses to sudden death vary from emotional withdrawal to outbursts of profound grief. Unexpected reactions commonly occur; for example, anger towards health-care providers who have done their best. Any response is appropriate, provided it does not threaten other people.

Brain death

Occasionally it becomes clear that a child who is dependent on mechanical ventilation is brain dead. In such a situation:

- The senior doctor needs to explain the meaning of brain death. Avoid the use of confusing words. The unambiguous message that death has occurred, together with the distinction between brain death and coma, needs to be clearly explained.
- It can be helpful to say that, although the child's body is still alive, the brain is dead and therefore the person is dead.
- It frequently helps parents to understand that their child has died by encouraging them to witness some or all of the brain death tests.
- The request for organ donation generally requires a separate interview, made in a positive manner, without coercion and with the clear acknowledgement of the family's vulnerability. Issues related to organ donation need to be discussed in order to receive an informed consent.

AFTER DEATH

The moment of death

Although usually anticipated, the moment of death is an important event and needs medical confirmation.

Mementos

Offer the family mementos such as photographs, locks of hair, hand and footprints together with personal belongings. Remember that:

- Black and white photographs of the dead child produce better looking pictures.
- If parents do not initially want mementos, these need to be stored as some families request them at a later date.

Viewing the body

This can be valuable for family members. It may eliminate the disbelief that death really occurred or, in the case of stillbirth, that the child was profoundly abnormal.

- A private area should be provided where the family can spend uninterrupted time with their child.

- Families should be offered the opportunity to wash and dress their child as a last act of love and care.

Autopsy

There has been a large amount of adverse publicity regarding the previous practice of organ retention without parental informed consent for autopsy procedures. Clear and accurate explanations need to be provided to families regarding the autopsy procedure and its purpose. Parents need to understand that the purpose of the autopsy is to seek full information regarding the cause of the child's death, the nature of the illness and the risk of recurrence of the illness in other family members or future children. If the healthcare professional is concerned about their ability to do this, support and assistance is available from senior colleagues. The autopsy may be limited to a system or area or be designated as a full autopsy. In particular, details need to be given regarding the removal, careful study and microscopic examination of tissues and organs and that some organs such as the heart and brain may need to be retained for a period of time before a proper examination can be performed. Informed consent needs to be given regarding the disposal of the removed organs, particularly if they are to be retained for teaching or training purposes. The parents should be informed that the autopsy will be performed on the next working day after the child's death and may interfere with the funeral arrangements depending on the choices they make when they consent to the procedure. The full results of the autopsy are usually not available until approximately six weeks after the autopsy procedure and this needs to be made clear to the family. Written consent forms need to be completed prior to the autopsy proceeding.

Many parents decide against an autopsy. They need to be reassured that a hospital autopsy will not be performed without their consent. However, there are occasions where a death needs to be reported to the coroner for further investigation and a coroner's autopsy can be performed without their consent.

Coroner's cases

A doctor must report a death to the coroner as soon as possible if:

- The cause of death is unable to be determined.
- The death appears to have been unexpected, unnatural or violent.
- The death appears to have resulted, directly or indirectly from accident or injury.

- The death occurs during an anaesthetic and is not due to natural cause.
- The deceased person was held in care immediately before death.
- The deceased person's identity is unknown.

The coroner then decides whether or not an autopsy is to be performed. Parents can request (on a special form) that the coroner does not direct that an autopsy be performed. In many cases where the cause of death is not in doubt (e.g. severe head injury), the coroner will respect the wish of the family.

Funeral options

These need to be discussed and the family assisted to make their own arrangements with a funeral director and religious personnel as appropriate. Encouragement is given to the family to involve siblings in this important ritual.

Sedation

Unless a parent has a well-defined psychiatric illness, sedation should be avoided for the acute stages of grief as it interferes with and suppresses the normal mourning process.

Breast-feeding

In the case of neonatal death or the death of an infant, advice needs to be given to the breast-feeding mother regarding suppression of lactation. Consultation with a specialist is recommended.

Surviving siblings

Children react in their own way to their sibling's death. They may blame themselves and will fear their own death. This fear is often unspoken. Parents often need help and support to understand the responses of their surviving children who need repeated reassurance.

Availability of the health-care team

The availability of the health-care team to the family after death needs to be assured and follow-up procedures arranged. It is usually important to both families and team members that farewells are made.

Notification of other professionals

Notify the health professionals who have been and who will continue to be involved with the family following the child's death, including the referring doctor or institution, the family's general practitioner and the maternal and child health nurse. This must be done as soon as possible.

Other families

The death of a child often affects the parents of other children in the hospital ward or local community. The acknowledgement of a child's death with these families is very important.

FOLLOW UP

Medical interview

Whether an autopsy is performed or not, it is essential that an appointment be made for the parents to see the child's treating doctor. Some parents are reluctant to attend, but most see the interview as a 'final farewell'. The discussion should include the autopsy results, the child's period of illness, future child bearing and issues related to bereavement. If a family is reluctant to attend this important interview, alternative interviews with other healthcare providers should be arranged.

If the child has died in hospital, the child's doctor should see the family for one or more follow-up visits, although they may not be the best person to conduct ongoing bereavement counselling. Families are more likely to attend if they receive both a written and verbal invitation and social workers may be helpful in facilitating attendance. Parents may find it helpful to discuss the reactions of siblings and ways in which to support them.

It is important the family be given information regarding potential sources of support and ongoing counselling if required.

Condolences

Communication such as a letter or card from the medical practitioner/ team involved with the care of the child can be important.

Ongoing support

Information needs to be provided to families about the support groups that are available both at the hospital and in the community. If someone is struggling more than expected, formal referral for psychotherapy should be considered. Medication is not a solution for grief.

SUDDEN INFANT DEATH SYNDROME

Sudden infant death syndrome (SIDS) is the sudden death of any infant or young child that is unexplained by history and in which a thorough post-mortem evaluation fails to demonstrate an adequate cause of death.

Epidemiology

Until 1990, about 550 babies a year died of SIDS in Australia, approximately 140 of these in Victoria, which correlated with the national and international average of 2 SIDS cases per 1000 live births. Following the 'Reducing the Risks' campaign initiated in 1990, the rate in Victoria has steadily fallen to 0.55 per 1000 live births in 1999. A drop in incidence has also been observed in Europe and New Zealand where similar campaigns have been promoted.

The decline in SIDS rates is due to changing babies sleeping position from lying on their front to lying on their back.

SIDS accounts for 28% of deaths that occur between the ages of 1 month and 1 year; 80% of cases occur in babies under 6 months of age and it is rare over the age of 12 months. It is rare in the first 2 weeks of life.

'Reducing the risks' campaign

The 'Reducing the risks' campaign advises that:

- Infants should be put on their back to sleep, not on their side or face down.

Table 15.1 Epidemiological features of SIDS

Epidemiological features of parents of SIDS infants	*Epidemiological features of infants who die from SIDS*
Younger mothers and fathers	Male-63%
Single and unsupported mothers	Lower birth weight
Higher maternal parity	Lower gestation
Lower family income	Lower Apgar score
Previous stillbirths	Admitted to a special care unit
Previous SIDS infant-approximately 1.6 times higher	Congenital abnormalities

The United Kingdom Confidential Enquiry for Stillbirths and Deaths in Infancy (CESDI) study into sudden unexpected deaths in infancy (SUDI). Reference: 'Sudden unexpected deaths in infancy: the CESDI SUDI Studies. Editors: Peter Fleming, Pete Blair, Chris Bacon, Jem Berry.

Table 15.2 Risk Factors for SIDS

Risk Factors for SIDS	*Items that were not confirmed as risk or protective factors for SIDS*
Sleeping positions-face down or on the side	**Breast feeding** – no independent factor found in the reduction of SIDS
Tobacco smoke-daily exposure of infant to smoke from either father, mother or other household members, is highly significant and dose related.	**Dummies** (pacifiers)-no increased risk.
The **cot environment**-infants dying from SIDS were found wrapped more warmly, wore hats, used quilts or 'dooners', had covers over their heads or were wrapped loosely.	**Aeroplane flights** – no evidence of risk.
Room sharing-evidence suggests that sharing a room with the baby in the first 6 months may be beneficial.	**Bed sharing** – no apparent increased risk in the absence of cigarette smoke, alcohol or drug abuse.
Bed sharing-when either parent has been smoking, drinking alcohol or using illegal drugs has been shown to be a risk factor.	**Cot bumpers**-no increased risk nor benefits
Sofa sharing-with an adult conveys a higher risk of SIDS	**Apnoea monitors**-no evidence of protection
Illness recognition-parents should be taught to recognise significant features of illness in babies	**Mattress type or age**- no relationship
Immunisation-infants who are fully immunised are at lower risk of SIDS than those who are not immunised	

The United Kingdom Confidential Enquiry for Stillbirths and Deaths in Infancy (CESDI) study into sudden unexpected deaths in infancy (SUDI) Reference: 'Sudden unexpected deaths in infancy: the CESDI SUDI Studies. Editors: Peter Fleming, Pete Blair, Chris Bacon, Jem Berry.

- Cigarette smoking during pregnancy should be avoided and a smoke-free home should be maintained.
- The infant's head should remain uncovered during sleep.

Further information on the campaign can be obtained from the appropriate SIDS organisations.

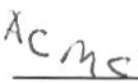

APPARENT LIFE-THREATENING EPISODE

Apparent life-threatening episode (ALTE) is defined as an episode that is frightening to the observer and that is characterised by some combination of apnoea, colour change, marked change of muscle tone, choking or gagging. The terms 'near miss SIDS' or 'aborted cot death' should not be used as it implies a close association between ALTE and SIDS.

- Up to 13% of infants who die from SIDS have a preceding history of ALTE.
- No cause for the ALTE is found in over 50% of cases presenting under the age of 6 months.

Associations that have been found with ALTE are:

- Gastro-oesophageal reflux – a small number of infants with this common condition experience coughing and choking episodes, and occasionally apnoea. These episodes occur most frequently when the infant is awake and are often recurrent. Most resolve within a month of onset but some persist for several weeks. The chest X-ray of these infants rarely shows signs of aspiration.
- Respiratory syncytial virus – can cause apnoea. Other upper airway viruses and pertussis can also be associated with apnoea.
- Upper airway obstruction – due to Pierre Robin syndrome, mid-nasal narrowing or adenoidal hypertrophy. It is usually suspected by a history of inspiratory stridor, snoring and sleep disturbance.
- Epilepsy – usually suggested by a good history. Investigations of ALTE by electroencephalogram (EEG) are usually fruitless unless accompanied by a history and examination suggestive of a seizure disorder.
- Cardiac arrhythmia – this is an uncommon cause but should be suspected in severe recurrent episodes. Obtain an electrocardiogram (ECG).

Most infants with ALTE need minimal resuscitation. However, some need cardiopulmonary resuscitation. These infants have at least a 10% chance of further episodes, which almost always occur in the first month after the previous episode.

A cause will often be found in infants presenting with ALTE over the age of 6 months. If no cause is found in this age group and the episodes are recurrent, formal investigation including sleep polysomnography should be performed. Munchausen's syndrome by proxy should be considered as a possibility when no other cause can be found, but remember no cause is found in over 50% and Munchausen's syndrome by proxy is very rare.

All infants presenting with ALTE should be admitted to hospital for monitoring, investigation and counselling of the parents. However minor the episode may appear to health-care professionals, the parents usually believe that their infant's life was endangered by the episode.

HOME APNOEA MONITORING

No study has demonstrated that home apnoea monitoring programs reduce the incidence of SIDS.

Home apnoea monitoring is not routinely recommended, however, there is a community awareness of its availability. Many baby goods stores sell monitors over the counter without any backup or counselling. Advice regarding home monitoring should concentrate on the lack of its proven efficacy together with the positive message about the falling incidence of SIDS. Frequently families are given inaccurate advice regarding frequency of false alarms, although this is not an issue for the majority. The following are recommendations for consideration of home apnoea monitoring:

- Infants with a history of SIDS in the family.
- ALTE – particularly if cardiopulmonary resuscitation has been used.

There are families who demand monitors and in this situation they are best used under medical supervision after appropriate counselling. Some examples of these are:

- Siblings of a previous SIDS victim.
- Extremely low birth weight infants.
- Infants with minor ALTE episodes.
- Previous family bereavement.
- Extreme family anxiety about apnoea and SIDS.

Counselling and instruction in cardiopulmonary resuscitation, together with complete medical and device back-up, are essential to a home monitoring program.

CHAPTER 16
ALLERGY AND IMMUNOLOGY

Mimi Tang
Andrew Kemp

ALLERGIC DISEASES

Allergic disease is a common problem in the community. It affects up to 30% of children. The allergic conditions include asthma, eczema, allergic rhinitis, and allergies to food, insects or drugs. Children who have allergic diseases are often atopic, that is, they produce IgE antibodies to common allergens such as house dust mite, animal dander, pollens and foods. The presence of IgE antibodies to these allergens does not necessarily cause disease; however, exposure to an allergen to which a patient is sensitised may exacerbate or precipitate symptoms (e.g. inhalant, food, insect or drug allergy).

Allergy tests: What are they, who should have them and what do they tell us?

Skin-prick tests (SPT) and radioallergosorbent tests (RAST) detect specific IgE antibodies against allergens.

Skin-prick tests

- Preferred because they are highly sensitive, inexpensive, simple and rapid.
- May be affected by medications. Antihistamines should be withheld for 2–4 days. Inhaled β-2 agonists, oral theophylline and corticosteroids do not interfere with skin-prick tests.
- Age is not a contraindication to skin-prick testing. Skin-prick testing can be performed from early infancy.
- Dermatographism may complicate the interpretation of skin-prick tests.

Radioallergosorbent tests

- Have reduced sensitivity, are expensive and slow – these are best used to assess sensitivity to a single allergen (e.g. cats).

- Are useful alternatives to skin testing if there is dermatographism, widespread skin disease, or the inability to discontinue antihistamines.

Skin-prick and RAST tests are available for numerous allergens. Testing should be individualised for each clinical situation.

Interpretation

- When ordering these tests the question that is being asked is: 'Are there IgE antibodies present?'. These tests will not necessarily answer the question: 'Is this antigen causing the patient's symptoms?'
- A positive SPT or RAST only identifies the presence of specific IgE against an allergen.
- **A positive test does not prove that an allergic illness exists, nor does it necessarily predict that the patient will develop symptoms on exposure to that substance**. For example, only 50% of individuals with a positive SPT to a food allergen will develop symptoms when exposed to that food. Skin-prick test results must be correlated with history and examination findings.

Indications for skin-prick testing

- Any patient with asthma or rhinitis who requires maintenance steroid therapy to control symptoms, including patients with frequent episodic asthma.
- Patients with moderate or severe eczema despite appropriate medical therapy. Skin-prick testing can identify major allergic factors that may exacerbate or contribute to symptoms and can guide the application of appropriate environmental modification.
- Evaluation of suspected IgE-mediated food reactions. A negative SPT almost eliminates the possibility that a food will induce an IgE-mediated immediate reaction. A positive SPT must be correlated with the history. When there is a clear history of reaction to a specific food, a positive SPT can confirm food allergy. If the history is uncertain, a positive test only indicates the possibility of food allergy and food challenge may be required to confirm the presence or absence of allergy.

In vivo challenges

- *In vivo* challenges are primarily used for diagnosis of food allergy.

- The clinical relevance of a positive SPT should generally be confirmed by a challenge unless the history clearly implicates a food or there is a history of anaphylaxis.
- Less than half of the patients with a positive SPT to a food will react to the food during a challenge.
- Diagnosis of delayed non-IgE-mediated reaction to foods requires a formal food challenge, as there are no skin-prick or blood tests for this type of food reaction.
- *In vivo* challenges are also used for the evaluation of antibiotic reactions.

ALLERGIC RHINITIS

Allergic rhinitis refers to nasal symptoms of paroxysmal sneezing, itching, congestion and rhinorrhoea caused by sensitivity to environmental allergens. It can have a major impact on the quality of life and school performance and appropriate recognition and treatment is important.

- Symptoms may be present throughout the year (perennial rhinitis), related to a particular season (seasonal rhinitis/hay fever) or related to a specific allergen (e.g. cats or horses).
- Diagnosis requires the demonstration of an allergic basis for symptoms. Other causes of rhinitis should be considered: non-allergic rhinitis with eosinophilia (NARES), infective rhinitis, vasomotor rhinitis, hormonal rhinitis or rhinitis medicamentosa (rhinitis induced by excessive use of topical decongestants).

Perennial allergic rhinitis

- Can occur at any age and is more common than seasonal rhinitis in preschool and primary school children.
- Sneezing and congestion are prominent especially on waking in the morning. There may be significant nasal obstruction and snoring at night.
- House dust mite is the major allergen involved but concurrent sensitivity to pollens is also common.
- Consider the possibility of perennial allergic rhinitis in any atopic child– this diagnosis is frequently missed.

Seasonal rhinitis

- More frequent in teenagers and young adults.

- Seasonal sneezing, itching and rhinorrhoea are prominent. Nasal symptoms are frequently associated with symptoms of itchy, red and watery eyes.
- Symptoms occur in the relevant pollen season.
- In general, trees pollinate in early spring, grasses in the late spring and summer, and weeds in the summer and autumn, although there is some overlap. Rye grass is the commonest provoking antigen in Australia, but multiple sensitivities to tree, grass and weed pollens are also seen.

Examination

- Assess airflow, the nasal airway and nasal mucosa.
- Pale oedematous mucosa and swollen turbinates indicate ongoing rhinitis. In seasonal rhinitis, examination may be normal outside the relevant pollen season.

Management

- Topical corticosteroid nasal sprays (e.g. beclomethasone or budesonide) are the treatment of choice for perennial and seasonal allergic rhinitis, as well as perennial non-allergic rhinitis.
- Continuous topical corticosteroid therapy for perennial rhinitis has not been shown to cause suppression of the hypothalamic-pituitary-adrenal axis. In seasonal rhinitis, commence treatments 1 month prior to the relevant pollen season and continues over the symptomatic period.
- Topical sodium cromoglycate is generally not effective.
- Topical anti-inflammatory treatment must be taken regularly for benefit. Improvement may not be apparent for 3–4 weeks and an initial course of treatment should last for 2–3 months.
- Allergen avoidance measures should be considered for patients placed on topical anti-inflammatory therapy. These consist of avoidance of relevant allergen triggers (e.g. pets with animal dander sensitivity, house dust mite allergen in perennial rhinitis with dust mite sensitivity). Dust mite reduction measures involve the use of appropriate allergen impermeable covers for mattress pillow and doona in conjunction with washing of bedding in hot water weekly, removal of soft toys and soft furnishings from the bedroom, vacuuming carpet weekly, and damp dusting of hard surfaces (including hard flooring) weekly. Avoidance of grass pollens is generally not possible.

Table 16.1 Antihistamine medications

Type of Antihistamine	*Brand Name*	*Doses*
Non-sedating		
Loratadine*	Claratyne Lorastyne	1–2 years: 2.5 mg/dose once daily 3–6 years: 5 mg/dose once daily >6 years & adults: 10 mg/dose once daily
Fexofenadine	Telfast	>6 years: 30 mg/dose twice a day Adults 60 mg/dose twice a day
Cetirizine*	Zyrtec	>1 years: 0.125 mg/kg/dose twice a daily 2–5 years: 2.5–5 mg/day in 2 doses 6–12 years: 5–10 mg/day in 1–2 doses Adults: 10–20 mg/day in 1–2 doses
Sedating		
Trimeprazine	Vallergan	>2 years (allergy): 0.1–0.25 mg/kg/dose 6-hourly (Sedation) dose: 1–2 mg/kg nocte Adults: 10 mg/dose 3 times a day (max 100 mg/day)

* Second generation

- Antihistamines are not helpful in relieving nasal obstruction and are not indicated as first-line treatment for rhinitis. They may be used in seasonal rhinitis (see Table 16.1) for control of break through sneezing, itching or rhinorrhoea while on topical corticosteroid therapy or prophylactically prior to allergen exposure in allergen-specific rhinoconjunctivitis (e.g. cats or horses). Second-generation non-sedating antihistamines (loratadine and cetirizine) are well tolerated. Terfenadine and astemizole should be avoided as they may cause cardiac arrhythmia when taken with other medications.

FOOD ALLERGY

Food allergy is commonest in infancy. Milk, egg, wheat, soy, peanut, tree nuts, fish and shellfish are responsible for 90% of food allergies in children and adults. Most food allergies resolve by 5 years of age. The exceptions are peanut, tree nut and shellfish allergies, which frequently persist.

Allergic reactions to food fall into two broad groups:

IgE-mediated food reactions

- Are common.
- Occur within 1–2 h of food ingestion.
- Typically occur in young infants and frequently resolve by the age of 3–5 years.
- Common foods that provoke reactions are milk, eggs and peanuts.
- Common symptoms are erythema where food touches the skin; urticaria, which may be facial or generalised; angioedema, which is usually facial; and vomiting immediately after the ingestion of the food.
- More severe reactions (anaphylaxis) involve the respiratory tract (stridor, wheezing, or hoarse voice) and/or the cardiovascular system, with hypotension and collapse (see Medical emergencies, chapter 1).

Management

- Patients with a suspected food allergy should be referred for specialist allergy advice.
- Practitioners should advise patients to avoid the suspected food until further evaluation.
- Parents should not challenge children with a suspected food at home as severe reactions and even death have occurred.
- Suspected IgE-mediated immediate food reactions are investigated with skin-prick testing. A negative SPT almost eliminates the possibility of an immediate IgE-mediated reaction to that food. A positive SPT may confirm food hypersensitivity if there is a convincing history. However, if the history is uncertain, further evaluation by formal challenge is required. In an infant with a suspected reaction to one food, SPT should also be performed with the other common food allergens, as reactions are often multiple.
- In IgE-mediated milk hypersensitivity cow's milk products should be eliminated. In infants and young children, who require formula, a soy-based milk can be used if the child is not sensitive to soy. In cases of cow's milk and soy protein sensitivity, a formula in which the milk proteins are broken down into hypoallergenic fragments (protein hydrolysate) should be used. Rarely children may react to the hydrolysed milk proteins in these formulas and in such cases an elemental amino acid formula (Neocate) is indicated.

Non-IgE-mediated and mixed IgE/non-IgE mediated food reactions

- Generally are delayed reactions occurring within 24–48 h of food ingestion, although some infants may have immediate non-IgE-mediated food reactions that occur within 1–2 h of food ingestion.
- Non-IgE-mediated food reactions are much less common and will often need specialist consultation to confirm.
- Typically, gastrointestinal symptoms are prominent with vomiting, diarrhoea and abdominal cramps. Occasionally there may be malabsorption, weight loss or failure to thrive.
- In severe cases there may be cardiovascular collapse.
- A worsening of eczema may also occur.
- Cow milk and soy proteins are the most common foods implicated.
- Diagnosis requires elimination of the suspected food followed by formal food challenge. Skin-prick testing is not helpful.

ALLERGIC FACTORS IN ATOPIC DERMATITIS (ECZEMA)

See also Dermatologic conditions, chapter 20.

Atopic dermatitis has a major impact on the lives of patients and their families. Allergic factors may play an important role in the exacerbation of eczema and this possibility should always be considered in moderate or severe disease. Avoiding the relevant allergic factors can improve symptom control, however, allergic factors are not the sole cause of the disease and allergen avoidance is only one component of overall management. An important triggering factor is *Staphylococcus aureus* infection and colonisation. Treatment of acute staphylococcal infection and reduction of staphylococcal loads on the skin can provide significant improvement of eczema control. Staphylococcal infection or colonisation, or both, must be controlled before the benefits of other allergen-avoidance measures can be assessed.

House dust mite sensitivity is an important exacerbating factor in atopic dermatitis. Dust mite allergen is ubiquitous in the home environment, particularly in the bedroom where a child spends up to 10 h each day. In patients with sensitivity to house dust mite allergen, instituting the appropriate avoidance measures may be beneficial (see Allergic rhinitis, page 243).

Immediate food hypersensitivity reactions can act as exacerbating factors, particularly in young children with severe atopic dermatitis and generalised erythema. Investigation is as outlined in the section on food allergy above. In a small number of the more severe cases, there may be delayed reactions to foods. There are no skin or blood tests that can reliably identify whether a delayed reaction to a food is occurring. The implementation of a restricted diet and a systematic reintroduction of suspected foods is used to assess this. These dietary manipulations are often complex and difficult to interpret. Specialist advice is required in the administration of the diet and in the interpretation of results. Appropriate case selection is important. Dietary restrictions should not be instituted in children with mild atopic dermatitis that can be readily controlled with the appropriate topical medication.

ALLERGIC FACTORS IN ASTHMA

See also Respiratory conditions, chapter 33.

Allergic factors may contribute to the symptoms of asthma, particularly in cases of chronic persistent asthma. Investigation for allergens to which a patient is sensitised should be pursued in any patient requiring maintenance anti-inflammatory corticosteroid therapy, particularly those with interval symptoms.

The avoidance of relevant allergic factors represents a simple, inexpensive and non-pharmacological approach to anti-inflammatory therapy. However, allergen avoidance only represents one component of the overall management of asthma. Patients should understand that allergic factors are not the sole cause of asthma. The major allergens implicated are the indoor inhalants (house dust mite, cat and dog dander). Pollens may also contribute to seasonal exacerbations of asthma, especially if the patient also suffers from seasonal allergic rhinitis. Moulds may trigger asthma symptoms in arid climates.

Allergic rhinitis can exacerbate asthma and untreated persistent rhinitis may be one of the reasons for a failed response to standard anti-asthma therapy. The possibility of allergic rhinitis should be considered in all patients with asthma – it is common and treatable.

Foods generally do not induce asthma symptoms in isolation. They may cause asthma symptoms as part of an immediate hypersensitivity reaction when cutaneous eruptions are usually also observed. In some patients with chronic asthma, the preservative metabisulphite can provoke acute exacerbations of asthma. Confirmation of this requires specialist consultation. Non-steroidal anti-inflammatory medications (e.g. Aspirin) may exacerbate asthma symptoms in some patients with chronic asthma. Specialist consultation is required to confirm this.

URTICARIA AND ANGIO-OEDEMA

Urticarial rashes

- Raised areas of erythema and oedema, which move over several hours.
- Usually itchy.
- Classified as acute (<6 weeks duration) or chronic (>6 weeks duration).

Acute urticaria

- Often only lasts a few days.
- In the vast majority of cases, no precipitating factor is identified.
- The most important step is to take a careful history to look for possible exposure to drugs (especially antibiotics) or foods that may have induced an immediate hypersensitivity reaction. If a precipitating factor cannot be identified on history, skin-prick tests and RAST tests will generally not provide additional information.
- Some cases follow viral or streptococcal infections.

Chronic urticaria

- Can persist or occur intermittently for months or years.
- The possibility of a physical urticaria (e.g. heat, cold or cholinergic) should be considered.
- In protracted cases, it is important to consider the possibility of an underlying connective tissue or autoimmune disorder that may (rarely) present as chronic urticaria. In these cases, there are usually other suggestive features such as arthritis or vasculitis. Biopsy of lesions for histologic analysis may be helpful in identifying vasculitis.

- Chronic urticaria is rarely caused by specific allergic factors and therefore investigation with skin-prick testing and RAST testing is not helpful.

Angio-oedema

- Swelling of deeper tissues that often involves areas of low tension, such as the eyelids, lips and scrotum.
- Not necessarily itchy.

Treatment of both acute and chronic urticaria

- Symptomatic – treat with second-generation antihistamines. Cetirizine is particularly effective (for doses see Table 16.1).
- Manipulation of the diet is generally not helpful and is not indicated in children. A small number of subjects may respond to a preservative and colouring-free diet; however, this should only be considered if symptoms are particularly troublesome. The institution of such a diet and the interpretation of the result require specialist advice.
- In resistant cases, the combined use of an H_2 antihistamine (cimetidine) with standard H_1 antihistamines may be considered but success is limited.

ANTIBIOTIC SENSITIVITY

Reported sensitivity to antibiotics in children is common, however, many patients are incorrectly labelled as 'antibiotic sensitive'. Careful history is required to identify those patients who are likely to have experienced true antibiotic reactions. Reactions may be IgE mediated or non-IgE mediated. The most common presentation is a cutaneous eruption, either urticarial or maculopapular. More severe reactions are anaphylaxis with angio-oedema and bronchospasm or laryngeal oedema, exfoliative dermatitis, Stevens-Johnson syndrome, or serum sickness with arthralgia. Multiple antibiotic sensitivities where a child is reported to react to a significant number of antibiotics are not uncommon.

The commonest reactions are to the penicillin family. Allergy to penicillin or its derivatives is associated with a 10% risk of reaction (through cross-reactivity) to the first and second-generation cephalosporins. This does not extend to third generation cephalosporins as reactions to these are usually directed to side chains.

Management

- No completely adequate *in vitro* or *in vivo* tests diagnose drug allergy.
- The detection of IgE antibodies by RAST or SPT may be helpful in the evaluation of penicillin or amoxicillin reactions.
- A negative SPT indicates that a patient is unlikely to react on re-exposure and any reaction is likely to be mild.
- A positive SPT is less helpful as the presence of IgE antibodies does not necessarily indicate a reaction after re-exposure.
- Skin-prick testing regimens have been established for the penicillin metabolites; however, this is not widely performed in Australia, as the test reagents are not readily available. Skin testing for other antibiotics is less helpful.
- In most cases, an oral challenge initiated under observation and then continued on an outpatient basis is required to confirm or exclude sensitivity.
- An assessment should be made of the severity of the reaction. Each case must be judged on its merits.
- If there has been significant anaphylaxis with respiratory problems or hypotension, or both, the patient should not be challenged with the drug again except in exceptional circumstances and after an appropriate evaluation.
- Other contraindications to challenge include severe mucocutaneous reactions such as Stevens–Johnson syndrome or exfoliative dermatitis and serum sickness. In these instances, an alternative class of antibiotic should be selected. In deciding whether to proceed with a challenge, a judgement should also be made regarding the importance of the antibiotic in question. In the vast majority of cases with the question of multiple antibiotic sensitivities, a challenge is performed with a single antibiotic selected as being appropriate for future use and the challenge is completed without reaction.

LATEX SENSITIVITY

Latex products contain two types of compounds that can cause reactions: chemical additives that cause dermatitis and natural proteins that induce immediate hypersensitivity reactions. The majority of reactions to latex in the hospital setting involve disposable gloves; however, other items including catheters, dressings and bandages, intravenous tubing, stethoscopes and airways may contain latex. Common latex products used in the community include balloons, baby bottle teats and dummies, elastic bands and condoms. Reactions to latex products may be irritant or immune mediated.

Irritant dermatitis

Irritant dermatitis is the most common problem encountered with the use of latex gloves. This is a non-allergic skin rash characterised by erythema, dryness, scaling and cracking. It is caused by sweating and irritation from the glove or its powder, or by irritation as a result of frequent washing with soap and detergents.

Immediate hypersensitivity to latex

Type I hypersensitivity reactions to latex are the most serious reactions; they are potentially life threatening. They are caused by IgE antibodies to latex proteins. Reactions may occur after contact with latex (e.g. gloves and catheters) or the inhalation of airborne powder particles containing allergenic latex proteins. Sensitisation may occur following direct exposure of mucosal surfaces to latex (e.g. catheterisation). The severity of the reaction may vary widely, ranging from isolated allergic rhinoconjunctivitis, urticaria or asthma, to anaphylaxis and death. Certain populations are at high risk for developing latex allergy: children with spina bifida or other urogenital anomalies and individuals undergoing multiple surgical procedures, particularly if they are atopic. Skin-prick testing and/or RAST testing is useful in confirming suspected hypersensitivity. Skin-prick testing is more reliable than RAST, however, well-standardised skin-prick test extracts are not widely available. There is no cure for latex allergy. The best approach is to avoid exposure. There may be cross-reactivity between latex and certain foods, in particular avocado and banana. If latex-allergic individuals experience discomfort in the mouth or throat while eating these foods, such foods should be avoided.

Contact dermatitis

This is a delayed Type IV hypersensitivity to chemical additives used in processing latex. Reactions are limited to the site of contact. Use of rubber gloves results in eczematous lesions on the dorsum of the hands. The skin may become dry, crusted and thickened. Oral reactions caused by dental appliances or balloons, and genital reactions caused by condoms have been described. The use of cotton-lining gloves inside latex gloves or a change to gloves that do not contain the chemicals contained in latex gloves usually reduces the problem. Patients with irritant and contact dermatitis are at an increased risk of developing immediate hypersensitivity to latex and exposure to latex should be minimised.

Management

- Patients at high risk for latex sensitivity should be referred to a paediatric allergist/immunologist for further evaluation.
- Patients who are confirmed to have latex allergy (either immediate or delayed) should undertake strict latex avoidance including having latex free precautions during surgery.

IMMUNOTHERAPY

- There are relatively few indications for immunotherapy in paediatric practice.
- Immunotherapy with purified bee venom is indicated for life-threatening anaphylactic reactions to bee stings in children. Referral should be made to a paediatric allergist/immunologist for allergy testing and further management.
- Severe local reactions are not an indication for immunotherapy and do not require further investigation with skin-prick testing.
- Immunotherapy may be an option in severe seasonal allergic rhinitis if the symptoms are not controlled with allergen avoidance and maximal medical therapy (topical anti-inflammatory medication and antihistamines), particularly if a limited number of allergens can be identified.
- Extreme caution is required in administering immunotherapy to unstable asthmatic patients, as deaths have resulted.

GUIDELINES FOR THE INVESTIGATION AND TREATMENT OF IMMUNODEFICIENCY

When to suspect immunodeficiency

Normal, immunocompetent children average 5–10 viral upper respiratory tract infections per year in the first few years of life (even more if the child attends child care or has older siblings). Recurrent viral infections in a well, thriving child do not suggest immunodeficiency. Immune deficiency should be suspected when there is a history of severe, recurrent, or unusual infections.

- Recurrent or chronic bacterial infections (e.g. persistently discharging ears or purulent respiratory secretions) or more than one severe pyogenic infection may indicate antibody deficiency.
- Severe or disseminated viral infections, persistent mucocutaneous candidiasis, chronic infectious diarrhoea and/or failure to thrive in infants suggest a severe T-cell deficiency. These children should be investigated for Severe Combined Immune Deficiency (SCID).
- The presence of autoimmune cytopenias, together with recurrent sinopulmonary infections, raises the possibility of less severe forms of combined immune deficiency.
- Recurrent pyogenic infections affecting lymph nodes, skin, lung and bones suggest a neutrophil defect.
- Recurrent meningococcal disease suggests a late component complement deficiency. Early component complement deficiencies may present with clinical features that are similar to antibody defects, or with autoimmune disease.

Which tests to order

Basic immunodeficiency screen

- An FBE with differential and Immunoglobulin levels (IgG, IgA and IgM) will identify the vast majority of treatable primary immunodeficiencies (e.g. Agammaglobulinaemia, Common Variable Immune Deficiency, selective IgA deficiency and SCID).
- If these tests are normal and the clinical suspicion of immune deficiency persists, referral to a clinical immunologist for further evaluation is indicated.

Specific antibody responses and IgG subclasses

- Only consider when there is evidence of persistent or recurrent suppurative upper or lower respiratory tract infection, or both, and hypo-gammaglobulinaemia has been excluded.
- Ask the question: 'If an antibody defect is found, does this clinical condition warrant regular gammaglobulin therapy?'

- Specific antibody responses should generally be performed in conjunction with IgG subclasses. Reduced absolute levels of IgG subclasses do not necessarily indicate abnormal antibody production. The most important question is whether appropriate antibodies can be made to specific protein and polysaccharide antigens. Abnormal IgG subclass levels may be a clue to an evolving antibody deficiency. However, isolated abnormalities of IgG subclasses with normal specific antibody responses rarely result in clinical problems. In general, regular gammaglobulin therapy is only indicated for severe recurrent infections when a specific antibody defect has been identified.

T-lymphocyte numbers and function

- The use of delayed hypersensitivity skin tests and a chest X-ray to look for absent thymic shadow may be helpful when a T-lymphocyte defect is suspected.
- Specialised T lymphocyte function tests are used to help in the diagnosis of SCID and Di George syndrome (absent thymus, hypocalcaemia and cardiovascular anomalies). Referral to a specialist is recommended if these conditions are suspected.

Neutrophil function tests

- Specific defects of neutrophil function (e.g. Chronic Granulomatous Disease and Leucocyte Adhesion Deficiency 1) are very rare. They are almost always associated with gingivitis and careful examination of the mouth is important when considering abnormalities of neutrophil function.
- Markedly elevated circulating neutrophil counts and delayed separation of the umbilical cord suggest the possibility of an adhesion molecule deficiency.
- Suspected cases of defective neutrophil function should be referred to a specialist for further evaluation.

Complement studies

- Deficiencies of complement are rare.
- The best screening test for congenital deficiency is a CH50, which measures the function of the classical complement pathway.

HIV tests

- HIV testing should be considered in the setting of recurrent, severe or unusual infections, particularly if there is hypergammaglobulinaemia.
- Specialised immune function testing is best undertaken in consultation with a clinical immunologist.

Immunodeficiency treatment

Immunisation

See also Immunisation, chapter 8.

- As a general rule all live virus vaccines should be avoided in immunodeficiency unless advised by a specialist.
- Patients with a T-cell defect and their immediate family should receive the killed polio (Salk) vaccine in place of the standard live oral polio vaccine.
- In certain circumstances, measles immunisation may be given to patients with a T-cell defect (e.g. Di George syndrome or paediatric HIV infection) as the risks of wild-type measles infection are considerable, while adverse reactions to the vaccine are largely theoretical.
- In cases of antibody deficiency, T-cell deficiency and combined immunodeficiency, immunisation with killed vaccines will not promote a significant antibody response.
- If the patient is on immunoglobulin replacement therapy, passively acquired antibody will prevent virus infections such as measles and chickenpox.
- Patients of any age with asplenia should be immunised with Hib, pneumococcal and meningococcal vaccines.

Immunoglobulin therapy

- Immunoglobulin therapy (400–600 mg/kg i.v. monthly) is given when a significant deficiency of antibody production is demonstrated in a patient with clinically significant infections (usually affecting the sinopulmonary tracts).
- In hypogammaglobulinaemia, immunoglobulin therapy is generally life-long.
- In patients with combined immunodeficiency, immunoglobulin treatment may be discontinued once normal B-cell function can be demonstrated following bone marrow transplantation.

- In patients with IgG subclass deficiency, immunoglobulin therapy is only indicated if a significant functional antibody deficit is demonstrated and the patient has significant symptoms. In this instance, a trial of immunoglobulin therapy may be used for a restricted period of time to determine if there is clinical benefit. This should only be instituted in conjunction with a clinical immunologist.
- The finding of a low immunoglobulin subclass level alone is not a sufficient indication for immunoglobulin therapy. Immunoglobulin therapy is not indicated for selective IgA deficiency. These patients should be referred to a specialist for further evaluation and/or follow up.

Antibiotics

- As immunoglobulin therapy does not provide significant levels of IgA antibody (the mucosal surface antibody), aggressive treatment of respiratory infections in patients with antibody deficiency is important in order to prevent bronchiectasis and permanent damage to the lungs.
- In severe cases, prophylactic rotating antibiotics are used to prevent recurrent severe sinopulmonary infections.
- Antibiotic prophylaxis with cotrimoxazole 2.5/12.5 mg/kg (max 80/400) p.o. b.d. 3 days per week, is indicated in patients with T-cell or combined immune deficiency to prevent infection with Pneumocystis.

Use of blood products

- If it is suspected or known that the patient has a significant T-cell deficiency, blood products that contain cells (e.g. whole blood, packed red cells or platelets) should be irradiated to prevent graft versus host disease.
- In infants with SCID, attempts should be made to provide cytomegalovirus (CMV) antibody-negative blood, as CMV infection can be a significant problem in such patients. If this is not possible, the blood product should be filtered to remove contaminating white blood cells as it is delivered to the patient. If possible, Epstein-Barr virus (EBV) antibody-negative blood should also be given, as EBV can induce lymphoproliferative states in severely immunodeficient subjects.

- Patients with IgA deficiency may develop IgE antibodies to IgA and have an anaphylactic reaction to blood products containing IgA (intravenous immunoglobulin, packed red cells, platelets). Immunoglobulin preparations that are depleted of IgA should be used and packed cells or platelets should be washed 4 times in physiologic saline prior to infusion.

Bone marrow transplantation

- Bone marrow transplantation is the definitive treatment for severe combined immunodeficiency. It may also be useful for the treatment of other T-lymphocyte immune deficiencies (e.g. Chronic Granulomatous Disease, Hyper IgM syndrome).
- The cure rate can be of the order of 80% if the transplant is from a matched sibling or a parent.
- Survival is slightly less, of the order of 50%, if the transplant is only partially matched and from an unrelated donor.

CHAPTER 17
BURNS

Russell Taylor

TREATMENT AIMS

- To prevent and treat burn shock.
- To provide adequate analgesia.
- To prevent infection.
- To obtain early skin cover.
- To prevent hypertrophic scar formation.
- To restore function and correct cosmetic defect.
- To prevent recurrence of injury and promote accident prevention.

ASSESSMENT

Age

The younger the child, the more likely shock will occur for a given extent of burn.

Estimating the surface area burned

The usual adult formula (rule of nines) is not applicable to children, because the proportions contributed by the head and limbs vary at different ages. The burned areas should be plotted accurately on the body chart and the area calculated with the aid of the Lund-Browder chart (see Figure 17.1). The extent of the burn is only rarely underestimated, but overestimation is common and frequently leads to excessive fluid administration.

Assessment of the depth of burn

In most burns, there are varying grades of injury (see Table 17.1).

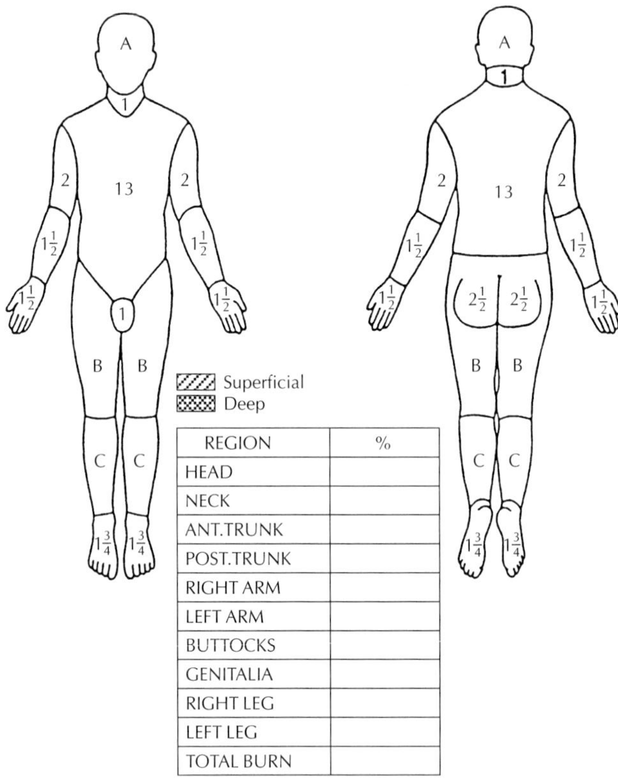

REGION	%
HEAD	
NECK	
ANT.TRUNK	
POST.TRUNK	
RIGHT ARM	
LEFT ARM	
BUTTOCKS	
GENITALIA	
RIGHT LEG	
LEFT LEG	
TOTAL BURN	

Relative percentage of areas affected by growth

Age (years)	0	1	5	10	15	Adult
A – $\frac{1}{2}$ of head	$9\frac{1}{2}$	$8\frac{1}{2}$	$6\frac{1}{2}$	$5\frac{1}{2}$	$4\frac{1}{2}$	$3\frac{1}{2}$
B – $\frac{1}{2}$ of one thigh	$2\frac{3}{4}$	$3\frac{1}{4}$	4	$4\frac{1}{4}$	$4\frac{1}{2}$	$4\frac{3}{4}$
C – $\frac{1}{2}$ of one leg	$2\frac{1}{2}$	$2\frac{1}{2}$	$2\frac{3}{4}$	3	$3\frac{1}{4}$	$3\frac{1}{2}$

Fig. 17.1 Lund–Browder chart

Table 17.1 Assessment of burn depth

Depth	*Cause*	*Surface/colour*	*Pain/sensation*	*Treatment*
Superficial (partial loss of skin)	Sun, flash, minor scald	Dry, minor blisters, erythema	Painful	Expose
	Scald	Moist, reddened with broken blisters	Painful	Non-adherent dressing
Deep partial	Scald, minor flame contact	Moist white slough, red mottled	Painless	Graft otherwise scarring
Deep (complete loss of skin)	Flame, severe scald or contact	Dry, charred whitish	Painless	Graft

FIRST AID

Instantly remove clothing or smother the flame and apply cold water.

In a minor burn, continue the cold water application in a bowl or by compressing for up to 30 min. In a major burn, bathe for 20 min while awaiting transport to the hospital. Cover to guard against hypothermia or cold injury. Never use ice or ice slush.

Major burns are covered in a special foam transport dressing (if available) or plastic cling wrap, with a blanket for warmth. These patients should be given intravenous fluid, oxygen and morphine, if necessary, before admission to hospital.

Check the tetanus immunisation status and boost with tetanus toxoid +/– tetanus immunoglobulin as appropriate (see Procedures, chapter 4).

MINOR BURNS

Superficial burns of less than 5% of the body surface are suitable for outpatient treatment, unless they occur on the face, neck, hands, feet or perineum. Infants under the age of 12 months are more likely to require admission.

Initial management

- Blisters should be left intact.
- Gently cleanse and remove loose skin.
- Dress with tulle gras and an absorbent dressing (e.g. gauze). Do not use Hypofix-type dressing directly on the burn.
- Immobilise with a crepe bandage, plaster slab or sling, if indicated.

Subsequent management

- Leave the initial dressing for 5–8 days. If the dressing is soaked by exudate, redress as necessary without disturbing the adherent tulle.
- Consider grafting to the residual areas if the healing process is not complete by the end of the second week. Graft deep second-degree burns by 5–10 days.

- Pain, fever and soiled or offensive dressings indicate that the dressing should be changed earlier than anticipated, then assessed and treated for infection if necessary.

MAJOR BURNS

Superficial burns to greater than 5% of the body surface area, and deep burns, require admission to hospital. **For any child with burns to greater than 10% of the body surface area, transfer to a specialist paediatric burns centre should be considered**. Older children with more extensive superficial burns, such as sunburn, may be managed as outpatients (see Table 17.1).

General

- A brief history should document the time, causative agent and circumstances of the burn, the therapy already given and the child's general health. If the history is inconsistent with the injury, consider child abuse.
- Carefully estimate and chart the extent and depth of the burn.
- Weigh the patient if possible – otherwise estimate weight.
- Insert an intravenous line in patients with burns greater than 10%. If a central venous line is needed, a specialist burn centre should be involved. Plan intravenous therapy (see below) and commence treatment with Hartmann's solution.
- Draw blood for baseline laboratory studies, including haemoglobin and haematocrit, serum electrolytes and, in severe burns, blood grouping and cross-matching.
- Insert a silastic urethral catheter for hourly urine volume in all patients with burns greater than 15%.
- Analgesia or sedation should be administered as necessary (see Pain management, chapter 3).
- Prevent infection. Care should be taken in ward management to guard against cross-infection. Antibiotics should not be prescribed routinely.
- Observations of general condition, pulse, respiration rate, temperature, BP and fluid balance (including hourly urine output estimations) are necessary.

- With severe burns to the face, consider early endotracheal intubation. As the face swells, airways obstruction may occur, making intubation very difficult.
- Observe for effects of smoke inhalation that lead to acute respiratory distress syndrome (ARDS) where ventilation perfusion defects result in hypoxaemia, alveolar collapse, shunting and decreased lung compliance.
- Carboxyhaemoglobin (COHb) and cyanide concentration should be measured in all burn/smoke inhalation patients. Symptoms of hypoxaemia will be manifested at levels greater than 30% COHb. Treatment is simple oxygen therapy as CO binding to Hb is reversible.

Fluid resuscitation

See Figure 17.2.

Fluid volume

Use 3 mL/kg bodyweight per 1% burn surface area (BSA) for the first 24 h. In less severe burns 2 mL/kg bodyweight per 1% BSA may be sufficient.

Type of fluid

Use 4% normal serum albumin solution (NSAS) and Hartmann's solution, 50% of each type of solution is used concurrently.

Fluid maintenance

Type of fluid

Use 0.45% saline in 5% dextrose to provide extra sodium.

Rate of infusion (first 24 hours)

- First 8 h: one-half resuscitation fluid plus one-third maintenance fluid.
- Second 8 h: one-quarter resuscitation fluid plus one-third maintenance fluid.
- Third 8 h: one-quarter resuscitation fluid plus one-third maintenance fluid.

The 24 h period commences from the time of burning, not from the time of admission.

BURNS SURFACE AREA (BSA)......%
TIME OF BURN.........24 h CLOCK
WEIGHT IN KG...............................

TIME IV COMMENCED......24 h CLOCK
DATE.......................................

A BURN RESUSCITATION * 3 × kg × % = ...mL	1st 24 h (volume)	1st 8 h (volume)	2nd 8 h (volume)	3rd 8 h (volume)
TYPE OF INFUSION ** **1 4% Normal Serum Albumin Solution (NSAS)** *** **2 Remainder as Hartmann's Solution** 50% of each type solution is used concurrently	______mL ______mL	$\frac{1}{2}$ of 24 h vol. ______mL ______mL	$\frac{1}{4}$ of 24 h vol. ______mL ______mL	$\frac{1}{4}$ of 24 h vol. ______mL ______mL
B MAINTENANCE FLUID **See oral fluids information below** 0.45% saline in 5% dextrose (estimated volume on bodyweight in kg)	______mL	$\frac{1}{3}$ of 24 h vol. ______mL	$\frac{1}{3}$ of 24 h vol. ______mL	$\frac{1}{3}$ of 24 h vol. ______mL
TOTAL A & B BURN RESUSCITATION + MAINTENANCE FLUID				

URINARY OUTPUT EXPECTED 0.75 mL/kg per h = ____ mL

ORAL FLUIDS: Most children with burn injuries tolerate oral fluids. Initially all children may be offered small amounts of milk and, if tolerated, the quantity is increased at hourly intervals. Usually after a few hours the patient is receiving most maintenance fluid by mouth, except for those patients with very severe burns.
IF ORAL FLUIDS ARE NOT TOLERATED SEE (B) ABOVE.

NOTES: * In less severe burns 2 mL × kg × 1% in the first 24 h may be sufficient.
** Normal Serum Albumin Solution (NSAS) is interspersed and not given as one bolus.
*** If no Hartmann's available use normal saline.

2nd 24 h: After the initial 24 h of fluid replacement, the type of fluid replacement will depend on urinary output, serum electrolytes and haemoglobin. The volume of burn resuscitation fluid is approximately $\frac{1}{2}$ that given for the first 24 h.

Fig. 17.2 Resuscitation of a burnt child during the first 24 h

Adjustments are made according to the hourly urine output, which is the best guide to the adequacy of fluid replacement. Expected flow is 0.75 mL/kg per h in children; in the infant and toddler, a urine output of up to 1 mL/kg per h is required. Record the urine specific gravity and serum and urine osmolality if renal function is poor.

Repeated haemoglobin, haematocrit and electrolyte estimations are made, the frequency depends on the severity of the injury. Restlessness may indicate inadequate fluid replacement.

Rate of infusion (second 24 hours and onwards)

- Replacement fluid: approximately one-half of the volume for the first 24 h.
- Maintenance fluid as before.
- Total volume is given at an even rate over 24 h.
- The volume and type of fluid given are adjusted according to urine flow and electrolyte estimations, then decreased as the shock diminishes over the succeeding days. Diuresis occurs 2–3 days post-burn.

Oral fluids

Most children will tolerate small amounts of milk (30–60 mL/h) after 4–8 h. If this is tolerated, increase the quantity to 4-hourly. In minor burns, oral fluids may be commenced earlier. If gastric dilatation associated with vomiting occurs, a nasogastric tube should be inserted.

After 48 h, the majority of fluid intake is usually oral. Children who refuse to drink, or who have burns to the face and mouth may require nasogastric feeding.

Blood

Whole blood is not required initially except in severe, deep burns, and then usually only 24 h post-burn, when the haemoglobin concentration is falling.

Local wound care

Minimal debridement of loose skin is performed initially and management continued by exposed or closed methods.

Escharotomies should be considered if the peripheral circulation to a limb is jeopardised. Before commencing this procedure contact with a paediatric burns unit is desirable.

Respiratory difficulties require particular attention; intensive care or escharotomy to the trunk may be required.

Exposed

- Indications: for burns on the face, perineum, or one surface of the trunk.
- Treatment: allow eschar to form if superficial, or apply topical silver sulphadiazine (SSD) cream. A daily bath is given with warm water and mild soap, followed by the application of SSD cream.

Closed

- Indications: for small children and burns on extremities. Except for burns to the face or perineum, nearly all children are ultimately nursed with closed dressings.
- Treatment: an antiseptic tulle gras and gauze for superficial burns, or topical SSD cream and Melolin for deep burns. Fingers and toes are separated with non-adherent tulle and wrapped together (not separately). Before the dressing, a daily bath is given with warm water and mild soap.

Fever in patients with burns and antibiotic choice

On admission, swabs should be taken of the burn area, nose, throat and rectum. The burn area should be re-swabbed twice weekly. In major burns, multiple 3 mL punch biopsy specimens are the most reliable method of detecting infection.

Antibiotics are usually only given for proven infection and on the basis of sensitivity tests.

If septicaemia is suspected clinically, blood culture should be performed and antibiotics such as gentamicin 7.5 mg/kg (max 240 mg) i.v. daily and flucloxacillin 50 mg/kg (max 2 g) i.v. 4–6 hourly are commenced.

Nutrition

All children with burns should receive a high-calorie diet containing adequate protein, and vitamin and iron supplements. In severe burns there is a marked increase in metabolic rate and gastric tube feeding with a complete fluid diet (e.g. Isocal or Osmolite) should be instituted early and adjusted to maintain or increase bodyweight. The involvement of a dietitian is recommended.

Room temperature

It is desirable that this is in the range of 22–26°C. If a child is partly exposed and nursed in a cool environment, metabolic requirements will increase.

Special therapy

Physiotherapy and occupational therapy should be commenced early and continue throughout the course of burn care. Splints and pressure dressings are necessary to control hypertrophic scar formation. The play therapist also has an important role.

Social rehabilitation is important, as many burned children come from disadvantaged homes. **Maltreated children constitute approximately 6% of admissions to the burns unit**. Psychological and psychiatric consultation is often required. The hospital teacher should also liaise with the child's schoolteachers.

Follow up

Healed burns and grafts are kept soft with emollient. Pressure therapy and supervision of splints should be continued by a physiotherapist and occupational therapist. Parents and children need continuing support. Further operations are sometimes necessary to correct contractures and relieve cosmetic defects.

CHAPTER 18
CARDIAC CONDITIONS

Marina Hughes
Dan Penny

WHEN TO INVESTIGATE A MURMUR

Background

At least 50% of school age children have a systolic cardiac murmur with no structural or physiological cardiac problem. Chest X-ray (CXR) and electrocardiogram (ECG) are specific, but not sensitive tests for cardiac disease.

Features of a physiological, functional or 'innocent' murmur

History:

- Benign family history.
- Asymptomatic.
- Normal growth.

Examination:

- Normal general physical examination.

Murmur characteristics:

- Continuous murmur, which varies with posture.
- Soft, systolic murmur with:
  - Normal second heart sound.
  - Separate, audible heart sounds.
  - A musical, vibratory quality.

When to refer

A cardiac murmur associated with any of the following requires clinical assessment by a specialist.

History:

- Family history of cardiomyopathy.
- Family history of sudden unexplained death.
- Maternal diabetes.
- Chromosomal disorder.
- Congenital malformation of other organs.

Examination:

- Cyanosis.
- Breathlessness.
- Failure to thrive not clearly due to other causes.
- Unequal pulses.

Murmur characteristics:

- Thrill.
- Diastolic murmur.
- Continuous murmur with no postural variation.
- Pan-systolic murmur.
- Loud murmur (amplitude Grade 3/6 or greater).
- Murmur harsh or high pitched.
- Murmur heard best at left upper sternal border.
- Abnormal second heart sound.
- Early or mid-systolic click.

Worrying CXR

- Enlarged heart.
- Abnormal cardiac contour.
- Pulmonary plethora.
- ↓ Pulmonary vascular markings.

Worrying ECG

- Abnormal QRS axis.
- Increased voltages.
- Abnormal intervals.
- ST/T wave changes.

THE UNWELL NEONATE

Congenital heart disease is a differential in any neonate with:

- Shock.
- Respiratory distress.
- Cyanosis.
- Poor pulses.

Severe sepsis has very similar manifestations to critically obstructed systemic circulation (e.g. hypoplastic left heart, critical aortic stenosis, coarctation).

Use of prostaglandin (PGE_1)

- There are no congenital cardiac lesions for which PGE_1 is absolutely contraindicated (initial dose PGE_1 0.01 mcg/kg/min i.v. = 10 ng/kg/min).
- The risk-benefit is in favour of PGE_1 infusion if:
  - Patient is in extremis.
  - Cyanosis with murmur.
  - Abnormal pulses.

Early ECG and paediatric echocardiography should be sought for infants with any of the above symptoms.

NEONATAL CYANOSIS

Cyanosis in any neonate must be investigated.

Consider congenital heart disease (right sided obstructive lesions and mixing defects), parenchymal lung disease and persistent fetal circulation.

Initial assessment

- Chest X-ray – look at cardiac silhouette, pulmonary vascularity and parenchymal lung disease.
- Arterial blood gases – look for acidosis, pCO_2.
- A 12 lead ECG should be performed. A normal ECG should have a rate 100–150 and a P-wave, which should be upright in leads I and aVF, preceding each QRS complex.
- Echocardiography remains the diagnostic test of choice.
- Nitrogen washout test:
  - After 10 min breathing 100% O_2, take right radial arterial blood gas.
  - A $P_aO_2 > 150$ mmHg suggests cyanosis is **not** due to structural heart disease.
  - A $P_aO_2 < 70$ mmHg will occur with most major cyanotic defects.
- Trial of inhaled nitric oxide.
  - May benefit the term neonate with persistent fetal circulation (PFC).
- Trial of prostaglandin (PGE_1).
  - Will result in considerable improvement with duct-dependent congenital heart disease.

HEART FAILURE AFTER THE NEONATAL PERIOD

Main causes

- Congenital heart defects with pressure or volume overload (+/– cyanosis).
- Cardiomyopathies – anthracycline medications, infectious, metabolic, muscle disorders.
- Myocardial dysfunction after repair or palliation of heart defects.
- Tachyarrhythmia.
- Rheumatic heart disease.

Manifestations

Infants and young children have non-specific symptoms and signs:

- Dyspnoea, fatigue, difficulty in feeding, perspiration.
- Failure to thrive, exercise intolerance.
- Gallop rhythm, hepatomegaly, cardiomegaly on chest X-ray.

Older children may have signs more like those in adults:

- Breathlessness, fatigue, exercise intolerance, orthopnoea.
- Nocturnal dyspnoea, venous distension, peripheral oedema.

Management principles

- Seek an anatomical and functional diagnosis as early as possible with echocardiography.
- Oxygen for hypoxia related to pulmonary congestion or respiratory infection.
- Pharmacological measures:
  - Diminish pulmonary and systemic venous congestion
    - Frusemide – 1 mg/kg per dose (8-hourly, 12-hourly or daily).
    - Spironolactone (dose by weight) 0–10 kg 6.25 mg/dose oral (12 or 24-hourly), 11–20 kg 12.5 mg/dose oral (12 or 24-hourly) and 21–40 kg 25 mg/dose oral (12 or 24-hourly).
  - Decrease loading conditions.
    - Captopril – 0.1–1 mg/kg/dose (max 50 mg) oral 8-hourly.
    - Lisinopril – 0.1 mg/kg/dose (max 5 mg) oral daily.
    - Commence ACE inhibitor in hospital to monitor blood pressure.
    - Monitor serum potassium if using spironolactone.

   - Inotropes for acute, low-output cardiac failure:
     - Dobutamine – Initially 5 mcg/kg/min i.v.
     - Dopamine – Initially 5 mcg/kg/min i.v.
     - Milrinone – 50 mcg/kg over 10 mins i.v. then 0.375–0.75 mcg/kg/min.
   - Correct severe acidosis (pH <7.0)
     - Sodium bicarbonate (see Pharmacopoeia).
- Positive pressure ventilation
- Attend complicating factors:
   - Infection.
   - Anaemia.
   - Arrhythmia.
   - Malnutrition.

HYPERCYANOTIC SPELLS ('TETRALOGY SPELLS')

Severe cyanotic spells are a characteristic feature of Fallots tetralogy but may occasionally occur with other cyanotic lesions.

Background

- Severe cyanosis with agitation and breathlessness.
- Mechanism probably involves increased right ventricle (RV) outflow tract contractility, peripheral vasodilatation and hyperventilation.
- The RV outflow tract murmur becomes softer and may become inaudible.
- Often precipitated by exertion, feeding or crying, but can be spontaneous.
- Spells usually occur in the morning, during summer months and during intercurrent illness.
- Most episodes are self-limiting, lasting 15–30 minutes, but can be prolonged or result in loss of consciousness.

Management

Initial

- Avoid exacerbating distress.
- Try to console the child by cradling, soothing or nursing in knee-chest position.

- Give high flow oxygen via mask or head box.
- Morphine 0.2 mg/kg i.m. may help in severe cases.
- Continuous ECG and oxygen saturation monitoring, frequent BP monitoring.
- Correct any underlying cause, e.g. arrhythmia, hypothermia, hypoglycaemia.

If prolonged

- Intravenous fluids – 0.9% normal saline 10 mL/kg bolus followed by maintenance fluids.
- Correct acidosis – sodium bicarbonate 1–2 mmol/kg i.v.

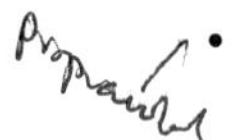

- Beta-blocking drugs – i.v. esmolol 0.5 mg/kg over 1 min, then 50–200 mcg/kg/min for up to 48 h.
- Intubation and positive pressure ventilation may be required in extreme cases.

A hypercyanotic spell is, in most cases, an indication for palliative or corrective surgery. Propranolol (orally) may be given prophylactically to prevent spells in a child awaiting surgery.

SUPRAVENTRICULAR TACHYCARDIA (SVT)

Seek urgent specialist advice if any tachycardia is broad complex or irregular, or fails to respond to the management advised below.

Definition

Supraventricular tachycardia is usually a regular, narrow complex tachycardia, with heart rate (HR) around 160–300 beats/min.

Differential diagnosis

Sinus tachycardia up to 230 beats/min may occur in the neonate with:

- Hypovolaemia.
- Hypoventilation.
- Pain.
- Fever.
- Pulmonary hypertension.

Note: Ventricular tachycardia in the neonate can have a relatively narrow QRS complex.

Clinical features

- In utero – may cause hydrops.
- Infancy – irritability, pallor, dyspnoea, poor feeding.
- Older children – palpitations, chest discomfort.
- Hypotension may be present.
- Congestive cardiac failure may occur in infants.

Initial management

- Physical examination: pulse, BP, murmur, heart failure.
- 12 lead ECG to check tachycardia is narrow complex.

Patient normotensive and well perfused

Infant and young child

- Ice water in bag or icepack to face for a few seconds only.
- Oropharyngeal suctioning.
- Gag with spatula.

Older child (if co-operative)

- Try vagal manoeuvres: Valsalva manoeuvre (e.g. forced blow through straw).
- Intravenous adenosine:
  - Need full resuscitation facilities available.
  - Intravenous access in a large, proximal vein.
  - Record a continuous ECG rhythm strip throughout administration, to monitor the pattern of reversal.
  - Begin with adenosine dose 0.1 mg/kg as an initial bolus (max 6 mg), then double (0.2 mg/kg) and repeat once (max 12 mg).
  - Dilute small doses of adenosine with saline to allow rapid infusion.
  - Give adenosine quickly, followed immediately with a 2–5 mL normal saline flush.
  - Wait 2 minutes between doses and check patient's vital signs.
  - Side effects of adenosine: facial flush, chest pain, bronchospasm.

Patient shocked (hypotensive, poor perfusion, impaired mental state)

- Ensure child is given oxygen and has intravenous access.
- The airway should be managed by experienced staff.
- Administer midazolam 0.2 mg/kg (max 10 mg) i.v. to minimise awareness
- D/C revert using a **synchronised** shock of 1 Joule/kg.

Subsequent management

After stabilisation of SVT, specialist review is required for:

- 12 lead ECG in sinus rhythm (pre-excitation and other abnormality)
- Echocardiogram (structural associations of atrioventricular re-entry SVT e.g. Ebstein's anomaly, cardiomyopathy)
- 24-hour Holter monitor (intermittent pre-excitation and initiating triggers such as premature atrial contractions)
- Decisions regarding prophylaxis, electrophysiological study

INFECTIVE ENDOCARDITIS

For infective endocarditis to develop, two independent events are normally required: a damaged area of endothelium and bacteraemia caused by adherent organisms.

Presentation

- Usually insidious and non-specific presentation.
- Often suggestive of intercurrent viral illness.
- Fever, anorexia, myalgia, arthralgia, headache, general malaise.

Splenomegaly, splinter haemorrhages, petechiae and other peripheral stigmata are rarely seen in children.

Diagnosis

- Multiple blood cultures (from separate sites and at different times), prior to antibiotic administration.

Table 18.1 Children at risk of infective endocarditis

Children at high risk	*Children at risk*	*Not usually at risk*
Cyanotic heart defects Prosthetic valves Conduits Shunts Previous endocarditis Intravenous drug use	Structural congenital heart defects (except isolated secundum ASD) Operated heart defects (except repaired secundum ASD and PDA) Acquired valve disease Endocardial pacemakers Intra-vascular lines / shunts	Physiologic, functional or 'innocent' murmurs Non-structural problems (e.g. arrhythmia, cardiac pacemaker) Previous Kawasaki disease without valvular dysfunction

- Full blood count.
- ESR and CRP.
- Echocardiogram.
  - Transoesophageal echo may be more sensitive than trans-thoracic echo.
  - The sensitivity or specificity of echocardiography are not 100%, thus **a normal echocardiogram does not exclude endocarditis**.

Management

- Admission to hospital.
- Commence empiric antibiotis.
  - Native valve/homograft: benzylpenicillin 60 mg/kg (max 2 g) i.v. 6-hourly and gentamicin 2.5 mg/kg i.v. (synergistic dose) 8-hourly and flucloxacillin 50 mg/kg (max 2 g) i.v. 6-hourly.
  - Prosthetic valve: vancomycin 15 mg/kg (max 500 mg) i.v. 6-hourly and gentamicin 2.5 mg/kg i.v. 8-hourly.
- Prolonged antibiotic therapy and specialist consultation are required.
- Close monitoring of clinical and cardiovascular status including serial echocardiographs, serial blood cultures and inflammatory markers.
- Close monitoring for evidence of other embolic phenomena.

Endocarditis prophylaxis

- Children at risk should establish and maintain the best possible oral health to reduce potential sources of bacteraemia.
- Antibiotic prophylaxis is recommended for children at risk, undergoing procedures likely to cause a bacteraemia (see Antimicrobial guidelines).

CHAPTER 19
DENTAL CONDITIONS

Nicky Kilpatrick
James Lucas

DENTAL DEVELOPMENT

Primary dentition

Teeth start to form from the 5th week in utero and may continue until the late teens or early twenties. The first teeth to erupt are usually the lower central primary incisors at around 7 months of age. Table 19.1 summarises the mean eruption dates for primary teeth.

If an infant shows no sign of any primary teeth by the age of 18 months they should be referred to a paediatric dentist.

By the age of $2\frac{1}{2}$ years most children will have a complete primary dentition consisting of 20 teeth; 8 incisors, 4 canines and 8 molars (see Figure 19.1). In most cases all primary or deciduous teeth are ultimately replaced, however, some individuals are missing permanent teeth and primary teeth may be retained into adulthood.

Permanent dentition

The permanent teeth start to form in the jaws around birth. At around the age of 6 years the primary incisors become mobile and fall out. The tooth fairy then comes to visit. The permanent dentition begins to develop starting with the eruption of the lower first permanent molars behind the second primary molars (Table 19.2). Permanent teeth are much larger than the primary predecessors and often look more yellow

Table 19.1 Eruption sequence of primary dentition (months after birth)

Central Incisors	*Lateral Incisors*	*Canines*	*First Molars*	*Second Molars*
6–12	9–16	16–23	13–19	23–33

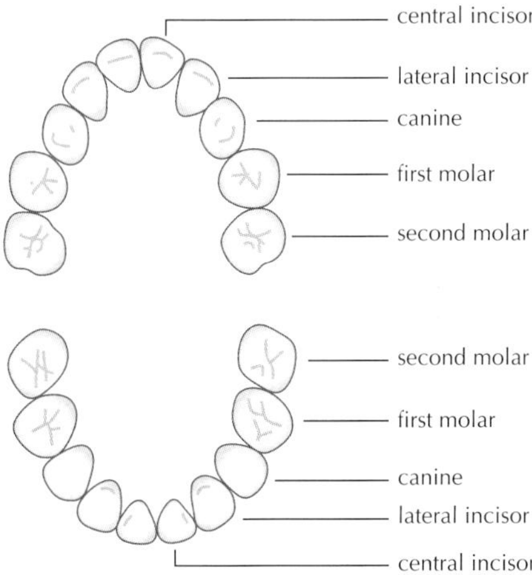

Fig. 19.1 Primary Dentition

Table 19.2 Eruption sequence of permanent dentition (years of age)

Central incisors	*Lateral Incisors*	*Canines*	*First premolars*	*Second Premolars*	*First molars*	*Second Molars*	*Third Molars*
6–8	6.5–8.5	9–13	9.5–11.5	10–13	5.5–7.0	11–13	17+

or cream in colour. The period that follows, referred to as the mixed dentition phase, is highly variable. Some second primary molar teeth are replaced by the second premolars as late as 14 years of age. The first, second and third permanent molars have no primary predecessors. Figure 19.2 shows the permanent dentition.

The simultaneous presence of primary and permanent teeth in the same site during the mixed dentition stage is common and is not a cause for concern.

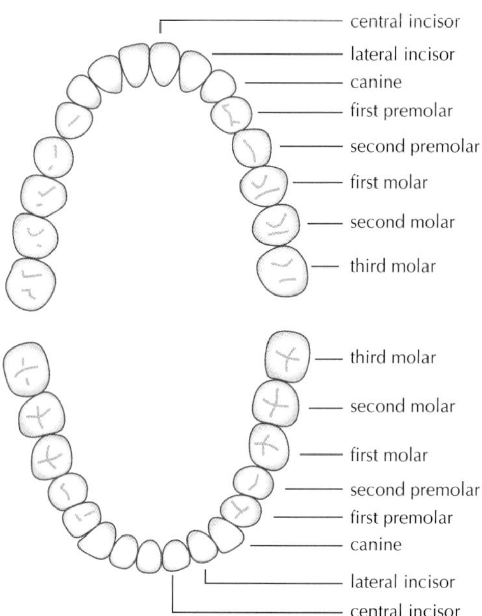

Fig. 19.2 Permanent Dentition

DENTAL CARIES

Dental caries (or decay) remains one of the most common childhood diseases. While in Australia just over 60% of 5 year-olds and 55% of 12 year-olds are decay free, 80% of all decay is experienced by 20% of children. It is therefore important to identify children at high decay risk and specifically target them for prevention both on a community and individual level (Table 19.3).

Dental decay can occur as soon as teeth erupt.

Early childhood caries (ECC) is a particular form of dental decay that is seen in infants as young as 18 months of age. It affects over 6% of Australian infants and has a characteristic appearance in which the upper front teeth are affected on their labial (or lip) surfaces. The

Table 19.3 Common risk factors for dental caries assessable by medical practitioners

Risk factor	*Influence*
Sugar exposure	Infant feeding habits are very important with frequency of exposure being most relevant. High risk associated with prolonged on demand night time feeds and day time grazing patterns
Family oral health history	Poor parental oral health places child at risk of decay as cariogenic bacteria are transmitted from the primary care giver.
Fluoride exposure	Exposure to fluoridated water source and the regular use of fluoridated toothpaste are two key factors that reduce caries risk.
Social and family practices	Low SES, ethnic and migrant groups have higher levels of dental disease.
Medical history	Medically compromised children are more at risk of dental decay and are less likely to receive appropriate treatment.

cariogenic bacteria causing ECC are transmitted from primary care giver to child and decay is closely associated with infant feeding habits.

Prevention

The prevention of dental decay should start as soon as the first teeth erupt.

There are 4 aspects to preventing decay:

Diet

- Minimise the total amount and reduce frequency of intake of sugary foods and drinks.
- Limit sugary snacks to meal times when salivary flow is optimal.
- Minimise intake of drinks with high acidity (e.g. carbonated, fruit and sports drinks); they cause erosion of the teeth.
- Increase water intake.
- Encourage drinking from feeder cup.
- Avoid demand feeding at night-time.

Oral hygiene

- Toothbrushing should commence within 6 months of the eruption of the first tooth.

- Parents should supervise toothbrushing until around 8 years of age.
- Use toothbrush with small head for infants and use only a 'smear' of toothpaste.
- For under 5 year olds use a low fluoride (Junior) toothpaste.

Fluoride

- Fluoride enhances the ability of teeth to resist demineralization caused by sugar acids.
- Apart from systemic water fluoridation, the most common source of fluoride is from toothpaste.
- Most adult toothpastes contain around 1000 ppm.
- Junior toothpastes contain a lower concentrations of fluoride – around 400 ppm.
- The use of additional topical fluoride supplements (tablets or drops) can be of benefit on an individual basis but should only be prescribed by an appropriate dental professional.

Regular dental check ups

- Children should see a dental professional within 6 months of the eruption of the first tooth.
- The first visit is a 'well baby' visit aimed at providing 'anticipatory guidance'.
- Children should have a dental check up at least annually.
- The frequency of dental attendance will vary according to disease risk assessment.

DENTAL EMERGENCIES

Toothache

- Assess level and nature of pain (e.g. intermittent pain on eating or in response to hot/cold or spontaneous pain at night).
- Provide analgesia (paracetamol should be adequate).
- Refer to dentist for assessment and treatment of the affected tooth.

Dental abscess

Presentation

- History of spontaneous pain particularly at night, pain may be constant.

- May or may not have recently had fillings placed.
- Swelling evident intra-orally near teeth.
- Red swollen face, unilateral and often spreading up under the orbit or under the mandible.
- Limited mouth opening.
- Elevated temperature and a generally unwell child.
- Tender teeth on side of the swelling.
- Enlarged lymph glands.

Investigations

- Orthopantogram (OPG) – will show dental pathology and usually decay.

Management

- Consider oral amoxicillin for early infection.
- Admit to hospital if red swollen face, fever and generally unwell.
- Intravenous antibiotics (benzylpenicillin in the first instance) and i.v. fluids.
- Extraction of the tooth is almost always indicated.
- Occasionally additional soft tissue drainage is required, however, dental abscesses in young children usually manifest with cellulitis rather than a collection of frank pus.

DENTAL TRAUMA

Traumatic injuries to the facial region can affect the teeth, soft tissues and jaw bones.

Assessment

Consider:

- How the injury occurred?
- Were there any other injuries?
- Time of the injury?
- Where are the teeth or fragments of teeth?
- How much of the tooth is broken off or how far is the tooth displaced?
- Can the patient bite their teeth together or does the displaced tooth get in the way?
- Are there associated soft tissue (mucosal) injuries?
- Is the avulsed tooth stored in milk?

Table 19.4 Dental trauma – Primary dentition

Injury	*Management*
No tooth displacement	Non urgent referral to dentist for review
Intrusion – tooth upwards and inwards	Needs dental review within 24 h to accurately locate the tooth Probably will re-erupt Otherwise will need to be extracted
Luxation – tooth palatal or sideways	Needs dental referral within 12 h Will need extraction sooner rather than later
Avulsion – knocked out completely	**Do not** replant primary teeth Needs dental review within 24 h

Locate all teeth or tooth fragments because;

- Most permanent teeth and tooth fragments can be replaced/recemented.
- 'Missing' teeth may have been intruded (pushed in) rather than knocked out.

Primary dentition

Never replant a primary tooth.

Injury (particularly intrusion) to a primary incisor can damage the permanent successor, therefore a dental review for all injuries is important (see Table 19.4).

Mucosal injuries should be assessed as they may require suturing. Refer to a dentist.

Permanent dentition

Whenever possible an OPG is useful as it allows a full review of the jaws, jaw joints and teeth. A chest X-ray is useful if the tooth or fragments cannot be located. Many injuries can be managed under local anaesthesia depending on the co-operation of the child and the presence of associated soft tissue or other bony injuries (see Table 19.5).

An avulsed permanent tooth is a genuine emergency and should be triaged as such. The longer the tooth is out of the mouth the worse the prognosis.

The impact on a young person of loosing a front tooth psychosocially, as well as economically, in the long term should not be underestimated. Correct emergency management can make a significant difference to the prognosis of any injured tooth.

Table 19.5 Dental trauma – Permanent dentition

Injury	*Management*
Fracture	
– < 1/3 crown	Non urgent referral to dentist
– > 1/3	Locate fragments, store in milk. Needs dental review within 24 h Some fragments can be stuck back on to broken teeth
Mobile but not displaced	Soft diet and analgesia Needs dental review within 12 h May need dental splint
Displacements	All these injuries should be referred to a paediatric dentist within 12 h.
– Intrusions	Locate teeth, using radiographs. Tooth may re-erupt or may require surgical or orthodontic repositioning
– Luxations	Use gentle finger pressure to reposition teeth, if in doubt leave alone. Loose splinting can be achieved using tin foil until patient sees dentist as soon as possible.
– Avulsions	**Urgent** referral to dentist Replace tooth in socket if possible. If not, store in milk at all times

Mucosal lacerations

Check carefully intra-orally for degloving injuries. This is where the gum tissue around the teeth is stripped away form the underlying bone. Unless the lips are retracted this injury is easily missed. These injuries need suturing under general anaesthesia.

Many tongue and intra-oral lip lacerations do not need suturing and heal well when left.

Extra-oral lacerations, particularly those crossing the vermilion border on to the skin, should be referred to a plastic surgeon.

In all cases of dental trauma – Lift the lips and look in!

Fractures to the jaw bones

Whenever a jaw fracture is suspected, a maxillofacial surgeon should be called. If teeth are also obviously displaced or lost, a paediatric dentist should also be called.

An OPG, lateral cephalometric view and/or a variety of occipitomental/antero-posterior radiographic views can be useful in inspecting the facial complex for fractures.

Commence antibiotics and consider tetanus prophylaxis should be considered in any compound fractures opening to mouth or skin (see Procedures, Chapter 4).

BLEEDING FROM THE MOUTH

If child has been bleeding for some time, assess haemodynamic status.

Clean the mouth with cold water or saline and remove any debris, blood, tissue etc. Identify source of bleeding – usually an extraction socket.

Bleeding socket

- Compress the sides of the socket together using finger pressure.
- If child is co-operative place a slightly damp gauze pack over the socket and have child bite down on to it for 20 minutes. Parents may be asked to assist. Do not pack anything into the socket.
- Refer to a dentist.

CHAPTER 20
DERMATOLOGIC CONDITIONS

Rod Phillips
John Su
George Varigos

INTRODUCTION

The key to accurate diagnosis and hence to appropriate management of skin disorders in children is a careful history and astute observation of rashes, particularly focusing on their appearance, site and pattern of development. During the examination consider a few key questions (see also Figure 20.1).

- Are there any vesicles, i.e. fluid-filled lesions? Finding these narrows greatly the range of possible diagnoses. Small circular erosions may be the only signs of an underlying vesicular process.
- Is the rash raised (papular) or flat (macular)?
- Is the rash red? Redness is from haemoglobin. Most red rashes blanch, i.e. the redness disappears with pressure. If not, the haemoglobin is outside the blood vessels (purpura).
- Is the rash scaly? If so, the epidermis may be broken (eczematous) to give weeping, crusting or bleeding, or it may be intact (papulosquamous).

VESICULOBULLOUS RASHES

Vesicles are usually caused by infections (herpes simplex virus (HSV), varicella zoster virus (VZV), enterovirus, tinea, scabies or impetigo) or contact dermatitis. Also, consider drug reactions and erythema multiforme. Larger blisters may be from Staphylococcal infections, Stevens-Johnson syndrome, arthropod bites, contact dermatitis, burns or trauma.

Impetigo (school sores)

Cause

Staphylococcus aureus or *Streptococcus pyogenes*, or both.

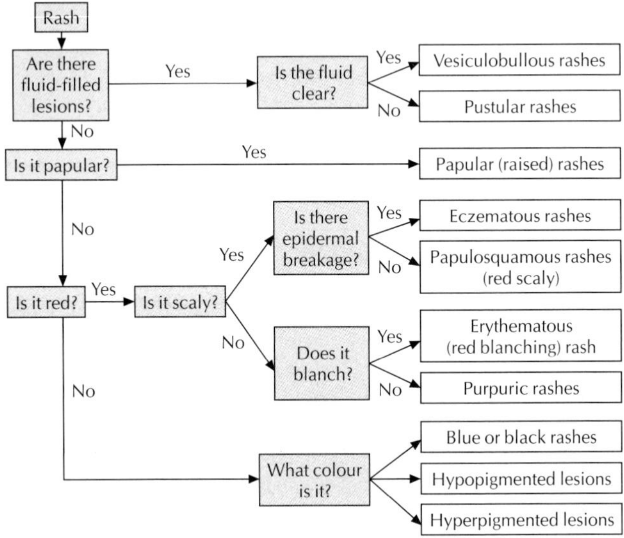

Vesiculobullous rashes
- Impetigo (school sores)
- Eczema herpeticum
- Erythema multiforme
- Single blisters

Pustular rashes
- Acne

Papular (raised) rashes
- Scabies
- Urticaria/serum sickness
- Papular urticaria
- Keratosis pilaris
- Papular acrodermatitis
- Molluscum
- Warts

Eczematous rashes
- Atopic eczema

Red scaly rashes (papulosquamous)
- Seborrhoeic dermatitis
- Psoriasis
- Tinea corporis
- Pityriasis rosea

Red blanching rashes (erythematous)
- Fever and exanthem
- Erythema infectiosum

Red blanching rashes (erythematous)
- Roseola infantum
- Kawasaki disease

Purpuric rashes
- Enteroviral infection
- Septicaemia
- Leukaemia
- Henoch–Schoenlein purpura
- Child abuse
- Idiopathic thrombocytopenic purpura (ITP)
- Trauma and vasomotor straining

Blue or black rashes
- Vascular malformations
- Haemangiomas

Hypopigmented lesions
- Tinea versicolor
- Pityriasis alba
- Vitiligo
- Post-inflammatory hypo- and hyperpigmentation

Hyperpigmented lesions
- Congenital pigmented naevi
- Acquired pigmented naevi

Fig. 20.1 Classification of skin disorders in children

Clinical features

Impetigo presents as areas of ooze and honey-coloured crusts on the face, trunk or limbs. Occasionally, the primary lesions are bullous. Lesions are rounded and well demarcated and may be single, grouped or widespread. Their onset and spread may be rapid or occur over days. In more chronic cases, there may be central healing with peripheral spread to give annular lesions.

Management

- Bathe off crusts.
- Apply topical mupirocin 2% ointment 8-hourly if localised, or flucloxacillin 15 mg/kg (max 500 mg) orally, 6-hourly if severe or extensive.
- Isolate the child from other children or from sick adults unless all lesions are covered or treated.
- Treat any underlying condition such as scabies (a common cause of widespread impetigo) or eczema.

Staphylococcal scalded skin syndrome

Clinical features

- Usually seen in younger children.
- Mediated by an epidermolytic toxin released from an often insignificant staphylococcal focus (e.g. eyes, nose or skin).
- Fever and tender erythematous skin are early features.
- Exudation and crusting develops, especially around the mouth.
- Wrinkling, flaccid bullae and exfoliation of the skin are seen – Nikolsky sign ('normal' skin separates if rubbed).
- Blisters are very superficial and heal without scarring.

Management

- Flucloxacillin 50 mg/kg (max 2 g) i.v. 6-hourly if there is evidence of sepsis or systemic involvement.
- Look for a focus of infection. Drain any foci of pus if present.
- Monitor temperature, fluids and electrolytes if large areas are involved.
- Handle skin carefully and use an emollient ointment.

Erythema multiforme

Clinical features

This is a specific hypersensitivity syndrome that occurs at any age. Lesions are usually symmetric and appear most commonly on the hands, feet and often the face. They can be found anywhere.

Typical target lesions have an inner zone of epidermal injury (purpura, necrosis or vesicle), an outer zone of erythema and sometimes a middle zone of pale oedema. They are not migratory. The involvement of mucous membranes is common and can be extensive. Most cases are caused by herpes simplex, some by other infections. Drugs are an uncommon cause.

Management

- Fluid maintenance.
- Apply emollient ointment to the lips, if needed.
- If the condition is recurrent, it is highly likely to be related to HSV. Prophylactic aciclovir should be considered if recurrences are frequent, severe and affecting the quality of life.

Stevens-Johnson syndrome/toxic epidermal necrolysis

Clinical features

- Stevens-Johnson syndrome and toxic epidermal necrolysis are believed by many to be variants of the one condition.
- They are characterised by widespread blisters on an erythematous or purpuric macular background, often with extensive mucous membrane haemorrhagic crusting.
- There may be tender erythematous areas with a positive Nikolsky sign ('normal' skin separates if rubbed).
- Conjunctivitis, corneal ulceration and blindness can occur.
- Anogenital lesions can lead to urinary retention.
- Fever, myalgia, arthralgia and other organ involvement can occur.
- Drugs are the most common cause, occasionally Mycoplasma.

Management

- Cease any drug that may be the cause.
- Fluid maintenance.
- Apply emollient ointment to the skin, lips and anogenital areas – this may be required many times a day.

- A regular eye examination with a specialist review for topical steroid drops if any eye involvement is noted.
- Corticosteroids may lessen the severity of the condition. Cyclosporin (5–6 mg/kg/day for a few days, then taper to 3–5 mg/kg for 2–3 weeks) is an alternative.

Note: Stevens-Johnson syndrome is not severe erythema multiforme (EM). They are distinct conditions with different aetiologies. Permanent sequelae are rarely seen in severe EM and concurrent drug use is unlikely to be the cause. Skin lesion morphology is the best discriminating factor; mucous membrane involvement can be seen in both conditions.

Eczema herpeticum

Clinical features

Herpes simplex virus infection in children with eczema is common, but many cases are misdiagnosed as either an exacerbation of the eczema or bacterial infection. Grouped vesicles may be prominent, but more often vesicles are rudimentary or absent and the infection presents as a group of shallow 2–4 mm ulcers on an inflamed base. The infected area may not be painful or itchy and does not respond to standard eczema therapy. If untreated, resolution usually occurs in 1–4 weeks, but dissemination may occur. Recurrences may occur at different sites.

Management

- Collect epithelial cells from the base and roof of the vesicles for herpes immunofluorescence and culture.
- Local disease in an otherwise well child requires regular observation but does not need antiviral therapy.
- A child with fever or multiple sites of cutaneous herpes infection may need admission to hospital and treatment with i.v. aciclovir 20 mg/kg per dose (2–12 weeks), 250 mg/m^2 per dose (12 weeks-12 years), 5 mg/kg per dose (>12 years) 8-hourly i.v. over 1 h.
- Milder cases demonstrating progression or facial involvement can be managed with oral acyclovir.
- Eye involvement should be managed with topical or systemic aciclovir, or both and urgent review by an ophthalmologist.
- The underlying eczema can be treated with moisturiser or wet dressings.

Single blisters

For a child who presents with a single blister as an isolated finding, consider mastocytoma, insect bite, cigarette burn, friction or spider bite. The latter can grow over days to become a non-tender blister with a diameter of many centimetres.

PUSTULAR RASHES

Consider acne, folliculitis, scabies and perioral dermatitis.

Acne

Clinical features

Acne mainly affects the forehead and face but can involve other sebaceous gland areas (neck, shoulders and upper trunk). Early lesions include blackheads, whiteheads and papules. In more severe cases there may be pustules or inflammatory cysts that can lead to permanent scarring. Undertreated acne is a cause of significant morbidity in adolescents and may be a factor in teenage suicide. Consider underlying endocrine disorders if acne begins before puberty.

Management

- Acne is treatable. No person with acne should just be told it is an inevitable part of adolescence. Effective acne therapies are now available and should be used to control the disease.
- For mild disease, use topical benzoyl peroxide 2.5–5%. Other topical agents include antibiotics (clindamycin, erythromycin or tetracycline), isotretinoin (not in pregnancy) or azelaic acid. These can be used singly or in combination. Improvement occurs over 1–2 months, not within days. All of these topical agents have side effects with which practitioners must be familiar.
- Treatment of moderate acne often involves the addition of oral antibiotic therapy (e.g. tetracycline 500 mg twice daily, erythromycin 500 mg twice daily, doxycycline 50–200 mg per day) for 3–6 months. Oral hormone therapy can help female patients.
- If antibiotics and topical treatment have not resulted in considerable improvement in 3 months, oral isotretinoin (Roaccutane) is indicated. Provided pregnancy is avoided, this is safe and highly

effective. Isotretinoin is also indicated if there is scarring, cyst formation, or significant depression. Treatment of severe acne with Roaccutane appears to decrease the risk of suicide. Assessment and treatment of any depression is also required.

PAPULAR (RAISED) RASHES

If the child is itchy, consider scabies, urticaria, serum sickness, papular urticaria or molluscum. If not, consider urticaria, molluscum, warts, melanocytic naevi, keratosis pilaris and papular acrodermatitis. For soft red, purple or blue swellings, consider haemangiomas or vascular malformations. For raised red circles or rings, consider urticaria.

Scabies

Clinical features

An intensely itchy papular eruption develops 2–6 weeks after first exposure to the *Sarcoptes scabiei* mite or 1–4 days after subsequent reinfestation. The characteristic lesion is the burrow that is several millimetres in length. Burrows are best seen on the hands, especially between the fingers, and on the feet. Early burrows may be vesicular. Papules can occur anywhere including the palms, soles and genitalia. Excoriations and secondary impetigo may be present. There is currently a worldwide pandemic of this contagious disease affecting both adults and children.

Management

- Treatment is expensive and upsetting. If diagnosis is unclear, confirm by scraping to find a mite, or refer before treating.
- Use permethrin 5% cream. An alternative for pregnant women or neonates is sulphur 2% in yellow soft paraffin. The following are *not recommended*: lindane 1% (contraindicated in infants or women who are pregnant or breast-feeding) or benzyl benzoate 25% (too irritating for children and ineffective if diluted).
- At the same time, treat all family members and any other people who have close skin contact with the affected individuals.
- Apply to dry skin (not after a bath) from the neck down to all skin surfaces. For infants, apply to the scalp as well (not face). Use mittens if necessary to prevent finger sucking.

- Leave the cream on for at least 8 h.
- Wash the cream off. Wash clothing, pyjamas and bed linen at this time.
- The itch takes a week or two to settle and can be treated with calamine lotion or an antihistamine, or both.
- Reinfestation is common. The family should notify all social contacts (e.g. crèche, school or close friends) to ensure that all those infected receive treatment.

Urticaria/serum sickness

See also Allergy and immunology, chapter 16.

Clinical features

Urticaria is characterised by the rapid appearance and disappearance of multiple raised red wheals on any part of the body. Individual lesions are often itchy and clear within 1 day. There may be central clearing to give ring lesions (these are not the so-called target lesions of erythema multiforme that persist for several days). The child is usually well. Urticarial episodes usually resolve over days or weeks and rarely last longer than 6 months. In most cases of short duration, the cause cannot be determined.

Some children develop fever and arthralgias in association with urticarial lesions that are more fixed and may bruise or be tender (serum sickness). In Australia, serum sickness is usually idiopathic or following a course of cefaclor.

Management

- Urticaria may be the first sign of anaphylaxis. If there is associated angio-oedema (prominent subcutaneous swelling) or wheeze, continued observation and appropriate treatment is required (see Medical Emergencies, chapter 1).
- Investigation is usually not required.
- Ask about medications.
- Treat the itch with oral antihistamine (Refer to Allergy and immunology, chapter 16, page 245). A few days of oral prednisolone (1mg/kg per day (max 50 mg)) may be beneficial in serum sickness but is rarely warranted in urticaria. Bed rest for joint involvement.

- For recurrent or chronic urticaria that persists for months, look for trigger factors. Consider mast cell degranulating drugs, foods, animals, parasitic infections, heat, cold and physical pressure. Consider investigating with a throat swab (for streptococcal carriage), full blood examination (for eosinophilia and anaemia), antinuclear antibodies, urine culture for bacteriuria, nocturnal check for threadworms and a possible challenge with any suspected agent. Adding cimetidine (10 mg/kg (max 200 mg) p.o. 6-hourly) to the antihistamine may help.
- If individual lesions last longer than 2 days or are tender or purpuric, consider investigation for cutaneous vasculitis.

Papular urticaria

Clinical features

This is a clinical hypersensitivity to insect bites. New bites appear as groups of small red papules, usually in warmer weather. Older bites appear as 1–5 mm papules, sometimes with surface scale or crust, or with surrounding urticaria. Vesicles or pustules may form. Individual lesions may resolve in a week or last for months and may repeatedly flare up after fresh bites elsewhere. The itch is often intense and secondary ulceration or infection is common.

Management

- Prevent bites (e.g. adequate clothing, modifying behaviour that leads to exposure, occasional repellent and the treatment of pets and house for fleas if necessary).
- Treat the itch with an agent such as aluminium sulphate 20% (Stingose), liquor picis carbonis 2% in calamine lotion, moderate potency steroid ointment or antihistamines (see Allergy and immunology, chapter 16, page 245). Protective dressings (e.g. Duoderm) can speed the healing of lesions.
- Treat secondary infection with topical mupirocin ointment 2% or oral antibiotics.

Keratosis pilaris

Clinical features

This is a rough, somewhat spiky papular rash on the upper outer arms, thighs, cheeks, or all three areas, with variable erythema. It is common at all ages.

Management

- Reassure the patient that this is rarely a problem. Soap avoidance and moisturisers can improve the feel. Steroids don't help.
- Older children may get some benefit from topical keratolytics (e.g. Dermadrate, Calmurid).
- Older children with troublesome facial redness can be treated with vascular laser (V beam)

Papular acrodermatitis

Clinical features

This is characterised by the acute onset of monomorphic red or skin-coloured papules mainly on the arms, legs and face.

It is usually asymptomatic. It can be caused by coxsackie virus, echovirus, mycoplasma, EBV, adenovirus and others.

Management

Reassure and advise that clearing can take a few weeks.

Molluscum

Clinical features

Uncomplicated molluscum lesions are easily recognised as firm, pearly, dome-shaped papules with central umbilication, however, presentation to a doctor is often prompted by the development of eczema in surrounding skin. In such cases, recognition can be difficult as eczematous changes can obliterate the primary lesions. A careful history of the initial lesions is usually diagnostic.

Management

- Education – molluscum is caused by a virus and is very common. A child may develop a few, or a great many lesions and individual lesions may last for months. Complete resolution will not happen until an immune response develops, which may take from 3 months to 3 years.
- Children with molluscum should not share towels but should not be restricted in their activities.
- The treatment depends on the age of the child, the location of the lesions and any secondary changes. Things to note include:
  - Treatment of the surrounding eczema may be all that is required.

- Uncomplicated lesions not causing problems and not spreading can be left alone.
- Isolated or troublesome lesions (e.g. on the face) can be physically treated. One method is gentle cryotherapy.
- Occasionally, children warrant curettage under topical anaesthesia. This is well tolerated and usually curative. Alternatively, the stimulation of an immune response can be attempted with aluminium acetate solution (Burrow's solution 1:30) for large areas, or benzoyl peroxide 5% daily to small areas and covered with the adhesive part of a dressing.
- Inflamed lesions rarely warrant antibiotic treatment.

Warts

Many serotypes of the papilloma virus can cause warts. Different serotypes have a predilection for different areas of the skin. No treatment is necessary unless the warts are causing a problem to the child (e.g. social embarrassment, or pain from a plantar wart). Avoid painful procedures unless chosen by older children. Resistant warts on the limbs often respond to contact sensitisation (e.g. Diphenylcyclopropenone (DCP) 0.1% cream after sensitisation with 2% solution). Diphenylcyclopropenone use requires caution, supervision and possible dose adjustment, as there is a wide variation in individual responses.

- *Ordinary warts* – if tolerated by the child, paring every 2–3 days with a razor blade or nail file will remove the surface horn. Apply a proprietary keratolytic agent that contains salicylic or lactic acid, or both, each day or two as directed.
- *Plantar warts* – these can be painful and can appear flat. Pare as for ordinary warts. Apply a proprietary keratolytic agent that contains salicylic or lactic acid, or both, each day or two. Alternatively, apply the affected area of sole for 30 min each night to a small pad of cotton wool soaked in 3% formalin and placed in a saucer on the floor. Cryotherapy and surgery are often ineffective and can lead to painful keloid scarring.
- *Plane (flat) warts* – these are smooth, flat or slightly elevated, skin-coloured or pigmented lesions. They may occur in lines or coalesce to form plaque-like lesions. If treatment is needed for plane warts on the hands, apply a formalin solution as for ordinary warts. Lesions on the face are often subtle and may not need treatment. Treatment may cause complications such as pigmentary changes and requires considerable caution.

- *Anogenital warts* – these are soft fleshy warts that occur at the mucocutaneous junctions, especially around the anus. They may be isolated flesh-coloured nodules or may coalesce into large cauliflower-like masses. Management options include awaiting resolution, topical podophyllotoxin, imiquimod, curettage and diathermy and carbon dioxide laser

Note: the presence of genital warts in a young child is not an indication for mandatory reporting to government protective services. Genital warts in children should lead to consideration of sexual abuse, but transmission is usually by normal intimate parent-child contact.

ECZEMATOUS RASHES

Consider atopic eczema, allergic contact dermatitis, irritant contact dermatitis, photosensitivity eruptions, molluscum, tinea corporis and scabies.

Atopic eczema

See also Allergy and immunology, chapter 16.

Clinical features

Eczema usually begins in infancy. It commonly involves the face and often the trunk and limbs as well. In older children the rash may be widespread or may be localised to flexures. Erythema, weeping, excoriation and rarely vesicles may be seen in acute lesions. Chronic lesions may show scale and lichenification. In some children, the lesions are more clearly defined, thickened discoid areas that may intermittently be itchy. There is usually a cyclical pattern of improvement and exacerbation. Weeping and yellow-crusted areas that do not respond to therapy may indicate secondary bacterial or herpetic infection.

Management

- *Hospitalisation* – if a child is missing school because of eczema, they should generally be in hospital for intensive treatment.
- *Education* – parents need to know that treatments are effective in controlling the disease. Environmental and food allergens may contribute to the exacerbation of symptoms in some patients. Allergen avoidance in these children may be of some benefit.

- *Avoid irritants* – the following may worsen eczema: soaps, bubble baths, prickly clothing, seams and labels on clothing, car seat covers, sand, carpets, overheating or contact with pets. Smooth cotton clothing is preferred.
- *Keep the skin moist* – use a moisturiser such as paraffin ointment (50:50 white soft paraffin/liquid paraffin) as often as several times a day if necessary.
- *Treat inflammation* – in mild or moderate cases, steroid creams can be used intermittently with good effect. Hydrocortisone 1% is usually adequate. If not, moderate potency (e.g. beta-methasone valerate 0.02%) or potent (e.g. mometasone 0.1% or methyl-prednisolone 0.1%) ointment can be used for exacerbations in areas other than the face or nappy area. Prolonged regular use of moderate potency steroids to the skin of young children can cause atrophy and adrenal suppression. Oral steroids are rarely indicated in eczema. For chronic eczema on the limbs, zinc and tar combinations are alternatives to steroids.
- *Control itch* – advise parents to avoid saying 'Stop itching' all the time and to distract the child instead. Avoid overheating, particularly at night. Wet bandaging is very helpful if warranted. Antihistamines are often unhelpful but may be tried if the itch is not controlled by other measures (see Allergy and immunology, chapter 16). Terfenadine (Teldane) and astemizole (Hismanal) should not be used because of occasional fatal interactions if erythromycin is also taken.
- *Treat infection* – take cultures and treat with simple wet dressings and oral antibiotics (e.g. erythromycin, cephalexin or flucloxacillin). Consider if herpes simplex is present (see p. 291). For recurrent bacterial infection, use antiseptic wash or bath oil (e.g. triclosan).
- *Diet* – a normal diet is usually indicated. If a child has immediate urticarial reactions to a particular food, that food should be avoided. In difficult cases, consider a more formal allergy assessment.

RED SCALY RASHES (PAPULOSQUAMOUS)

Consider seborrhoeic dermatitis (infants), psoriasis, tinea corporis, pityriasis rosea, pityriasis versicolor and atopic eczema. Ichthyosis vulgaris is a common cause of generalised scale without itch or redness.

Seborrhoeic dermatitis

Clinical features

- This condition presents in the first months of life, partly due to the activity of commensal yeasts.
- Red or yellow/brown scaly areas will commonly affect the scalp, forehead and napkin area. The folds behind the ears and around the neck, axillae, groin and gluteal clefts are also affected.
- Resolution by the age of 1 year is usual.

Management

- Paraffin or olive oil applied to scalp to loosen scale
- Imidazole creams with hydrocortisone 1% cream or with a mixture of salicylic acid (1%) and sulphur (1%) ointment, twice daily.
- Anti-yeast shampoos (e.g. selenium sulphide – Selsun) can be helpful. Use carefully to avoid irritation or toxicity.

Psoriasis

Clinical features

Psoriasis can occur at any age. Lesions begin as small red papules that develop into circular, sharply demarcated erythematous patches with prominent silvery scale. Common presentations include plaques on extensor surfaces, generalised guttate (small) lesions, red scaly scalp lesions or moist red anogenital rashes. Itch can be a problem. Nail changes are often seen in childhood.

Management

- The treatment depends on the site and extent of disease and the age of the child. Adolescents are less tolerant of tar creams.
- Treat isolated skin plaques with either topical steroids (e.g. intermittent mometasone with clinical monitoring) or tar-based creams (e.g. liquor picis carbonis 3%, salicylic acid 2% in sorbolene cream). Generally avoid tars on the face, flexures and genitalia.
- Use hydrocortisone 1% ointment on the face and anogenital region. Topical steroids are not used for large areas in childhood psoriasis because of the possible development of rebound pustular disease.
- Thick scalp plaques can be softened overnight with a similar tar cream and removed with a tar shampoo.

- Topical calcipotriol can be used in children older than 12 years.
- Widespread psoriasis may need treatment with one or more of dithranol, etretinate, methotrexate, cyclosporin or ultraviolet therapy, all of which are effective.

Tinea corporis

Clinical features

The typical lesion is a slow-growing erythematous ring with a clear or scaly centre, however, tinea corporis can present in a wide variety of ways, particularly if previously treated with steroid ointments. It can be pustular or vesicular, or spread to many sites within days. Tinea should be considered in any red scaly rash where the diagnosis is unclear.

Management

- If in doubt about the diagnosis, confirm by scraping the scale for microscopy and culture.
- Lesions are treated with terbinafine cream (twice daily for 1 week), an imidazole cream (e.g. clotrimazole, miconazole or econazole 2–4 times per day, for 4 weeks) or oral griseofulvin for widespread lesions.

Pityriasis rosea

Clinical features

The condition is common between the ages of 1–10 years.

Initially, a pink scaly patch appears, followed a few days later by many pink/red scaly oval macules mainly on the trunk. It is usually asymptomatic.

Management

Reassure the patient. The condition can persist for weeks.

RED BLANCHING RASHES (ERYTHEMATOUS)

Macular erythematous lesions are most commonly caused by viral infections (e.g. coxsackie, echovirus, Epstein-Barr virus, adenovirus, para-influenza, influenza, parvovirus B19, human herpes virus 6 (HHV6), rubella and measles) or drug reactions. Consider also septicaemia, scarlet fever, Kawasaki disease (see Infectious diseases, chapter 27) and Mycoplasma infection.

Fever and exanthem

The onset of fever and exanthem is usually due to a viral illness, often enterovirus. Some infections have specific clinical features that aid diagnosis; for example measles and erythema infectiosum. However, in most instances a diagnosis cannot be made with certainty. To manage such a child, consider:

- Is the child sick? Is the child lethargic, cold peripherally or young? Consider meningococcal disease, other bacterial sepsis and Kawasaki disease. Investigate and treat.
- Are they taking any medication? Consider ceasing medication.
- Are there other people at risk? If relatives are immunosuppressed or pregnant, consider serology, stool viral culture and advising the at-risk person to consult their doctor.
- Is the rash papular? Consider papular acrodermatitis.

If the answer to all the above is 'no', reassurance and review is probably appropriate.

Erythema infectiosum and Kawasaki disease

See Infectious diseases, chapter 27.

Roseola infantum

This condition is seen every day in paediatric emergency departments. Typically, an infant has had a high fever for 2–4 days and has often been put on antibiotics. The fever then goes but a widespread erythematous rash appears. The family need reassurance that the rash is not a drug reaction. See Infectious diseases, chapter 27.

PURPURIC RASHES

Consider viral infections, meningococcal sepsis, platelet disorders, vasculitis, drug reactions and trauma.

Septicaemia

Suspect septicaemia (usually meningococcal) in a child with recent onset of fever and lethargy. Skin lesions may be erythematous macules progressing to extensive purple purpura. If in doubt, take blood cultures, give antibiotics and arrange admission (see also Medical emergencies, chapter 1).

Enteroviral infection

Scattered petechiae are common in children who have fever from enteroviral infections. These children are usually well. If in doubt, or if the child appears unwell, investigate (full blood examination, blood cultures) and consider treatment for septicaemia.

Leukaemia

Suspect leukaemia in a child with generalised petechiae or purpura in the absence of trauma. Look for tiredness or pallor. Obtain an urgent full blood examination (see Haematologic conditions and oncology, chapter 26).

Henoch-Schönlein purpura

See also Rheumatologic conditions, chapter 34.

Non-itchy, painless macules, papules or urticarial lesions with purpuric centres occur in a symmetrical distribution mainly on the buttocks and ankles, occasionaliy on the legs, arms and elsewhere. There may be associated abdominal pain, arthralgia, arthritis or haematuria. Renal involvement leading to chronic renal failure is rare, but can occur irrespective of the severity of the rash and other symptoms and may be delayed until weeks or months after the onset of the illness.

Idiopathic thrombocytopenic purpura

See also Haematologic conditions and oncology, chapter 26.

Bruises, petechiae or purpuric lesions appear over a period of days or weeks, mainly in sites of frequent mild trauma. The child is otherwise well. Full blood examination will show a low platelet count.

Child abuse

Twisting, compression, pinching and hitting can all cause petechial or purpuric lesions (see Child abuse, chapter 14). Look for bruises of bizarre shapes and different ages, evidence of bony fractures and an abnormal affect.

Trauma and vasomotor straining

In some ethnic groups it is common to treat a febrile or unwell child by rubbing or suctioning the skin with a variety of implements. This produces bizarre circular and linear patterns of petechiae that can alarm the unwary.

Petechiae can appear around the head and neck in normal children after coughing or vomiting. Restraining a small child for a procedure such as a lumbar puncture or venepuncture can also lead to the development of petechiae on the upper body.

BLUE OR BLACK RASHES

Consider vascular malformations, haemangiomas, Mongolian spots, blue naevi and melanoma.

Vascular malformations

- These can be blue, red, purple or skin coloured. They are developmental defects and do not resolve.
- Such malformations can involve any mix of capillaries (e.g. port-wine stain), veins, arteries (e.g. arteriovenous malformation) and lymphatics (e.g. cystic hygroma).
- Extensive malformations can be associated with pain, soft tissue or bony hypertrophy, bone erosion, haemorrhage, infection and platelet trapping.
- Management requires a multidisciplinary approach using expertise from surgical, paediatric, dermatological and radiological fields.

Haemangiomas

Clinical features

Superficial haemangiomas begin as macular erythematous lesions in the first weeks of life and become soft, partly compressible, sharply defined, red or purple swellings that can occur anywhere on the body. Deeper haemangiomas may appear as blue or skin-coloured swellings. Most haemangiomas are not present at birth; they grow for several months and resolve fully over several years.

Management

Parents need reassurance about the inherently benign nature of these lesions. Most haemangiomas are best left alone and allowed to involute spontaneously. In some sites, however, haemangiomas can rapidly lead to problems such as ulceration, blindness, destruction of cartilage, respiratory obstruction or death.

Urgent assessment by an experienced clinician is needed if any developing haemangioma:

- Is ulcerating and potentially disfiguring.
- Is on the eyelid or adjacent to the globe of the eye.
- Deforms structures such as the lip, ear cartilage or nasal cartilage.
- Begins as an extensive macule that grows thicker.
- Is associated with stridor, thrombocytopenia or multiple lesions.

Corticosteroids are usually used, occasionally with vascular laser, surgery or interferon.

HYPOPIGMENTED LESIONS

In hypopigmented lesions, look for a fine scale. If it is scaly, consider pityriasis versicolor or pityriasis alba. If it is not scaly, consider pityriasis versicolor, post-inflammatory loss of pigment, halo naevi or vitiligo.

Pityriasis versicolor

- This is common in adolescents and probably caused by an increased activity of commensal yeasts.
- Multiple oval macules, usually covered with fine scale, appear on the trunk or upper arms. The lesions may appear paler or darker than the surrounding skin.
- Treatment with anti-yeast shampoos is effective. For example, apply selenium sulphide 2% (Selsun shampoo). Leave on for 2 h, if tolerated, rinse and treat weekly for 4 weeks and then monthly. The recovery takes weeks and relapses are common.

Pityriasis alba

This condition is common in prepubertal children. Single or multiple, poorly demarcated hypopigmented 1–2 cm macules are seen on the face or upper body. Lesions are not itchy but often have a fine scale. Reassure and treat with hydrocortisone 1%. Resolution takes weeks.

Vitiligo

This condition is characterised by sharply demarcated, often symmetrical areas of complete pigment loss. Eventual repigmentation in childhood vitiligo is common and is helped by topical steroids. In troublesome cases refer to a specialist for advice regarding treatment (e.g. corrective cosmetics or psoralen therapy).

Post-inflammatory pigmentation changes

This condition occurs particularly in dark-skinned people. Many inflammatory skin disorders may heal leaving diffuse, hypo- or hyper-pigmented macules that can persist for months or years. No treatment is satisfactory.

HYPERPIGMENTED LESIONS

If they are flat, consider junctional melanocytic naevi, café-au-lait spots, naevus spilus, pityriasis versicolor and post-inflammatory hyper-pigmentation. If raised, consider compound melanocytic naevi, Spitz naevi and warts.

Congenital pigmented naevi

Congenital melanocytic naevi that cover large areas or are likely to cause concern need very early assessment by a skin specialist and plastic surgeon, preferably in the first week of life, for diagnosis, surgery, laser treatment and/or long-term follow up.

Acquired pigmented naevi

- During childhood, most children develop multiple pigmented lesions, which may be freckles, lentigines, naevus spilus, acquired melanocytic naevi or very rarely, melanoma.
- Immune-suppressed children and those who have had chemo-therapy are at greater risk of skin malignancy.

ANOGENITAL RASHES

Most anogenital rashes seen in infants that wear nappies are primarily caused by reaction with urine or faeces (irritant napkin dermatitis) or by seborrhoeic dermatitis. Soaps, detergents and secondary yeast infection may contribute. In older children, threadworms (*Enterobius vermicularis*) are a common cause of an itchy anogenital rash. Look for the worms at night and treat with mebendazole 50 mg (<10 kg), 100 mg (>10 kg) (not in pregnancy or less than 6 months) or pyrantel 10 mg/kg (max 500 mg) once oral. A repeat dose 2 weeks later helps reduce the high rate of reinfestation.

Consider also less common causes such as malabsorption syndromes (diarrhoea, erosive dermatitis and failure to thrive), zinc deficiency (a sharply defined anogenital rash with associated perioral, hand and foot 'eczema'), Langerhans' cell histiocytosis, psoriasis and Crohn's disease.

Irritant napkin dermatitis

Clinical features

This is the most common cause of napkin dermatitis in infants and typically presents as confluent erythema that spares the groin folds. Variant presentations include multiple erosions and ulcers, scaly or glazed erythema and satellite lesions at the periphery. Satellite lesions are suggestive of Candida infection.

Management

- Keep the area clean and dry. Leave the nappy off whenever possible.
- Gel-based disposable nappies or a non-wettable under-napkin can be helpful. Cloth nappies should be thoroughly washed and rinsed.
- Use topical zinc cream or paste for mild eruptions.
- Add hydrocortisone 1% cream if inflamed. Do not use stronger steroids.
- Consider mupirocin 2% cream if not settling. Antifungal therapy is often not needed, even if Candida is present.

Candida napkin dermatitis

This occurs secondary to irritant napkin dermatitis and antibiotic use. Treat the underlying cause as above and use topical imidazole cream.

Perianal streptococcal dermatitis

Streptococcus pyogenes infection.

Clinical features

- A localised, well-demarcated erythema that covers a circular area of 1–2 cm radius around the anus.
- If not treated, it may persist for months.
- May have painful defaecation, fissures and constipation.

Management

- Take perianal and throat cultures to confirm the presence of *Streptococcus pyogenes*.

- Apply paraffin ointment three times daily to the perianal area for symptomatic relief. Treat with oral antibiotics (phenoxymethylpenicillin 15 mg/kg (max 500 mg) 6-hourly) for a minimum of 2 weeks. Several weeks of therapy may be required. Intramuscular penicillin can be used if there are concerns about compliance.
- Keep stools soft with oral liquid paraffin for several weeks.

Lichen sclerosis

This condition presents as an area of atrophy with white shiny skin, purpura or telangiectasia in the perivulval region of girls aged 3 years or older. It may be itchy. Cases have been misdiagnosed as sexual abuse. Management is with moisturisers and brief courses of moderately potent steroid ointment. About 50% of cases resolve spontaneously.

HAIR PROBLEMS

Consider alopecia areata, traumatic alopecia, tinea capitis, kerion and head lice.

Alopecia areata

Clinical features

Typically one or more oval patches of hair loss develop over a few days. Some hairs may remain within the patches. Occasionally, the hair loss is diffuse. The scalp appears normal and does not show scaling, erythema or scarring. Most cases in childhood resolve spontaneously but progression to total scalp or body hair loss or recurrent alopecia can occur. Regrowth can occur decades later.

Management

- For isolated small patches present for weeks without further progression, no treatment is needed.
- For recent or progressive hair loss, treatment with moderate potency topical steroids for a few weeks may help. In difficult cases, other therapies including contact sensitisation, irritant agents and pulsed corticosteroids need to be considered.

Traumatic alopecia

Clinical features

This condition is usually caused by rubbing (as on the occiput of many babies), cosmetic practices (e.g. tight braiding) or hair pulling as a habit (trichotillomania). Trichotillomania may be largely nocturnal and parents are often unaware of it. The affected areas are usually angular and on the anterior or lateral scalp. The areas contain hairs of different lengths and are never completely bald.

Management

- Recognition of the problem and a careful explanation to the family is often sufficient.
- Trichotillomania in younger children does not usually indicate that significant psychological problems are present. It is a habit similar to thumb sucking or nail biting and a low-key approach similar to that used in those conditions is appropriate.

Tinea capitis

Clinical features

In Australia, tinea capitis is usually caused by *Microsporum canis* contracted from cats or dogs. It is characterised by patches of hair loss with some short, lustreless, bent hairs a few millimetres in length. Redness and scaling are present in the patch. Hair loss without any of these features is not likely to be fungal.

Management

Confirm the diagnosis, if possible, by greenish fluorescence of the hair shafts with Wood's light (not present with some fungi) or by microscopy and culture of hair and scale. Treatment usually comprises griseofulvin orally 10–15 mg/kg (max 0.5–1 g) daily for 4–6 weeks or until non-fluorescent. Pulse therapy (1 week treatment, 3 weeks off, then repeat) with newer antifungals (terbinafine, itraconazole) is also effective. Children may attend school provided that they are being treated.

Kerion (inflammatory ringworm)

This represents an inflammatory scarring immune response to tinea. It is an erythematous, tender, boggy swelling that discharges pus from multiple points. The swellings appear fluctuant but skin incision should be avoided. Treatment is with oral antifungals, often with antibiotics for secondary infection, and a brief course of oral steroids to suppress the immune response. Other inflammatory granulomas can mimic kerions.

Head lice

Clinical features

Infestation of the scalp with *Pediculus capitis* is associated with itching. Eggs (nits) can be seen attached to the hairs just above the scalp surface. Epidemics of head lice regularly sweep through primary schools in all areas.

Management

- Suitable treatments include pyrethrin 0.165% (e.g. Pyrifoam), maldison 0.5% and permethrin 1% (e.g. Nix and Lyclear cream rinse).
- Wash the hair with soap and water. Thoroughly moisten the hair with the treatment and leave for 10 min. Rinse well and comb out with a fine-toothed comb. Reapply 1 week later to kill any eggs that have subsequently hatched.
- Reinfestation is common. A regular physical inspection, use of conditioner and combing of the hair are as important as chemical treatment.

NAIL PROBLEMS

Congenitally abnormal nails are usually atrophic and can be the presenting feature of rare inherited conditions such as ectodermal dysplasias, dyskeratosis congenita, pachyonychia congenita, congenital malalignment of the great toenails and the nail-patella syndrome.

Acquired nail disease is usually a result of fungal infection, psoriasis, ingrown toenails or 20-nail dystrophy. It may also be seen in association with diseases such as alopecia areata and lichen planus. Nail biting and picking can lead to marked deformity of involved nails.

Tinea unguium (onychomycosis)

Clinical features

- Dermatophyte infection may affect one or more nails.
- White or yellow patches develop at the distal and lateral nail edges. The rest of the nail may become discoloured, friable and deformed with accumulation of subungual debris.
- Tinea is often also present on the adjacent skin.

Management

- Always confirm the diagnosis by microscopy and culture of nail clippings.
- In mild cases, treatment with physical debridement and antifungal nail lacquer (e.g. amorolfine) may be effective.
- Most cases require oral therapy for months – oral griseofulvin 10–20 mg/kg (max 1 g) or griseofulvin ultramicrosize 5.5 mg/kg (max 330 mg). Oral terbinafine is more effective, can be given for shorter periods (often only 4–6 weeks) and is better tolerated.

CHAPTER 21
EAR, NOSE AND THROAT CONDITIONS

Robert Berkowitz
Michael Marks

UPPER RESPIRATORY TRACT INFECTIONS

The average child has 4–12 upper respiratory tract infections (URTI) a year, the peak incidence being between 1–6 years. Risk factors include exposure to other young children (either at home, childcare or school) and passive tobacco smoke exposure.

Causes

Viruses are responsible for at least 90% of upper respiratory tract infections. Bacterial causes include Group A streptococcus and *Mycoplasma pneumoniae*.

Local symptoms include coryza, cough, sore throat and ears. There may be fever, lethargy and decreased feeding. Infants and young children with an URTI may appear quite unwell. It is important to exclude serious bacterial infections in children who have severe constitutional symptoms.

Management

Symptomatic if necessary.

- Ensure adequate fluid intake.
- Give paracetamol if the child is distressed.
- The following may be administered for temporary relief of nasal congestion interfering with feeding or sleeping: saline nasal drops/spray, eucalyptus inhalant (e.g. chest rub), or ephedrine nose drops (maximum duration of therapy is 48 h).

Beware of using antihistamines in children under 2 years.

OTITIS MEDIA

This term covers a spectrum of conditions, which are characterised by the presence of fluid in the middle ear. Fluid may be recognised by tympanic membrane appearance or by assessment of tympanic membrane mobility. Otitis media may be classified according to clinical presentation as either:

- Acute suppurative otitis media (ASOM).
- Otitis media with effusion (OME).

ACUTE SUPPURATIVE OTITIS MEDIA

This condition is characterised by both:

- Middle ear effusion;
  - Otoscopic features include loss of the normal tympanic membrane translucency, loss of the light reflex and yellowish discolouration rather than the usual grey colour of the tympanic membrane.
  - Tympanic membrane motility is reduced – assess by pneumatic otoscopy and/or tympanometry.
- Features of inflammation clinically, that are either:
  - Localised (e.g. ear pain) *or*;
  - Generalised (e.g. fever, irritability) and where no other cause is apparent to explain these generalised features of inflammation. **Be cautious of accepting ASOM as the sole diagnosis in an unwell infant with a fever. There may be a coexistent serious bacterial infection. Consider a septic work-up or very careful observation**. The degree of redness of the tympanic membrane is relatively unhelpful in deciding whether or not bacterial infection is present.

Acute suppurative otitis media is very often preceded by a viral upper respiratory tract infection. The causative bacteria are usually;

- *Streptococcus pneumoniae.*
- Non-typeable *Haemophilus influenzae.*
- *Moraxella catarrhalis.*

Management

Initial management

- Adequate analgesia.
  - Paracetamol – 15 mg/kg oral 4–6-hourly (max 90 mg/kg per day) as required.
  - Topical application of lignocaine 1% (2–3 drops in the external canal) is advocated by some but is of unproven benefit.
- Consider antibiotics
  - Acute symptoms resolve without antibiotics within 24 h in most cases.
  - Withhold in children >12 months who are mildly unwell.
  - Commence if distress continues beyond 24–48 h or if the child is more unwell initially; amoxicillin 15 mg/kg (max 500 mg) orally, 8-hourly for 5 days or erythromycin 15 mg/kg (max 500 mg) orally, 8-hourly for 5 days if allergic to penicillin.
  - Antibiotics do not reduce the incidence of recurrent ASOM or otitis media with effusion (below).

Follow up

The key features of ASOM, clinical inflammation and middle-ear effusion, need to be followed up separately.

Clinical inflammation

Review in 48 h if there is no resolution of the symptoms of inflammation. Possible explanations include:

- Wrong diagnosis (most commonly a viral URTI).
- Failure to take the medication (either the antibiotics were not given or they were vomited).
- Inappropriate antibiotic was prescribed (i.e. bacterial resistance: switch to amoxicillin with clavulanic acid 15 mg/kg (max 500 mg) orally, 8-hourly).
- Antibiotic itself is responsible for the child remaining unwell.
- Suppurative complication of ASOM has developed (e.g. mastoiditis, labyrinthitis, intracranial infection). These complications are rare in a first world setting.

If the medical treatment has been unsuccessful and the child remains symptomatically unwell, early drainage of the ear (myringotomy) with or without insertion of a tympanostomy tube may need to be considered. Refer to a paediatric ear, nose and throat (ENT) surgeon.

Middle ear effusion

A middle-ear effusion is present for a variable period of time following ASOM and may be associated with noticeable hearing loss, particularly if bilateral. A middle ear effusion will be present in approximately;

- 80% of cases at 2 weeks following ASOM.
- 40% at 1 month.
- 20% at 2 months.
- 10% at 3 months.

Review at 3 months is recommended, particularly if symptomatic hearing loss is present. Management – see below (otitis media with effusion).

Recurrent ASOM

ASOM is common in the first 3 years of life and is generally a seasonal condition with a peak incidence in winter and early spring, parallelling the incidence of viral URTI. Prevention of recurrent ASOM may need to be considered during this period, depending on the frequency, severity and duration of infections. Prophylactic measures include:

- Limiting exposure to viral URTI (e.g. by avoiding excessive attendance at large child care groups).
- Long-term prophylactic antibiotics (e.g. cotrimoxazole for 6 weeks).
- Insertion of tympanostomy tubes, which should be considered particularly if infections are associated with morbidity and are thought likely to persist for a significant period of time.

OTITIS MEDIA WITH EFFUSION

This presents as a persistent middle-ear effusion (which has been present for a variable period of time) without clinical features of inflammation. Otitis media with effusion tends to resolve spontaneously with time. Factors contributing to persistence include recurrent upper respiratory tract infection, recurrent ASOM, underlying poor Eustachian tube function and exposure to tobacco smoke.

Management

For symptomatic cases that have not resolved in 3 months, a prolonged course of antibiotics (amoxicillin 15 mg/kg (max 500 mg) 8-hourly for 3 weeks) will result in resolution of a significant proportion. Medical treatment apart from antibiotics is not of proven benefit (except for steroids, although their use in treatment of OME is not recommended). Eustachian tube exercises are of limited value.

Tympanostomy tubes

If OME is symptomatic and thought likely to be present for a significant period of time in the future, insertion of tympanostomy tubes should be considered. Insertion of tympanostomy tubes does not cure the underlying Eustachian tube dysfunction responsible for OME, but only temporarily removes the symptoms by providing an alternative means for middle ear ventilation. Adenoidectomy may be beneficial in addition (by removing a reservoir of infection from the nasopharynx), but it adds significant morbidity to an otherwise very minor procedure.

The prerequisites for tympanostomy tubes are:

- Middle-ear effusion present for at least 3 months (90% of effusions will resolve within the first 3 months) and appears likely to persist long term.
- Symptoms must be present: either recurrent ASOM or functionally significant hearing loss (e.g. speech delay, behavioural disturbance or poor school performance). Otitis media with effusion and ASOM are commonly related to URTI and are therefore more common in winter and early spring. Inserting tubes towards the end of this period should be avoided in the expectation that there may be a resolution with the onset of warmer weather.

The long-term value of insertion of tympanostomy tubes (i.e. language, literacy and cognitive function) is the subject of debate. The benefits of the temporary alleviation of symptoms of OME by the insertion of tympanostomy tubes need to be balanced against the disadvantages:

- Need for general anaesthesia and surgery.
- Tubes usually remain *in situ* for only 6–9 months (although longer-stay tubes are available) and the reinsertion rate of tubes is approximately 25%.

- Tympanic membrane perforation rate of approximately 1% per year that the tube is *in situ*. A range of other tympanic membrane and middle ear complications are associated with tubes.
- Otorrhoea occurs in up to 25% of cases. It is often associated with an URTI, and may also occur because of external contamination (e.g. swimming or bathing without ear protection).

In a child with tympanostomy tubes, discharging ears should be treated by ear toilet (gentle removal of excess discharge and debris from the outer external canal using cotton wool) and topical antibiotics (e.g. soframycin). Discharge refractory to treatment can be managed by 3% hydrogen peroxide ear washes; however, the possibility of an underlying immunodeficiency or cholesteatoma should be considered. Refer to an ENT surgeon.

OTITIS EXTERNA

Clinical features

Commonly occurs due to water contamination following swimming or in children with dermatitis of the external auditory canal. It is characterised by pain, which is often severe, together with:

- Inflammation of the ear canal, which may include the tympanic membrane (mobility of the tympanic membrane on pneumatic otoscopy excludes otitis media).
- Pre-auricular tenderness.

Management

- Ear toilet.
- Topical antibiotics (e.g. soframycin).
- An ear wick should be inserted when the ear canal is very oedematous (to maintain patency of the ear canal and allow topical antibiotics to enter the ear canal) and moistened frequently with topical antibiotics.
- Hospital admission for administration of (anti-pseudomonal) intravenous antibiotics may be necessary when ear pain is severe and not relieved by regular analgesics, or where cellulitis has extended beyond the ear canal. See Antimicrobial guidelines.

ACUTE PHARYNGITIS/TONSILLITIS

The combination of fever and sore throat is a common presenting problem in children. Determining the aetiology and deciding whether to treat with antibiotics can be difficult.

Background

- Most sore throats are due to a viral infection (almost entirely in children under 4 years of age).
- The only clinically important bacterial pathogen is group A β-haemolytic streptococcus (GABHS).
- GABHS is found in around 20–30% of older children presenting with an acute sore throat.
- GABHS colonises the throat in some normal children (up to 1 in 5).
- Distinguishing colonisation from acute infection is a major problem. A child with a sore throat may be colonised with GABHS and therefore have a positive throat swab (or a positive antigen test), yet the cause of the episode may be a viral infection.
- GABHS is more likely if the child has tenderness and enlargement of the tonsillar cervical lymph nodes, inflammation of the tonsils and the rest of the pharynx (pharyngotonsillitis), unilateral signs or a generalised erythematous (scarlatiniform) rash.
- The presence of tonsillar exudate is not helpful in distinguishing viral infection from GABHS.
- GABHS is less likely if the child also has coryza, cough or generalised lymphadenopathy or splenomegaly.
- Streptococcal serology (ASOT, antiDNase-B titre) can only be used to make a retrospective diagnosis (rise in titre between baseline and 3 weeks later).
- Penicillin reduces the duration of symptoms, possibly by up to a day or more. Penicillin reduces the incidence of uncommon suppurative complications (e.g. quinsy) and acute rheumatic fever. These problems are now rare except in some developing countries and in indigenous groups.

Practical management

Children who probably **do not** need antibiotics are those aged less than 4 years and/or those with associated cough or coryza.

Children who are most likely to benefit from antibiotics are those aged over 4 with marked pharyngotonsillitis, tender tonsillar cervical nodes, and without cough and coryza. Send a throat swab for culture and give oral phenoxymethylpenicillin 250 mg (500 mg if >10 years) 12-hourly. Erythromycin 15 mg/kg (max 500 mg) 8-hourly or roxithromycin 2.5 mg/kg (max 150 mg) 12-hourly may be used for children with true penicillin allergy. If the throat swab does not grow a GABHS (the result is normally available 48–72 hours later) the antibiotics can be stopped. If GABHS is grown, continue antibiotics for a total of 10 days.

In populations with high rates of acute rheumatic fever (e.g. Aboriginal Australians in remote/rural settings), all sore throats should be treated with antibiotics and throat swabs are not needed.

Infectious mononucleosis is a relatively common cause of acute pharyngitis in older children. The diagnosis often becomes apparent when there is no response to penicillin, other characteristic features develop (e.g. generalised lymphadenopathy, splenomegaly, mild jaundice and rashes) and the illness has a more prolonged course.

Recurrent acute pharyngitis/tonsillitis

Recurrent sore throats are a normal part of growing up for many children. Many of these children have recurrent viral pharyngitis. True recurrent GABHS pharyngotonsillitis is much less common but often over-diagnosed.

A variety of strategies have been used to reduce recurrences of GABHS pharyngotonsillitis:

- Use of another antibiotic to attempt eradication of GABHS (e.g. amoxicillin/clavulanic acid).
- Use of low-dose prophylactic penicillin.
- Treatment of culture-positive family members.
- Tonsillectomy.

None of these is universally effective in preventing recurrent episodes and each has its own disadvantages.

Tonsillectomy (with or without adenoidectomy) probably works by removing a reservoir of GABHS infection. It should be considered if the pattern of infection – i.e. frequency, severity and duration of infections – is such that significant morbidity is expected to continue for a prolonged and unacceptable period of time. Children with suspected recurrent GABHS pharyngotonsillitis should have a throat swab taken during an acute episode to aid in treatment decisions. Streptococcal serology may also be of value.

OBSTRUCTIVE ADENOTONSILLAR HYPERTROPHY

Pathophysiology

Upper airway obstruction occurs when there is an imbalance between the neuromuscular control, which supports the airways, and the negative inspiratory pressure, which tends to collapse the airways. The site of obstruction is generally in the oropharynx at the level of the tonsil and tonsillectomy therefore is beneficial in relieving upper airways obstruction. Removal of the adenoids improves the nasal airway and thereby decreases the negative pressure generated during inspiration.

Indications for surgery

Involution of the adenoids and tonsils will occur with time and is accompanied by the resolution of obstructive symptoms. With this in mind, the indications for surgical management depend on the severity of the symptoms, which can be classified according to the following hierarchy as follows:

- Snoring alone: this does not require surgical management.
- Sleep disturbance characterised by laboured respiration, restlessness and waking at night with daytime somnolence or chronic mouth breathing by day.
- Observed episodes of apnoea while asleep.
- Complications of obstructive sleep apnoea (OSA), which include failure to thrive, significant hypoxia and *cor pulmonale*.

Decisions regarding surgery are primarily based on parental observation and description of sleep patterns. Decision making may be assisted by overnight oximetry, although this test only documents episodes of desaturation; significant sleep disturbance and CO_2 retention are not detected. A formal sleep study should be considered if uncertainty persists.

Adenotonsillectomy is associated with a 2 week recovery period and there is a 2–3% risk of secondary haemorrhage occurring during this time, particularly at 5–10 days postoperatively. Adenoidectomy alone, which is associated with much less morbidity than adenotonsillectomy, can be considered for relief of nasal obstruction and sleep disturbance in the absence of tonsillar hypertrophy. Mirror examination of the post-nasal space is often impossible in children. Nasal endoscopy under local anaesthetic or lateral neck X-ray may have a place in assessing adenoidal size.

EPISTAXIS

This is usually due to bleeding from the anterior nasoseptal vessels, often in association with nasal crusting or nose picking. Acute bleeding usually settles with local pressure to the lower nasal septum, but occasionally the application of a cotton wool pledget soaked with a topical decongestant is necessary.

Recurrent bleeding can be treated by the application of an antibiotic ointment if there is significant nasal crusting present, or by cautery if enlarged blood vessels are seen. Nasal cautery can be performed as an office procedure following the application of a topical anaesthetic and decongestant (e.g. cophenylcaine spray – lignocaine/phenylephrine) using a silver nitrate stick. Epistaxis is very unlikely to be due to a nasal tumour or a previously undiagnosed coagulopathy, but further evaluation is necessary if there are suggestive symptoms or signs.

TRAUMA

Nasal trauma

Treatment is required for either cosmesis or drainage of septal haematoma.

- *Cosmesis.* A nasal deformity due to a displaced nasal fracture should be reduced within 7–10 days of injury. The presence of a bony deformity due to a nasal fracture is best determined at about 5 days following the injury, once the soft tissue swelling has resolved. The decision to reduce the nasal fracture is based on clinical grounds and radiology is unhelpful.
- *Septal haematoma.* This can occur after nasal trauma, regardless whether a fracture is present or not. It invariably leads to septal abscess formation with cartilage destruction and nasal collapse.

A septal haematoma presents with nasal obstruction associated with a bulge of the septum that can be confirmed by palpating with an instrument (e.g. wax curette) following the application of a topical anaesthetic. Treatment involves incision and drainage, nasal packing to prevent recurrence and anti-staphylococcal antibiotics.

Oral/oropharyngeal trauma

This invariably occurs after a fall with a stick or similar object in the mouth and may sometimes be associated with a significant injury.

Admit and evaluate if:

- Unable to feed.
- Upper airway obstruction.
- Significant laceration, requiring debridement, closure or both.
- Significant retropharyngeal injury.
- Suspicion of injury to the internal carotid artery.

Involvement of the retropharynx may not be obvious by oral examination, particularly for injuries that penetrate the soft palate. The retropharynx is ideally examined by flexible nasopharyngoscopy. In addition, a lateral cervical spine X-ray is required to rule out the presence of gas in the soft tissues, the presence of a foreign body and any associated cervical spine injury. Widening of the retropharynx may also be demonstrated, but this may be misleading unless the radiological features are confirmed by nasopharyngoscopy. A significant retropharyngeal injury requires intravenous antibiotics and a period of nasogastric feeding to prevent abscess formation.

The internal carotid artery lies posterolateral to the tonsil. An injury to this region may be associated with injury to the internal carotid artery whether the trauma is blunt or sharp. Internal carotid artery injuries are rare; they are usually due to blunt trauma causing intimal disruption and progressive thrombosis and they typically present with neurological signs over a period of 24 h.

Aural trauma

Trauma to the external auditory canal is usually associated with bleeding, but it is an insignificant injury and requires no treatment. The tympanic membrane can be perforated by direct trauma or a pressure wave (e.g. a slap across the ear or diving). Acute tympanic membrane perforations usually heal within weeks and do not require acute intervention. Topical antibiotics are recommended for water-related injuries. Direct trauma may rarely cause ossicular disruption, facial paralysis or inner ear damage (with complete deafness and vertigo).

FOREIGN BODIES

The first attempt at foreign body removal is always the easiest and should be performed by an experienced clinician with the appropriate instruments and good illumination. Take into account the child's developmental stage and their level of anxiety in planning this procedure. Failure of the initial removal may lead to an otherwise unnecessary general anaesthetic.

Ear

Foreign bodies in the external auditory canal are best removed by a hook-shaped instrument, which is passed behind the foreign body and then used to pull it out. Grasping instruments, such as forceps, should not be used as they invariably lead to the foreign body being displaced further medially. Suction may also be useful.

Nose

The technique for the removal of nasal foreign bodies is the same as for foreign bodies in the external auditory canal. A topical anaesthetic (e.g. cophenylcaine) should be applied prior to the attempted removal. The risk of inhalation of a nasal foreign body is minimal and therefore acute removal should be deferred until appropriate personnel and equipment are available.

Fish bone in pharynx

A fish bone usually lodges in the tonsil or at the base of the tongue and therefore can be seen on oral examination and removed following the application of a topical anaesthetic. If the fish bone cannot be seen during the oral examination, a more thorough examination by nasopharyngoscopy is required. Fish bones rarely reach the oesophagus and so oesophageal evaluation is usually unnecessary. Where a fish bone is not found, despite a suggestive history, the child should be reviewed until symptoms resolve and an examination under general anaesthetic considered. Although fish bones are radiolucent, radiology (particularly CT) may be helpful to detect the presence of complications when symptoms have persisted.

Oesophagus

The vast majority of swallowed foreign bodies pass without difficulty. If a foreign body becomes lodged in the oesophagus, it usually does so in the upper oesophagus, at the level of the cricopharyngeus. Lower oesophageal foreign bodies suggest the presence of underlying oesophageal pathology (e.g. stricture).

If a swallowed object reaches the stomach it will almost always pass without incident. Two types of object, however, may cause problems: (i) long thin objects (e.g. hair pins and locker keys) may impact at the duodenojejunal flexure and (ii) button batteries, if held up at any point in the alimentary canal, may release alkali, causing local necrosis and perforation. X-rays (including neck, chest and abdomen) should be taken if there are symptoms suggestive of oesophageal impaction (e.g. drooling and dysphagia), or if long thin objects or button batteries have been swallowed. Oesophageal foreign bodies impact in the coronal plane, whereas tracheal lodgement occurs in the sagittal plane. Radiolucent foreign bodies may be imaged by barium swallow. If an object is impacted in the oesophagus, endoscopic removal is required.

Tracheobronchus

See Respiratory conditions, chapter 33.

CHAPTER 22
ENDOCRINE CONDITIONS

Margaret Zacharin
Garry Warne
Fergus Cameron
George Werther

TYPE 1 DIABETES MELLITUS

Diagnosis

Diagnosis is made by either:

- Random blood glucose >11 mmol/L, *or*
- Fasting blood glucose >7 mmol/L.

Note: there is no need for oral glucose tolerance testing.

Clinical features

Typical symptoms are polyuria, polydipsia or weight loss. Glycosuria and ketonuria are often present.

Children presenting with diabetes may range from being mildly unwell to severely unwell in diabetic ketoacidosis. Management varies according to presentation.

Differential diagnosis

(i) Transient hyperglycaemia

Transient elevation of blood glucose and glycosuria (and possibly ketonuria) may occur in children with an intercurrent illness or with therapy such as glucocorticoids. The risk of later developing diabetes mellitus is about 3%, but is approximately 30% if these findings are picked up in an otherwise well child. Check HbA1c and diabetes-related autoimmune markers (antibodies against insulin, glutamic acid decarboxylase (GAD) and islet cells) and discuss with a specialist.

(ii) Type 2 diabetes mellitus

This form of diabetes is rare in children. It is being seen increasingly in children who are overweight, those with a family history of type 2 diabetes mellitus and in some ethnic minority groups.

NEW PRESENTATION, MILDLY UNWELL

Assessment

Less than 3% dehydration, no acidosis and not vomiting.

Management

Initial Treatment

- 0.25 units/kg of quick-acting insulin s.c. stat.
- If within 2 h of a meal give mealtime dose only (see below). Halve dose if <4 years old.
- Before breakfast and lunch give 0.25 units/kg of rapid-acting insulin. Before the evening meal give 0.25 units/kg rapid-acting insulin and 0.25 units/kg of intermediate-acting insulin. If this is the first insulin dose give 0.25 units/kg rapid-acting insulin only, then a further 0.25 units/kg rapid-acting insulin at midnight followed by a snack. Continue until normoglycaemia and negative ketonuria are achieved.
- Encourage fluid intake with sugar free fluid and a normal diet according to appetite, but exclude foods with quick acting sugars.

Ongoing Treatment

- Once normoglycaemia is achieved and ketonuria disappears, change insulin to twice daily mixture of short and intermediate insulins.
- The usual initial total dose is 1 unit/kg /day. This is given as:
  - 2/3 in morning and 1/3 at night.
  - 2/3 of each dose intermediate-acting and 1/3 as rapid-acting.
- Occasionally older adolescents go onto a basal bolus regimen: 30–40% intermediate acting insulin given at 2200 h, rest given as quick-acting insulin in 3 equal doses before meals.

HYPERGLYCAEMIA, MILDLY UNWELL (KNOWN DIABETIC)

Usually advised to take 10% of total daily dose as rapid acting insulin every 2 h until normoglycaemic (in addition to normal insulin). Consult with a specialist if uncertain.

DIABETIC KETOACIDOSIS

This is the mode of presentation in >30% of newly diagnosed diabetes in childhood and adolescence. Diabetic ketoacidosis (DKA) may occur in any child or adolescent with established type 1 diabetes. Rapid onset is more likely in patients with poor underlying control or in patients on an insulin pump.

Definition

- Hyperglycaemia >14 mmol/L.
- Metabolic acidosis (pH <7.3 or bicarbonate ≤15 mmol/L).
- Hyperketonaemia or moderate to severe ketonuria.

Causes

- Delayed diagnosis of insulin-dependent diabetes mellitus (IDDM).
- Omission of insulin (especially in adolescents with recurrent DKA).
- Acute stress (infection, trauma, psychological).
- Poor management of intercurrent illness.

History

- Polyuria, polydipsia, loss of weight and lethargy. These symptoms are usually of 1–3 weeks duration in newly diagnosed patients. Symptoms are either absent' or of shorter duration in patients with established diabetes.
- There may be a family history of diabetes or other auto-immune disease.

Examination

- Degree of dehydration (often overestimated).
  - Mild/nil (<4%): no clinical signs.
  - Moderate (4–7%): easily detectable dehydration (e.g. reduced skin turgor, poor capillary return).
  - Severe (>7%) poor perfusion, rapid pulse, reduced blood pressure, i.e. shock.
- Level of consciousness.
- Body temperature – hypothermia is common.
- The presence of a precipitating cause (e.g. infection).

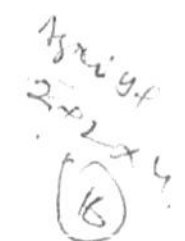

Investigations

- Blood glucose, urea and electrolytes.
- Arterial or capillary acid/base.
- Urine – ketones, culture.
- Check for precipitating cause e.g. infection (urine, FBE, blood cultures; consider chest X-ray).
- In newly diagnosed patients: islet cell antibodies, insulin antibodies, GAD antibodies, total IgA, antiendomyseal IgA antibodies and thyroid function tests.

> Calculated values
> Serum osmolality = $Na^+ \times 2$ + glucose + urea
> Adjusted Na^+ = plasma $Na^+ + 0.3 \times$ (plasma glucose – 5.5)

Management

1. Initial fluid requirements

- If hypoperfusion is present, give normal saline at 10 mL/kg stat.
- Repeat until perfusion is re-established (warm, pink extremities with rapid capillary refill).
- Commence rehydration with normal saline (see Table 22.1).
- Keep nil by mouth (except ice to suck) until alert and stable. Insert a nasogastric tube if patient is comatose or has recurrent vomiting; leave on free drainage.
- Rehydration may be completed orally after the first 24–36 h if the patient is metabolically stable.

2. Fluids once insulin is commenced

- If the blood sugar falls very quickly, i.e. within the first few hours, change to normal saline with 5% dextrose.
- When the blood sugar reaches 12–15 mmol/L, use 0.45% NaCl with 5% dextrose. Aim to keep the blood sugar at 10–12 mmol/L.
- If the blood glucose falls below 10–12 mmol/L and the patient is still sick and acidotic, increase the dextrose in the infusate to 7.5–10%.
- **Do not turn down insulin infusion.**

Table 22.1 Diabetic ketoacidosis fluid rates (mL/h) including deficit and maintenance fluid requirements, to be given evenly over 48 h.

Weight (kg)	*Mild/Nil*	*Moderate*
5	24	27
7	33	38
8	38	43
10	48	54
12	53	60
14	58	67
16	64	74
18	70	80
20	75	87
22	78	91
24	80	95
26	83	100
28	86	104
30	89	108
32	92	112
34	95	116
36	98	120
38	101	125
40	104	129
42	107	133
44	110	137
46	113	141
48	116	146
50	119	150
52	122	154
54	124	158
56	127	162
58	130	167
60	133	171
62	136	175
64	139	179
66	142	183
68	145	187
70	148	191

3. Insulin

- Commence after treatment of shock.
- Add 50 units of clear/rapid-acting insulin (Actrapid or Humulin R) to 49.5 mL 0.9% NaCl (1 unit/mL solution).
- Ensure that the insulin is clearly labelled.

- Start at 0.1 unit/kg per h in newly diagnosed children and those already on insulin who have glucose levels ≥15 mmol/L.
- Children who have had their usual insulin and whose blood sugars are <15 mmol/L should receive 0.05 units/kg/h.
- Adjust the concentration of dextrose to keep blood glucose 10–12 mmol/L.
- Adequate insulin must be continued to clear acidosis (ketonaemia).
- The insulin infusion can be discontinued when the child is alert and metabolically stable (blood glucose <10–12 mmol/L, pH >7.30 and HCO3 >15 mmol/L). The best time to change to s.c. insulin is just before meal time.
- The insulin infusion should only be stopped 30 minutes after the first s.c. injection of insulin.

4. Potassium

- Add potassium chloride (KCl) to the i.v. fluid at the time of starting the insulin infusion.
- Start KCl at a concentration of 40 mmol/L if body weight <30 kg, or 60 mmol/L if ≥30 kg.
- Measure levels 2 h after starting therapy and 2–4-hourly thereafter.
- Specimens should be arterial or venous. Do not give K^+ if the serum level is >5.5 mmol/L or if the patient is anuric.

5. Bicarbonate

- This is usually not necessary if shock has been adequately corrected. Continuing acidosis usually means insufficient resuscitation.
- In extremely sick children (with pH <7.0 ± HCO3 <5 mmol/L), small amounts may be given.
- Give over 30 min with cardiac monitoring. Reassess acid base status. Remember risk of hypokalaemia.
- The HCO3 dose (mmol) = 0.15 × body weight (kg) × base deficit.

6. Other instructions

- Intensive care is required if: age <2 years, coma, cardiovascular compromise or seizures.
- Patient should remain nil orally until alert and stable.
- Nurse the patient in a head-up position and in good light.

Clinical monitoring should include:

- Strict fluid balance.
- Check all urine for ketones.
- Hourly observations: pulse, BP, respiratory rate and neurological observations.
- Hourly glucose (glucometer) while on insulin infusion.
- 4-hourly temperature.

Note: **Any headache or altered behaviour that may indicate impending cerebral oedema.**

Biochemical monitoring should include:

- 2–4-hourly laboratory blood glucose levels (with hourly bedside glucometer readings).
- Serum sodium (adjusted for hyperglycaemia), potassium, chloride.
- Serum osmolality.

Beware of falling adjusted sodium levels as glucose declines – hyponatraemia may herald cerebral oedema.

If the sodium level falls, consider decreasing the rate of fluid administration to replace over 72–96 h.

COMPLICATIONS OF DIABETIC KETOSIS

Hypernatraemia

Measured serum sodium is depressed by the dilutional effect of the hyperglycaemia. If Na is >160 mmol/L, discuss with a specialist. Sodium should rise as the glucose falls during treatment. If this does not happen or if hyponatraemia develops, it usually indicates overzealous volume correction and insufficient electrolyte replacement. This may place the patient at risk of cerebral oedema.

Hypoglycaemia

If blood glucose ≤2.2 mmol/L give i.v. 25% dextrose 2 mL/kg over 3 minutes or 10% dextrose 5 mL/kg. **Do not discontinue the insulin infusion**. Continue with a 10% dextrose infusion until stable.

Hypokalaemia

Monitor frequently and adjust potassium concentration in the infusate. Children at particular risk of this complication are those who are very acidotic or have low potassium levels at presentation.

Cerebral Oedema

This is an uncommon (0.5–3.0%) but extremely serious complication of diabetic ketoacidosis in children, usually occurring 6–12 h after commencement of therapy. This condition is often fatal. If the patient survives there may be profound neurological impairment.

Prevention

Slow correction of fluid and biochemical abnormalities. Optimally, the rate of fall of blood glucose and serum osmolality should not exceed 5 mmol/L/h, but in children there is often a quicker initial fall in glucose. Patients should be nursed head up.

Risk factors

- Newly diagnosed diabetes young age, poorly controlled diabetes.
- Excessive fluid rehydration, particularly with hypotonic fluids.
- Severe initial acidosis.
- Hyponatraemia or hypernatraemia and negative sodium trend during the therapy.

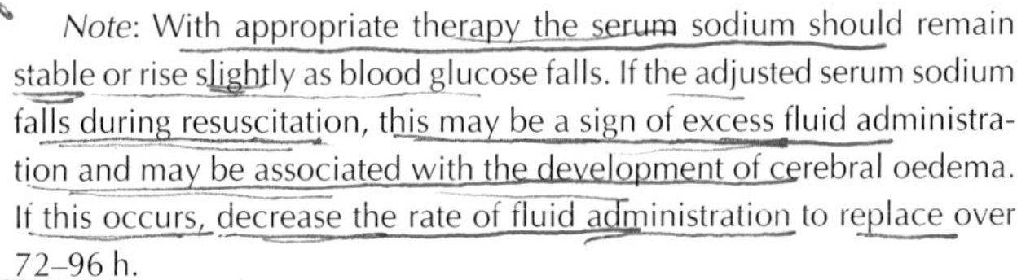

Note: With appropriate therapy the serum sodium should remain stable or rise slightly as blood glucose falls. If the adjusted serum sodium falls during resuscitation, this may be a sign of excess fluid administration and may be associated with the development of cerebral oedema. If this occurs, decrease the rate of fluid administration to replace over 72–96 h.

Signs

- *Early* – negative sodium trend, headache, behaviour change (sudden irritability, depression of conscious state) and incontinence.
- *Late* – bradycardia, elevated blood pressure and depressed respiration.

Treatment

This is a medical emergency.

- Administer 20% mannitol i.v. as a bolus dose at 0.25–0.5 g/kg (1.25–2.5 mL/kg of 20%). This can be repeated if the response is inadequate.
- Nurse the patient in a head-up position, maintain the airway.
- Severely restrict fluids.

- Transfer to an intensive care unit for intubation, intermittent positive pressure ventilation and further management.
- **Do not delay treatment for radiological confirmation – diagnosis is clinical.**

HYPOGLYCAEMIA IN CHILDREN WITH DIABETES

Common causes

- Missed meal/snack.
- Vigorous exercise (can be during exercise or hours afterwards).
- Alcohol.
- Too much insulin.

Table 22.2 Management of hypoglycaemia in children with diabetes

Awake	Sugar, e.g. 1 cup lemonade/orange/apple juice; jellybeans; honey (1 tbs); condensed milk in tube. Repeat in 5–10 min if no improvement, follow with 'sustaining serve'; e.g. milk, bread.
Drowsy/uncooperative/ unconscious/fitting	Glucagon* i.m. injection 1 mg (1 ampoule) >2 years, blood sugar rises in 5–10 minutes, sips of sugar containing fluid when awake
Uncooperative/ unconscious/fitting	Glucose –2 mL/kg of 25% dextrose i.v. over 2 min then 3–5 mg/kg/min until awake and able to drink/eat.

Note: Glucagon can cause headache/vomiting

SICK DAY MANAGEMENT DURING INTERCURRENT ILLNESS IN THE CHILD WITH DIABETES

Principles

- Frequent testing of blood sugar and urine ketones.
- The meal plan may temporarily be dropped – replace with fluids and easily digested carbohydrates.
- Ensure good fluid intake – alternate sugar and non-sugar-containing fluids depending on blood sugar levels (water is best if high).
- Insulin doses usually need to be increased; never omit insulin.
- Keep in touch with medical staff.

Table 22.3 Sick day management

Problem	*Danger*	*Fluids*	*Meals*	*Insulin*	*Monitor*	*Further action*
1. BSL high urine ketones 0–trace vomiting +/–		Ensure good intake (to thirst)	Normal meal plan	Increase normal dose by 10%	4–6-hourly BSL and urine ketones	If ketones increasing – as per group 2
2. BSL high Urine ketones >1+ Vomiting –/occasional	DKA	Increase intake++	Can drop normal meal plan	Give rapid acting insulin at 10–20% total daily dose. Repeat 4-hourly (2-hourly if 3+ ketones or mild vomiting	2–4-hourly	If not improving – admit
3. BSL normal/low Urine ketones 0–trace Vomiting +/–	Hypoglycaemia	Ensure good intake		Reduce normal insulin by 10–25%. May drop intermediate insulin if giving quick insulin 4–6-hourly	2–4-hourly	If BSL low – manage as for hypoglycaemia, if high – as per groups 1 or 2

MANAGEMENT OF CHILDREN WITH DIABETES UNDERGOING SURGERY

The main aims are to prevent hypoglycaemia before, during and after surgery and to provide sufficient insulin to prevent the development of ketoacidosis.

Factors that must be considered are:

- Time of surgery.
- Duration of surgery.
- Urgency of surgery.

Minor elective morning surgery

- Admit the child on the evening prior to surgery.
- Aim for the patient to be first on the operating list.
- Administer normal food and insulin until midnight on the night before surgery.
- At 0600 h perform blood glucose. If blood glucose is <10 mmol/L give lemonade or sugar-containing clear fluid at 5–10 mL/kg (max = 200 mL) and inform the anaesthetist.
- Monitor blood glucose every 2 h and immediately before surgery. If blood glucose is less than 6 mmol/L insert intravenous line and give i.v. glucose.
- Give rapid-acting insulin equal to 1/10th of the total daily insulin dose (rapid-and intermediate acting) at the usual time.
- An intravenous line with glucose will be inserted in the operating theatre (if not required pre-operatively).
- Perform regular blood glucose every 2–4 h postoperatively, and adjust the i.v. glucose infusion as necessary. Give extra insulin 0.25 units /kg every 4–6 h to keep glucose between 5 and 10 mmol/L.
- When the patient can tolerate oral fluids stop the intravenous infusion and resume the normal insulin regimen.

Minor elective afternoon surgery

- Continue normal food and insulin until midnight on the night before surgery.
- Provide a light breakfast at the usual time.
- Give rapid-acting insulin equal to 1/10th of the total daily insulin dose half an hour before breakfast.

- Monitor blood glucose every 2 h (commence i.v. glucose if BSL is <6 mmol/L, otherwise i.v. glucose can be commenced in theatre).
- Give additional insulin at the same dose at 1200 h.
- Adopt same regimen as previous postoperatively.

Minor surgery/short anaesthetic

- Intravenous glucose may not be necessary, provided that the oral intake can be resumed soon after surgery and that the pre-operative blood glucose concentration does not fall below 6 mmol/L. If in doubt, it is safer to follow the routines outlined above.

Emergency and major surgery

- Urgent clinical and biochemical assessment as for diabetic ketoacidosis.
- Rehydrate and start i.v. insulin as required.
- Maintain i.v. 0.45% saline with 5% dextrose and insulin infusion at 0.05–0.1 units/kg per h pre- and postoperatively until the patient is able to resume oral feeding.

SHORT STATURE

Stature must be assessed in the context of parental heights and pubertal status. Growth velocity must be compared with normal children and assessed with regard to pubertal status; that is, is a growth spurt occurring at an expected time for this child?

Stature

Measure the child and, wherever possible, both biological parents. Plot all three heights on appropriate height percentile charts, and compare the percentiles (see Appendix 2). The child's height percentile should approximate the mean of the parents' percentiles.

Questions that need to be asked:

- Is the child short in relation to other children the same age (i.e. below the third percentile)?
- Is the child unexpectedly short for their family?

Growth rate

Ask for any previous height measurements and plot them on the percentile chart. If no previous measurements are available, review at 3-month intervals and after 6 months, calculate the height velocity and check this against a growth velocity (GV) chart. Growth velocity can only be reliably calculated from measurements taken over 6–12 months.

In normal children GV tends to fluctuate and only a consistently low GV will lead to a falling off in height percentile. The criterion for further investigation in a short child is a GV below the 25th percentile.

Questions that need to be asked:

- Is the child growing slowly?
- If the child's growth really is slow, what is the reason?
- Is the child growing at the rate expected for pubertal status? A growth spurt should always accompany puberty.

Causes

Physiological

Constitutional delay in maturation

This is a common (and often familial) normal variant. Characteristically, growth slows at about 2 years of age, producing a fall in the height percentile. Thereafter, growth is parallel to the 3rd percentile, but the prepubertal decline in growth is exaggerated and the onset of the growth spurt is later than average. Bone age is delayed. The final height is likely to be in keeping with the height of other family members.

Familial short stature

Several adult family members are short. Skeletal proportions and GV are normal. Bone age is equivalent to the chronological age.

Some children from short families also have constitutional delay in maturation. Parents who have suffered protein calorie malnutrition as children may not have achieved their own genetic potential and may be on a lower percentile than their children.

Organic

Organic causes of short stature are classified in Table 22.4.

Clues to the diagnosis may emerge from the history and the child's general appearance. Some serious medical conditions (e.g. chronic renal failure, coeliac disease, inflammatory bowel disease, craniopharyngioma) may present with slow growth as the only abnormal sign.

Table 22.4 Organic causes of short stature

	Examples	*Clues to diagnosis*
Intra-uterine	Russell–Silver syndrome	Birth length <third centile for gestational age
Skeletal	Bone dysplasia (e.g. achondroplasia)	Skeletal dysproportion (short limbs)
	Spinal irradiation	Low upper : lower segment ratio
Nutritional	Rickets	History of poor nutrition
	Calorie–protein malnutrition (world no. 1)	Low weight-for-height (not if chronic)
	Malabsorption (e.g. coeliac disease)	Abdominal distension
	Chronic illness (e.g. renal failure, Crohn's disease)	Anaemia, high ESR
Iatrogenic	Corticosteroid therapy	Cushingoid features
Chromosomal and genetic	Turner, Down, Prader–Willi, Noonan, Cornelia de Lange, Rubinstein–Taybi syndromes	Specific dysmorphic features
	Inborn errors of metabolism: storage disorders (MPS[†], Gaucher)	Peculiar odour
	Organic/amino acidopathies (e.g. MMA*, MSUD**)	Metabolic acidosis
Endocrine	Hypothyroidism, Cushing disease, growth hormone deficiency, pubertal arrest, parathyroid disorders, AHO[#]	Height centile < weight centile (i.e. short and plump) Associated examination findings

[†] MPS, mucopolysaccharidosis
* MMA, methylmalonic aciduria
** MSUD, maple syrup urine disease
[#] Albright hereditary osteodystrophy

Important clues include:

- Dysmorphic features (e.g. Turner syndrome).
- Cutaneous changes (e.g. café au lait markings).
- Hand changes (e.g. short $4^{th}/5^{th}$ metacarpals, narrow deep set nails).
- Fundal changes (e.g. optic atrophy).

Measure the skeletal proportions (arm span/height and upper/lower segment ratios).

- The lower segment should be >1/2 the height beyond the age of 8 years.
- The arm span should be within a few centimetres of height at all ages.

Investigations

Check the bone age initially. If the GV is <25th percentile for bone age then tests are indicated.

- Thyroid function tests – thyroid stimulating hormone (TSH) is the usual screening test, check free T4 (FT4) if central dysfunction is considered.
- Haemoglobin and erythrocyte sedimentation rate (ESR) (inflammatory bowel disease).
- Renal function and urine MC&S.
- Serum calcium, phosphate and alkaline phosphatase.
- Consider testing for coeliac disease.
- Chromosomes (all short girls; lack of dysmorphism does not exclude Turner syndrome).
- Skeletal survey (if disproportionate).
- Consider growth hormone (GH) studies as a second step (always performed fasting):
  - Exercise.
  - Glucagon stimulation (the current definitive test).

Interventions

Growth hormone therapy

Recombinant human GH is government controlled in Australia; it costs an average of $20 000–$30 000 per year per child.

To qualify, children must meet certain criteria:

- The height is below the 1st percentile.
- The GV is below the 25th percentile for bone age.
- The bone age is <13.5 years for girls, or <15.5 years for boys.
- They must be free of any condition known not to respond to GH (e.g. high-dose steroid therapy or thalassaemia) or that could be worsened by GH therapy (e.g. insulin-dependent diabetes mellitus (IDDM), Fanconi anaemia or active malignancy).

Children with GH deficiency or Turner syndrome respond to growth hormone with an increase in final height. Use of growth hormone for other conditions without biochemical growth hormone deficiency will increase growth velocity in the short term but usually does not result in significant increase in final height.

The dose of growth hormone is 14–22 units/m^2 per week divided into 6–7 doses/week.

TALL STATURE

Cause

- Familial.
- Precocious puberty.
- Hyperthyroidism.
- Syndromes: Marfan, Klinefelter, triple X, homocystinuria and Sotos.
- Pituitary gigantism (juvenile acromegaly).

Assessment

Height must be considered in the context of mid parental expectation and pubertal status, e.g. if puberty is 2–3 years earlier than average, the child may appear to be very tall for chronological age but have a perfectly normal final height expectation for the family.

Investigations

Consider:

- Thyroid function.
- Karyotype.
- Urine metabolic screen/antithrombin III/coagulation/lipids (homocystinuria).
- 3 hour oral glucose tolerance test for growth hormone/IGF 1.

Management

Management of any underlying disorder, for example, precocious puberty. High-dose oestrogen is sometimes used in selected very tall girls and tall boys may be similarly treated with testosterone. Treatment is managed by a paediatric endocrinologist.

HYPOTHYROIDISM

Hypothyroidism may be congenital or acquired.

Congenital hypothyroidism

Incidence

- 1:3200 births.

Causes

- Absent thyroid 40–45%.
- Thyroid arrested in line of normal descent (lingual) 40–45%.
- Abnormal function (dyshormonogenesis) 10–15%.
- Maternal iodine deficiency.

Clinical

- Unusually sleepy baby.
- Jaundice.
- Large anterior fontanelle, persistent posterior fontanelle.
- Coarse features.
- Dry skin.
- Peri-orbital oedema.
- Umbilical hernia.
- Harsh or hoarse cry.
- Slow feeding.
- Distal femoral epiphysis that is not ossified.

Investigations

- Most cases are detected by neonatal screening (high thyroid stimulating hormone (TSH)). Confirmation of the diagnosis on whole blood thyroid function tests (TFT) is essential.
- Technetium (Tch) scanning for position, function, size (presence of goitre, Tch uptake).

Management

- Thyroxine therapy (8–12 mcg/kg/day) must be started as early as possible – before 2 weeks. Evidence suggests better outcome if treatment started at 10 days and T4 in upper range.
- Aim for:
  - FT4 at the upper limit of normal range for age or just above.
  - Normalisation of TSH.

Acquired hypothyroidism

Acquired hypothyroidism is called primary when the thyroid gland itself is abnormal (e.g. ectopic thyroid dysgenesis, auto-immune chronic lymphocytic thyroiditis and dyshormonogenesis) and secondary when the abnormality is a deficiency in pituitary TSH.

Clinical features

Hypothyroidism is often very difficult to detect clinically in children. Growth retardation may be the only sign, often with a relatively excess weight for height. The classical signs are usually absent when the cause is hypothalamic–pituitary.

- Growth retardation.
- Weight gain.
- Lethargy.
- Constipation.
- Cold intolerance.
- Goitre.
- Dry cool skin, dry hair.
- Prolonged ankle jerk relaxation time.

Investigations

- TSH as screening test.
- FT4 for degree of deficit and for primary diagnosis when cause is central.
- Thyroid auto-antibodies.
- Urinary iodine (early morning).
- Technetium thyroid scan.
- Thyroid ultrasound where indicated (for assessment of gland structure).

Referral to a specialist is important for the management of hypothyroidism.

HYPERTHYROIDISM

Hyperthyroidism is usually due to Graves' disease in children and adolescents (different spectrum to adults). Six times as many girls are affected as boys, most commonly during puberty. A family history of thyroid disease (hyper- or hypothyroidism) is common. A family history should be sought for: IDDM, vitiligo, pernicious anaemia, Addison disease or premature gonadal failure, as part of the spectrum of autoimmune polyglandular syndrome types I and II.

Other causes to consider:

- Toxic phase of Hashimoto thyroiditis (usually 4–6 weeks duration and usually not detected clinically).
- Thyroid adenoma (rare in childhood).
- Factitious (thyroxine consumption for weight loss).

Clinical features

- Goitre (nearly all), diffuse, with bruit.
- Weight loss, heat intolerance, tiredness.
- Warm sweaty hands, tremor, tachycardia.
- Irritability and restlessness.
- Proximal muscle weakness and wasting, accelerated ankle jerk relaxation time.
- Lid lag; exophthalmos, peri-orbital oedema, extra-ocular muscle trapping causing diplopia on upward and lateral gaze.
- Accelerated growth velocity.

Investigations

- FT4, FT3. TSH should be suppressed to undetectable (<0.01 mU/L).
- TSH receptor antibodies.
- Bone age (usually advanced).
- Technetium thyroid scan – expect diffuse increased uptake.
- Thyroid ultrasound if adenoma suspected.

Management

Antithyroid drugs are used for long-term treatment in childhood and adolescence. The long-term remission rate in this age group is 40%. Management by a specialist is necessary.

Antithyroid drugs

- Carbimazole – 0.4 mg/kg (max 30–60 mg/day depending on age, size), oral 8–12-hourly, for 2 weeks. Then reduce dose to 0.1 mg/kg (max 5 mg) oral 8–24-hourly for at least 18–24 months, until remission is achieved. Short courses of treatment result in low remission rates.

- Propylthiouracil (PTU) – 4 mg/kg oral 8-hourly with similar reduction in dose after 2 weeks. Propylthiouracil prevents conversion of T4 to T3 and is the preferred treatment in severe toxicity.

Idiosyncratic reactions may occur to either drug with urticaria and/or neutropaenia. This can occur at any time during treatment but is more common with high doses early in treatment. There is approximately 40% crossover intolerance.

Surgery

Used for:

- Non-compliance.
- Allergy to drugs.
- Large goitre, increasing in size.
- Long-term patient choice.

Radioactive iodine

The use of radioactive iodine in children and adolescents is controversial and is not advocated. It is considered safe by WHO by age 17 years. It is the treatment of choice for adults.

Thyroid storm

Thyroid storms are a rare complication of untreated primary hyperthyroidism or non-compliance with thyroid medication. It is characterised by tremor, anxiety, tachycardia, fever and confusion. It requires treatment (usually in ICU), with intravenous beta blockade, sedation, Lugol's iodine and propylthiouracil.

DELAYED PUBERTY

Delayed puberty is defined as the absence of pubertal changes over 13–14 years for girls and over 15 years for boys. There is no absolute age for diagnosis; later than average and inappropriately late in a family being common reasons for referral (see Appendix 2 for pubertal stages charts/diagrams).

Cause

With normal or low serum gonadotrophins

- Constitutional delay (usually familial) is the most common cause. It is associated with slow growth and a delayed bone age in an otherwise healthy child.
- Chronic illness/poor nutrition (e.g. inflammatory bowel disease, anorexia nervosa, cystic fibrosis).
- Endocrine causes:
  - Hypopituitarism (gonadotrophin and possibly GH and other hormonal deficiencies).
  - Kallmann syndrome (isolated gonadotrophin deficiency with anosmia).
  - Hyperprolactinaemia (prolactinoma, secondary to medication (e.g. anti-psychotics), functional (e.g. post cranial irradiation).

With elevated serum gonadotrophins

This signifies primary gonadal failure, which may be due to:

- A genetic abnormality associated with gonadal dysgenesis (e.g. Turner, Klinefelter and Noonan syndromes).
- Anorchia.
- Gonadal destruction secondary to vascular damage, irradiation, infection, torsion or autoimmune disease.

Investigations

- Serum follicle-stimulating hormone (FSH), luteinising hormone (LH), testosterone or oestradiol; serum prolactin; other pituitary function tests (e.g. GH studies), as indicated by growth.
- Full blood examination, erythrocyte sedimentation rate (ESR).
- Urea, creatinine, serum proteins.
- Thyroid function test (TFT).
- Chromosomes.
- Bone age.

Management

Referral to a specialist is advised. Testosterone may be used in boys and oestradiol in girls, however, excess or too early use of sex hormones for pubertal management will result in rapid advancement of bone age, epiphysial fusion and stunting of final height in both sexes. Growth hormone therapy may be offered to girls with Turner's syndrome (see Short stature, page 339).

PRECOCIOUS PUBERTY

Precocious puberty is defined as the onset of pubertal changes under 8 years in girls and under 9.5 years in boys. For pubertal staging, refer to Appendix 2.

Cause

Gonadotrophin dependent ('central' or 'true' precocious puberty)

- True precocious puberty is 20 times more common in girls than boys.
- Girls are less likely to have an underlying pathological cause than boys.
- Girls with this disorder have accelerated growth, development of both pubic hair and breasts and the vaginal mucosa has a pale, shell-pink colour with increased mucus secretion due to the effects of oestrogen.
- Boys with true precocious puberty have enlargement of both testes, as well as accelerated linear and genital growth.
- The commonest pathological cause is hypothalamic hamartoma. Practically all intracranial pathologies (malformation, trauma, tumour, infection and haemorrhage) are associated with an increased prevalence of precocious puberty. After cranial irradiation, puberty occurs on average 2 years earlier than usual in both boys and girls.
- Investigations are designed to demonstrate the premature activity in the hypothalamic-pituitary-gonadal axis and to exclude intracranial pathology.

Gonadotrophin independent ('pseudo' precocious puberty)

- Congenital adrenal hyperplasia.
- Adrenal, testicular or ovarian neoplasms.
- Tumours that secrete non-pituitary gonadotrophin such as chorionic gonadotrophin (hCG).
- McCune-Albright syndrome.
- Familial male precocious puberty.

Investigation of precocious puberty (both types)

- Serum FSH and LH.
- Gonadal steroid (testosterone or oestradiol).
- β HCG where indicated.
- Bone age.
- Magnetic resonance imaging (MRI) of the head, if increased FSH or LH is found. All boys with central precocious puberty must have an MRI. In girls with central precocious puberty MRI is less likely to yield an intracranial organic lesion and is not commonly performed if puberty occurs at >5 years, unless there is a specific clinical indication (e.g. headache, visual change).
- Pelvic ultrasound in girls for ovarian cyst or tumour.
- Testicular ultrasound if indicated.

Management

A referral should be made to a specialist, who may use medroxyprogesterone acetate, cyproterone acetate or a luteinising hormone releasing hormone superagonist (LHRH agonist). Not all cases require treatment.

Conditions resembling precocious puberty

Premature thelarche

- Isolated breast development is common in girls under 2 years of age (8–10%) and can be expected to regress spontaneously in most cases.
- Simple observation is usually sufficient but if the condition is associated with rapid growth velocity, consider true oestrogen excess of any cause and investigate (as above).

Premature adrenarche

- The isolated appearance of pubic hair (usually in a girl) under the age of 8 years may occur as a normal variant, but it may also signify non-classical congenital adrenal hyperplasia.
- Appropriate investigations are bone age, basal serum dehydroepiandrosterone sulphate (DHEA-S), androstenedione, testosterone and 17–hydroxyprogesterone (17–OHP). The measurement of 17–OHP at 30 and 60 min after intramuscular Synacthen (synthetic adrenocorticotrophic hormone (ACTH)) is recommended to diagnose non-classical congenital adrenal hyperplasia.
- Referral to a specialist is recommended.

PUBERTAL GYNAECOMASTIA

- In true gynaecomastia there will be a palpable disc of breast tissue; this is to be distinguished from adiposity of the breast area.
- Breast development occurs transiently in many boys mid-way through puberty and is usually physiological.
- If associated with testicular volumes <6 mL, Klinefelter syndrome must be excluded by a chromosomal analysis (boys with Klinefelter syndrome are usually tall (>50th percentile), but this is not universal).
- Adrenal and gonadal tumours can cause gynaecomastia, but this is rare.
- Prolactinoma must be considered, particularly if gynaecomastia is associated with galactorrhoea.
- Many drugs, notably cimetidine, digoxin, spironolactone and i.m. testosterone can induce breast development, as can heavy marijuana use.
- Prepubertal gynaecomastia also occurs, but in most cases no cause can be found.

Assessment

Most require no investigation, refer if concerned about diagnosis.

Management

Ninety percent of gynaecomastia disappears spontaneously within 2 years of onset. Refer boys with significant breast enlargement to a plastic or general surgeon for subareolar mastectomy.

OBESITY

See also Weight related problem, chapter 7 and Table 22.5.

Nutritional obesity is associated with growth acceleration and advancement of bone age. Endocrine obesity is associated with growth retardation and a delay in bone age.

Table 22.5 Endocrine causes of obesity

Cause	*Clinical features*	*Screening investigation*
Cushing disease	Growth retardation, hypertension, hirsutism, striae, typical facial changes, bruising	24 h urinary free cortisol
Hypothyroidism	Growth retardation, tiredness, constipation, cold intolerance, dry skin	Thyroid function tests (TSH)
Growth hormone (GH) deficiency	Growth retardation	GH studies
Prader–Willi syndrome	Neonatal hypotonia, growth retardation, developmental delay, hyperphagia, hypogonadism, typical facial appearance, small hands and feet	Specific DNA test

AMBIGUOUS GENITALIA

An underlying endocrine or genetic cause should be sought in:

- Any infant with ambiguous genitalia.
- Boys with perineal hypospadias.
- Boys with any combination of the following: micropenis, hypospadias, short stature, dysmorphic features or undescended testis.
- Girls with inguinal herniae containing gonads.

Note: Clitoral enlargement of any degree is abnormal.

Cause

In decreasing order of frequency:

- Gonadal dysgenesis.
- Congenital adrenal hyperplasia.
- Androgen insensitivity syndrome.
- Testosterone biosynthetic defects.

Investigations

- Electrolytes, urea and blood glucose.
- Serum 17–hydroxy progesterone and 24 h urine steroid profile.
- Chromosomes.
- Pelvic ultrasound.

Management

- Refer urgently to an experienced paediatric endocrinologist and surgeon.
- Inform the parents about the problem and show them the genitalia; tell them that the infant appears otherwise healthy and that the true sex will be ascertained within a few days. Do not attempt to predict the child's sex.
- Offer emotional support (refer to a social worker or an experienced mental health professional).
- Transfer the baby to a tertiary-referral centre without delay.
- Call a meeting of all nursery staff and discuss policy about communication with the parents about the baby. Keep detailed notes about communication with the parents.

ADRENAL HYPOFUNCTION

Primary adrenal insufficiency

This is rare in childhood and adolescence. It should be considered in the presence of vomiting, weight loss, pigmentation, chronic tiredness, low serum sodium and high serum potassium of unknown cause.

X-linked adrenoleukodystrophy

This is the commonest cause of primary adrenal insufficiency in school-age boys.

- Clinical hyperpigmentation of the skin (ACTH-mediated), tiredness, nausea, anorexia and weight loss.
- Adrenal features are usually preceded by the development of a neurological disability (e.g. memory loss, sleep disturbance or ataxia).
- Test blood and skin fibroblasts for very long-chain fatty acids.
- Dietary modification and bone marrow transplantation may be helpful in cases with normal MRI.

Autoimmune destruction (Addison disease)

This is usually part of the autoimmune polyglandular syndrome (in combination with either chronic mucocutaneous candidiasis, primary hypoparathyroidism, or both). Presenting in later childhood or adolescence, it may also be associated with thyrotoxicosis, diabetes mellitus, Hashimoto's thyroiditis, coeliac disease, Graves disease, Sjögren syndrome, rheumatoid arthritis and less commonly with T or B cell deficiency.

Congenital adrenal hyperplasia

- 21–Hydroxylase deficiency.
- Other rare types.
- Signs of androgen excess are usually obvious- with ambiguous genitalia and precocious sexual development.

Investigations

- Serum electrolytes (low sodium and high potassium).
- Simultaneous serum cortisol and plasma ACTH.
- Specific investigations if congenital adrenal hyperplasia (CAH) is suspected; 17OH progesterone, urine steroid profile.

Management

- Hydrocortisone 20 mg/m^2 BSA per day in divided doses.
- Fludrocortisone 0.05–0.2 mg daily, orally.
- Steroid cover for stress (see below).

'Secondary' adrenal insufficiency (due to ACTH deficiency)

Causes

Hypothalamic pituitary failure due to tumour, trauma, post surgery, cranial irradiation (where it may be subtle) or histiocytosis.

Clinical

- Not usually associated with salt-wasting.
- No hyperpigmentation of the skin.
- Treat with hydrocortisone alone; fludrocortisone is unnecessary.

Steroid cover for stress (1° and 2° adrenal insufficiency)

- **All patients with adrenal insufficiency of any cause are at risk for adrenal crisis during periods of severe stress.**
- **All need extra steroid cover.**

- In cases of acute medical illness (e.g. gastroenteritis, influenza), any surgery requiring general anaesthetic and any major fracture:
  - **Hydrocortisone 25–100 mg i.m./i.v. stat.**
  - Repeat every 4–6 h until recovery.
  - Follow by triple the usual daily doses of hydrocortisone for 2 days, then double for 3 days.

ADRENAL HYPERFUNCTION

Adrenocortical tumours

- This may manifest as Cushing syndrome, virilisation, hypertension, abdominal mass or pain.
- These tumours are very rare.

Adrenocortical hyperplasia

- This is usually secondary to a pituitary adenoma secreting ACTH (Cushing disease).
- The primary micronodular form (genetic cause) is rarely seen.

Cortisol excess in children is more difficult to detect clinically than in adults. It is characterised by poor growth velocity and excessive weight gain. The child usually looks obese but the clinical features of moon face, thin limbs and striae may be absent.

Investigation

- 24 h urinary free cortisol. Plasma cortisol is often abnormal in obesity and may give a spurious result.
- Overnight dexamethasone suppression (1 mg dexamethasone given at 2400 h and a plasma cortisol at 0800 h the following day) will differentiate Cushing syndrome from obesity.

Further investigation for origin and type of cortisol excess is by a specialist. Treatment is surgical.

Adrenal medullary tumours

- Neuroblastoma usually occurs in very young children, but may present in adolescence.
- Phaeochromocytoma in older children (leading to hypertension).

DISORDERS OF CALCIUM METABOLISM

Hypocalcaemia

Table 22.6 Causes of hypocalcaemia

Neonatal presentation	*Infant/childhood presentation*
Prematurity/IUGR/birth asphyxia Hypoparathyroidism +/– Di George syndrome Phosphate load (high phosphate milk) Low magnesium Maternal gestational diabetes	Vitamin D deficiency Groups at risk: • Families where covering clothing is worn at all times, especially breast fed infants in such families • Dark skin colour • Indoor lifestyle • Anticonvulsants (alter vitamin D metabolism/calcium absorption) • Chronic immobilisation • Malabsorption, liver disease Hypoparathyroidism • Association with autoimmune polyglandular syndrome. Look for mucocutaneous candidiasis and/or Addison disease in a young child Pseudohypoparathyroidism • Albright hereditary osteodystrophy Chronic renal failure Pancreatitis Organic acidaemia Critical illness 1–α hydroxylase deficiency (rare) Vitamin D resistant rickets

Clinical features

- Rachitic changes in long bones (swollen wrists etc), rachitic rosary.
- Tetany (may be demonstrated using sphygmomanometer cuff above systolic pressure for up to 2 min).
- Laryngeal stridor.
- Fitting.
- Weakness, tiredness, irritability.

Even extreme hypocalcaemia may be asymptomatic in an infant.

Investigations

- 25 OH vitamin D.
- Renal function, lipase, albumin.
- Magnesium, phosphate.
- Alkaline phosphatase.
- Parathyroid hormone (PTH).
- Total and ionised calcium.
- 1,25 diOH vitamin D if hypophosphataemic rickets is suspected.
- X-ray wrist, knee (metaphyseal splaying).
- Malabsorption studies.
- ECG (prolonged QT interval).

Treatment

Emergency

- Intravenous calcium chloride 10% (infusion 1 mmol/kg/24 hours in 5% dextrose) monitor calcium levels 6-hourly.
- Occasionally i.v. calcium chloride 10%, 0.2 mL/kg stat may be required for severe tetany.
- Correct magnesium if low.
- ECG monitor.
- 25 OH vitamin D if nutritional rickets is suspected: 4000 IU/day for 2 weeks then maintenance (see below).
- 1,25 diOH vitamin D if parathyroid disorders suspected: 0.01–0.02 mcg/kg/day starting dose may need to be increased.
- Treatment of underlying condition.

Note: 'hungry bones' for first days-weeks after treatment started for rickets – large doses of calcium supplement may be required to maintain normocalcaemia and prevent carpopedal spasm once vitamin D is started.

Maintenance

- Adequate calcium intake, preferably as dairy products, 600–1500 mg/day depending on age.
- 500 IU/day 25 OH vitamin D for months-years depending on cause (for infant rickets, usually treat to age 4).
- 1,25 diOH vitamin D (Rocaltrol) for vitamin D resistant rickets, hypoparathyroidism, patients on anticonvulsants.
- 1,25 diOH vitamin D and phosphate for hypophosphataemic rickets (high dose).

Hypercalcaemia

Table 22.7 Causes of hypercalcaemia

Neonatal	*Infant/childhood*
Hyperparathyroidism (rare) Iatrogenic Subcutaneous fat necrosis Familial hypocalciuric hypercalcaemia – severe form Hypophosphatasia Bartter syndrome William syndrome (with elfin face, supravalvular aortic stenosis)	Primary hyperparathyroidism Familial hypocalciuric hypercalcaemia Vitamin D 1,25 diOH D excess (nutritional, inflammatory disease e.g. sarcoidosis, leukaemia) Neoplasia (lytic bone lesions or humoral hypercalcaemia PTHrP) Immobilisation e.g. burns (severe), quadriplegia – can be very severe and cause renal calculi, pancreatitis Drugs (lithium, thiazides) Endocrine disorders: Hyperthyroidism (mild, usually asymptomatic), phaeochromocytoma, adrenal insufficiency

Clinical features

- Polyuria, polydipsia.
- Vomiting, dehydration.
- Failure to thrive.
- Abdominal pain (constipation, renal stones, pancreatitis).
- Confusion, apathy (if severe).

Investigation

- Total and ionised calcium, phosphate.
- Magnesium, albumin.
- Alkaline phosphatase.
- 25 OH vitamin D +/– 1,25 diOH vitamin D.
- Thyroid function.
- Chest X-ray +/– skeletal survey.
- Parathyroid imaging.
- Renal ultrasound (nephrocalcinosis).
- ECG (short QT interval).

Management of severe hypercalcaemia

- Rehydration with 0.9% saline/5% dextrose. For infants <2 years use 0.45% saline/5% dextrose.
- Diuretics (thiazide) to decrease urinary calcium excretion and/or reduce oedema.
- Bisphosphonates, particularly for increased bone resorption (e.g. immobilisation).
- Steroids for vitamin D excess (Prednisolone 2 mg/kg/day, reducing).
- Low calcium diet.
- Surgery if indicated, treatment of underlying condition.

CHAPTER 23
EYE CONDITIONS

James Elder
Peter Barnett

IMPORTANT PRINCIPLES

- Always test and record vision as the first part of any eye examination. In infants, observe following and other visual behaviour and listen to the parents' impressions of their child's vision.
- Transient malalignment of the eyes is common up to 6 months of age. A child with a constant squint at any age or any transient squint after 6 months of age should be referred promptly to an ophthalmologist. True squints rarely improve spontaneously.
- Never pad a discharging eye.
- Pad an eye into which a local anaesthetic has been instilled until the effect of the local anaesthetic has worn off or keep the child indoors until the local anaesthetic has worn off (10–20 min).
- Do not use local steroid drops unless corneal ulceration has been excluded by fluorescein staining. Only use steroids for short periods (2 days or less), unless an ophthalmologist directs otherwise.
- In cases of photophobia or watery eyes in the first year of life, when there is no significant discharge, consider the possibility of congenital glaucoma.
- All children with a white-red reflex or white masses in the retina must be referred immediately to an ophthalmologist to exclude retinoblastoma.
- Instilling eye drops/ointment in a young child: carer sits on the floor with legs extended; lay child between carer's legs with child's arms under the carer's thighs and the child's feet near the carer's feet. This leaves the child's head secured and the carer with both hands free to hold open the child's eyelids and instil eye medication.

TRAUMA

Trauma to the eye can take many forms. Physical trauma to the eye and surrounding structures may be blunt or sharp. Trauma can also result from radiation (thermal and electromagnetic) and chemical agents.

Foreign bodies

Foreign bodies on the surface present with a painful, watery eye. If a foreign body or corneal ulcer is suspected, instil 1 drop of local anaesthetic to ease the pain and facilitate examination. Suitable local anaesthetics are proxymetacaine 0.5%, amethocaine 0.5 or 1%, or benoxinate 0.4%. **Do not use local anaesthetics for the continuing treatment of ocular pain under any circumstance**.

Conjunctival foreign bodies are common and are often found on the posterior surface of the upper lid. Therefore, eversion of the lid is essential. Most foreign bodies are easily removed with a moist cotton wool swab. If they are embedded or difficult to remove, refer the patient to an ophthalmologist. Beware of an iris naevus or iris prolapse through a perforating injury of the cornea mimicking a corneal foreign body.

Intraocular foreign bodies are generally from high-velocity fragments. Suspect them if the history involves an explosion, metal(s) striking on metal, or any other situation that involves high-speed objects (e.g. power tools or a lawn mower). If the history is at all suggestive, even in the absence of local signs, an X-ray of the orbit (AP and lateral) is necessary. If an intraocular foreign body is demonstrated, immediate referral to an ophthalmologist is mandatory.

Eyelid injuries

All eyelid lacerations except the most minor should be repaired as an in-patient procedure. Suspect canalicular injury in all lacerations involving the medial aspect of the eyelids and refer to an ophthalmologist. All lacerations involving the lid margin should be referred to an ophthalmologist.

Hyphaema (blood in the anterior chamber)

This is the result of blunt trauma to the eye. This generally requires admission to hospital. All cases require referral to an ophthalmolgist, as there is a potential for secondary haemorrhage and loss of vision.

Fracture of the orbital bones

A blowout fracture through the wall of the orbit is suspected if one or more of the following 3 cardinal signs are present:

- Restricted movement of the eye, particularly in a vertical plane, with double vision.
- Infra-orbital nerve anaesthesia.
- Enophthalmos – this may be difficult to assess initially because of eyelid haematoma.

Diagnosis is usually clinical. Refer to an ophthalmologist before organising a CT scan. A CT scan is used to demonstrate the fracture of the orbital wall and entrapped orbital tissue (the classic sign is a tear drop 'polyp' hanging from the roof of the maxillary antrum).

Penetrating injury (including intraocular foreign body)

This should always be considered in patients with lacerations involving the eyelids, particularly after motorcar accidents. This should be suspected if the pupil is distorted, the iris is prolapsing through the cornea, or pigmented tissue is seen over the sclera. If suspected, protect the eye with a cone or shield that does not place pressure on the eyelids or eye and admit. Prevent vomiting with an anti-emetic as vomiting may cause extrusion of eye contents. Refer to an ophthalmologist immediately.

Chemical burns

Irrigate the eye with saline or water copiously for 15 min using an i.v. giving set. The instillation of local anaesthetic first will facilitate this. Refer all chemical burns to an ophthalmologist.

Thermal burns

The ocular surface is rarely involved. Check for ulceration with fluorescein staining. Butesin picrate ointment is suitable for use on lid burns. Secondary lid swelling may result in corneal exposure and ocular lubricants are then required.

THE ACUTE RED EYE

Common causes of the acute red eye are conjunctivitis, corneal ulceration, corneal or conjunctival foreign bodies (see previously), less common causes are pre-septal and orbital cellulitis. Table 23.1 gives a

Table 23.1 The causes of red, watery and sticky eyes

Problem	*Pain*	*Itch*	*Photophobia*	*Reduced Eye Movements*	*Epiphora*	*Discharge*	*Erythema*	*Other*
Neonatal conjunctivitis (ophthalmia neonatorum)	+++				++	+++	++ to ++	
Congenital nasolacrimal duct obstruction	–				+ to ++	+ to +++	–	
Infantile glaucoma			++		++	–	+	Enlarged & cloudy cornea
Viral conjunctivitis	++				++	+	+ to ++	
Bacterial conjunctivitis	++ to +++				++	+++	++ to +++	
Allergic conjunctivitis		++ +++			++ to +++	Stringy	+	
Chemical conjunctivitis	+++				+++	+	++ to +++	
Corneal abrasion	+++				++	–	Variable	
Foreign body	+++				++	–	Variable	Variable fluorescein staining
Preseptal cellulitis	++				+	Variable	+++ Swelling of eyelids	Conjunctiva not inflamed
Septal cellulitis	+++			+ to +++	+	Variable	+++ Swelling of eyelids	Eye is often inflamed and proptosed

brief outline of the presenting features of red, sticky and watery eyes, which have a large number of causes and whose clinical presentations may overlap.

Conjunctivitis

Aetiology

- Bacterial – generally pus is present.
- Viral – generally there is watery discharge.
- Allergic – history of atopy and 'itchy eyes'.

Neonatal conjunctivitis (ophthalmia neonatorum)

Neisseria gonorrhoeae

Acute severe, purulent discharge associated with marked conjunctival and lid oedema (the clinical appearance is of 'pus under pressure'). It occurs within a few days of birth. This is an ocular emergency because of the risk of corneal perforation.

- *Diagnosis.* Urgent Gram stain for Gram-negative intracellular diplococci and direct culture to appropriate culture media.
- *Treatment.* Admit and give i.v. cefotaxime 50 mg/kg 8-hourly for 7 days (dose may need adjustment according to age and birthweight). Penicillin (same duration) is an alternative if the organism is known to be susceptible. In all cases local measures such as ocular lavage and topical antibiotics (chloramphenicol or neomycin) may be of help.
- Investigate and treat the mother and partner.

Chlamydia

Usually occurs at 10 to 14 days of age. Fails to respond to routine topical antibiotics. If left untreated, there is a risk of pneumonitis.

- *Diagnosis.* Giemsa stain of conjunctival scraping for intranuclear inclusions. Also antibodies in tears and immunofluorescent stains of conjunctival scrapes. Use a chlamydia kit, ensuring conjunctival cells are collected.
- *Treatment.* Erythromycin 10 mg/kg oral 8-hourly for 21 days and eye toilet.
- Investigate and treat the mother and partner.

Other bacteria

Other causes of conjunctivis are *Staphylococcus, Streptococcus* or diphtheroids. Culture and treat with neomycin or chloramphenicol eye drops/ointment. A rapid clinical response is anticipated. Occasionally *Neisseria meningitidis* can cause conjunctivitis and should be treated as for invasive infection (see Infectious diseases, chapter 27).

Blocked nasolacrimal duct

A mucopurulent discharge with a watery eye. On waking the discharge is worse and conjunctiva is not inflamed (see Watering eyes, p. 365).

Conjunctivitis in older children

Management of this condition depends on the aetiology.

Bacterial

Severe: Chloramphenicol eye drops: 2-hourly by day and ointment at night. Less severe: Chloramphenicol eye drops or ointment 3 times a day.

Viral

This condition usually clears spontaneously. If it is unclear whether the infection is viral or bacterial, Neomycin eye drops may be given.

Herpes simplex conjunctivitis

Suspect if the child has vesicles. Check for corneal ulceration and treat with 4-hourly aciclovir ointment if ulceration is present. Refer to an ophthalmologist.

Allergic

In mild cases use an astringent (phenylephrine 0.12% or naphazoline 0.1%). In moderate cases use a topical antihistamine (antazoline 0.5%). In severe cases refer to an ophthalmologist. Topical steroid or sodium cromoglycate should only be given under the supervision of an ophthalmologist.

Corneal ulceration

Cause

- Trauma (with or without a foreign body).
- Herpes simplex (dendritic ulcer).

Diagnosis

- The symptoms are pain, photophobia, lacrimation and blepharospasm.
- Fluorescein stain after the instillation of a local anaesthetic.

Management

- If traumatic: chloramphenicol ointment (1%) and pad if possible. Review in 24 h. If the condition has not healed in 48 h, refer to an ophthalmologist. When ulcer has healed, continue chloramphenicol ointment twice daily for 1 week.
- Herpes simplex: aciclovir eye ointment (1 cm inside of the lower conjunctival sac) 5 times a day for 14 days and refer to an ophthalmologist.

PERIORBITAL AND ORBITAL CELLULITIS

Both periorbital and orbital cellulitis present with erythematous, swollen lids in a febrile child. In periorbital cellulitis, the lid swelling frequently prevents the eye from opening. The lids must be separated (a Desmarres' lid retractor may be used) to exclude proptosis and limitation of eye movement. These are important signs of orbital cellulitis.

Periorbital (preseptal) cellulitis

Periorbital (preseptal) cellulitis refers to infection in the soft tissues of the eyelids; which may come from purulent conjunctivitis, dacryocystitis, or gain entry via local trauma or insect bite.

It is important to distinguish this condition from a *periorbital allergic reaction.* A well child, who has no fever and eyelid swelling without much redness, tenderness and local warmth, is quite likely to have an allergic reaction to an allergen that has been blown or rubbed into the eye, or secondary to an insect bite. An oral antihistamine may be used. In this case no specific radiological imaging is required. The child should be reviewed if the swelling does not settle in a few hours or if signs of inflammation develop.

Recommended antibiotics

In children who are systemically unwell it may be reasonable to use both cefotaxime and flucloxacillin initially. Any child in whom there is a reasonable suspicion of primary skin infection, or who is not improving on cefotaxime alone should have flucloxacillin added. Failure to respond in 24–48 h may indicate orbital cellulitis or underlying sinus disease. Treat as for orbital cellulitis.

Table 23.2 Recommended antibiotics in periorbital cellulitis

Mild	Amoxicillin/clavulanate (400/57 mg per 5 mL) 12.5–22.5 mg/kg/dose/p.o. 12 h
Moderate	Flucloxacillin 50 mg/kg (2 g) i.v. 6 h
Severe or under 5 years of age and non Hib immunised (treat as for orbital cellulitis)	Flucloxacillin 50 mg/kg (2 g) i.v. 6 h and Cefotaxime 50 mg/kg (2 g) i.v. 6 h

Orbital (septal) cellulitis

Orbital (septal) cellulitis occurs when infection is present around and behind the globe of the eye. It is usually due to spread from sinus infection (especially in the ethmoid sinuses) and occurs particularly in children beyond the age of 2 years. Orbital cellulitis is a medical emergency and should be treated with the same level of urgency as meningitis or a brain abscess. The potential for loss of vision and suppurative intracranial complications is significant.

Orbital cellulitis is differentiated from periorbital cellulitis by the presence of:

- Chemosis.
- Proptosis.
- Ophthalmoplegia.
- Decreased visual acuity.
- Systemic symptoms.

If the features of orbital cellulitis are present, a CT scan is required to determine if the sinusitis is complicated by abscess formation. This is most commonly a subperiosteal abscess on the medial wall of the orbit adjacent to the ethmoid sinus, which requires surgical drainage (usually by an external ethmoidectomy approach). If no abscess is present, treatment is by intravenous antibiotics alone; however, CT scanning may need to be repeated if there is a progression of symptoms and signs, or if there is a lack of improvement following medical treatment.

Intravenous antibiotic therapy is required; flucloxacillin 50 mg/kg (max 2 g) 4–6-hourly and cefotaxime 50 mg/kg (max 2 g) 6-hourly. See also Antimicrobial guidelines.

Urgent ENT and ophthalmology consultation are ı . suspected orbital cellulitis.

WATERING EYES

Watery eyes are common in children and are the result of poor tear drainage or the over-production of tears. The latter is usually the result of eye irritation and causes include: foreign bodies, corneal ulcer, conjunctivitis and infantile glaucoma (these are discussed elsewhere).

Nasolacrimal duct obstruction is the commonest cause of watery eyes and discharge that persists after the first 2 weeks of life. The discharge is worse on waking and the conjunctiva is not inflamed. It usually resolves spontaneously, due to an opening of the lower end of the nasolacrimal duct. Local eye cleaning is usually the only treatment indicated. If the eye is red and inflamed, topical neomycin eye drops may be given (avoid repeated courses of chloramphenicol). If the discharge and watering have not settled by 12 months of age, refer to an ophthalmologist for probing.

STRABISMUS OR SQUINT (TURNED EYE)

Refer all children with squint or suspected squint to an ophthalmologist. This will allow early detection (and possibly prevention) of amblyopia and detection of any underlying pathology such as retinoblastoma or cataract. Examine the red reflex of all children suspected to have a squint, if the reflex is abnormal (very dull or white) urgent referral to an ophthalmologist is required to exclude cataract or retinoblastoma.

A child does not 'grow out of' a squint. However, in the first few months of life babies may have an intermittent squint, especially when feeding. A child of any age with a constant large angle squint or a child over 6 months with any squint (constant or intermittent) should be referred to an ophthalmologist. All children with a first-degree relative with a squint should be seen by an ophthalmologist at about 3–3½ years of age, even if there is no squint, as they may have a refractive error alone.

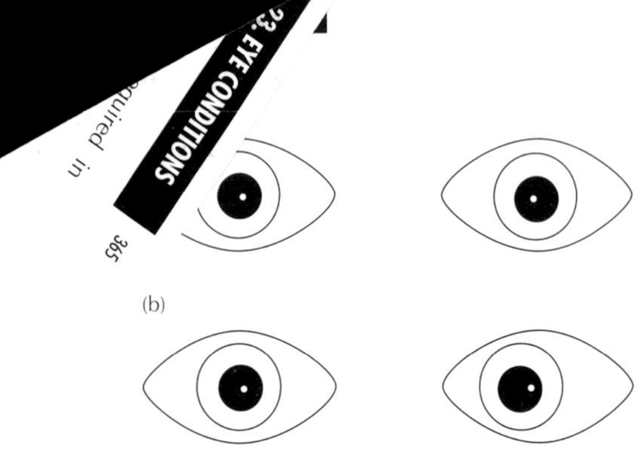

Fig. 23.1 Corneal light reflex. Shine a light at the child's eyes and observe the reflection. (a) Eyes are straight and the corneal light reflex is symmetrical. (*Note*: it is displaced slightly to the nasal side of the centre in each eye.) (b) Left convergent strabismus. The reflection from the deviated eye is displaced laterally.

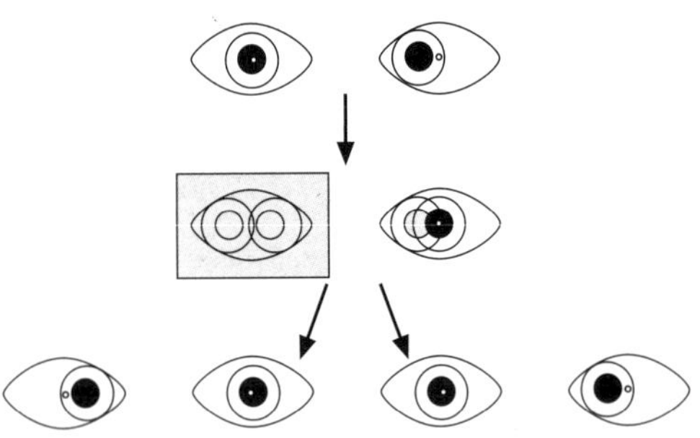

Fig. 23.2 The cover test. The child's attention is attracted with a toy. The eye that appears not to be deviating is covered. The uncovered eye is then observed for movement. If there is a convergent squint, the eye will move outwards (top and middle). The uncovered eye should also be observed when the cover is removed from the fellow eye. In an alternating squint there will be no movement of the uncovered eye and the previously covered eye will now be deviated (bottom left). In non-alternating or constant squint (vision is usually reduced in the deviating eye), there will be a rapid return to the original situation (bottom right). If no movement is detected, the test should be repeated but cover the other eye first.

A pseudo-strabismus (pseudo-squint) is due to a broad nasal bridge or epicanthic folds, or both. This results in the appearance of a squint, but corneal light reflexes are central and there is no movement on cover testing (see Figs 23.1 and 23.2). Only make the diagnosis of pseudo-strabismus if absolutely certain. Refer doubtful cases to an ophthalmologist.

EYELID LUMPS AND PTOSIS

Styes are acute bacterial infections of an eyelash follicle. They occur at the eyelid margin and are red and tender. Removing the lash directly related to the stye will often result in discharge of pus and hasten its resolution. Local antibiotics are sometimes indicated. Systemic antibiotics are rarely needed.

A chalazion is an obstructed tarsal (or Meibomian) gland. These glands are situated within the substance of the eyelid and thus a chalazion will present as a lump within the eyelid. There may be no associated symptoms. Redness associated with a chalazion is usually the result of sterile inflammation due to leakage of the contents, rather than a bacterial infection. Thus local or systemic antibiotics seldom influence the natural history of these lesions. Warm compresses may hasten resolution. If the chalazion is persistent (more than 6 months), large or causes discomfort, incision and drainage under a general anaesthetic may be indicated.

Ptosis is a droopy or lowered upper eyelid. In children it is usually the result of a minor and isolated anomaly in the development of the levator muscle. It may be unilateral or bilateral, and it is sometimes inherited in a dominant manner. If the lowered eyelid obstructs the pupil in a young child, visual loss will occur secondary to amblyopia. Urgent referral to an ophthalmologist is appropriate in such cases. In more minor degrees of ptosis, surgical intervention is for cosmesis and is less urgent.

RARE BUT IMPORTANT EYE CONDITIONS

Iritis

Acute iritis is very rare in children and presents with an acute red eye similar to the symptoms for a corneal ulcer. The pupil is small and does not react well to light. Refer to an ophthalmologist. Consider iritis in children with juvenile chronic arthritis (JCA). This form of iritis is chronic and painless.

Infantile glaucoma

The presenting features are:

- A hazy cornea.
- An enlarged cornea.
- Watery eyes.
- Photophobia.

This is a rare condition, but early recognition is vital. Prompt surgery offers a chance of cure and preservation of vision. All infants with suspected glaucoma require urgent referral to an ophthalmologist for examination under anaesthesia to measure corneal diameter, optic disc cupping and intraocular pressure.

Congenital cataracts

Congenital cataracts are rare, but early detection and removal with subsequent optical correction (contact lenses or spectacles) offers a good chance of visual preservation. All newborn infants should have their red reflexes examined prior to discharge from hospital. Check the red reflexes and fundi in any infant with poor visual performance (fixation and following). Nystagmus is a late sign for congenital cataracts. A unilateral cataract will often present as a squint. Any child suspected of having a congenital cataract must be referred urgently.

Retinoblastoma

This is a rare childhood cancer of the retina and presents with squint, a white pupil (cat's eye reflex), poor vision or a family history of the tumour. Prompt recognition is vital to maximise the possibility of preserving vision. Untreated this is a fatal disorder. If suspected refer urgently to an ophthalmologist.

CHAPTER 24
GASTROINTESTINAL CONDITIONS

Mark Oliver
Lionel Lubitz

ACUTE INFECTIOUS GASTROENTERITIS

This condition is most commonly caused by rotavirus infection with a seasonal peak period of infection in the autumn and winter in Australia. Adenovirus infection causes between 7–17% of cases requiring admission to hospital. Bacterial gastroenteritis is less common, causing 5–10% of all cases, causes include: *Salmonella* spp., *Campylobacter jejuni, Yersinia enterocolitica* and *Escherichia coli*. Parasites, such as *Cryptosporidium*, are also a known cause of acute gastroenteritis.

The two most important issues in the management of acute infectious diarrhoea are:

- Exclusion of other important causes of vomiting and diarrhoea.
- Adequate assessment and treatment of dehydration.

Differential diagnoses of vomiting and diarrhoea

- Appendicitis.
- Urinary tract infection.
- Other sepsis (including meningitis).
- Other surgical conditions including intussusception, enterocolitis associated with Hirschsprung disease and malrotation of the bowel.
- Haemolytic uraemic syndrome.

Clinical features

Presenting symptoms of acute infectious gastroenteritis include poor feeding, vomiting and fever, followed by diarrhoea. Stools are frequent and watery in consistency. The passage of blood and mucus, with frequent small volume stools and abdominal pain is suggestive of bacterial gastroenteritis. Be cautious of diagnosing gastroenteritis in the child with vomiting alone who is dehydrated or unwell.

It is essential that all children with acute onset of vomiting, diarrhoea and fever are re-evaluated regularly so as to confirm the diagnosis of acute gastroenteritis and adequacy of rehydration therapy.

Assessment of dehydration

- Risk of dehydration is increased with younger age, with infants (<6 months) having an increased surface area: body volume ratio resulting in increased insensible fluid losses.
- Recent change in body weight provides the most accurate indication of fluid depletion. Starvation produces no more than 1% body weight loss per day.
- Decreased skin turgor and peripheral perfusion accompanied by deep (acidotic) breathing are the only signs proven to discriminate between dehydration and hydration.
- Actual degree of dehydration may be underestimated with obesity and overestimated with wasting or sepsis.

<4% body weight loss represents no or mild dehydration
4–6% body weight loss represents moderate dehydration
≥7% body weight loss represents severe dehydration

Note: these percentages are approximate and given only as a guide.

Guidelines to management of dehydration and nutrition

General (see Table 24.1)

- For children/infants with dehydration, rapid hydration over 4–6 hours is now suggested (see Table 24.2). Past regimens aimed at gradual rehydration over 24 hours were not evidence based.
- Most children/infants with dehydration can be safely and adequately rehydrated using oral rehydration solutions (ORS). If these are not tolerated by the oral route, nasogastric administration is an alternative. Vomiting is not a contraindication to a nasogastric tube.
- Oral rehydration solutions use the principle of glucose-facilitated sodium transport in the small intestine. The solutions currently used in Australia are outlined in Table 24.3.

Table 24.1 Guidelines to assessment and management of dehydration

Assessment of dehydration	*Management*
Mild ≤4% body weight loss decreased peripheral perfusion* thirst, alert and restless	Rehydrate over 6 h with ORS/water in children/infants with mild dehydration. Oral rehydration solution only is preferred in high risk patients (infants <6 months). Infants and children in the moderate group may require rehydration via the nasogastric route.
Moderate 4–6% body weight loss all of the above signs (mild group) plus rapid pulse sunken eyes and fontanelle dry mucous membranes deep acidotic breathing* pinched skin retracts slowly (1–2 seconds)*	Re-assessment (including body weight and clinical examination) is required at 6 h. If fluid replete, maintenance age appropriate fluids can then be used. Weigh inpatients every 6 h during the first 24 h of admission. Introduce food intake after rehydration if dehydration has been corrected.
Severe 7% or greater of body weight loss all of above signs (mild-moderate group) plus in infants – drowsy, limp, cold, sweaty, cyanotic limbs and altered conscious level children – apprehension, cold, sweaty, cyanotic limbs, rapid feeble pulse and low blood pressure	If shock is present, give normal saline 20 mL/Kg i.v. (repeated fluid boluses may be required until organ perfusion is restored). Can start ORS once initial resuscitation is completed – give over 6 h. Following rehydration the same general principles as those for mild-moderate group apply.

* These are the only signs proven to discriminate between hydration and dehydration (4% or greater)

Table 24.2 Recommended hourly oral or nasogastric rehydration rate for children

Weight (kg)	*Maintenance (per h)*	*Moderate dehydration (4–6%) (mL/h)*		*Severe dehydration (≥7%) (mL/h)*	
		1st 6 h	*Next 18 h*	*1st 6 h*	*Next 18 h*
5	20	45	35	70	35
10	35	85	55	135	55
15	50	125	70	200	70
20	60	140	80	220	80
30	70	190	95	300	95
40	80	250	110	400	110
50	90	300	120	500	120

The daily water requirement is relatively high in neonates (150 mL/kg per day), reducing to 100 mL/kg per day in older infants and 80 mL/kg per day between 1 and 5 years.

Table 24.3 Oral rehydration preparations available for use in Australia

	Na	*K*	*Cl*	*Citrate*	*Glucose*
Gastrolyte	60	20	60	10	90
Repalyte	60	20	60	10	90
Hydralyte	45	20	35	30	80

Concentration expressed as mmol/L of made up solution.

- Early re-feeding (after rehydration) has been shown to enhance mucosal recovery in children/infants with acute gastroenteritis and reduces the duration of diarrhoea. Therefore continue breast-feeding or in formula fed infants, start oral intake with formula after rehydration and in children, introduce complex carbohydrates (e.g. rice, wheat, bread and cereals), yoghurt, fruit and vegetables.
- Transient lactase deficiency with acute gastroenteritis is not common in infants <6 months, so lactose free diets are rarely required after acute gastroenteritis.
- Drug avoidance: anti-diarrhoeals have no place in the treatment of infants or young children with acute gastroenteritis and antibiotics have only a limited role (see later).

Table 24.4 Suitable fluids for non-dehydrated children

Solution	*Dilution*
Sucrose (table sugar)	1 teaspoons in 200 mL boiled water
Fruit juice	1 in 6 with tap water
Cordials	1 part in 16 parts water
Lemonade	1 part in 6 parts water

Do not use undiluted or low calorie lemonade or fruit juice

- Parent education is vital, especially in the outpatient management of children. The important message is the need to drink more fluid more often, which is best given in small volumes and frequently (see Table 24.4). It should be emphasised that home-made solutions and ORS should be carefully prepared according to instructions provided, as they can be potentially dangerous if made up incorrectly.

Specific Recommendations

Admission to hospital

- Infants/children who have moderate or severe dehydration.
- Patients at a high risk of dehydration on the basis of young age (<6 months) with a high frequency of diarrhoea (8 per 24 h) and vomiting (>4 per 24 h) should be observed for 4–6 h to ensure adequate maintenance of hydration.
- High-risk infants/children (e.g. ileostomy, short gut, cyanotic heart disease, chronic renal disease, metabolic disorders and malnutrition).
- Infants/children whose parents and carers are thought to be unable to manage the child's condition at home.
- If the diagnosis is in doubt.

Biochemical investigations

Electrolyte and acid-base studies are required in children with:

- A history of prolonged diarrhoea with severe dehydration.
- A disturbance of conscious state or convulsions.
- Short bowel syndrome, ileostomy, chronic cardiac, renal and metabolic disorders.
- Infants <6 months of age who are judged as being dehydrated.

Nutritional management

- Breast-feeding should continue through rehydration and maintenance phases of treatment.
- Formula fed infants and children should re-start oral age appropriate formula or food intake after completion of rehydration.
- If there is persistent diarrhoea after re-introduction of feeds, evidence for lactose intolerance should be sought (stool pH <5 and more than 0.5% reducing substances). A lactose free formula can be used if the patient is lactose intolerant.

Pharmacotherapy

- Infants and children should not be treated with anti-diarrhoeal agents, as there is no substantial clinical evidence to suggest that this treatment alters symptoms.
- Most bacterial infections do not require antibiotics.
- *Salmonella* or *Campylobacter* gastroenteritis may require antibiotic treatment (see Infectious diseases chapter 27).
- *Shigella* dysentery requires antibiotic treatment.

Hypernatremic dehydration (sodium >150 mmol/L)

- Results from severe water and sodium depletion with greater loss of water. This can lead to severe neurological sequelae if rehydration is not carried out appropriately.
- Oral rehydration therapy is preferred to intravenous rehydration. If the patient is in shock, give a bolus of normal saline 20 mL/kg i.v., repeat until organ perfusion is restored.
- Following this, 'slow ORT' aiming to complete rehydration over 12 hours is required, followed by maintenance fluids.
- Serum electrolytes should be monitored on a 4-hourly basis. As a guideline, serum sodium should not fall by more than 1 mmol/L per h (on average).
- Consultation with an intensive care unit is recommended for these patients.

Hyponatraemic dehydration (serum sodium <130 mmol/L)

- Can cause seizures and coma, and requires consultation with an intensive care unit.
- Be aware of iatrogenic hyponatraemia due to fluid (hypotonic) overload.

SUGAR INTOLERANCE

Lactose intolerance

Following infectious diarrhoea, infants may have temporary lactose intolerance. This sequelae of acute gastroenteritis used to be prominent in infants <6 months of age, however, it is now uncommon. This may be due in part to early oral feeding which aids mucosal recovery.

Clinical features of sugar intolerance include:

- Persistently fluid stool.
- Excessive flatus.
- Excoriation of the buttocks.

Typically, these infants appear well.

Diagnosis

Collect the fluid stool in napkins lined with plastic. Dilute 5 drops of stool with 10 drops of water. Add a Clinitest tablet. A colour reaction corresponding to 0.5% or more reducing substance indicates that sugar intolerance is present.

Management

- Breast feeding should continue unless there are persistent symptoms with buttock excoriation and failure to gain adequate weight.
- Formula fed infants should be placed on a lactose-free formula for 3–4 weeks.

Note: A clinical response after change to soy formula may indicate either post-infectious lactose intolerance or allergy to cow milk protein, as soy formulae available in Australia are lactose-free.

Monosaccharide intolerance

Infrequently, infants with severe bowel damage secondary to gastroenteritis may be unable to absorb normal amounts of monosaccharide such as glucose or fructose. Diarrhoea will continue even with a lactose-free formula. Monosaccharide intolerance requires specialist consultation.

CHRONIC DIARRHOEA

An increase in stool frequency or fluid content is often of concern to parents, but does not necessarily imply significant organic disease, although this needs to be excluded. In every child who presents with chronic diarrhoea, the decision must be made as to whether further investigation is required.

The algorithm in Figure 24.1 outlines an approach to the child with chronic diarrhoea.

Toddler diarrhoea

- This is a clinical syndrome characterised by chronic diarrhoea often with undigested food in the stools of a child who is otherwise well, gaining weight and growing satisfactorily. Stools may contain mucus and are passed between 3 and 6 times a day; they are often looser towards the end of the day.
- Onset is usually between 8 and 20 months of age.
- Often there is a family history of functional bowel disease, such as irritable bowel syndrome.
- The treatment consists of reassurance and explanation. No specific drug or dietary therapy has been shown to be of value in toddler diarrhoea. Some toddlers on a high-fructose intake (i.e. 'apple juice' diarrhoea) may have diarrhoea that responds to dietary change.

COELIAC DISEASE

Coeliac disease is an autoimmune enteropathy triggered by the ingestion of gluten in genetically susceptible individuals. The prevalence of this disorder amongst first-degree relatives is in the order of 10%. The clinical expression of this disorder is more heterogeneous than previously thought and onset may be at any time after years without symptoms.

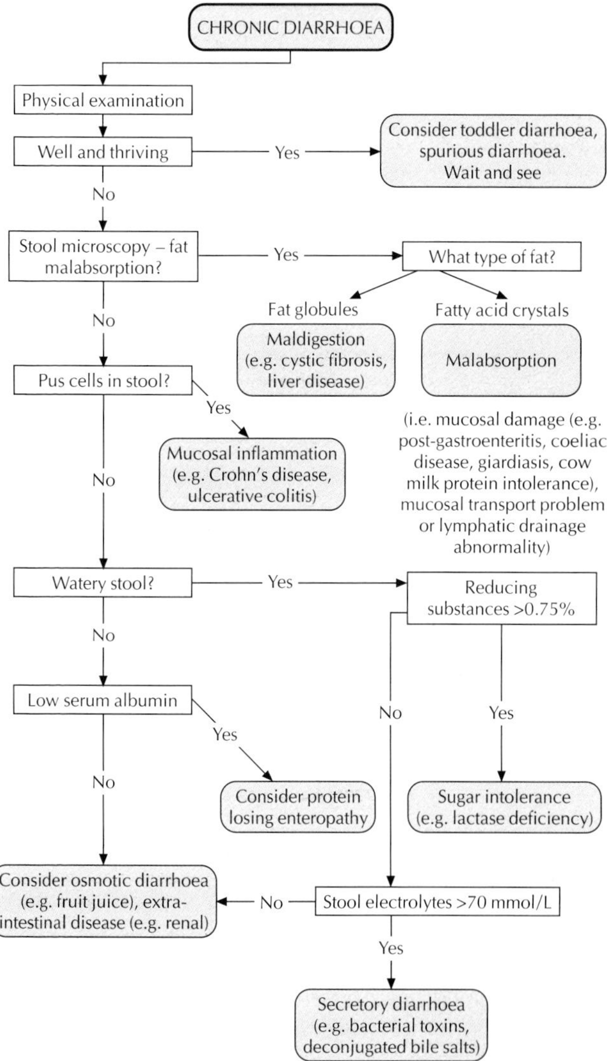

Fig. 24.1 Investigation of chronic diarrhoea

Table 24.5 Presentations of coeliac disease

Classical presentation	First 2 years of life poor weight gain Chronic diarrhoea Anorexia, apathy and abdominal distension
Atypical presentation	Growth retardation/pubertal delay only Amenorrhoea Arthritis Recurrent spontaneous foetal loss Peripheral neuropathy Cerebellar atrophy Hepatitis Recurrent mouth ulcers
Associated disorders	Insulin dependent diabetes mellitus Addison disease Down syndrome Selective IgA deficiency

Serological screening tests

- Combined use of an IgG antigliadin antibody (high sensitivity) and IgA antigliadin antibody (high specificity). False positive results (of both) can occur in other gut conditions including cow milk protein intolerance, Crohn's disease and post-infectious gastroenteritis.
- An anti-endomysial antibody test is more specific and sensitive than the antigliadin tests, however, false negative results can occur if the patient is IgA deficient.
- An IgA antibody to tissue transglutaminase (result of enterocyte damage) is 98% specific and sensitive, and may replace the anti-gliadin test in the future. False negative results can occur in IgA deficient patients.

Diagnosis

- Small bowel biopsy remains the gold standard.
- The need for subsequent biopsies to confirm or refute the diagnosis is dependent upon the clinical response of the patient to a gluten-free diet or if the patient is <2 years of age.

Management

A gluten free diet excluding wheat, barley, rye and oats.

COW MILK PROTEIN INTOLERANCE

Symptoms related to the ingestion of food or milk may be induced by any one of several components (see also Allergy and immunology, chapter 16). These may be due to immune or non-immune effects.

Cow milk protein intolerance predominantly affects young infants, prospective studies suggest a prevalence of 2% in this group.

Allergic responses to cow milk protein may result in a rapid or delayed onset of symptoms. Rapid onset responses are less common, often characterised by the sudden onset of vomiting and rarely by acute anaphylaxis. Delayed onset responses may be more difficult to diagnose and present with diarrhoea, malabsorption or failure to thrive, as well as occasion intestinal loss of protein or blood.

- Cow milk protein intolerance can only be diagnosed with a complete and thorough history, and with **unequivocal reproducible reactions to elimination and challenge.**
- Blood tests and skin prick testing may help, but are not substitutes for clinical assessment.
- After a definitive diagnosis is established, cow milk protein should be removed from the diet and replaced with a soy or a hydrolysed/elemental formula. A full soy formula is not recommended in young infants with severe enteropathy, as soy allergy can occur in 15–20% of such patients.
- Most food allergies in infants improve or resolve with increasing age.

Note: Hydrolysed and elemental milk formulas are expensive and should only be prescribed following specialist review.

RECTAL BLEEDING

See Figure 24.2.

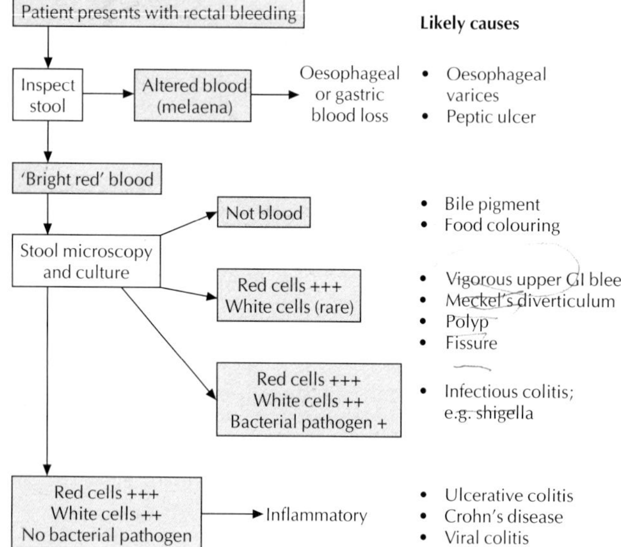

Fig. 24.2 Assessment of lower gastrointestinal blood loss

INFLAMMATORY BOWEL DISEASE

The incidence of Crohn's disease has increased dramatically in Australian children since the 1970's. In contrast ulcerative colitis shows an annual fluctuation without an upward trend.

- Crohn's disease can present in several ways including recurrent abdominal pain, weight loss, chronic diarrhoea, mouth ulcers and perianal disease. It may also present with isolated growth failure without any gastrointestinal symptoms.
- Ulcerative colitis is associated with bloody diarrhoea, which extends beyond the time frame of infective colitis.
- Extra-intestinal manifestations can occur in both disorders and include arthritis, erythema nodosum, hepatitis and ophthalmological complications (uveitis, episcleritis and conjunctivitis).

- Initial laboratory investigations should include a full blood count (anaemia and thrombocytosis), ESR (often raised) and albumin level (low with active disease). Stool cultures for bacterial pathogens and *Clostridium difficile* and toxin should collected.
- Evaluation and management should occur under specialist guidance.

CONSTIPATION/ENCOPRESIS

Constipation is defined as the infrequent passage of stool (less than 3 per week) associated with pain on defaecation, rectal bleeding, straining and soiling.

Holding back defaecation (functional constipation) is the most common cause of constipation in infants and toddlers. Important but rare organic causes of constipation include: Hirschsprung disease, ano-rectal malformations, metabolic conditions (hypothyroidism, hypercalcaemia and hypokalaemia), drugs (codeine, antacids, phenytoin) and perianal bacterial infection.

Encopresis refers to faecal soiling in the presence of functional constipation (i.e. constipation not secondary to organic or anatomical causes or intake of medication) after a child has reached 4 years of age.

The majority of children with encopresis have significant faecal retention. This causes rectal dilatation and insensitivity to the normal urge to pass stool and results in secondary adjustment difficulties, which improve with resolution of soiling.

History

- A careful history can aid in excluding an important organic cause of constipation and check the adequacy of fibre and fluid intake.
- Toddlers with functional constipation extend the body, contract the anal and gluteal muscles, hold their legs and buttocks stiffly and often rock back and forth while holding onto a piece of furniture.
- School aged children will often present with encopresis secondary to a megarectum.
- Daytime incontinence of urine is present in 20% of encopretic children, bed wetting in 30% and recurrent bladder infections in 10% of girls.

Examination

- Check growth percentiles and assess for hypothyroidism and lower spinal abnormalities.
- Abdominal palpation will usually reveal abnormal amounts of firm faeces.
- External examinations of the perineum and perianal areas are important as a bacterial infection in this region can cause erythema and acute constipation.
- Digital examination of the rectum is helpful in establishing anal tone and the consistency of stool. This is usually not necessary unless a local cause for constipation is suspected or if the child is not responding to prescribed treatment.

Investigations

- Are almost never required unless either the history or physical examinations suggest an organic cause for onstipation.
- An abdominal X-ray is not indicated unless there is some doubt about the diagnosis. Digital rectal examination is a much more sensitive indication of constipation.
- Rectal biopsy is indicated to exclude Hirschsprung's disease if there is a history of delayed passage of meconium, failure to thrive or abdominal distension.

Management

The aim of treatment is to:

- Empty the colon.
- Prevent re-accumulation of abnormal amounts of faeces by regular toileting and use of laxatives.

Patient education

- Attention to toilet: with the child sitting on the toilet 2–3 times per day, preferably after a meal to make use of the gastro-colic reflex. During this time the child is asked to 'push', with feet well supported, allowing the generation of adequate intra-abdominal pressure.
- Normal diet, adequate fluids and regular exercise (as this promotes normal colonic motility).
- Punitive methods used by parents to deal with either constipation or encopresis do not work.

Disimpaction

- Can usually be achieved by using oral laxatives (Table 24.6).
- Enemas can also be used, however, this can be traumatic for both child and parent. Phosphate containing enemas can cause dangerous electrolyte abnormalities if used in young children.
- In the worst cases, consider admission to hospital for bowel washout.
- Infants – usually disimpaction is achieved by using prune juice and increased cereals in the diet. If this is not successful, lactulose is effective and safe.
- Older children – use a stimulant laxative such as Senna (granules or tablet) or alternatively, bisacodyl may be used in children over the age of 4 years. A stool softener such as mineral oil is usually used in combination with a stimulant laxative in children with moderate constipation, but is not recommended in infants <12 months old, due to the risk of aspiration.

Maintenance therapy

- Ongoing use of a laxative agent (usually a stool softener) to control symptoms of constipation and encopresis and prevent recurrence. A common mistake is to give intermittent short courses of treatment, which does not allow adequate readjustment of colonic size and sensation. Stimulant laxatives may be necessary for short periods if a patient relapses while on a stool softening agent.
- The laxative dose may need to be modified until the child is achieving the passage of at least one soft stool per day.
- The longer constipation has been a problem, the longer it takes to achieve this aim.

Behavioural modification

- Using a star chart with daily recording of toilet sitting and defaecation provides positive reinforcement for the child. This retraining of the bowel is of vital importance to achieving resolution of encopresis associated with constipation. This can be a very useful adjunct to laxative therapy and is important in emphasising to both the child and the family the importance of attention to toilet.

Table 24.6 Medications commonly used to treat constipation

Laxative	*Dosage*	*Side effects*
Lubricant • Mineral oil (e.g. Parachoc, Agarol)	12 months–6 years, 15 mL/day 7–12 years, 20 mL/day	Not recommended for children <12 months of age (or children with vomiting) as it can result in lipoid pneumonia. Possible malabsorption of fat soluble vitamins can occur at all ages.
Osmotic • Lactulose (e.g. Actilax, Duphalac)	<12 months, 5 mL/day 1–5 years, 10 mL/day 6–12 years, 15 mL/day	Flatulence and abdominal cramps.
Stimulants • Senna (e.g. Senekot)	2–6 years, 1/2-1 tablet or 1/4– 1/2 teaspoon/day 6–12 years, 1–2 tablets/day or 1/2-1 teaspoon/day	Abdominal pain, melanosis coli, idiosyncratic hepatitis.
• Bisacodyl (e.g. Durolax, Bisalax)	5–10 mg in older children (>4 years)	Abdominal pain, diarrhoea, hypokalaemia.

GASTRO-OESOPHAGEAL REFLUX

Oesophageal reflux of gastric contents occurs normally and is more frequent after meals. It is regarded as pathological if associated with frequent regurgitation, or if it results in clinically significant adverse sequelae. The number of reflux episodes is normally increased in infants compared with older children.

Reflux of gastric acid with heartburn may result in episodic irritability, but this is usually associated with obvious regurgitation and is rarely 'silent'. Although gastro-oesophageal reflux may cause infant distress, it is important to consider other possible causes. Both infant distress and frequent regurgitation are common in the first 6 months of life. Coexistence does not prove cause and effect. Investigations such as 24-hour oesophageal pH monitoring can be useful to correlate any episodes of reflux with irritability.

It is important to recognise that vomiting in infants may result from other causes, such as urinary tract infection, metabolic disturbances, bowel obstruction and increased intracranial pressure. These need to be excluded on the basis of history, physical examination and further tests (if clinically indicated).

Complications

- *Peptic oesophagitis* – this is usually correlated with an increase in the number and duration of reflux episodes. Blood-flecked vomitus and anaemia may result.
- *Peptic strictures* – these are well recognised in childhood and present with dysphagia and failure to thrive.
- *Failure to thrive* – severe cases of gastro-oesophageal reflux may cause the loss of calories and anorexia.
- *Pulmonary complications* – recurrent or persistent cough and wheeze may be present and can occur without marked vomiting. These symptoms may result from aspiration of refluxed material (inhalation pneumonia) or through reflex bronchospasm. This mode of presentation requires a high degree of clinical suspicion to make the diagnosis.

Specialist advice should be sought if complications are present.

Management

Regurgitation of gastric contents is common in infancy. In most cases this 'possetting' does not result in any adverse sequelae and the most appropriate therapy is parental reassurance. 'Physiological' gastro-oesophageal reflux with regurgitation usually resolves by the age of 9–15 months.

Simple measures

In the absence of signs of significant oesophagitis, aspiration or growth failure, the following should be suggested:

- The avoidance of excessive handling.
- Posturing after feeds: the infant should be placed in a cot in the head-up position at or near 30°.
- Thickening of feeds: use a proprietary thickening agent or a pre-thickened formula if formula-fed.

Medication

Note: Medications are not indicated in otherwise healthy, thriving infants with frequent regurgitation.

- Mylanta may offer relief from symptoms of heartburn (0.5–1.0 mL/kg per dose given 3–4 times a day). There are some concerns about its long-term use because of its mineral content.
- H_2 receptor antagonists such as ranitidine (2–3 mg/kg per dose given 2–3 times a day before meals) will reduce gastric acidity. There may be role for a brief empirical trial of anti-reflux therapy in infants in whom it is thought reflux is the cause of their distressed behaviour. However, these agents are not without risk and should not be prescribed for prolonged periods without evidence to substantiate the severity of reflux.
- Proton pump inhibitors are prescribed to infants and children with severe oesophagitis that is unresponsive to an H_2 receptor antagonist.

Surgery

Fundoplication is indicated for reflux with complications when medical therapy has failed or is inappropriate.

RECURRENT ABDOMINAL PAIN

Recurrent abdominal pain affects about 10% of school-age children. There is usually no specific identifiable cause though it has been speculated that this condition may be a result of dysmotility of the bowel. Occasionally it can result from a significant emotional problem.

Recent evidence suggests there may be a subgroup with migrainous abdominal pain (associated with pallor and family history). Emotional factors, life-style and temperamental characteristics can modulate the child's response to pain, irrespective of its cause.

Assessment

- It is essential to take a careful history, including psychosocial details. It may be helpful to interview the parents alone, the child alone and the family together. Onset of pain after the consumption of dairy products in older children and young adolescents should be sought, as lactase deficiency can present in this manner. Constipation needs to be excluded. 'Red flags' in the evaluation of chronic abdominal pain include pain localised away from the umbilicus, accompanying vomiting, diarrhoea, poor weight gain or linear growth and pain awakening the patient from sleep.
- A thorough physical examination is essential.
- Urine microscopy and culture is an appropriate baseline investigation.

Management

- The two major causes in childhood are constipation and dysfunctional pain.
- The treatment of underlying constipation is essential and management of non-organic issues may be required.
- 'Dysfunctional' pain may be related to variation in the perception of visceral sensation in the absence of an identifiable organic cause. A detailed explanation to the child and reassurance is often all that is required.
- The diagnosis of psychogenic recurrent abdominal pain cannot be made simply in the absence of positive findings for an organic disorder. Positive evidence of emotional maladjustment is required separately. If present, it should be managed appropriately.

LIVER DISEASE

Infants

Infants (1–3 months of life) may present with:

- Jaundice (usually conjugated hyperbilirubinaemia).
- Passage of pale grey or white stools and dark tea coloured urine.
- Hepatosplenomegaly.
- Failure to thrive.
- Bleeding diathesis.
- Hypoglycaemia.

Biliary atresia is the most common cause of obstructive jaundice in young infants. Infants with this condition will present with jaundice in the first 4–6 weeks of life. They appear well on clinical examination with conservation of growth. The degree of jaundice may be variable, but onset is usually from birth. They will consistently pass acholic (pale white) stool. If untreated, the outcome is fatal. However, the natural history of this condition can be modified by early surgery, which must be performed prior to 70 days of age for success.

Apart from this condition there are several other causes of early onset liver disease, many of which may have dire consequences if not recognised or treated adequately, including galactosaemia, tyrosinaemia, fructosaemia and other metabolic conditions. Therefore, **prompt referral of infants with liver disease to a specialist is essential**.

Table 24.7 Causes of liver disease in children

Infection:	Viral (hepatitis A, B, C, D, CMV, EBV), bacterial sepsis.
Inflammatory:	Autoimmune hepatitis, sclerosing cholangitis
Metabolic:	Galactosaemia, tyrosinaemia, fructose intolerance, Wilson disease, α1 antitrypsin deficiency
Drugs	Particularly paracetamol
Structural	Gallstones, choledochal cyst
Malignancy	Histiocytosis x, leukaemia, lymphoma
Others	Cystic fibrosis

Children

May present acutely with a sudden onset of jaundice, cholestasis (dark urine and pale stools), pruritus, irritability and vomiting. Signs of chronic liver disease should be sought and include poor growth, delayed puberty, dilated abdominal veins and palmar erythema. In general, prompt specialist consultation for acute and chronic liver disorders is required, as both forms of liver disease require urgent investigation and treatment.

CHAPTER 25
GYNAECOLOGIC CONDITIONS

Sonia Grover

PREPUBESCENT PROBLEMS

Vaginal Discharge

Most newborn girls have some mucoid white vaginal discharge. This is normal and disappears by about 3 months of age.

Vulvovaginitis

This is the commonest gynaecologic problem in childhood, usually occurring in girls aged between 2 years and puberty. The vaginal skin in childhood is thin and atrophic. Overgrowth of mixed bowel flora occurs in this environment and the resultant discharge can be an irritant to the vulval area, which is also atrophic. The moist environment between the opposed skin surfaces may also be exacerbated by urine dribbling, particularly in the obese young girl.

Presentation

- Erythema/irritation of the labia and perineal skin.
- Itch and dysuria may also be present.
- +/− offensive vaginal discharge.

Management

Investigations are usually not required. If urinary symptoms are present check the urine to exclude urinary tract infection (UTI).

- Explanation and reassurance.
- Vinegar (1 cup white vinegar in a shallow bath) or the use of a simple barrier, or both, and soothing cream to the labial area (e.g. zinc-castor oil or nappy rash cream).
- Toileting/hygiene advice: avoid potential irritants such as soaps and bubble bath.

Rarely, if the problem persists, further action may be required. The natural history is for recurrences to occur up until the age when oestrogenisation begins.

- If a heavy discharge persists or marked skin inflammation is present, take swabs from the perineum in case of an overgrowth of one organism (e.g. group A Streptococcus) and treat it with the appropriate antibiotics (usual culture findings are mixed coliforms).
- Do not take vaginal swabs, as it is painful and distressing. If swabs for culture are required, introital area swabs will do.
- If itch/irritation is the main complaint, consider pinworms.
- If eczema occurs elsewhere on the body, this can be superimposed on the irritation. Combined treatment of the vulvovaginitis (as above) and hydrocortisone may be indicated.
- Foreign bodies are a potential cause for a persistent, unresolving, often blood-stained discharge. An examination under anaesthesia with vaginoscopy is required to exclude this.
- Consider sexual abuse.

Thrush is very uncommon in this age group unless there has been significant antibiotic use. Thrush thrives in an oestrogenised environment, not in the atrophic setting.

Vaginal pessaries should never be prescribed to this age group.

Vaginal Bleeding

Many girls will have some vaginal bleeding in the first week of life, caused by the withdrawal of maternal oestrogens. This is normal. In older girls blood stained discharge may indicate:

- Vulvovaginitis – associated with atrophic changes (see vulvovaginitis).
- A foreign body – particularly if it is persistent despite management of vulvovaginitis.
- Trauma (including straddle injuries and sexual abuse).
- Excoriation secondary to threadworms or eczema.
- Haematuria.
- Urethral prolapse.

Labial adhesions

- Labial adhesions are seen in infancy and usually resolve by about 8 years. They may occasionally persist through to puberty but will resolve by the time of menarche.
- The adhesion is not congenital, but acquired from a secondary adherence of the atrophic surfaces of the labia minora, presumably as a result of irritation.

- **Uncomplicated labial adhesions in girls do not need division.** Refer to a specialist if the child has difficulty voiding or recurrent UTI. Treat vulvovaginitis or nappy rash if present. Parents should be reassured that the labia will separate when oestrogenisation occurs as the child grows. Although it is possible to divide the adhesions with lateral traction this is frequently distressing for the child and the parents. Recurrence is common.
- The use of topical oestrogen cream is unnecessary and is associated with significant failure and recurrence rates.

MENSTRUAL PROBLEMS

Dysmenorrhoea

Clinical features

- Cramping lower abdominal pain, lower back pain and pain radiating to the anterior aspects of the thighs with menses (these may begin a few days before menstruation).
- Associated symptoms such as nausea, vomiting, change in bowel actions (usually softer bowel actions or diarrhoea, but occasionally constipation), headaches and general lethargy may occur. These symptoms should be looked for as they support the diagnosis of a prostaglandin-induced dysmenorrhoea. Occasionally these symptoms, occurring in an intermittent pattern, may begin a few months prior to menarche.
- Stress will often precipitate more severe episodes of dysmenorrhoea.
- Vaginal examination is not performed if the young woman is not sexually active. Occasionally in young women who are using tampons a vaginal examination may be possible, but alternatives such as a pelvic ultrasound examination will usually provide all the required information (e.g. obstructive congenital anomalies and ovarian cysts).

Management

- General measures: assess and manage other adolescent issues (see Adolescent health, chapter 12) and encourage exercise.
- Antiprostaglandins (e.g. mefenamic acid, naproxen, ibuprofen; see Pharmacopoeia) ideally should be commenced prior to the

onset of any symptoms. The failure to respond to one type of antiprostaglandin warrants the trial of an alternative type.

- If the menstrual cycle is too irregular for prophylactic use of anti-prostaglandins, it can be regulated with hormonal treatment. The oral contraceptive pill (OCP) can also be used for dysmenorrhoea. This may be the first-line treatment in a sexually active teenager.
- Non-responsive or worsening dysmenorrhoea will require investigation. Pelvic ultrasound can usually identify an obstructive congenital anomaly and detect significant endometriosis (e.g. an endometrioma).
- Diagnostic laparoscopy may identify mild endometriosis. However, the value of treating this with specific hormonal therapy or operative laser diathermy is unclear from both the short-term and long-term perspective. Therefore, this operative investigation should be withheld until optimal management with anti-prostaglandin therapy or OCP, or both, has been tried and failed, and other adolescent issues explored.

Amenorrhoea

Primary

See Delayed puberty, Endocrine conditions, chapter 22.

Secondary

Consider the following diagnoses:

- Pregnancy.
- Weight loss/anorexia nervosa.
- Strenuous exercise.
- Stress (e.g. exams, social-family or travel).
- Polycystic ovaries: associated problems of hirsutism and obesity are usually present. These patients often have irregular, infrequent periods rather than amenorrhoea. Investigations can help confirm or support the diagnosis (e.g. follicle-stimulating hormone, luteinising hormone and pelvic ultrasound).

Amenorrhoea itself does not need treatment but associated problems may require intervention (e.g. obesity – dietary/nutritional, exercise; hirsutism – the oral contraceptive pill, particularly Diane 35, which contains cyproterone acetate, an antiandrogen). The use of hormonal treatment to cause withdrawal bleeds has the advantage of making periods lighter and more regular, rather than infrequent and heavy.

Prolonged amenorrhoea associated with low oestrogen levels potentially leads to a negative effect on bone mineral density and the addition of hormonal treatment may then be indicated.

Metrostaxis (severe heavy loss)

- Check haemoglobin (Hb).
- Check clotting profiles (PT, KPPT, vWF, collagen-binding assay (CBA), platelet function assay (PFA100)).
- Exclude pregnancy.
- The young woman having her first or second period usually requires oestrogen therapy (Fig. 25.1). In the young woman who has been menstruating for some time progestogen therapy will be more appropriate (Fig. 25.2).

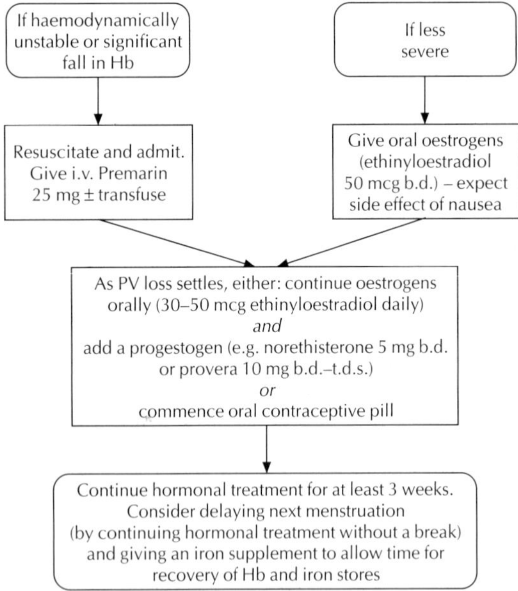

Fig. 25.1 Heavy loss at first or second period

Ongoing management – see menorrhagia section

If a transfusion is required treatment should be continued for at least 3–6 months before a trial without hormonal therapy is considered.

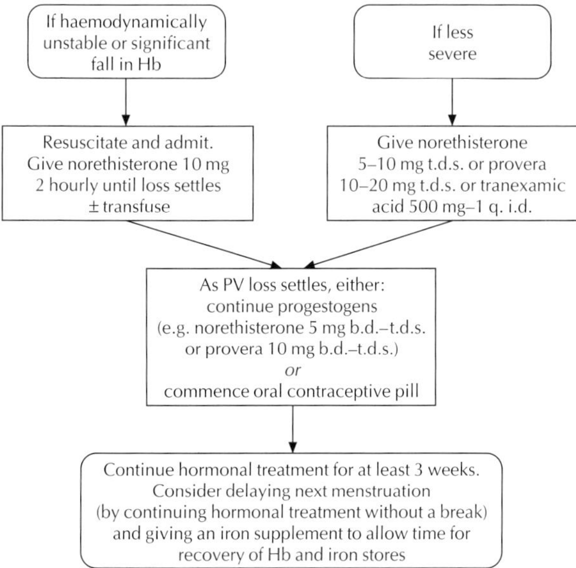

Fig. 25.2 Heavy loss in the young woman who has been menstruating for some time

Menorrhagia

- Menstrual history.
- FBE, iron studies.
- Clotting screen if good history for heavy loss (changing soaked pads <3 hourly), ask for other bleeding history – epistaxis, bruising, family history).
- βHCG (β human chorionic gonadotrophin) if sexually active and delayed menses (possible threatened abortion or ectopic pregnancy).

Management

Non-hormonal

- If anaemic, use iron supplements.
- NSAIDs can reduce flow by 30% if taken regularly (see dysmenorrhoea section and Pharmacopoeia).
- Antifibrinolytic agents (tranexamic acid 500 mg 1–2 tablets q.i.d.) can reduce flow by 50%.

Hormonal

The alternatives are:

- Cyclical progesterones (Primolut = norethisterone 5 mg, or Provera = medroxyprogesterone acetate 10 mg daily or twice daily for 14 or 21 days/month).
- Combined oral contraceptive pill (can reduce flow by 50%).
- Depo Provera (75% amenorrhoea after 1 year use).

PELVIC PAIN: GYNAECOLOGICAL CAUSES

See Figure 25.3 Adolescent gynaecology – assessment of lower abdominal pain.

Midcycle pain (Mittelschmerz)

This occurs in midcycle; therefore, it can often be diagnosed on history.

Ovarian cysts

Most ovarian cysts detected from a scan will be normal follicles and reassurance that these are physiological and represent healthy functioning ovaries is important. Presume that all cysts less than 6 cm are physiological unless specific features are present to suggest otherwise. Repeating a scan 4–6 weeks later to prove the resolution of cysts less than 6 cm can prevent operative intervention.

Torsion of the ovary is very uncommon, but it usually occurs in the presence of an ovarian cyst. The history is of a sudden onset of severe pain with associated nausea, vomiting and dizziness. A diagnostic laparoscopy is the best way of excluding this condition, although if an immediate ultrasound can be performed and the ovaries are normal the diagnosis is most unlikely.

Pelvic inflammatory disease

- This only occurs in females who have been sexually active.
- A history of dyspareunia, discharge and fever may be associated with the pelvic pain.
- Chlamydial pelvic inflammatory disease (PID) may cause endometritis with intermenstrual bleeding, menorrhagia or metrostaxis.
- As these young females are sexually active it is appropriate that cervical swabs be taken, including specific swabs for Chlamydia culture, or utilise urine or cervical PCR testing for Chlamydia.

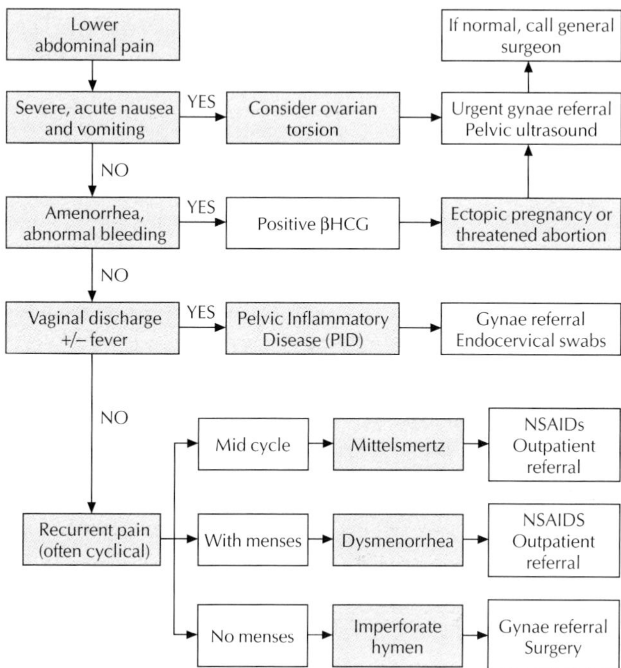

Assess menstrual history, sexual activity, associated symptoms and consider performing βHCG in all patients. Always consider urinary or gastrointestinal causes.

Fig. 25.3 Adolescent gynaecology – Assessment of lower abdominal pain

Management

- If febrile (severe infection) admit for i.v. antibiotics (cefotaxime 1 g i.v., 8-hourly (or ceftriaxone 1 g i.v. daily) and metronidazole 500 mg i.v., 12-hourly, plus doxycycline 100 mg orally, 12-hourly).
- For mild to moderate infection use ceftriaxone 250 mg (in 1% lignocaine), i.m. as a single dose, plus doxycycline 100 mg orally, 12-hourly for 14 days and metronidazole 400 mg orally, 12-hourly, for 14 days.
- In the sexually active teenager Papanicolaou (PAP) smears should be taken annually, commencing approximately 6 months after intercourse began.

- Discuss contraception. If PID is suspected it generally implies that condoms are not being used. Discuss the benefits of condoms for protection against sexually transmitted diseases (STD).

Ectopic pregnancy

- A recent 'period' does not exclude this diagnosis.
- The use of contraception does not exclude this diagnosis. Suspicion is increased if an intra-uterine device (IUD) is used (although unlikely in an adolescent) and decreased with the use of the oral contraceptive pill.
- Perform a pregnancy test and organise a pelvic ultrasound unless the clinical situation (i.e. shock) necessitates immediate resuscitation and surgical intervention.
- Contraception and PAP smear need to be discussed.

Congenital obstructive anomalies

- May cause acute onset pain or progressively increasing dysmenorrhoea (if there is unilateral obstruction) or progressively increasing pelvic pain without menstruation (if there is complete obstruction – most common is an imperforate hymen.).
- Pelvic mass may be palpable. Perineal examination may reveal an imperforate hymen.
- Pelvic ultrasound or other imaging techniques will help clarify the anatomy.
- Associated renal agenesis on the side of the obstructed genital tract may occur.

BREAST PROBLEMS

- The asymmetrical development of the breast bud may lead to a presentation with a 'breast lump'. Biopsy at this early stage is contraindicated. Reassure during the time of breast growth and development. Growth that is initially asymmetric may correct itself.
- Persistent unequal breast size can cause considerable embarrassment and distress to the teenager, and referral to a specialist (usually a plastic surgeon with an interest in breast surgery) may be appropriate. Eventually, surgical correction may be required, but this would not be undertaken until growth has ceased.

CONTRACEPTION: BEST OPTIONS FOR YOUNG WOMEN

Other issues pertinent to adolescence and health risk behaviours must be explored (see HEADSS approach, Adolescent health, chapter 12).

Condoms

Condoms offer the advantage of protection from STD, as well as fairly good contraception. They may not be a reliable form of contraception if alcohol and drug-taking are issues.

Oral contraceptive pill

Contraindications

- Thromboembolic disease.
- Liver disease.
- Oestrogen-dependent tumours.

Short-term side effects

- Nausea.
- Breakthrough bleeding (this should resolve with continuing usage).
- Migraines.

Types

- *Sequential pills* (e.g. Triquilar and Triphasil): these are generally the first choice.
- *Constant dose* (e.g. Microgynon 30ED and Nordette): for the patient who suffers erratic, heavy periods, premenstrual moodiness or irregular lifestyle routines (there is a slightly greater leeway in the time of taking such pills).
- *Higher oestrogen content*: if using anticonvulsants or if there is persistent breakthrough bleeding.

Other forms of contraception

- *Implanon*: Hormonal implant inserted under the skin in the upper arm. Very effective contraception that lasts 3 years. Often associated with a reduction in menstrual loss, although irregular periods and amenorrhoea do occur.
- *Depo-Provera*: a 150 mg, 3-monthly injection. This often causes irregular bleeding initially but amenorrhoea after 6–9 months usage. This is a very reliable form of contraception. Long-term usage in teenagers may have some impact on bone density.

Intra-uterine contraceptive (IUD) devices and diaphragms are generally not appropriate for young women.

The progesterone-only pill is also generally not appropriate – it needs to be taken at the same time every day to be effective and it is less reliable than the combination OCP.

Emergency contraception: the morning-after pill

- Can be used up to 72 h after unprotected intercourse.
- Some evidence for its use up to 1 week – although reduced efficacy.
- Contraindications are as for OCP.
- Two versions are available:
  - Postinor 2 (levonorgestrel 750 mcg tablet) 2 × one tablet, then a second tablet 12 h later.
  - Any OCP that contains 50 mcg of ethinyloestradiol and 125 mcg of levonorgestrel (e.g. Nordiol, Microgynon 50) two tablets, then 2 further tablets 12 h later.
- As nausea and vomiting may occur, administer an oral anti-emetic (e.g. metoclopramide 10 mg) 30 min before the 'pill' tablets.

These treatments are effective (>90%), but do not provide continuing contraception. Discuss and plan ongoing contraception and PAP smears and plan follow-up strategies to ensure that the emergency treatment has worked.

CHAPTER 26
HAEMATOLOGIC CONDITIONS AND ONCOLOGY

Karen Tiedemann
Mike South
Paul Monagle

ANAEMIA

Anaemia is defined as having a haemoglobin (Hb) less than the lower limit of the reference range for age.

Table 26.1 Haemoglobin reference ranges for age

Age	*Lower limit of normal range of Hb (g/L)*	
2 months	90	
2–6 months	95	
6–24 months	105	
2–11 years	115	
>12 years	girls – 120	boys – 130

Clinical features suggestive of anaemia

- Pallor
- Pale conjunctivae
- Flow murmur
- Lethargy
- Poor growth
- Signs of cardiac failure
- Listlessness
- Shortness of breath

Investigation

If anaemia is suspected, begin with a full blood examination (FBE), blood film, ferritin and reticulocyte count. The initial classification is based on the mean corpuscular volume (MCV) (see Fig. 26.1).

Iron deficiency

Iron deficiency is common among Australian children. However, it may be subclinical and lead to anaemia only in those with more severe deficiency. Iron deficiency may be present in 10–30% of children in

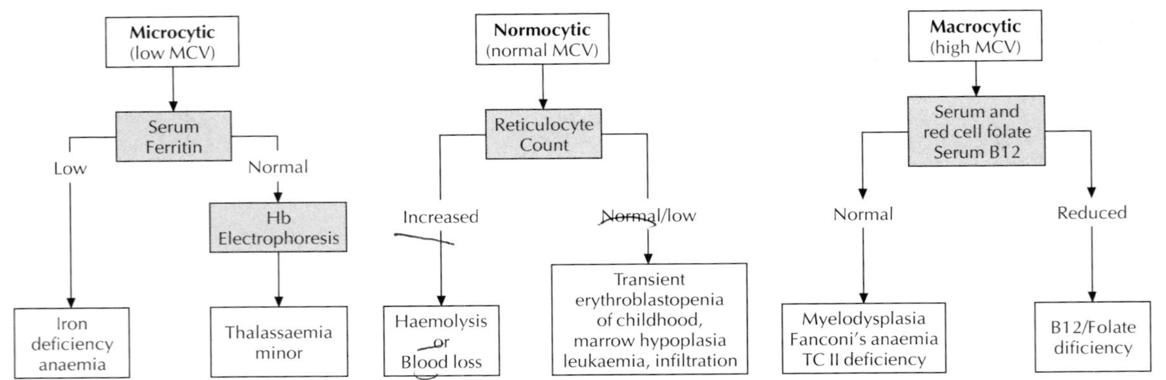

Fig 26.1 Classification of anaemia
* TCII, transcobalamin II deficiency.

high-risk groups. Iron deficiency (see Table 26.1) may lead to impaired cognitive and psychomotor performance, even in the absence of anaemia.

Most cases of iron deficiency anaemia in young children are due to inadequate dietary intake. Blood may be lost through cow milk provoked faecal blood loss in infants and menstruation in adolescent girls.

Table 26.2 Children at high risk for iron deficiency anaemia

Group	*Additional risk factors*	*Mechanisms*
<6 months of age	Prematurity Low birth weight Multiple births Maternal iron deficiency	Inadequate stores
6–24 months of age	Exclusive breast feeding after 6 months. Delayed introduction of iron-containing solids. Excessive cow milk	Inadequate intake Cow milk may cause microscopic gut blood loss
Adolescents	Females Poor diet	Menstruation Rapid growth spurt
Aborigines Migrant families Socially disadvantaged Vegetarian / fad diets	Poor diet Excessive cow milk	Inadequate intake

In iron deficiency anaemia, the ferritin, Hb, mean corpuscular volume (MCV) and mean corpuscular Hb concentration (MCHC) are low. In mild iron deficiency, the FBE is normal but the ferritin is reduced, which demonstrates low iron stores. Ferritin is an acute phase reactant and may be misleadingly normal/high during an acute febrile illness. In such circumstances, a repeat measurement a month later or an empiric trial of iron therapy are alternative strategies.

Remember that iron deficiency anaemia caused by a poor diet may be associated with other macro- or micro-nutrient deficiencies.

Prevention of iron deficiency

- Introduce iron-containing solids from 4–6 months.
- Avoid cow milk in the first 12 months (small amounts allowed in custards and cereals, etc.).

- Cow milk should only form a small part of the diet up to 2 years of age.
- Ensure that formulas (if used) and cereals are iron fortified.
- Consider supplementation in high-risk groups (see Table 26.2).

Good sources of iron for children

See also Nutrition, chapter 6.

- Infant milk formulas.
- Fortified breakfast cereals.
- Meat (including red meat, chicken and fish).
- Green vegetables (especially legumes, e.g. peas and beans).
- Dried beans and fruit.
- Egg yolk.

Note: Foods high in Vitamin C, including citrus fruit, strawberries, cauliflower and broccoli, will increase iron absorption from non-meat sources.

Management

- Dietary advice must be given in all cases. This includes increasing the amount of iron containing foods and limiting the intake of cow milk.
- Supplemental iron should be recommended for any child with reduced haemoglobin, because it takes a long time to replenish iron stores by dietary change alone.
- For young children, supplemental iron is usually given as ferrous gluconate mixture (daily dose 1.0 mL/kg of the 300 mg/5 mL preparation) and should be continued for 3 months after the Hb has returned to normal to replenish stores. The stools may become black/grey. **An iron overdose can be fatal and supplements should be stored in a locked cabinet.**
- Parenteral iron supplementation is rarely indicated in children. Blood transfusion is also rarely indicated. It may be used if a very anaemic child requires urgent surgery or if cardiac failure is present. A transfusion should be slow and only raise the Hb to 60–80 g/L (see Calculating the blood transfusion volume p. 413).

B_{12} deficiency

B_{12} deficiency in childhood most commonly presents during the first two years of life. The most common cause is nutritional, due to undiagnosed maternal B_{12} deficiency in a fully breast-fed child. Transcobalamin II deficiency is uncommon, but is associated with normal serum B_{12} levels, despite severe tissue B_{12} deficiency. Any child with failure to thrive or neurodevelopmental abnormalities who also has a haematological abnormality (any cytopenia, macrocytosis or hypersegmented neutrophils) should be suspected of B_{12} deficiency and investigated urgently. The urgency relates to the propensity for rapid neurological deterioration (seizures, apnoea, choreoathetosis) and the lack of reversibility of these symptoms if treatment is delayed. Bone marrow aspirate can confirm megaloblastosis within an hour to allow therapy to commence immediately.

Haemoglobinopathies

β-globin thalassemia

β thalassemia minor is very common and causes hypochromic microcytosis without significant anaemia and clinical symptoms. Clues on a FBE include an elevated red cell count. The diagnosis is confirmed by Hb electrophoresis (or High Performance Liquid Chromatography, HPLC) demonstrating an elevated HbA_2. Children with thalassemia minor are often treated unnecessarily with iron therapy. Iron deficiency may cause reduced HbA_2, obscuring the diagnosis of thalassemia minor.

Thalassemia major is uncommon now due to the increased use of antenatal screening and prenatal termination. However, the diagnosis should be considered for a hypochromic microcytic anaemia presenting during the second 6 months of life (i.e. after β globin chain switch has occurred at 6 months). Hepatosplenomegaly, marked erythroblastosis and bizarre red cell forms on the blood film are usually diagnostic.

Alpha globin thalassemia

Alpha thalassemia traits are relatively common in Asian populations. Hb Barts (4 gene deletion) classically presents with hydrops fetalis at birth. Children with HbH disease (3 gene deletion) usually have a mild to moderate microcytic anaemia but are asymptomatic when well, potentially becoming significantly anaemic when physiologically stressed. Children with alpha thalassemia traits (1 or 2 gene deletions) may be microcytic (from birth) but not anaemic and are asymptomatic throughout life.

Sickle cell anaemia

Homozygous SS or double heterozygous (HbS/β thalassemia trait) usually presents after 6 months of age (after β globin chain switch).

Clinical presentations include:

- Anaemia (haemolysis or aplasia).
- Joint pains (especially small hand and foot joints).
- Acute chest syndrome (pneumonia like with prominent hypoxia).
- Arterial ischaemic stroke.
- Acute splenic sequestration (rapidly progressive anaemia and splenic enlargement).
- Painful crisis (usually bone or abdominal pain).
- Asymptomatic diagnosis when parents are known carriers.
- Sepsis, especially encapsulated organisms in young infants.

Diagnosis

Diagnosis is made by blood film examination, sickle solubility tests and Hb electrophoresis.

Management

Long-term management includes folate supplementation, penicillin prophylaxis and transfusion support as required. Acute management of crisis includes hydration, analgesia, transfusion and often antibiotics. Chest syndrome and stroke usually require exchange transfusion. Specialist consultation is required for each presentation.

Haemoglobin C/E

HbC and E are common in Asian populations and in the hetero and homozygous forms are asymptomatic. Blood films may show many target cells and the MCV is often normal. Thalassemia minor and HbC or E double heterozygotes present clinically as thalassemia major.

Haemolysis

Acute haemolysis in childhood is a life threatening disorder that usually requires admission, thorough investigation and potentially transfusion support. Severe anaemia can develop quickly and frequent clinical review of vital signs and monitoring of Hb is required.

The diagnostic features of haemolysis include anaemia, polychromasia on the blood film, reticulocytosis and hyperbilirubinaemia. Haptoglobin is unhelpful in infants.

Investigations

The first line investigations include:

- Blood film examination:
  - Spherocytes – hereditary spherocytosis, Coombs positive, ABO, G6PD.
  - Fragments – microangiopathic haemolysis.
  - Blister/bite cells – oxidative haemolysis (drug or G6PD).
  - Sickle cells.
- Direct Coombs test.
- Heinz body preparation.
- Hb electrophoresis/isopropanol test for unstable Hb.
- G6PD assay.
- Acidified glycerol lysis time (AGLT) screening test for hereditary spherocytosis.

Further investigation is often required once the acute episode has resolved, and usually requires input from a specialist.

The potential aetiology of acute haemolysis is shown in Figure 26.2.

Transient erythroblastopenia of childhood

This is a form of acquired red cell aplasia predominantly affecting children under 7 years of age. There may be a history of a viral illness in the previous 3 months.

The anaemia is normochromic, normocytic and there is no reticulocyte response until the recovery phase commences. Bone marrow aspirate may show red cell aplasia with preservation of other cell lines. The prognosis for previously normal children is excellent, with recovery for most within 2 months. No specific therapy is warranted and blood transfusion is best avoided if possible (consider if Hb <50 g/L and no reticulocyte response). The differential diagnosis is Blackfan–Diamond Syndrome, which usually occurs at a younger age, but may be indistinguishable on peripheral blood and bone marrow aspirate findings.

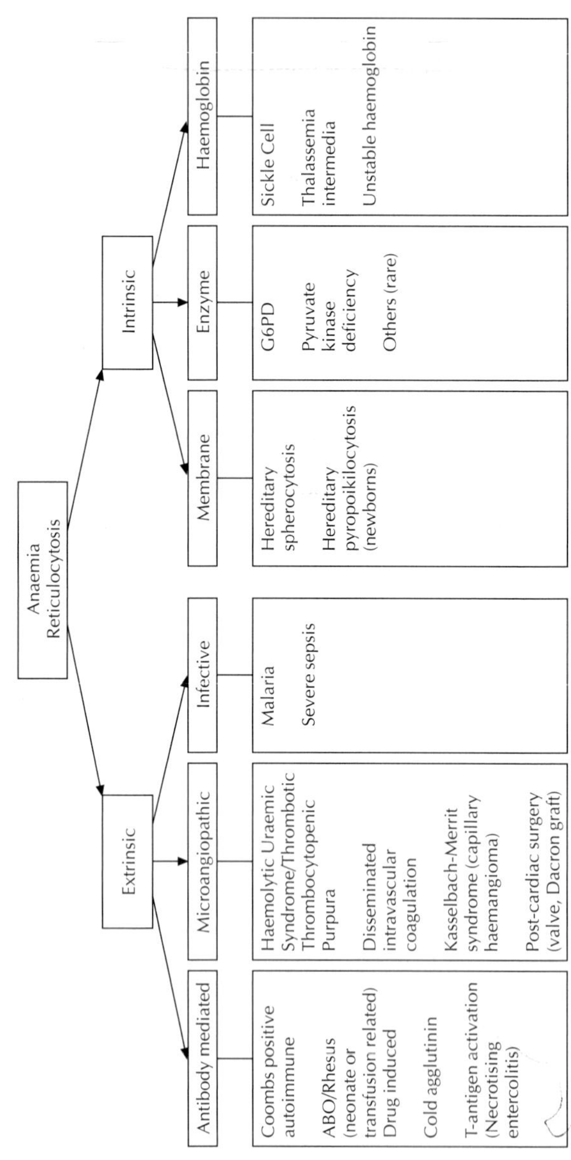

Fig 26.2 Acute haemolysis

COAGULATION ABNORMALITIES

Severe bleeding disorders in childhood usually present in the newborn period, although they can present at any time. Spontaneous bleeding or bruising of multiple ages in unusual sites should raise suspicions of a bleeding tendency. Often coagulopathy screening is required to differentiate a bleeding diathesis from non-accidental injury. Family history, drug history and history of previous surgical challenges (including tooth extraction) are important. Routine coagulation screening preoperatively in well children is rarely indicated and coagulation testing should be guided by the clinical history.

Investigation

First line investigations of a suspected bleeding disorder include:

- Platelet count and blood film.
- Activated partial thromboplastin time (APTT).
- Prothrombin time (PT) or international normalised ratio (INR).
- Fibrinogen.

Interpretation of these investigations is shown in Table 26.3. Further investigations should usually be performed following discussion with a haematologist.

Fibrinogen is an acute phase reactant. In severe sepsis, when fibrinogen should be elevated, a normal level is still consistent with disseminated intravascular coagulation (DIC).

If the above investigations are normal in the setting of clinically abnormal bleeding, consider Factor XIII deficiency, Von Willebrand disease, platelet function defects or a capillary fragility syndrome, specific investigations will be required.

If the diagnosis of a bleeding disorder is in doubt, 10–20 mL/kg of fresh frozen plasma (FFP) +/– platelets may be required to treat acute bleeding.

In general, children presenting acutely with bleeding disorders should discussed with a haematologist. Haemophilia A or B, von Willebrand disease and other bleeding disorders are complex disorders that require specialist management.

Table 26.3 Investigation of coagulation abnormalities

Screening Test Result	*Causes*
Low platelet count	Immune thrombocytopenia purpura (ITP) Neonatal alloimmune thrombocytopenia (NAITP) Congenital thrombocytopenia syndromes Chemotherapy / marrow replacement
Isolated prolonged APTT	Factor XI, IX, VIII deficiency Von Willebrand disease Heparin Factor XII (no clinical bleeding)
Isolated prolonged PT/INR	Factor VII deficiency Warfarin
Prolonged APTT, PT Low Fibrinogen	Vitamin K Deficiency Liver disease Disseminated intravascular coagulation (DIC) – also low platelets Factor II, V, X deficiency (normal fibrinogen)

General measures

These are applicable to all congenital bleeding disorders.

- Analgesia: do not give aspirin and avoid narcotic analgesics.
- Do not give intramuscular injections. Do not perform arterial puncture.
- The splinting of limbs reduces pain.

Consult with a haematologist about the need for joint aspiration. Beware of the risk of Volkmann's ischaemic contracture in forearm bleeds and of femoral nerve palsies with retroperitoneal bleeds tracking underneath the inguinal ligament.

Haemophilia A (factor VIII deficiency)

Management of bleeding

In general, the factor VIII dose (desired levels of factor VIII to control haemorrhage) is 1 unit/kg of factor VIII (raises levels by 2%). Thus, 15 units/kg will increase factor VIII by 30% and 25 units/kg by 50%.

Most bleeding can be controlled with a single dose calculated to increase the factor VIII level to 30–50%.

Note: a minor head injury can become serious: the factor VIII level should be raised to 100% and the child admitted for observation.

Recombinant human factor VIII (Kogenate/Recombinate) has recently become available; it is used for all patients without previous exposure to human derived factor VIII.

Patients with factor VIII inhibitors are now treated with recombinant factor VIIa (Novoseven). The usual dose is factor VIIa 90–100 mcg repeated in 2 h.

Mouth bleeding

Use tranexamic acid tablets (see Pharmacopoeia).

Von Willebrand disease

Responds to cryoprecipitate, or less predictably, to factor VIII. Many patients respond to desmopressin. The half-life of von Willebrand factor is approximately 4 h, but factor VIII levels continue to be increased for 48–72 h after the infusion of cryoprecipitate. Further doses are given if bleeding recurs.

Christmas disease – Haemophilia B (Factor IX deficiency)

Bleeding is treated with Factor IX concentrate (Monofix).

- Requirements: as in haemophilia.
- Dose: in general 1 unit factor IX/kg increases the factor IX level by 1.6%.
- Frequency: injections at 24 h intervals (the half-life for factor IX is 24 h).

Idiopathic thrombocytopaenic purpura

Idiopathic thrombocytopaenic purpura (ITP) is an acquired thrombocytopaenia due to shortened platelet survival (immune mediated) in the absence of other disturbances of haemostasis or coagulation.

In young children, ITP usually presents with bruising and petechiae, often with a history of recent viral infection. In some instances there is oral bleeding, epistaxis, rectal bleeding or haematuria.

If the clinical presentation, FBE and blood film suggest ITP (i.e. no hepatosplenomegaly or lymphadenopathy; no anaemia, leucopenia or blasts), a bone marrow biopsy is not necessary.

Although the bruising and petechiae are sometimes quite dramatic in appearance, morbidity in ITP is usually minimal. Intracranial haemorrhage is the most serious risk but probably has an incidence much less than 1%.

Management

The indications for treatment and the best form of treatment for children with acute ITP, remain controversial. Without active treatment, most patients' platelet counts will return to a satisfactory level within a month.

Careful observation without specific treatment may be appropriate in milder cases. Patients with active bleeding (e.g. mucosal and gastrointestinal) should receive treatment to increase their platelet count more rapidly. Some authorities also recommend treating patients with a platelet count <10–20 × 10^9/L and a florid petechial rash (especially mucosal petechiae).

When treatment is indicated, corticosteroids are usually the first line therapy. High dose intravenous immunoglobulin is reserved for the most severe or refractory cases. Various steroid regimens have been used. The following has been demonstrated to raise the count almost as quickly as intravenous immunoglobulin: prednisolone 4 mg/kg for 1 week (maximum 75 mg/day), then 2 mg/kg for 1 week followed by 1mg/kg for 1 week.

While the platelet count is very low, the child should rest quietly at home. As the count rises, more activity is allowed, but contact sports, cycling and rough physical activity should be avoided until the count is normal. Aspirin, non-steroidal anti-inflammatory drugs and intramuscular/subcutaneous injections (including immunisations) should be avoided until thrombocytopenia remits.

It is quite common for thrombocytopenia to recur with further viral infections in the year after diagnosis. Chronic ITP (lasting more than 6 months) occurs in less than 10% and requires specialist management.

TRANSFUSION THERAPY

Blood transfusion is common in the tertiary paediatric setting. The commonest blood product transfused is packed red cells (PCC). Packed red cells are indicated when acute restoration of oxygen carrying capacity is required (i.e. to relieve symptomatic or predictably progressive anaemia) or to achieve marrow suppression in chronic ineffective erythropoiesis (e.g. thalassemia major, sickle cell anaemia). Nutritional anaemia rarely, if ever requires transfusion.

In order to calculate the desired transfusion volume, the following formula can be used:

$$\text{Packed red cells (mL)} = (\text{desired Hb} - \text{actual Hb}) \times \text{weight (kg)} \times 4$$

Adverse reactions

There are many potential adverse reactions from blood transfusions. Statistically, the most likely life threatening adverse event from blood transfusion is an acute haemolytic reaction due to an incompatible transfusion. This occurs due to mistaken identification of either the cross match sample or the unit being transfused to the patient and is most likely to occur when children of similar names are on the same wards, or in multiple emergencies. Fastidious adherence to identification procedures is required at all times.

Directed donations from parents are reportedly no safer than anonymous homologous transfusions. However, the family may prefer them. Directed donations can only be arranged electively as they require 5 days to process.

Non-haemolytic febrile transfusion reactions are the most common adverse events and are due to release of cytokines from white cells within the PCC. Slowing the transfusion rate and premedicating with promethazine (Phenergan) and paracetamol may be helpful. Leukodepletion (via filters) reduces the risk of non-haemolytic febrile transfusion reactions and can also be used to prevent cytomegalovirus transmission.

Irradiation of blood products is required prior to transfusion in all immunocompromised children, including neonates, oncology patients and some cardiac surgical patients to reduce the possibility of transfusion associated graft versus host disease. Irradiation reduces the shelf life of PCC so is usually performed immediately prior to release from the blood bank.

Bacterial infection can present as an acute haemolytic reaction with catastrophic hypotension and fever. Bacterial infection from blood transfusion is much more likely if the PCC has been unrefrigerated for more than 4 h and so a unit of PCC should not be infused over longer than this time.

Viral infections from blood transfusions are rare. In Victoria, since the introduction of nucleic acid testing, the risk of:

- HIV from a blood transfusion is approximately 1 in 9 million.
- Hepatitis C is 1 in 1 million.
- 'Mad cow disease' transmission by transfusion has not been documented, although this is theoretically possible.

The most important preventative measure to keep blood safe from viral infection is not laboratory testing, but the use of volunteer donors and the accurate completion of the donor declaration form.

ONCOLOGY

Malignancy in childhood is rare. Approximately 1:600 children will develop a malignancy before the age of 14 years. The expeditious investigation and management of the child with a malignancy is a

Table 26.4 Age distribution of common tumour types

	0–4 years	*5–9 years*	*10–14 years*
% **Total tumours**	46	29	25
CNS and Eye	44	30	26
Leukaemia	49	30	21
Neuroblastoma	84	11	5
Wilm's tumour	81	18	1
Soft tissue sarcomas	40	34	26
1° Bone tumours	5	27	68

specialised field and should be undertaken under the supervision of a paediatric oncologist.

Many paediatric malignancies occur over a relatively restricted age range. A broad understanding of the peak age of occurrence of different tumour types is useful when considering the possibility of malignancy in a child with unusual symptoms or signs.

Presentation of childhood malignancies

The possibility of malignancy should be considered in children presenting with any of the following symptoms or signs:

- Combinations of pallor, bruising or petechiae, fever and bone pain.
- Lymphadenopathy – marked, progressive or persistent, localised or generalised.
- Hepatosplenomegaly.
- Any unusual mass or swelling.
- Ataxia, cranial nerve palsies, or other neurological signs, particularly when associated with headache or back pain.
- Recurring morning headache particularly if associated with vomiting or visual disturbance.
- New onset of dry cough, stridor or wheeze, without other symptoms of respiratory infection, particularly if associated with orthopnoea.
- Unexplained weight loss.
- Persistent severe unexplained pain, especially bone or joint pain.

Prompt referral is appropriate.

Emergency presentations

The majority of children with suspected malignancy can have investigations and diagnostic procedures scheduled electively during normal working hours without compromising outcomes. There are however some malignancies which may threaten life or organ function at presentation because of their site and biological behaviour. It is vital that children with the following presentations are referred urgently.

Anterior mediastinal mass

Symptoms:

- Cough, stridor, wheeze, orthopnoea, (tracheal/bronchial compression).
- Facial /neck oedema, suffusion (superior vena caval obstruction).

Minor increase in size of mass, sedation or anaesthesia may result in respiratory obstruction or right ventricular outflow tract obstruction

Differential diagnoses:

Most commonly T cell Non-Hodgkin's lymphoma (NHL), Hodgkin's disease, Germ cell tumour, Carcinoid tumour.

Leukaemia with WCC $>100 \times 10^9$/L

High WCC is typically found in T cell acute lymphocytic leukaemia (ALL) and infant leukaemias.

Patients are at risk of:

- Cerebral leukostasis (avoid transfusion >70 g/L to prevent further increase in haematocrit).
- Uric acid nephropathy.

Leukaemia with severe coagulopathy

New patients with clinical features suggestive of leukaemia, with active bleeding or gross bruising should have coagulation screening performed promptly. Evidence of active disseminated intravascular coagulation (DIC) suggests acute promyelocytic leukaemia and urgent therapy with heparin, fresh frozen plasma (FFP) and platelets is required. Coagulation factor concentrates might occasionally be life saving. Gross bruising and active bleeding secondary to thrombocytopenia alone is relatively rare unless the platelet count is $<5 \times 10^9$/L.

Rapidly enlarging abdominal mass with ascites and/or pleural effusion

- Typical of mature B cell NHL.

Extremely rapid cell turnover may result in **tumour lysis syndrome** with renal failure and hyperkalaemia even before therapy commences. Attention to hyperhydration, alkalinisation of urine, allopurinol or urate oxidase therapy are vital in prevention of tumour lysis syndrome.

Children with symptoms/signs of raised intra-cranial pressure

- Headache, vomiting, cranial nerve palsy or papilloedema.
- Urgent CT/MRI evaluation is required.
- Emergency shunting may be required before tumour biopsy/removal.

Symptoms or signs of nerve root or cord compression

Many of the tumours that can result in cord or nerve root compression respond very rapidly to chemotherapy. Prompt radiologic and haematological investigation and biopsy before frank cord compression occurs may enable conservative management without the need for a decompression laminectomy.

Emergencies during therapy

Fever in a patient receiving chemotherapy

Risk factors for infection in immunocompromised patients are:

Neutropaenia: A neutrophil count of $<0.5 \times 10^6$/L, is associated with a significantly increased risk of bacteraemia and focal infection. This risk is markedly increased with a neutrophil count $<0.2 \times 10^9$/L. The longer the duration of neutropenia, the higher the risk of infection.

Lymphopaenia is associated with increased risk of opportunistic infection such as *Pneumocystis carinii* and reactivation of Herpes Simplex and Herpes Zoster viruses.

Steroid therapy is a risk factor for invasive fungal infection.

Central venous catheters: The majority of children receiving chemotherapy now have either Hickman catheters (externalised central venous catheter (CVC)) or infusaports (completely subcutaneous) inserted. Infection may occur at the exit site of a Hickman catheter, along the subcutaneous tunnel or within the lumen of the catheter. The reservoir of the port and associated catheter lumen may become colonized.

Breaches of the normal skin and mucosal barriers particularly in heavily colonised sites around the perineum, in the mouth, nose and lower gastrointestinal tract allow organisms access to the blood stream.

Most children with solid tumours receive intensive myelosuppressive chemotherapy regimens resulting in recurrent neutropenia 1–2 weeks post chemotherapy. Children with acute myeloid leukaemia (AML) have prolonged periods of neutropenia throughout their therapy. Children with ALL are likely to have several phases of treatment in the first 6–8 months of treatment that are myelosuppressive but often have reasonably stable blood counts during maintenance therapy.

Any child receiving an intensive therapy regimen, who develops a fever (>38.5°C on one occasion or 38.0°C on two occasions at least an hour apart), should be presumed to be neutropaenic and assessed promptly, with respect to:

- Cardiovascular stability.
- Respiratory status.
- Signs associated with anaemia and thrombocytopenia.
- Possible sites of infection:
  - Upper respiratory tract infection.
  - Dental sepsis.
  - Mouth ulcers including herpetic.
  - Cuts, abrasions, skin sores.
  - Inflamed Hickman/CVC site.
  - Anal fissures.
  - Embolic phenomena of septicaemia / bacterial endocarditis (especially if central line is *in situ*).
  - Lower respiratory tract infections especially *Pneumocystis carinii* pneumonia (fever, cough, tachypnoea, desaturation; clear chest to auscultation; interstitial infiltrate on chest X-ray).
  - Gastrointestinal tract infection including typhlitis (colonic wall inflammation especially caecum).

Investigations

- FBE and differential.
- Blood cultures (from both barrels of a dual lumen CVC).
- Swabs of local lesions.
- Urine culture.
- Sputum culture in older children.
- Chest X-ray (may be no changes when neutropaenic).
- Cross-match.
- Stool for M/C/S and viral studies.

Note: Lumbar puncture is contraindicated, as there is often a co-existent thrombocytopenia.

An initial dose of antibiotics should be given without delay. Delay in administering antibiotics until neutropenia is confirmed may result in progression from bacteraemia to septic shock.

Antibiotic choices must be determined by the infection profile of the unit as well as recent previous infections experienced by the patient, particularly if a CVC is in situ.

In the absence of focal signs, one example of an empiric antibiotic regimen is:

- Timentin 50 mg/kg i.v. 6-hourly (dose divided between the barrels of a dual lumen CVC device) and;
- Gentamicin 7.5 mg/kg i.v. daily (dose divided between the barrels of a dual lumen CVC device).

Most febrile neutropaenic patients will be admitted to hospital and continue i.v. antibiotics until blood cultures have been reported as negative after 48 h.

Children on maintenance therapy for ALL, with previously stable blood counts, who present with a mild fever, are assessed as being well and have signs of a respiratory infection or other focal infection may await the results of a blood count before making a decision regarding oral versus i.v. or no antibiotics.

Other issues during treatment

Nausea and Vomiting

Nausea and vomiting are common side effects of chemotherapy. They can now be successfully prevented or ameliorated in most children with the use of a 5HT-receptor antagonist such as ondansetron (0.15 mg/kg) pre-chemotherapy and 8–12-hourly during a course of treatment. Highly emetogenic chemotherapy combinations, such as high dose doxorubicin combined with high dose cyclophosphamide or cisplatin may require the addition of dexamethasone, given pre- and post-chemotherapy. If this combination fails, consider chlorpromazine (0.3 mg/kg) i.v., given over 30 min to minimise the risk of hypotension and dysphoria.

Constipation

Constipation is a side effect of vincristine therapy and can be particularly troublesome when the drug is used weekly for some weeks (as in induction for ALL, Wilm's tumour, rhabdomyosarcoma, and Ewing's sarcoma). Prophylaxis with lactulose or another stool softener should be instigated at the beginning of therapy. If despite prophylaxis and the addition of other agents if necessary, severe constipation develops, Golytely may be administered by nasogastric tube and is usually successful in relieving constipation. **Suppositories and enemas must not be used** because of the risk of small abrasions with secondary local infection or septicaemia.

Pain

See also Pain management, chapter 3.

There are many potential causes of pain and distress in children with malignancy. Assessment of the cause will usually allow appropriate therapy to provide adequate relief of symptoms. Pain caused by the underlying malignancy at presentation usually responds rapidly to the commencement of chemotherapy, though analgesia may be required while investigations are being carried out, the diagnosis established and treatment commenced.

Pain in patients with cancer is complex and multi-factorial; refer for appropriate specialist advice promptly.

Infectious disease contacts in immunosuppressed patients

Varicella and measles may lead to very severe illness in immunocompromised children. There is no effective anti-viral agent available for measles and it may cause fatal pneumonitis. Although immunity may wane during chemotherapy, prior vaccination or infection is usually protective. If the patient's immune status is not known or negative, give Herpes zoster immunoglobulin (ZIG) for varicella contact or human immunoglobulin for measles contact within 72 h. Contact must have been directly between the patient and the affected individual during the period extending from 48 h before the appearance of the rash to 7 days after the appearance of the rash.

Zoster Immunoglobulin dose for varicella contact

- Weight up to 20 kg or <5 yrs of age: 250 mg i.m. (1 × 2 ml vial).
- Weight 20–40 kg or 5–10 yrs of age: 500 mg i.m. (2 × 2ml vial).
- Weight >40 kg or age >10 yrs: 750 mg i.m. (3 × 2 ml vials).

Immunoglobulin for measles contact

- 0.25 ml/kg i.m. daily for 2 days.

Immunisation during and after therapy

Responses to routine immunisations will not be optimal during therapy. It is therefore recommended that routine immunisation programmes be interrupted while the child is on therapy. If required for treatment of a tetanus prone wound, tetanus toxoid can be safely given but concurrent use of tetanus immunoglobulin should also be considered.

- **Live virus vaccines must not be given to immunocompromised children.**
- **Siblings of patients should not receive Sabin; give injectable polio vaccine inactivated instead.**
- It is strongly advised that unimmunised, non-immune siblings receive MMR and Varicella vaccine.
- All family members including the immunocompromised child should be encouraged to have annual influenza vaccination.
- Approximately 6 months after completion of chemotherapy, interrupted immunisation programmes should be completed. A booster dose of ADT or CDT, Sabin and MMR should be given to those who have previously been fully immunised. Hepatitis B immunisation should be commenced if not previously given.
- Consult with a specialist regarding immunisation after an allogeneic bone marrow transplant.

CHAPTER 27
INFECTIOUS DISEASES

Nigel Curtis
Jonathan Carapetis
Mike Starr

RATIONAL ANTIMICROBIAL PRESCRIBING

- Unnecessary antibiotic use for viral illnesses contributes to the increasing problem of antibiotic resistance. Most respiratory tract infections in children, including tonsillitis and otitis media, are self-limiting and do not require antibiotic therapy. If the diagnosis is unclear, it is preferable to perform repeated clinical evaluations and simple laboratory tests than to use empiric antibiotic therapy 'just in case'.
- Antibiotics do not prevent secondary bacterial infection in viral illnesses.
- The use of antibiotics may make definitive diagnosis and subsequent decisions about management more difficult.
- Empiric antibiotic therapy (i.e. not based on specific aetiological diagnosis) should only be prescribed when a *serious* bacterial infection is suspected (e.g. meningitis) *and* it is not safe or possible to obtain definitive culture specimens or culture results are pending.
- Empiric therapy should be based on the likely cause, local antibiotic resistance patterns and individual host factors (e.g. immunocompromise) in accordance with local guidelines.
- For mild infections, the safest and best-tolerated antibiotic with the narrowest spectrum against the most likely pathogens should be chosen (e.g. trimethoprim for urinary tract infection).
- For serious infections, broad-spectrum agents are chosen until the pathogen and its susceptibility is identified (e.g. cefotaxime for meningitis).
- Theoretical benefits of new antibiotics based on *in vitro* data do not necessarily translate into greater efficacy. Newer antibiotics often offer no advantages, might be expensive with more side

effects and have a greater likelihood of leading to resistance or superinfection.

ANTIBIOTIC RESISTANCE

Although many bacteria are still susceptible to long-established treatments, antibiotic resistance is an increasing problem worldwide. Examples of particular clinical concern include:

- Penicillin (and cephalosporin)-resistant *Streptococcus pneumoniae* (PRP).
- Methicillin (multi-drug)-resistant *Staphylococcus aureus* (MRSA).
- Vancomycin-resistant (glycopeptide intermediate) *Staphylococcus aureus* (GISA).
- Vancomycin-resistant *Enterococcus* (VRE).
- Multi-drug-resistant *Mycobacterium tuberculosis* (MRTB).
- Bacteria that produce inducible β-lactamases (IBL, e.g. some *Pseudomonas* spp. and *Enterobacter* spp.).
- Bacteria that produce extended-spectrum β-lactamases (ESBL, e.g. some *Klebsiella* spp.).
- Multi-drug-resistant *Salmonella* spp.
- Macrolide-resistant *Streptococcus pyogenes*.

Strategies to deal with infections caused by these organisms include the use of new or broader spectrum antibiotics or the use of two or more antibiotics concurrently. The choice for empiric therapy becomes increasingly difficult.

APPROACH TO THE FEBRILE CHILD

Fever is the most common presenting symptom in children in the primary care setting. Although there is no universally accepted definition, fever is generally considered to be present if:

- Rectal (or tympanic) temperature >38°C.
- Oral temperature >37.5°C.
- Axillary temperature >37°C.

Although tympanic thermometers provide certain advantages over other thermometers (ease of use, rapid results and convenience), several studies have found that they are not as accurate or sensitive for the detection of fever. This is particularly the case in infants <3 months of age.

Self-limiting viral infections are the most common cause of fever in children. However, the challenge to the clinician is to identify those children with a more serious cause. Fever in children may be classified into three groups:

- Fever with localising signs.
- Fever without focus.
- Fever of unknown origin.

Fever with localising signs

A careful history and examination will identify the source of infection in most patients. These children should be managed according to the individual condition and its severity.

Fever without focus

In a small number of children presenting with fever, no focus is found. While most will have a viral infection, a more serious illness such as a urinary tract infection (5–8%), occult bacteraemia (3–5%) or meningitis may be present. Infants with rectal temperature >38.0°C have an 8–15% risk of occult bacteraemia.

Most children who present with fever and no identifiable focus appear otherwise well. History should include details about immunisation status, infectious contacts, travel, diet and contact with animals or insects. A thorough physical examination should be performed, paying particular attention to:

- General appearance: the level of activity and social interaction; peripheral perfusion and colour.
- Vital signs: pulse; respiration; blood pressure.
- Possible clues to source: full fontanelle, neck stiffness; respiratory distress (tachypnoea; grunt; nasal flare; retractions), abnormal chest signs; rhinitis, pharyngitis, otitis or mastoiditis; lymphadenopathy; abdominal distension, tenderness or masses; hepatosplenomegaly; bone and joint tenderness or swelling; skin rashes, petechiae or purpura, or skin infection.

Always consider Kawasaki disease in any child with a persistent fever.

Patients with unexplained fever with a higher likelihood for serious infection include the following patient groups or conditions:

- Neonates and infants under 3 months of age.
- Immunocompromise (e.g. congenital immunodeficiency, HIV, neutropaenic and other oncology patients, cytotoxic drugs and steroids).
- Asplenic children (congenital, post splenectomy or functional, e.g. sickle cell disease).
- Children with central venous or arterial catheters, or other foreign bodies, including shunts.
- Multiple congenital abnormalities.
- Other specific illnesses (e.g. sickle cell disease, cystic fibrosis or structural cardiac defects (endocarditis)).
- Toxic-appearing children (e.g. those with an altered conscious state, decreased peripheral perfusion or blood pressure or purpuric rash).
- Children under 6 months of age (higher chance of UTI).
- Children under 12 months of age with febrile convulsion (consider LP to exclude meningitis).

These children require admission to hospital, with culture of blood, urine and CSF ('full septic screen') and a chest X-ray if indicated. Antimicrobial therapy should be based on the patient's clinical illness and the local epidemiology of potential pathogens and their antibiotic susceptibility (see Antimicrobial guidelines).

In the absence of the above risk factors, a well-appearing febrile child (over 6 months of age) without a focus of infection does not require laboratory testing or treatment. There is no evidence that oral or parenteral antibiotics prevent the rare occurrence of focal infections from occult bacteraemia; instead, they result in delayed diagnosis, drug side effects, additional costs and the development of resistant organisms. What is required is a careful clinical assessment, review within 24 h and parental education. See Table 27.1 and Box 27.1.

Occult bacteraemia

Some infants with bacteraemia clear the bacteria spontaneously. This is particularly true for pneumococcal bacteraemia. Patients who grow *Streptococcus pneumoniae* in their original blood culture do not require further investigation or treatment if they are now well, remain afebrile

Table 27.1 Management of fever without focus

Age	*Investigations*	*Management*
<1 month	FBE; blood, urine and CSF cultures; CXR	• Admit • Empiric i.v. benzylpenicillin and gentamicin, *plus* cefotaxime if meningitis is suspected (see Antimicrobial guidelines)
1 to 3 months	As above (CXR may be omitted if no respiratory symptoms or signs present)	• If WCC 5–15 × 10^9 /L with other investigations normal: discharge and review within 12 h, or sooner if deterioration occurs • If child is unwell, or any results are abnormal: admit and consider empiric antibiotics (see Antimicrobial guidelines)
3 months to 3 years *and well*	Consider urine culture (mandatory if <6 months)	• If <6 months and UTI is suspected from dipstick urine testing: admit for i.v. benzylpenicillin and gentamicin (see Antimicrobial guidelines) • Otherwise: discharge and review within 24 h, or sooner if deterioration occurs
3 months to 3 years *and unwell*	FBE; blood, urine and CSF cultures; CXR if respiratory symptoms or signs present	• Admit and start empiric antibiotics: – if CSF normal: i.v. flucloxacillin and gentamicin – if CSF abnormal or unavailable: i.v. cefotaxime (see Antimicrobial guidelines)

Notes:

- Fever = rectal temperature >38°C (>38.9°C over 3 months of age)
- FBE = full blood examination, including film; CSF = cerebrospinal fluid; WCC = white cell count; CXR = chest X-ray
- Urine specimens should be obtained by suprapubic aspiration or catheter drainage. Bag specimens are useless in this context
- Lumbar puncture should not be performed in a child with impaired conscious state or focal neurological signs (See Medical Emergencies, chapter 1, Procedures, chapter 4)
- Ceftriaxone can be substituted for cefotaxime (see Antimicrobial guidelines)

Box 27.1 Advice for parents about fever

When caring for your child:

- Make the child comfortable; e.g. dress in light clothing.
- Give small, frequent drinks of clear fluid; e.g. water and diluted juice.
- Fever does not necessarily require treatment with medication. Finding the cause and treating it is often more important.
- Paracetamol should be given only if the child is irritable, miserable or appears to be in pain (15 mg/kg p.o. 4-hourly when required to a maximum of 90 mg/kg per day).
- Giving paracetamol has not been shown to prevent febrile convulsions
- Do not continue giving regular paracetamol for >48 h without having the child assessed by a doctor.
- Aspirin and other non steroidal anti-inflammatory drugs (NSAIDs) should be avoided.

Seek immediate medical attention if there is no improvement in 48 h or if the child:

- Looks 'sick': pale, lethargic and weak.
- Suffers severe headache, neck stiffness or light hurting eyes.
- Has breathing difficulties.
- Refuses to drink anything.
- Persistently vomits.
- Shows signs of drowsiness.
- Suffers pain.

and have not received antibiotics, as they have cleared the organism themselves. Parents should, however, be asked to bring children back for immediate review if they develop further fever within the following 7 days. Refer for specialist advice if uncertain.

Other pathogens causing occult bacteraemia should be treated with appropriate antibiotics.

Partially treated bacterial infection

Patients presenting with fever who have received prior antibiotics should be assessed with a high index of suspicion. Although the child may have a viral illness, partial treatment with antibiotics may mask the typical clinical presentation of a serious bacterial infection, such as meningitis. A full septic screen should be considered in most cases even if the child looks well.

Fever (pyrexia) of unknown origin

This is defined as prolonged fever (2 weeks or longer is the commonest definition) for which history, examination and routine tests have failed to reveal a cause. In general, pyrexia of unknown origin (PUO) in children is more likely to be due to chronic, non-infectious conditions, such as juvenile chronic arthritis and other collagen vascular diseases, inflammatory bowel disease or malignancy. Infectious causes include systemic viral syndromes (such as infectious mononucleosis), upper or lower respiratory infections (e.g. sinusitis), urinary tract infection, central nervous system (CNS) infection, bone infection, tuberculosis, abscess (e.g. parameningeal, intra-abdominal), endocarditis and enteric infections (e.g. typhoid fever). The term PUO is often *incorrectly* applied to patients who are suffering a series of simple viral infections.

Febrile neutropenia

See Haematologic conditions and oncology, chapter 26.

BACTERIAL INFECTIONS

Group A Streptococcus

Group A beta haemolytic streptococci (GABHS or *Streptococcus pyogenes*) cause a variety of diseases including pharyngotonsillitis (see Ear, nose and throat conditions, chapter 21), impetigo, cellulitis, scarlet fever, otitis media, streptococcal toxic shock syndrome, necrotising fasciitis, glomerulonephritis and rheumatic fever. Group A beta haemolytic streptococci infection usually occurs in school-age children.

Scarlet fever

Transmission	Droplet, direct contact.
Incubation period	2–5 days.
Infectious period	10–21 days (24–48 h, if adequate treatment).
Clinical features	*Prodrome*: sudden onset high fever, vomiting, malaise, headache and abdominal pain. *Rash*: appears within 2 h of prodrome, diffuse

	red flush involving torso and skin folds, blanches, circumoral pallor, strawberry tongue (initially white, then red day 4–5), pharyngotonsillitis, tender cervical / submaxillary nodes.
Complications	Otitis media, rheumatic fever, glomerulonephritis.
Diagnosis	Culture of throat swab may confirm clinical impression.
Treatment	Phenoxymethylpenicillin (Penicillin V) 250 mg p.o. (<10 years), 500 mg p.o. (>10 years) 12-hourly for 10 days.
Control of case	Exclude from school until treated for longer than 24 h.

Acute rheumatic fever

Incubation period	7–28 days after group A streptococcal infection.
Clinical features	Jones criteria (1992) for initial diagnosis: two major or one major and two minor manifestations and evidence of preceding group A streptococcal infection (culture or serological). *Major manifestations*: carditis (usually mitral regurgitation murmur), polyarthritis, chorea, subcutaneous nodules, erythema marginatum. *Minor manifestations*: fever, prolonged PR interval on ECG, raised inflammatory markers. Recurrences can be diagnosed without major manifestations if there are no other more likely diagnoses.
Complications	Increased risk of recurrent disease, particularly for first 5 years after last attack. Heart valve damage may be permanent – especially after severe or recurrent disease – leading to rheumatic heart disease.
Diagnosis	Clinical features (Jones criteria) + culture/serology. Echocardiography may be useful in detecting subclinical lesions or typical rheumatic valvular involvement.
Treatment	Admission to hospital. Phenoxymethylpenicillin (Penicillin V) 250 mg p.o. (<10 years), 500 mg p.o. (>10 years) 12-hourly for 10 days or a single

i.m. injection of benzathine penicillin G (900 mg, or 450 mg if <30 kg). Aspirin 25 mg/kg oral 6-hourly (4–8 g/day total in adults) initially, reducing to 15 mg/kg oral 6-hourly after 2 weeks for a further 2 weeks, may be used to relieve arthritis or fever and leads to resolution of symptoms within 1–2 days (sometimes this response is diagnostic of rheumatic fever). There is no evidence that aspirin affects the long-term outcome. Corticosteroids (usually prednisolone 2 mg/kg/day, tapering after 2 weeks) are often used when carditis with cardiac failure is present, although there is no definitive evidence that they improve long-term outcome. Haloperidol, sodium valproate or other major tranquillisers have been used to control severe chorea, with mixed success.

Follow-up

Secondary prophylaxis is essential to prevent subsequent group A streptococcal infections, which may cause recurrences. Phenoxymethylpenicillin (Penicillin V) 250 mg p.o. twice daily, or benzathine penicillin G 900 mg i.m. every 3 or 4 weeks. Duration is until 21 years if age or 5 years after last attack (whichever is later) or to age 35 years if moderate or severe carditis present. Prophylaxis may be lifelong if severe carditis or if patient has required cardiac surgery. Long term clinical and echocardiographic follow up is essential.

Post-infectious Glomerulonephritis

See Renal conditions and enuresis, chapter 32.

Streptococcus pneumoniae

Streptococcus pneumoniae (pneumococcus) is a Gram-positive diplococcus that causes a wide variety of infections including severe, invasive disease (e.g. meningitis, septicaemia, septic arthritis, peritonitis), or mild, often self-limited, invasive disease (occult bacteraemia), pneumonia, otitis media and sinusitis.

Transmission	Droplet.
Epidemiology	Ninety serotypes described. Most human disease caused by 23 serotypes. 7 serotypes cause about 85% of invasive disease in non-Aboriginal Australian children. Incidence of invasive disease is about 50–100 cases per 100,000 children aged <5 years. Incidence in central Australian Aboriginal children is the highest in the world (~1,000 to 2,000 per 100,000 aged <5 yrs). Antibiotic resistance becoming a problem worldwide – organisms classified as penicillin-susceptible, penicillin-non-susceptible (PNSP), and cefotaxime/ceftriaxone susceptible or resistant. The resistant groups include intermediate and high-level resistance.
Clinical features	Meningitis, pneumonia, septicaemia, otitis media.
Diagnosis	Meningitis, septicaemia and other sterile site infection confirmed by culture/Gram stain of appropriate specimen (blood, CSF, joint fluid, peritoneal fluid, etc.). Pneumococcal pneumonia is blood culture positive in only about 10–20% of cases.
Treatment	Penicillin is the drug of choice, except in CNS infection with cefotaxime/ceftriaxone-resistant pneumococci. If non-CNS infection with PNSP, treat with high-dose penicillin (benzylpenicillin 60 mg/kg (max 2 g) i.v. 4-hourly for invasive disease including pneumonia, or amoxicillin 90–120 mg/kg/day p.o. divided into 3 or 4 doses for otitis media or sinusitis). If CNS infection with cefotaxime/ceftriaxone-non-susceptible pneumococci, use vancomycin and cefotaxime (see Bacterial meningitis, following). Duration of treatment is 10 days for meningitis and usually 5 to 7 days for other infections.
Vaccines	Twenty-three-valent polysaccharide vaccine not effective in children aged <2 yrs and has questionable efficacy in preventing non-bacteraemic pneumococcal disease. It is used

routinely for elderly people and other high-risk individuals (e.g. post-splenectomy patients) and more recently as a booster in some recipients of the conjugate pneumococcal vaccine. Seven-valent conjugate vaccine protects at all ages >6 weeks, against the 7 most common serotypes causing invasive disease in Australia. Its efficacy against serotype-specific invasive disease is 89–97%. Its efficacy in preventing X-ray confirmed pneumonia is approximately 20% and against acute otitis media is about 6% (although it may be more effective against frequent recurrent otitis media and in preventing tympanostomy tube placement). The vaccine is expensive, but provided free of charge to certain high-risk groups (see Immunisation, chapter 8). The conjugate vaccine is recommended for all Australian children <2 (and possibly up to 5) yrs of age.

Neisseria meningitidis

Neisseria meningitidis (meningococcus) is a Gram-negative diplococcus that mainly causes meningitis or septicaemia, or both. Less commonly, it may cause other infections including conjunctivitis, septic arthritis, pharyngitis, pneumonia, occult bacteraemia. For recommendations specific to meningitis see bacterial meningitis p. 452.

Transmission	Droplet.
Incubation period	Hours to 3 days usually
Infectious period	As long as carried – may be months. Most virulent within days of acquisition.
Epidemiology	Peak age groups <2 years and 15–24 years. Serogroups B and C are most common in Australia (A, Y and W135 usually confined to travellers). Incidence is particularly high in Victoria and rising in recent years. Traditionally, group B most common in young children and group C more common in adolescents. Recently, group C increasing in incidence (~50% of Victorian cases in 2001) and virulence (case fatality rate 5% for group B, 14% for group C).

Clinical features	Meningitis – see following. Septicaemia: often non-specific prodrome suggestive of viral upper respiratory infection. Rapid progression with any or all of fever, rash (classically purpuric or petechial, but can be less specific), malaise, myalgia, arthralgia, vomiting, headache, reduced conscious state. Chronic meningococcaemia occurs rarely – particularly if terminal complement deficiency.
Diagnosis	Initially based on clinical features. To confirm, take blood for culture and perform LP unless contraindicated (see Procedures, chapter 4), preferably before first dose of antibiotics. Do not delay antibiotics while attempting to collect blood. Additional tests may include shave biopsy of skin lesions (for Gram stain and culture), PCR on blood and throat swab.
Treatment	Immediate intravenous antibiotics (cefotaxime 50 mg/kg/dose (max 2 g) 6-hourly, or if unavailable, use benzyl penicillin G 60 mg/kg/dose (max 2 g) 4-hourly). Can give antibiotics and fluids intraosseously if intravenous access is not possible. Usually require fluid resuscitation (20 mL/kg normal saline i.v., repeated as necessary) and may require inotropic support. Intensive care unit should be consulted. Duration of antibiotics – usually 7 days. Can revert to i.v. benzyl penicillin when isolate identified as meningococcus.
Other aspects	All cases should be notified immediately to statutory health authorities. Family and household contacts >1 month old should receive prophylaxis with rifampicin 10 mg/kg p.o. 12-hourly (max 600 mg) for 2 days. Infants <1 month should receive rifampicin 5 mg/kg p.o. 12-hourly for 2 days, and pregnant women should receive ceftriaxone 250 mg i.m. as a single dose.

Vaccines — Tetravalent polysaccharide vaccine (A, C, Y, W135) protects for a short time (3–5 yrs) and only in those aged >2 years. Therefore, this vaccine is reserved for travellers (e.g. to African "meningitis belt" or attending the Haj) and for controlling outbreaks. Meningococcal group C conjugate vaccine is effective at all age groups and recommended for all children >6 weeks old, adolescents and young adults (see Immunisation, chapter 8).

Staphylococcus aureus

Staphylococcus aureus is a Gram-positive coccus that causes a wide variety of invasive and non-invasive disease.

Epidemiology — *Staphylococcus aureus* is a common commensal, being present in the nose of about one third of individuals. Both hospital- and community-acquired multi-resistant *S. aureus* (MRSA) are an increasing problem.

Clinical features — Causes a variety of diseases including impetigo, boils and abscesses, cellulitis (including periorbital cellulitis), osteomyelitis, septic arthritis, endocarditis, pneumonia, food poisoning, bacteraemia, septicaemia and toxic shock syndrome. *Staphylococcus aureus* is responsible for scalded skin syndrome in younger children. Staphylococcal infection may be accompanied by significant constitutional symptoms (e.g. myalgia) in addition to localising features.

Diagnosis — Sterile site infection is confirmed by appropriate culture/Gram stain.

Treatment — Surgical drainage may be necessary for abscesses and other foci of infection. Anti-staphylococcal antibiotics include flucloxacillin, cephalexin, cephazolin and clindamycin. Vancomycin is necessary to treat MRSA but is not as effective as flucloxacillin for the treatment of susceptible *S. aureus* (MSSA). Prolonged duration of treatment is often required to prevent recurrence.

Mycoplasma pneumoniae

Transmission	Droplet.
Incubation period	1–4 weeks.
Infectious period	Unknown, likely to be many months; typically infects all members of a family over a period of weeks/months.
Clinical features	*Pneumonia*: malaise, fever, headache, non-productive cough for 3–4 weeks (may become productive); 10% have rash (usually maculopapular); bilateral, diffuse infiltrates on chest X-ray; bronchitis, pharyngitis, otitis media. *CNS manifestations* (uncommon; likely post-infectious): aseptic meningitis, meningoencephalitis, encephalitis, polyradiculitis/ Guillain–Barré syndrome, acute cerebellar ataxia, cranial nerve neuropathy, transverse myelitis, acute disseminated encephalomyelitis and choreoathetosis.
Complications	Idiopathic thrombocytopaenic purpura.
Diagnosis	*Serology*: four-fold rise in IgG; IgM alone can be difficult to interpret, mycoplasma specific antibodies, polymerase chain reaction (PCR) of CSF.
Treatment	Roxithromycin 2.5–4 mg/kg (max 150 mg) p.o. 12-hourly for 10 days; role of antibiotics (e.g. azithromycin) in CNS infections is unclear.

VIRAL INFECTIONS

Cytomegalovirus

Cytomegalovirus (CMV) is a ubiquitous herpes virus. It persists in latent form after primary infection and reactivation can occur years later, particularly with immunosuppression.

Transmission	*Horizontal*: salivary contamination or sexual transmission; blood transfusion/organ transplantation.

	Vertical: transplacental, intrapartum by passage through infected genital tract and postnatal by ingestion of CMV-positive breast milk.
Incubation period	Unknown, infection usually manifests 3 weeks to 3 months after blood transfusion and 4 weeks to 4 months after tissue transplantation.
Clinical features	Vary with age and immunocompetence of child; asymptomatic infection is most common. *Cytomegalovirus mononucleosis*: cervical lymphadenopathy; hepatosplenomegaly in children, fever in adults. *Note*: clinical signs of CMV infection are similar to graft rejection in transplant patients. Both events peak 30–90 days after transplantation.
Diagnosis	Distinguishing CMV infection from active CMV disease can be difficult. The following tests on blood, urine, oral secretions or biopsy specimens can help make this distinction: *viral culture* (rapid enhanced tissue culture immunofluorescence) and *PCR*, *leucocyte antigenaemia assay* (degree of antigenaemia correlates with the severity of CMV disease and is therefore a good means of predicting disease and monitoring progression).
Complications	Encephalitis, myocarditis, pneumonia, haemolytic anaemia, thrombocytopaenia. Primary CMV infection has been described in conjunction with Guillain–Barré syndrome and other peripheral neuropathies. Pneumonia, retinitis, hepatitis and colitis in immunocompromised. *Congenital infection*: >90% appear normal at birth: CNS sequelae in 10–20% of these (mainly sensorineural hearing loss); 5% present early with petechiae, hepatosplenomegaly, microcephaly and thrombocytopaenia.
Treatment	Ganciclovir for active CMV disease in the immunocompromised. Cytomegalovirus hyperimmune globulin is also sometimes used in these patients.

Enterovirus (non-polio)

Coxsackie A, B and echoviruses are important causes of childhood infections, especially in the summer months. These include a wide range of clinical presentations, including non-specific febrile illness, pharyngitis, herpangina, hand, foot and mouth disease, gastroenteritis, aseptic meningitis, encephalitis, myocarditis, pericarditis and several forms of viral exanthem (maculopapular, vesicular, petechial). Infection in agammaglobulinaemic patients can cause particularly severe or persistent meningoencephalitis.

Hand, foot and mouth disease

Cause	Coxsackie A virus (A16) usually.
Transmission	Direct contact/droplet.
Incubation period	3–6 days.
Infectious period	Until blisters have gone.
Clinical features	Vesicles on cheeks, gums, sides of the tongue; papulovesicular lesions of palms, fingers, toes, soles, buttocks, genitals, limbs (may look haemorrhagic); sore throat; fever and anorexia.
Diagnosis	Tests are usually unnecessary as the clinical picture is sufficient for diagnosis.
Control of case	Exclusion is unnecessary (as virus is excreted in faeces for weeks).
Treatment	Symptomatic.

Epstein-Barr virus (infectious mononucleosis)

Incubation period	30–50 days.
Infectious period	Unknown, viral excretion from oropharynx for months.
Clinical features	Fever, malaise, exudative tonsillopharyngitis, generalised lymphadenopathy and hepatosplenomegaly. Highly variable clinical course: acute phase lasts 2–4 weeks and convalescence may take weeks to months. In immunocompromised (particularly transplant patients), can cause severe lymphoproliferative disease.
Diagnosis	Atypical lymphocytes in the peripheral blood. Monospot test in blood for heterophile antibody

	identifies 90% of cases in older children and adults, but lacks sensitivity in children under 4–5 years of age. Serology is the gold standard. PCR of blood or tissue may be helpful in transplant patients.
Complications	Upper airways obstruction; dehydration from poor oral intake (uncommon).
Treatment	*Symptomatic*: Prednisolone 1 mg/kg (max 50 mg) oral, daily may be considered in patients hospitalised for airways obstruction. Amoxicillin and ampicillin may cause a florid rash in children with Epstein-Barr virus (EBV) infection.

Herpes simplex virus

Manifestations of Herpes simplex virus (HSV) infection include skin and mucous membrane involvement, gingivostomatitis (mainly HSV-1), genital herpes (mainly HSV-2), eczema herpeticum (see Dermatologic conditions, chapter 20), herpetic whitlow and eye involvement. Herpes simplex virus encephalitis is an important treatable condition that must not be missed (see page 460 and Neurologic conditions, chapter 30). Pneumonia and disseminated infection occur in the immunocompromised. Congenital infection also occurs. Infection can be primary (e.g. gingivostomatitis) or from a reactivation of the latent virus (e.g. cold sores).

Primary herpes gingivostomatitis

Transmission	Droplet, direct contact.
Incubation period	2–14 days
Infectious period	Indeterminate; virus can be excreted for at least 1 week, occasionally months. Shed intermittently in the absence of symptoms for years afterwards.
Clinical features	Fever, irritability, cervical lymphadenopathy, halitosis, diffuse erythema and ulceration within the oral cavity (buccal mucosa, palate, gingiva and tongue) and mucocutaneous junction. Duration is 7–14 days.
Diagnosis	Immunofluorescence or culture of vesicular scrapings.
Complications	Poor oral intake; autoinoculation resulting in herpetic whitlow, keratitis or genital herpes;

	eczema herpeticum; dissemination (particularly in immunocompromised).
Treatment	Symptomatic: topical anaesthesia (e.g. 1–2% lignocaine gel), analgesia (paracetamol), fluids and a soft diet. Aciclovir should be given only if immunocompromised.

Herpes simplex virus in pregnancy

Primary infection during the first 20 weeks of gestation is associated with an increased risk of spontaneous abortion, stillbirth and congenital disease. Beyond 20 weeks, premature labour and growth retardation are more common.

Neonatal HSV

Transmission	*Intrapartum* (70–85%): perinatal acquisition from maternal genital tract; usually presents day 5–19. *Postnatal* (10%): usually presents day 5–19. *Intrauterine* (5%): transplacental; usually presents within 48 h of birth. Transmission is 10 times more likely to occur with primary than with recurrent infection, both of which may be asymptomatic in women. More than 70% of women who give birth to infants with neonatal HSV infection give no history of genital HSV in themselves or their partners. The risk to a baby of an asymptomatic woman with a history of recurrent genital herpes is <3%.
Clinical features	Neonatal infection presents in three ways: *Localised skin, eye and/or mouth ('SEM') disease* (45%). Onset 7–14 days. Death is rare; 30% or more of patients eventually develop evidence of neurological impairment. *Central nervous system disease* (50%). Onset 14–21 days, in the form of encephalitis or a more disseminated disease. Mortality is 15%; 50–60% of survivors have psychomotor retardation, with or without microcephaly, spasticity, blindness, etc.

	Disseminated disease (20%). The onset is at 5–10 days. Involves any organ but primarily liver and adrenals; encephalitis occurs in 70% or more of patients. Presentation includes irritability, seizures, respiratory distress, jaundice, coagulopathy, shock and characteristic vesicular rash. *Note*: About 20% of babies never have skin lesions. Mortality is 50–60% (in spite of treatment) and neurological sequelae in 40%.
Diagnosis	Viral isolation from neonatal vesicular fluid, mouth or conjunctival swabs, stool, urine, leucocytes and maternal genital tract swabs. Herpes simplex virus antigens are detected by immunofluorescence. Serology is not always helpful, as maternally acquired IgG confounds interpretation in the neonate and IgM may not be produced until 2 weeks after the onset of illness. Detection of viral DNA by PCR, (especially in CSF to detect subclinical CNS disease) is helpful. Changes on EEG, CT and MRI may all provide supporting evidence of HSV infection.
Complications	Overall mortality (following treatment) is 15–20% and 40–50% of infants have some neurological impairment.
Treatment	Aciclovir 20 mg/kg i.v. 8-hourly (see Antimicrobial guidelines) for at least 14 days (SEM disease) or 21 days (CNS or disseminated disease). Suppressive treatment with aciclovir, for 6–12 months, is usually recommended for CNS or disseminated disease.
Prevention	20% of newborns born to women with primary HSV will be infected, even if delivered by Caesarean section.

Herpes simplex virus encephalitis

See page 460 and Neurologic conditions, chapter 30.

Human herpes virus 6 (roseola infantum)

Ninety-five per cent of children are infected with human herpes virus 6 (HHV-6) by the age of 2 years. Up to 30% will present with the clinical features of roseola. Human herpes virus-7 has also been shown to be the cause in a small number of children. Human herpes virus 6 infection may also present as an acute febrile illness without a rash.

Transmission	Direct contact/droplet (asymptomatically shed).
Incubation period	9–10 days.
Infectious period	Unknown (greatest during period of the rash).
Clinical features	Fever, occipital lymphadenopathy; then rapid defervescence corresponding with appearance of a red, maculopapular rash over trunk and arms for 1–2 days. *Note*: Many children are started on antibiotics for the fever and then misdiagnosed as having a drug reaction when the rash appears.
Diagnosis	Investigations do not usually alter management, but serology and PCR are available.
Complications	Febrile convulsions (HHV-6 is thought to be the cause of up to 1/3 of febrile convulsions in children <2 years of age), aseptic meningitis, encephalitis (rare), hepatitis.
Treatment	Symptomatic.

Measles virus (rubeola)

As a result of widespread measles immunisation, this disease is now seen infrequently. However, outbreaks continue to occur in most parts of the world.

Transmission	Droplet, direct contact.
Incubation period	7–14 days (14 days to the appearance of a rash).
Infectious period	1–2 days before the onset of symptoms to 4 days after the onset of the rash.
Clinical features	*Prodrome*: fever, conjunctivitis, coryza, cough and Koplik spots (white spots on a bright red buccal mucosa). *Rash*: appears 3–4 days later; erythematous and blotchy; starts at hairline and moves down the

	body, then becomes confluent; lasts 4–7 days; may desquamate in the second week.
Diagnosis	Serology (IgM is usually detectable 1–2 days after onset of rash), nasopharyngeal aspirate immunofluorescence and culture.
Complications	Otitis media (25%), pneumonia (1/25), encephalitis (1/2,000), subacute sclerosing pan encephalitis (SSPE) (1/25,000).
Treatment	*Symptomatic*: Vitamin A should be considered for young infants with severe measles, the immunocompromised and those with vitamin A deficiency.
Control of case	Exclude from school for at least 5 days from the appearance of the rash.
Contacts	Measles, mumps, rubella (MMR) vaccine should be given within 72 h of exposure to unimmunised children over 6 months of age (needs to be repeated 3 months later for children <12 months of age). If MMR is contraindicated, or if longer than 72 h since exposure, normal immunoglobulin should be given i.m. within 7 days (see Haematologic conditions and oncology, chapter 26). Exclude from school for 2 weeks if unimmunised.

Parvovirus B19 (erythema infectiosum, slapped cheek disease, fifth disease)

Transmission	Droplet, direct contact.
Incubation period	4–21 days.
Infectious period	Highly infectious until rash appears (50% of adults are immune).
Clinical features	Fever in 15–30%; non-specific prodrome. The rash has three stages: *Slapped cheek appearance* (1–3 days). *Maculopapular rash*: on proximal extensor surfaces, flexor surfaces and trunk; fades over next few days, then central clearing, forming a reticular pattern (after 7 days). *Reticular rash*: reappears with heat, cold and friction (weeks/months).

Diagnosis	Mainly clinical. PCR on blood and serology.
Complications	Arthritis; aplastic crisis in children with chronic haemolytic anaemia; bone marrow suppression; foetal hydrops.
Treatment	*Symptomatic*: School exclusion is inappropriate. Pregnant contacts should seek advice regarding possibility of intrauterine infection (uncommon).

Rubella virus

Transmission	Droplet, direct contact.
Incubation period	14–21 days.
Infectious period	5 days before to 7 days after rash.
Clinical features	25–50% have no symptoms. *Rash*: small, fine, discrete pink maculopapules; starts on face and spreads to chest and upper arms, abdomen and thighs, all within 24 h. *Prodrome*: (1–5 days) low-grade fever, malaise, headache, coryza, conjunctivitis (more common in adults), postauricular/occipital/posterior triangle lymphadenopathy precedes rash by 5–10 days.
Diagnosis	Serology.
Complications	*Congenital rubella syndrome*: more than 25% affected if mother infected during 1st trimester; 10–20% have single congenital defect if infection occurs at 16–40 days.
Control of case	Exclude from school for at least 5 days from the onset of the rash.
Contacts	Check serology if pregnant. Immunoglobulin given after exposure in early pregnancy may not prevent infection or viraemia, but may modify risk of abnormalities in the baby.

Varicella zoster virus (chickenpox, shingles)

Incubation period	10–21 days. Shorter incubation in the immunocompromised. Zoster Immune Globulin (ZIG) may prolong incubation to 28 days.
Infectious period	1–2 days before appearance of the rash until the rash is fully crusted.

Clinical features	Fever, irritability, anorexia and lymphadenopathy. The rash develops over the next 3–5 days. Macular, papular, vesicular and crusted by 5–10 days. Scalp, face, trunk, mouth, conjunctivae and extremities. Central distribution, lesions appear in crops. Itchy.
Diagnosis	Immunofluorescence of vesicular scrapings for VZV antigen, or serology. PCR of CSF may be useful in suspected encephalitis.
Complications	Secondary bacterial infection of skin lesions (most commonly *Streptococcus pyogenes* or *Staphylococcus aureus*); neurological (cerebellitis, transverse myelitis, Guillain-Barré syndrome); dissemination (pneumonitis, hepatitis, encephalitis) in patients with abnormal T-cell immunity. *Herpes zoster ('shingles')*, resulting from a reactivation of the latent virus, is more common in children who have had chickenpox in infancy or who have been exposed *in utero*.
Treatment	Aciclovir in patients with impaired T-cell immunity. Aciclovir is **not** indicated in the immunocompetent child. Antibiotics for secondary bacterial skin infection (e.g. flucloxacillin). **Aspirin is contraindicated because of the association with Reye's syndrome.**
Prevention	ZIG within 96 h of exposure (6 mL for adults, 4 mL for children 6–12 years of age, 2 mL for children up to 5 years of age) for the following patient groups in contact with varicella or shingles: • Immunocompromised children (e.g. HIV, immunosuppressive therapy (including high-dose steroids; prednisolone 2 mg/kg or more per day) and patients with transplants, lymphoma, leukaemia or severe combined immunodeficiency syndrome).

- Newborn infants whose mothers have varicella within the 5 days before, or 2 days after delivery.
- Infants with varicella onset under 28 days of age.
- Hospitalised premature infants with no maternal history of varicella.
- Hospitalised premature infants under 28 weeks gestation or <1,000g, regardless of maternal history.

Varicella vaccine – see Immunisation, chapter 8.

GASTROINTESTINAL INFECTIONS

See also Gastrointestinal conditions, chapter 24.

Infectious diarrhoea

Infectious diarrhoea continues to cause significant morbidity in children in developed and developing countries. In Australia, approximately 20,000 children (15/1,000) <5 years of age are admitted to hospital each year with acute gastroenteritis. Rotavirus is the causal agent in up to 2/3 of children in whom a pathogen is identified. Other important pathogens in children hospitalised with diarrhoea include caliciviruses, enteric adenoviruses, astroviruses, *Salmonella* spp., *Campylobacter jejuni, Giardia intestinalis (lamblia), Cryptosporidium parvum*, Enteropathogenic (and other) *Escherichia coli, Shigella* spp. and *Yersinia enterocolitica.*

- Children <5 years of age with rotavirus-positive gastroenteritis are unlikely to have another pathogen isolated from their faeces.
- It is unusual to find a protozoal parasite in the setting of acute diarrhoea.
- Repeat stool investigations are not helpful except in patients with chronic diarrhoea, suspected *Salmonella* carriage or parasitic infection.
- The cause of infectious diarrhoea can often be identified by simple laboratory studies but rarely alters management.
- Most bacterial causes of diarrhoea are self-limiting and do not usually require antibiotic therapy. The primary aim of treatment, as with viral gastroenteritis, is to achieve and maintain adequate hydration.

- Nosocomial infection is common. The prevention of its spread by adequate infection control measures is an essential component of hospital management.

Rotavirus

Incubation period	Illness usually begins 12 h–4 days after exposure.
Infectious period	Most children shed the virus in the stools for up to 10 days, however, about 1/3 with severe primary rotavirus infection may continue to excrete the virus for >21 days.
Clinical features	Major cause of severe diarrhoea in children causing over 50% of hospitalisations for acute gastroenteritis in children <5 years. Also a common cause of nosocomial infection. Annual peak of infection and illness occurs in the winter-spring period. Presents with diarrhoea, vomiting (may precede diarrhoea) and fever lasting for up to 1 week. Respiratory symptoms are common. May be complicated by dehydration, electrolyte imbalance and acidosis.
Diagnosis	Enzyme immunoassay and latex agglutination assay.
Treatment	Supportive, with particular attention to hydration.
Vaccine	An oral vaccine has been shown to have protective efficacy in large-scale clinical trials. A possible association with intussusception resulted in the withdrawal of the vaccine in the United States.

Adenovirus

Similar presentation to rotavirus, but there is no seasonality. It is more common under 12 months of age. Diarrhoea and vomiting may last longer and high fever is less common.

Salmonella (non typhi)

Clinical features	Broad spectrum of clinical syndromes including asymptomatic carriage, gastroenteritis, bacteraemia and focal infections (e.g. bone and joint). Age-specific attack rates are highest in

	children <5 years of age (peak at <1 year of age) and the elderly. Invasive infections and mortality are more common in infants, the elderly and those with underlying diseases.
Diagnosis	Does not usually alter management, but serology and PCR are available.
Treatment	Antibiotic treatment is not usually indicated for uncomplicated gastroenteritis as it may prolong excretion. Antibiotic treatment is indicated for: bacteraemia, systemic involvement or infection in infants <3 months of age, those with underlying disease (e.g. immunocompromised) and the elderly. The choice and duration of treatment depends on the clinical manifestation and antibiotic susceptibility.

Campylobacter jejuni

More common >5 years of age. Causes diarrhoea with visible or occult blood, abdominal pain, malaise and fever. Antibiotic treatment is not usually necessary, except in special circumstances where the elimination of the carrier state is important, such as infection in food handlers.

Giardia intestinalis (lamblia)

Transmission	The most common parasite identified in stool specimens from children. More common in children (and staff) in childcare centres and returned travellers. The major reservoir and means of spread is contaminated water and, to a lesser extent, food. Person-to-person spread also occurs.
Clinical features	There is a broad spectrum of clinical manifestations, but the most common are: diarrhoea (usually persistent), abdominal distension, flatulence, abdominal cramps and weight loss/failure to thrive.
Diagnosis	Confirmed by microscopy of stool specimens. These do not usually contain blood, mucus or leucocytes. Repeat specimens may be necessary.

Treatment	Metronidazole 30 mg/kg (max 2 g) p.o. daily for 3 days *or* tinidazole 50 mg/kg (max 2 g) p.o. as a single dose are effective treatments for symptomatic giardiasis.

Dientamoeba fragilis

Transmission	This parasite is thought to be transmitted with the eggs of *Enterobius vermicularis* (pinworm).
Clinical features	Symptoms include acute or chronic diarrhoea and abdominal pain, although many infected children are asymptomatic. May be associated with eosinophilia.
Treatment	May be treated with metronidazole (dose as above) although treatment is unnecessary in asymptomatic patients where the organism is found incidentally.

Escherichia coli

There are at least five categories of diarrhoea-producing *E. coli*:

- *Enterohaemorrhagic E. coli* (EHEC): haemolytic uraemic syndrome (HUS) haemorrhagic colitis.
- *Enteropathogenic E. coli* (EPEC): watery diarrhoea in children <2 years of age in developing countries.
- *Enterotoxigenic E. coli* (ETEC): the major cause of traveller's diarrhoea (usually self-limiting).
- *Enteroinvasive E. coli* (EIEC): usually watery diarrhoea, but may cause dysentery.
- *Enteroaggregative E. coli* (EAEC): chronic diarrhoea in infants and young children.

Antibiotic treatment is not usually indicated for diarrhoea caused by *E. coli* and it is associated with a worse outcome in HUS.

Clostridium difficile

Transmission	Acquired from the environment or by faecal-oral transmission from a colonised host. Up to 50% of healthy neonates and infants <2 years of age are colonised, in contrast to 5% of those >2 years of age.

Clinical features	Rare cause of diarrhoea in those <12 months of age. Only clinically significant diarrhoea or colitis should be considered to be caused by *Clostridium difficile*. Pseudomembranous colitis usually occurs in patients on antibiotics (particularly penicillins, clindamycin and cephalosporins).
Treatment	Management includes the cessation of antibiotics and the use of **oral** metronidazole 7.5 mg/kg (max 400 mg) p.o. 8-hourly; (vancomycin should be avoided to decrease the emergence of resistance). Probiotics (*Saccharomyces* spp. – baker's or brewer's yeast – or *Lactobacillus* spp.) have been shown to be effective when added to antibiotics for treatment and may also be used for prevention in susceptible patients.

Enterobius vermicularis (threadworm, pinworm)

The most common worm infection in Australia. School-age children, followed by preschoolers, have the highest rates of infection. In some groups, nearly 50% of children are infected.

Transmission	Eggs survive up to 2 weeks on clothing, bedding or other objects. Eggs often remain under the fingernails. Reinfection by autoinfection is common. Infection often occurs in more than one family member.
Incubation period	At least 1–2 months from the ingestion of eggs until the adult female migrates to the perianal region to deposit eggs.
Infectious period	Eggs are infective within a few hours of being deposited on the perianal skin.
Clinical features	Causes pruritus ani and vulvae.
Diagnosis	Visualisation of worms in the perianal region (at night) or microscopy of eggs collected on sticky tape briefly applied to perianal skin in the morning.

Treatment	Mebendazole 50 mg (<10 kg), 100 mg (>10 kg) p.o. (not in pregnancy or in those <6 months of age) or pyrantel 10 mg/kg (max 750 mg) p.o. as a single dose, followed by a second dose 2 weeks later. All family members should be treated.

HEPATITIS

Hepatitis A

Hepatitis A (HAV) is the most common viral hepatitis; it is particularly prevalent in children.

Transmission	Faecal-oral route.
Incubation period	Usually about 4 weeks (2–7 weeks).
Infectious period	Viral shedding lasts 1–3 weeks; the highest titres in stool occur 1–2 weeks before the onset of illness, corresponding to the highest risk of transmission; lowest risk after onset of jaundice.
Clinical features	Usually an acute self-limited illness; mild, non-specific symptoms without jaundice in infants and preschoolers; fever, malaise, jaundice, anorexia and nausea in older children and adults.
Complications	Relapse (unusual), fulminant hepatitis (rare).
Diagnosis	Serology for HAV-specific IgM and IgG.
Treatment	Supportive.
Control of case	Cases should be excluded from child-care or school for 7 days from the onset of illness.
Prevention	Inactivated HAV vaccine (or immunoglobulin for short-term protection) should be considered for travellers to endemic areas and those with high occupational risk and chronic liver disease (e.g. hepatitis B infection) or transfusion dependent illness.

Hepatitis B

Hepatitis B (HBV) infection is endemic worldwide. The prevalence of HBV and carriage rates vary in different parts of the world. In Australia, the carriage rate in Caucasians is about 0.2%, and over 10% in some Aboriginal populations.

Transmission	Blood or body fluids that are HBsAg positive; vertical transmission occurs in infants born to HBsAg-positive mothers; there is a high risk of horizontal transmission in the first 5 years of life.
Incubation period	7 weeks–6 months.
Infectious period	From several weeks before the onset until the end of the period of acute illness.
Clinical features	Symptomatic acute hepatitis (jaundice, anorexia, malaise and nausea) in adults; usually asymptomatic in young children, particularly in those <1 year of age.
Complications	Twenty-five per cent of chronic carriers die later in life of primary liver cancer or chronic liver disease. Those infected as infants or young children are more likely to become carriers and to develop fatal complications as adults: 70–90% of infants infected at birth become chronic HBV carriers (particularly if the mother is HBeAg positive), in contrast to only 5% of adults. The remainder eliminate the virus and have no long-term effects.
Diagnosis	Serology for detection of HBsAg, HBeAg (also anti-HBsAb, anti-HBcAb, anti-HBeAb).
Treatment	No specific therapy for HBV is available; alpha-interferon and nucleoside analogues may resolve chronic infection but are less effective if infection is acquired during childhood. Hepatitis A vaccination is recommended.
Prevention	In Australia, recombinant HBV vaccine is currently recommended for all infants from birth, pre-adolescents, as well as those at high risk. Infants born to HBsAg-positive mothers and individuals exposed to HBsAg-positive blood or body fluids should be given HBV-specific immunoglobulin plus HBV vaccination. See needle stick injuries (p. 467).

Hepatitis C

Hepatitis C (HCV) causes at least 95% of cases of acute and chronic hepatitis that were previously classified as non-A, non-B. The carriage rate is about 0.3% in apparently healthy new blood donors in Australia, however, this probably underestimates the prevalence in the population, which may be around 1%.

Transmission	Parenteral exposure to HCV-infected blood and blood products; vertical transmission occurs from about 6% of HCV-positive mothers (higher if the mother is co-infected with HIV); breast-feeding is not believed to be a major route of transmission; sexual transmission is uncommon.
Incubation period	6–7 weeks (range 2 weeks–6 months).
Clinical features	Mild, insidious hepatitis; usually asymptomatic in children.
Complications	Persistent infection in >85% (most children with chronic infection are asymptomatic); 65–70% develop chronic hepatitis, 20% develop cirrhosis. Hepatitis C appears to have a role in primary liver cancer.
Diagnosis	Detection of anti-HCV antibodies using ELISA and/or recombinant immunoblot assay, PCR for HCV RNA.
Treatment	Patients must be monitored regularly (examination and liver function tests) for carriage and development of chronic liver disease. Optimal treatment regimens using alpha-interferon, ribavirin and other antivirals are under investigation. Hepatitis A and B vaccination is recommended.

BACTERIAL MENINGITIS

Bacterial meningitis is a medical emergency.

Clinical features

- Non-specific in infants e.g. fever, lethargy, irritability or vomiting.
- In older children, headache, vomiting, drowsiness, photophobia and neck stiffness may be present. Kernig sign (inability to extend the knee when the leg is flexed at the hip) and Brudzinski sign (bending the head forward produces flexion movements of the legs) may be positive.

Diagnosis

Diagnosis is confirmed by examination of the cerebrospinal fluid (CSF), unless lumbar puncture is contraindicated (see Procedures, chapter 4). If lumbar puncture is deferred or reveals no organism, identification of the pathogen will rely on other methods. These include:

- Blood cultures, which are positive in a high proportion of cases.
- PCR on blood or CSF for enterovirus, HSV and other viruses, TB and *N. meningitidis*.
- Blood smear for Gram stain.
- Skin scraping or aspirate from purpuric lesions, which may reveal meningococci on Gram stain or (less likely) culture.
- Throat swab.

Antibiotics must be given immediately after the collection of appropriate cultures, but they should not be delayed if the lumbar puncture is to be deferred. Antibiotics should be rationalised to more specific treatment based on CSF or blood culture results (but not on the basis of a Gram stain or PCR result alone).

Interpretation of cerebrospinal fluid findings

CSF findings should always be interpreted in the light of the clinical setting (see Table 27.2 and Box 27.2).

Box 27.2

Cell count

- **Perform microscopy without delay**. Cell lysis begins shortly after collection: neutrophils may decrease by up to 1/3 after 1 h and by 1/2 after 3 h (lymphocytes may decrease by about 10% after 2 h).
- Macroscopic appearance of CSF may be misleading: 200–500 × 10^6/L cells are necessary for the CSF to be cloudy to the naked eye.
- In early bacterial meningitis there may be no increase in the CSF cell count.

Continue overleaf

Box 27.2 *Cont'd*

- If the CSF is contaminated with blood (14% of neonatal taps), a ratio of one white blood cell to 500–700 red blood cells is allowable and 0.01 g/L protein for every 1,000 red blood cells. However, it is safer to be more cautious and interpret the CSF as if it has *not* been contaminated with blood.
- The CSF cell count may remain normal in up to 4% of younger infants and up to 17% of neonates with bacterial meningitis.
- The presence of neutrophils in the CSF should always raise concern (except in neonates, see Table 27.2).
- In early viral (typically enteroviral) meningitis, the CSF findings can mimic bacterial meningitis with a neutrophil predominance. This shifts to a lymphocytic picture after 6–8 h.
- In bacterial meningitis there can be a shift to a lymphocyte predominance after 48 h of therapy.
- Listeria infection is associated with a lower neutrophil rise than other causes of bacterial meningitis.
- Gram stain may be negative in up to 60% of cases of bacterial meningitis even without prior antibiotics.
- Antibiotics usually prevent the culture of bacteria from the CSF, but they do not significantly alter the CSF cell count or biochemistry in samples taken early. In 'partially treated meningitis' the CSF should be interpreted like any other CSF.
- Seizures do *not* cause an increased CSF cell count.
- Interpretation of CSF may be difficult in neonates. Normal values for CSF cell counts and biochemistry differ from those of older infants (typically higher cell count and protein and lower glucose, particularly in premature neonates) (see Table 27.2).

Biochemistry

- CSF protein is normal in about 40% of school-age children with bacterial meningitis.
- CSF glucose is normal in about 1/2 of school-age children with bacterial meningitis.
- CSF glucose may be decreased in mumps meningitis and lymphocytic choriomeningitis, as well as in bacterial and TB meningitis.

Table 27.2 Classical cerebrospinal fluid (CSF) findings

	Neutrophils ($\times 10^6$ */L)*	*Lymphocytes* ($\times 10^6$ */L)*	*Protein (g/L)*	*Glucose (CSF : blood ratio)*
Normal (>1 month of age)	0	≤5	<0.4	≥0.6 (or ≥2.5 mmol/L)
Normal term neonate	Higher than for older infant/child	<20–30	Higher than for older infant/child usually <1	Lower than for older infant/child
Bacterial meningitis	100–10 000 (but counts may be normal)	Usually <100	>1.0 (but protein may be normal)	<0.4 (but glucose may be normal)
Viral meningitis	Usually <100	10–1000 (but counts may be normal)	0.4–1 (but protein may be normal)	Usually normal
TB meningitis	Usually <100	50–1000 (but counts may be normal)	1–5 (but protein may be normal)	<0.3 (but glucose may be normal)
Encephalitis	Usually <100		0.4–1 (but protein may be normal)	Usually normal
Brain abscess	Usually 5–100		>1 (but protein may be normal)	Usually normal

Antibiotic treatment of meningitis

Age >2 months

The incidence of bacterial meningitis has fallen dramatically since the introduction of conjugated *Haemophilus influenzae* type b (Hib) vaccine. The major pathogens are now *Streptococcus pneumoniae* and *Neisseria meningitidis.*

Penicillin (and cephalosporin) resistant pneumococci (PRP) are an increasing problem worldwide. Local patterns of resistance dictate treatment.

In areas with a significantly high incidence of PRP, or when PRP are suspected, vancomycin 15 mg/kg (max 500 mg) i.v. 6-hourly should be added to a 3rd generation cephalosporin as empiric therapy. If there is prolonged or secondary fever, or where sensitivity testing indicates the pneumococcal isolate has reduced susceptibility to 3rd generation cephalosporins, a repeat lumbar puncture should be performed to detect treatment failure.

Initial therapy

Cefotaxime 50 mg/kg (max 2 g) i.v. 6-hourly.

Continued therapy

Antibiotic treatment is adjusted according to the culture and sensitivity results to complete (intravenous therapy):

- 7 days for *Neisseria meningitidis.*
- 10 days for *Streptococcus pneumoniae.*
- 7–10 days *Haemophilus influenzae* type b.

Benzyl penicillin 60 mg/kg (max 2 g) i.v. 4-hourly, or amoxicillin 50 mg/kg (max 2 g) i.v. 4-hourly, or continue with cefotaxime.

Age <2 months

The organisms responsible for meningitis in this age group can be either neonatal pathogens (e.g. group B streptococcus, *Escherichia coli* and *Listeria monocytogenes*), or those more commonly detected in older children (e.g. *Streptococcus pneumoniae, Neisseria meningitidis,* Hib).

Initial therapy

Benzyl penicillin, cefotaxime and gentamicin (see Antimicrobial guidelines).

Continued therapy

Treatment is adjusted according to the culture and sensitivity results. Gentamicin is used for its synergistic action with penicillin for the treatment of group B streptococcal and *Listeria meningitis*. Therapy is continued for 2–3 weeks for these two infections and for at least 3 weeks in Gram-negative coliform meningitis.

Meningitis associated with shunts, neurosurgery, head trauma and CSF leak

In addition to the organisms discussed above, meningitis in these circumstances can be caused by *Staphylococcus aureus*, *Staphylococcus epidermidis* and Gram-negative bacilli including *Pseudomonas aeruginosa*.

Initial therapy

Vancomycin 15 mg/kg (max 500 mg) i.v. 6-hourly and ceftazidime 50 mg/kg (max 2 g) i.v. 8-hourly.

Antibiotic prophylaxis for contacts of meningitis cases

See Table 27.3.

General measures

Requirement for intensive care

Admission to ICU should be discussed with a specialist in the following circumstances:

- Age <2 years.
- Coma.
- Cardiovascular compromise.
- Intractable seizures.
- Hyponatraemia.

Fluid management

Careful fluid management is important in the treatment of meningitis as many children have increased anti-diuretic hormone (ADH) secretion. The degree to which fluid should be restricted varies considerably from patient to patient depending primarily on their clinical state. Hypovolaemia should be corrected with 10 mL/kg of normal saline. A patient who is not in shock and whose serum sodium is in the normal range should be given 50% maintenance fluid requirements as initial management. If the serum sodium is <135 mmol/L give 25–50% of maintenance requirements. The serum sodium should be repeated every 6–12 h for the first 48 h and the total fluid intake adjusted accordingly.

Table 27.3 Prophylaxis regimens for contact of meningitis cases

Organism	*Antibiotic*	*Those requiring prophylaxis*
Haemophilus influenzae type b	Rifampicin 20 mg/kg (max 600 mg) p.o. daily for 4 days *Infants <1 month of age*: Rifampicin 10 mg/kg p.o. daily for 4 days *Pregnancy/contraindication to rifampicin*: Ceftriaxone 250 mg i.m. daily for 2 days	• Index case and all household contacts if household includes other children <4 years of age who are not fully immunised. • Index case and all household contacts in households with any infants <12 months of age, regardless of immunisation status. • Index case and all household contacts in households with a child 1–5 years of age who is inadequately immunised. • Index case and all room contacts, including staff, in a child care group if index case attends >18 h/week and any contacts <2 years of age who are inadequately immunised. • Children who are not up to date with Hib should be immunised.
Neisseria meningitidis	Rifampicin 10 mg/kg (max 600 mg) p.o. 12-hourly for 2 days *Infants <1 month of age*: Rifampicin 5 mg/kg p.o. 12-hourly for 2 days *Pregnancy/contraindication to rifampicin*: Ceftriaxone 250 mg (>12 y) or 125 mg (<12 y) i.m. as a single dose *or* Ciprofloxacin 500 mg (>12 y) or 250 mg (6–11 y) p.o. as a single dose	• Index case (if treated only with penicillin) and all intimate household or day care contacts who have been exposed to index case within 10 days of onset. • Any person who gave mouth-to-mouth resuscitation to the index case.
Streptococcus pneumoniae	Nil	• No increased risk to contacts

Notes:

- It is important that Rifampicin is given early to both the index case and contacts, especially for *N. meningitidis* disease, because of the rapidity with which secondary cases may develop.
- As prophylaxis is not infallible, any febrile household contact should seek urgent medical attention.
- Nasopharyngeal carriage of Hib is not eradicated by a single injection of ceftriaxone.
- Rifampicin interferes with the metabolism of several medications, including the oral contraceptive pill (alternative contraception should be instituted), anticonvulsants, warfarin and chloramphenicol.

Observations

Neurological observations including blood pressure should be performed every 15 min for the first 2 h and then at intervals determined by the child's conscious state. Weight and head circumference should be monitored daily.

Seizures

Control of seizures is vital and specialist consultation is advised.

Analgesia

Ensure adequate analgesia; children in the recovery phase may have significant headache.

Fever persisting for longer than 7 days

May be due to nosocomial infection, subdural effusion or other foci of suppuration. Uncommon causes include inadequately treated meningitis, a parameningeal focus or drugs.

Steroids

Although widely practised, routine administration of dexamethasone is controversial and is not routinely recommended. Studies using dexamethasone have drawn criticism and benefits have mainly been proven in Hib meningitis. Since the introduction of immunisation, Hib meningitis has become very uncommon. More recently there has been some evidence of steroids having a beneficial role in the treatment of adults with meningitis.

Outcome/follow up

All patients require a hearing assessment 6–8 weeks after discharge, or sooner if hearing loss is suspected.

More than one in four survivors have mild disabilities that adversely affect school performance and behaviour. Consequently, all children surviving bacterial meningitis should be regularly reviewed during their early school years.

Prevention

Many cases of meningitis are now preventable. All parents should be encouraged to have their children immunised with the new conjugate pneumococcal and meningococcal vaccines (see Immunisation, chapter 8).

OTHER CENTRAL NERVOUS SYSTEM INFECTIONS

Viral meningitis

The most common causes of viral meningitis or meningoencephalitis are enteroviruses (Coxsackie and echoviruses) and HHV-6 (see p. 441). Most cases are self-limiting and their importance lies in the fact that their clinical presentation can mimic bacterial meningitis. An enterovirus may be isolated from throat swabs and stools and PCR of the CSF may be positive. Treatment is symptomatic except in the rare instance of infection in the immunocompromised where IVIG may be used. A new antiviral drug with activity against enteroviruses, Pleconaril, may be useful in selected severe cases.

Tuberculous meningitis

Tuberculous meningitis is uncommon in Australia. It often presents in an insidious manner and can be difficult to recognise. Large volumes of CSF are required (at least 10 mL) for diagnosis by isolation and culture of mycobacteria and/or PCR. Treatment with multiple antitubercular antibiotics should be started early and requires specialist advice. Steroids may also play an important role in treatment.

Encephalitis

Encephalitis is most commonly caused by HSV-1 or 2, EBV, VZV, enterovirus, adenovirus, influenza virus or *Mycoplasma pneumoniae*. Encephalitis usually presents with one or more of the following: fever, headache, vomiting, change of behaviour, drowsiness, convulsions (particularly focal), focal neurological deficits and signs of raised intracranial pressure. Cerebrospinal fluid findings are non-specific (see Table 27.2). Computed tomography or MRI of the brain and EEG may be more helpful.

The recognition of herpes encephalitis is critical because treatment with acyclovir is indicated. Focal seizures and neurological signs are more typical of herpes encephalitis but clinical presentation, especially early in the disease, is not specific to any aetiological agent. Therefore, any child with encephalitis of an uncertain cause should be started on i.v. aciclovir (see Antimicrobial guidelines). If the patient does not regain consciousness over a short period of time, i.v. aciclovir should be continued until:

- An alternative diagnosis is reached; or
- Herpes encephalitis is excluded by:
  - Absence of typical clinical features.
  - Normal serial CT or MRI scans.
  - Normal serial EEG.
  - Negative CSF PCR for HSV.

Macrolides (e.g. azithromycin) are sometimes used in encephalitis due to *M. pneumoniae* but their benefit is uncertain.

Brain abscess

Brain abscess classically presents with fever, headache and focal neurological deficit. Although rare, early recognition is important because most cases are readily treated and delayed diagnosis can be disastrous. Diagnosis is by brain CT or MRI. Empiric treatment to cover the major aetiological pathogens is flucloxacillin 50 mg/kg (max 2 g) i.v. 4-hourly, cefotaxime 50 mg/kg (max 2 g) i.v. 6-hourly **and** metronidazole 15 mg/kg (max 1 g) i.v. stat., then 7.5 mg/kg (max 500 mg) i.v. 8-hourly (see Antimicrobial guidelines). Aspiration for diagnosis and neurosurgical intervention are sometimes necessary.

KAWASAKI DISEASE

Kawasaki disease (KD) is a systemic vasculitis that predominantly affects children under 5 years of age. Although the specific causal agent remains unknown, it is believed that KD is caused by an infectious agent, although it is not transmitted from person to person.

Diagnosis

Diagnosis is often delayed because the features are similar to those of many viral exanthems. The diagnostic criteria for KD are:

- Fever for 5 days or more; plus
- Four of the following five features:
  - Polymorphous rash.
  - Bilateral (non-purulent) conjunctivitis.
  - Mucous membrane changes; e.g. reddened or dry cracked lips, strawberry tongue, or a diffuse redness of oral or pharyngeal mucosa.

  - Peripheral changes; e.g. erythema of the palms or soles, oedema of the hands or feet and desquamation *in convalescence*, particularly involving skin of hands, feet or perineal region.
  - Cervical lymphadenopathy (larger than 15 mm in diameter, usually unilateral, single, non-purulent and painful).
- Exclusion of diseases with a similar presentation: staphylococcal infection (e.g. scalded skin syndrome and toxic shock syndrome), streptococcal infection (e.g. scarlet fever and toxic shock-like syndrome, but not just isolation from throat), measles, adenovirus and other viral exanthems, leptospirosis, rickettsial disease, Steven's Johnson syndrome, drug reaction and juvenile chronic arthritis.

The diagnostic features of KD can occur sequentially and may not all be present at the same time. Moreover, it is recognised that some patients with KD do not develop sufficient features to fulfil the formal diagnostic criteria. Clinical vigilance and recognition of this possibility are necessary to recognise these 'incomplete' or 'atypical' cases. Other relatively common features include arthritis, diarrhoea and vomiting, coryza and cough, and hydropic gall bladder.

Investigations

Laboratory features may include neutrophilia, raised erythro-cyte sedimentation rate (ESR) and C-reactive protein (CRP), mild normochromic, normocytic anaemia, raised transaminases, hypoalbuminaemia and marked thrombocytosis in the second week.

Complications

Up to 30% of untreated children develop coronary artery involvement, with dilation or aneurysm formation. This can occur up to 6–8 weeks after the onset of the illness. Echocardiography should therefore be performed at least twice: at presentation and, if negative, again at 6–8 weeks.

Management

Management includes early (preferably within the first 10 days of the illness) administration of intravenous immunoglobulin (IVIG) (single dose of 2 g/kg i.v. over 10 h) and aspirin (3–5 mg/kg p.o. once a day (antiplatelet dose) for at least 6–8 weeks). There is no evidence that using high (anti-inflammatory) dose aspirin decreases the risk of aneurysm development over and above that prevented by IVIG. However, some guidelines suggest using high dose aspirin (10 mg/kg p.o. 8-hourly) until defervescence. Paracetamol can be used for symptomatic relief.

Treatment with IVIG is highly effective in preventing the potentially devastating complication of coronary artery involvement. Treatment should still be undertaken in patients presenting after 10 days of illness if they have evidence of ongoing inflammation (fever, raised acute phase markers).

CERVICAL LYMPHADENITIS

This is usually caused by an infection or inflammation of the lymph nodes. Malignancy is much less common.

Infectious causes

Acute bilateral lymphadenitis

- Viral upper respiratory tract infections.
- Systemic viral infections (e.g. EBV and CMV: may have generalised lymphadenopathy and hepatosplenomegaly).
- Kawasaki disease: may present initially as cervical lymphadenitis alone (see above).

Acute unilateral lymphadenitis.

- Group A streptococcus or *Staphylococcus aureus*: 40–80% of acute unilateral lymphadenitis; occurs at 1–4 years of age; fever, tenderness, overlying erythema; may be associated with cellulitis.
- Anaerobic bacteria: older children with dental caries or periodontal disease.
- Group B streptococcus (neonates).

Subacute/chronic unilateral lymphadenitis

- *Bartonella henselae* (cat-scratch disease): occurs about 2 weeks after a scratch or lick from a kitten or dog, usually involves axillary nodes, tender nodes; there may be a papule at infection site.
- *Mycobacterium avium* complex (MAC – formerly known as MAIS): patient usually 1–4 years of age, afebrile, systemically well and not immunocompromised; node usually unilateral, slightly fluctuant, non-tender, sometimes tethered to underlying structures and with violaceous hue to overlying skin.
- *Toxoplasma gondii*: systemic features (fatigue, myalgia) there may be generalised lymphadenopathy.

- *Mycobacterium tuberculosis*: usually a contact history; affects older children; systemic symptoms (e.g. fever, malaise, weight loss), non-tender nodes.
- *Human immunodeficiency virus.*

Management

Acute bilateral lymphadenitis of viral cause usually needs no specific treatment. Acute unilateral lymphadenitis with a fluctuant node needs incision and drainage (contraindicated in suspected TB as may result in sinus formation). Otherwise acute unilateral lymphadenitis is treated with oral Flucloxacillin 25 mg/kg (max 500 mg) p.o. 6-hourly for 10 days (see Antimicrobial guidelines), with review in 48 h.

CELLULITIS

Clinical features

- An infection of cutaneous and subcutaneous tissue characterised by erythema, warmth, oedema and tenderness.
- Predisposing factors include a break in the skin (e.g. insect bite, trauma) or a pre-existing skin lesion.
- May be associated with regional lymphadenopathy, fever, chills and malaise.
- Usually caused by *Streptococcus pyogenes* or *Staphylococcus aureus.*
- *Haemophilus influenzae* type b is uncommon but should be considered in non-immunised children <5 years. It is often accompanied by bacteraemia or meningitis, or both.
- It may be associated with deeper involvement including necrotising fasciitis, osteomyelitis and septic arthritis.

Diagnosis

- Cultures of blood, skin aspirate or skin biopsy are positive in about 25% of cases.

Management

- Flucloxacillin 25 mg/kg (max 500 mg) p.o. 6-hourly.
- Parenteral therapy is needed if there is fever, rapid progression, lymphangitis or lymphadenitis. Non-immunised children <5 years with facial cellulitis should be treated with cefotaxime 50 mg/kg (max 2 g) i.v. 6-hourly **and** flucloxacillin.

TOXIN MEDIATED DISEASE

Gram-positive bacteria (group A beta haemolytic streptococci and *Staphylococcus aureus*) can cause disease as a result of production of protein (superantigen) toxins.

Clinical features:

Fever, erythematous rash, conjunctivitis, reddened mucus membranes, strawberry tongue and prolonged capillary refill time. A range of clinical presentations may be seen. At the most severe end of the spectrum, capillary leak leads to hypotension, shock and multi-organ failure (toxic shock syndrome).

Diagnosis

Early diagnosis depends on recognition of clinical features. Culture results may help to confirm the diagnosis later.

Management

A critical part of early management is to remove any focus of infection (including retained tampon). Early recognition of shock with appropriate fluid management and intensive care is important. Antibiotics should include an anti-staphylococcal agent (e.g. flucloxacillin 50 mg/kg (max 2 g) i.v. 4 h, see Antimicrobial guidelines). There also some evidence for the addition of clindamycin (to inhibit bacterial toxin and host cytokine production) and the use of intravenous immunoglobulin.

HIV INFECTION AND AIDS

Cause

Acquired immunodeficiency syndrome (AIDS) is caused by human immunodeficiency virus (HIV).

Transmission

Perinatal (vertical) transmission is the most common means of paediatric HIV infection.

Incubation period

It is important to distinguish between infection with HIV, which may be asymptomatic during a variable latent period, and the progressive immunological derangement that leads to AIDS. Perinatally infected infants may be asymptomatic for several months or years.

Risk groups

- Infants of mothers who are known to be HIV positive or who are members of a high-risk group (e.g. sex workers, intravenous drug users and those with bisexual partners).
- Intravenous drug users.
- Homosexual or bisexual males.
- Sexual contacts (including sexually abused children) of individuals with HIV.
- Transfusion recipients, particularly patients with congenital bleeding disorders who received blood products before 1985.
- Individuals from countries with a high prevalence of HIV infection.

Clinical features

Clinical presentations of HIV infection include: prolonged fever, failure to thrive or weight loss, generalised lymphadenopathy, hepatosplenomegaly, parotitis, chronic or recurrent diarrhoea, recurrent otitis, chronic candidiasis and chronic eczematous rash.

The indicator diseases for the diagnosis of AIDS in children include: candidiasis, lymphoid interstitial pneumonitis, recurrent episodes of serious bacterial infection, opportunistic infection (e.g. *Pneumocystis carinii* pneumonia and disseminated *Mycobacterium avium* complex disease), CMV retinitis, cerebral toxoplasmosis, progressive neurological disease and malignancy (e.g. primary brain lymphoma).

Diagnosis

Patients require counselling and informed consent before testing for HIV, which should be performed on a confidential basis. Specific antibody detection is a sensitive indicator of HIV infection in adults and children, but passively transferred maternal antibodies may persist for up to 18 months in infants. The presence of free viral protein (p24 antigen), a positive viral culture or PCR assay of non-cord blood, help confirm the diagnosis of HIV infection. The disease is monitored using a combination of CD4+ T-cell count and quantification of HIV RNA (viral load).

Patients may also have lymphopaenia, abnormal T-cell subsets and hypergammaglobulinaemia.

Management

A multidisciplinary approach by a specialised team is vital for the unique needs of these patients and their families. Medical management of HIV-positive patients includes:

- Antiretroviral drugs (highly active antiretroviral treatment, HAART).
- Prevention of opportunistic and other infections (immunisation and prophylactic antimicrobials).
- The early diagnosis and aggressive management of opportunistic infections.

Control

Antiretroviral therapy given to the HIV-infected woman during pregnancy and delivery, and to the newborn, together with other measures, can decrease the rate of transmission to the child from 25–35% to <2%. Recognition of HIV-infected pregnant women is therefore critical.

Antiretroviral therapy and other interventions (e.g. immunisation, *Pneumocystis* prophylaxis) can have a significant impact on disease progression. Human immunodeficiency virus can be transmitted in breast milk – wherever artificial feeding can be undertaken safely it is advised that HIV-infected women should not breast-feed.

NEEDLE STICK INJURIES

Community acquired needle stick injuries

The risk of seroconversion to human immunodeficiency virus (HIV), hepatitis B virus (HBV) or hepatitis C virus (HCV) from a community acquired needle stick injury (NSI) is low. Exposed individuals should be reassured. Hepatitis B virus status should be assessed, and HBV-specific immunoglobulin and vaccine given if indicated. Follow-up should be arranged for counselling.

Occupational needle stick injuries

Standard precautions

- All sharp objects and body fluids should be considered as potentially contaminated.

- Avoid contact with blood and other body fluids by:
  - Using protective barriers (e.g. gloves) if contact is likely.
  - Immediately cleaning up accidental spills.

Managing needle stick injury or exposure to blood/blood-stained body fluid

- Squeeze the puncture wound.
- Wash blood off the skin with soap and water.
- Rinse blood from the eyes and mouth with running water.
- Document the date and time of exposure, details of incident, names of the source and exposed individuals.
- Inform source individual of exposure.
- Assess the risk of HIV, HBV and HCV in the source individual (see below).
- If indicated, test known sources for HBV surface antigen (HBsAg), HCV antibody (anti-HCV Ab) and antibodies to HIV 1 and 2 (HIV Abs). Obtain consent from the source individual.
- If the source individual is not infected with a blood borne pathogen, baseline testing of the exposed person is not necessary.
- Follow-up should be arranged for counselling (of the exposed person).
- Give HBV-specific immunoglobulin +/– HBV vaccine if appropriate (see Table 27.4).
- Human immunodeficiency virus post-exposure prophylaxis is only required if source is HIV Ab positive, or if the source is unknown, but exposure to HIV is considered likely.

Table 27.4 Evaluation of needle stick injury sources

High risk of HIV and HBV	*High risk of HCV*
• Unsafe sex, particularly with multiple (or homosexual) partners • Intravenous drug users (IVDU) (particularly if they share equipment) and their sexual partners • Family members of an infected person • Individuals from communities with high HIV prevalence	• Recipients of blood products prior to 1985 • IVDU past or current (particularly if they share equipment)

Table 27.5 Management of needle stick injury

Exposure	*Virus*	*Bloods to take from the affected individual*	*Bloods to take from the source individual*	*What to give the affected individual*
High-risk	Hepatitis B	Anti-HBsAb (urgent)	HBsAg (urgent)	*HBV immune*: Nil *HBV non-immune*: • Source HBsAg positive/unknown ⇒ HBV immunoglobulin (*within 48 h*)* + HBV vaccine • Source HBsAg negative ⇒ HBV vaccine
	Hepatitis C	ALT + hold serum	Anti-HCV Ab (urgent)	Nil
	HIV	Hold serum	HIV Ab (urgent)	HIV prophylaxis† if HIV positive and/or risk of transmission is significant
Low-risk	*All viruses*	Anti-HBsAb (if unsure of mmunity) Hold serum	HBsAg	*HBV immune*: Nil *HBV non-immune*: HBV vaccine

* HBV immunoglobulin should be given as soon as possible, but can be deferred for 48 h, while awaiting results of serology to confirm affected individual's immunity (when checking whether a vaccinated individual has maintained immunity or whether the individual is immune from previous infection).

† Current HIV prophylaxis is zidovudine, lamivudine and indinavir (this may change with ongoing developments in antiviral drugs). The treatment should be started promptly, preferably within 1–2 h of the exposure.

Assessing risk

A significant exposure is considered to have occurred if there has been:

- An injection of blood/body fluid (particularly if >1 mL).
- A skin penetrating injury with a sharp that is contaminated with blood/body fluid.
- A laceration from a contaminated instrument.
- A direct inoculation in the laboratory with contaminated material.
- A contaminated wound or skin lesion.
- Mucous membrane/conjunctival contact with blood/body fluid.

The incidence of HBV, HCV and HIV in Victorian intravenous drug users is 1.8, 10.7 and 0.2 per 100 person years, respectively.

The estimated risk of virus transmission from an occupational NSI from a *known positive donor* (e.g. in Victoria) is:

- HBV: 6–30%
- HCV: 0–7%
- HIV: ~0.4%.

Note: These figures are for NSI from a positive source. When the source is unknown, the actual risk of infection for the affected individual depends on the probability of infection in the source population.

CHAPTER 28
METABOLIC CONDITIONS

Avihu Boneh
Glynis Price
Stephen Kahler
George Werther

Metabolic diseases, although generally rare individually, in aggregate are an important cause of illness in Western society. Some newborns admitted with a clinical presentation of 'neonatal septicaemia' will eventually be found to have an inborn error of metabolism.

- A high index of suspicion is the primary rule in the diagnostic approach to metabolic disorders.
- The presenting symptoms of metabolic diseases are non-specific (see Table 28.1).
- A careful history regarding the pregnancy, delivery, neonatal period, dietary history (food refusal or craving) and motor and cognitive development should be recorded.
- A review of the systems, including a record of medications is required.
- The family history should be recorded, with particular note of consanguinity, relatives with seemingly unrelated disorders (e.g. 'retardation'), maternal morbidity during pregnancy (e.g. severe chronic vomiting, liver disease and intercurrent infections), miscarriages, unexplained deaths of newborns and Sudden Infant Death Syndrome (SIDS), as well as other children having similar clinical signs in the family.

PHYSICAL EXAMINATION

Some findings on physical examination may be suggestive of a metabolic disease. These are summarised in Table 28.2.

Table 28.1 Clinical signs suggestive of a metabolic disease

Age	*Clinical signs*	*Possible diagnosis*
Day 1 of life	Seizures	Persistent – hyperinsulinaemia Mitochondrial – cytopathy Disorders of purines and pyrimidines
Neonatal period(*)	Vomiting, feed refusal, changes in respiration, prolonged jaundice, lethargy or irritability, movement disorder, seizures, hypo/hypertonia, changes in the level of consciousness	Organic acidaemias, non-ketotic-hyperglycinaemia Urea cycle defects Fatty acid oxidation defects Tyrosinaemia Galactosaemia Mitochondrial – cytopathy Disorders of purines and pyrimidines
1st year of life	Same as above, motor/cognitive developmental delay or regression	Organic acidaemias Urea cycle defects Fatty acid oxidation defects Lysosomal storage diseases
Early childhood	Mental retardation, seizures, behavioural abnormalities, learning difficulties, autistic features	Organic acidaemias Urea cycle defects Fatty acid oxidation defects Amino-acidopathies Lysosomal storage diseases Adrenoleukodystrophy
Any age group(**)	Acute decompensation: change in consciousness, seizures, movement disorder, change in respiration	Organic acidaemias Urea cycle defects Fatty acid oxidation defects Adrenal insufficiency

* Symptoms should be considered in relation to the child's age (in days), fasting, food intake (i.e. specific sugars, protein and fat) and changes in diet.
** May follow an intercurrent infection, prolonged fasting, a large meal with high protein content, and so on.

Table 28.2 Physical examination: potential signs of metabolic disease

General appearance	Growth parameters: height and weight
	Dysmorphism
Skin	Rash
	Odour
	Hyperkeratosis
	Signs of chronic scratching
Head and neck	Craniomegaly
	Dysmorphism
	Bulging fontanelle
	Signs of rickets
	Abnormal eye movements
Chest	Signs of lung disease
Heart	Cardiomegaly
	Signs of cardiac failure
Abdomen	Hepato ± splenomegaly
	Signs of liver disease
Genitalia	Ambiguous genitalia
Skeleton	Signs of rickets
	Bone or joint pain, contractures
	Abnormal spine posturing/vertebral disease
Muscles	Muscle mass, wasting
Neurological	Muscle strength, tone
	Sensation
	Reflexes (tendon and primitive)
	Movement disorders
	Ataxia

LABORATORY INVESTIGATIONS

Blood, urine and CSF samples collected at the time of presentation may be diagnostic and are invaluable. Always attempt to collect these samples **before** commencing treatment, but do not delay treatment in crisis situations.

There are four initial questions to be answered:

1. Is there acidosis and is it of metabolic origin?
2. Is there hypoglycaemia?
3. Is there hyper- or hypoketonaemia?
4. Is there hyperammonaemia?

Table 28.3 Investigation of suspected metabolic disease

	First-line tests	*Second-line tests**
Blood	Acid–base (arterial or capillary) Electrolytes Glucose (in 'lactate tube'; see below) Ammonia Lactate (1 mL blood in yellow lactate tube, place on ice.) Acylcarnitines (blood spots on a Guthrie ('PKU') Card) Insulin, cortisol, growth hormone (3mL blood min)	Full blood count Plasma amino acids (place on ice) Pyruvate (place on ice) FA/Ketones (specify: beta-hydroxy butyrate *and* acetoacetate) (place on ice) Liver transaminases Urea, creatinine, phosphate, calcium Uric acid Cholesterol Freeze additional plasma for further testing
Urine	pH, glucose, ketones, protein Reducing substances (ward test) Organic acids (keep frozen if not analysed immediately)	Freeze additional urine for further testing
CSF	Glucose, protein, lactate	Freeze additional CSF for further testing (amino acids, neurotransmitters, etc.)

* Check with the laboratory for the preferred sample.
* Do not discard any blood urine or CSF fluid taken at the time of metabolic decompensation and hypoglcaemia. Send any excess to the laboratory marked 'excess store'.

The investigations listed in Table 28.3 should be performed.

In addition to these tests, brain CT or MRI and abdominal ultrasound examination may be helpful in the diagnostic process.

See Table 28.4 for interpretation of laboratory results.

Table 28.4 Interpretation of laboratory results

Metabolic condition	*pH*	*Glucose*	*Ketones*	*Ammonia*
Urea cycle defects	N or ↑	N	N	↑↑
Organic acidaemias	↓	↑, N or ↓	N or ↑	↑
Ketolysis defects, MSUD*	N or ↓	N or ↑	↑↑	N
FA oxidation defects	N or ↓	N or ↓	N or ↓	N or ↑
Hyperinsulinaemia	N	↓↓	N	N or ↑
Pituitary/adrenal deficiency	N	↓	↑	N

N = normal
* MSUD = Maple Syrup Urine Disease

GENERAL TREATMENT GUIDELINES

There are 3 basic guidelines in the treatment of metabolic conditions:

- *Enhance the disposal of the accumulating toxic metabolites.* Adequate fluid intake is important, particularly as many of the toxic metabolites are excreted by the kidney. Correct dehydration and replace ongoing losses (diarrhoea, fever, etc). Haemofiltration should be considered in severe cases or when there are indications of rapid accumulation of toxic metabolites (rapid deterioration in the level of consciousness, increasing intracranial pressure, etc.).
- *Avoid catabolism, which might lead to an ongoing accumulation of these metabolites.* It is of the utmost importance to provide the patient with an adequate amount of calories for age and weight. Intravenous glucose infusion (10–20% solution) is usually a safe mode of treatment. Intravenous fat solutions (10% or 20% solutions) may serve as a good source of calories in a small fluid volume. Do not use intravenous fat solutions if a fatty acid oxidation disorder is suspected. Intravenous amino acids can usually be given at a low dose (e.g. 0.5 g/kg per day for a newborn) to enhance anabolism, unless there is hyperammonaemia.
- *Enhance enzymatic activity whenever possible.* Treatment with some vitamins and co-factors may be indicated to enhance the disposal of toxic metabolites or to enhance residual enzymatic activity. These are listed in Table 28.5.

Table 28.5 Vitamin treatments

Compound	*Dose (mg/day)*	*Indication*
Carnitine	50–100 mg/kg per day (oral) or 15–60 mg/kg per day (i.v.)	Organic acidaemias Fatty acid oxidation disorders
Thiamine (B_1)	50–100 mg t.d.s. (i.v. or oral)	MSUD, PDH deficiency MRC disorders
Riboflavin (B_2)	50–100 mg t.d.s.	Glutaric acidurias MRC disorders
Pyridoxine (B_6)	100–300 mg/day (i.v. or oral)	Homocystinuria Seizures
Cobalamin (B_{12})	1 mg/day as hydroxycobalamin (i.m.)	Homocystinuria and MMA, combined or separately
Biotin	10–20 mg/day (i.v. or oral)	Hyper-lactataemia Biotinidase deficiency Holocarboxylase synthetase deficiency
Vitamin C	250–500 mg/day (oral)	MRC disorders Organic acidaemias
Vitamin K (menadione)	10 mg/kg per day (oral) or 1 mg/kg per day i.m.	MRC disorders
Coenzyme Q	50–100 mg t.d.s.	MRC disorders
Folic acid	5 mg/day	MRC disorders with anaemia Some amino-acidopathies
Glycine	200 mg/kg per day	May be given in some cases instead of carnitine

PDH, Pyruvate dehydrogenase.
MRC, Mitochondrial respiratory chain.
MMA, Methymallonic aciduria.
MSUD, Maple syrup urine disease.

HYPOGLYCAEMIA

Definition

A blood sugar level of <2.5 mmol/L. If suspected clinically and on a glucose reflectance meter, it must be confirmed with a true blood glucose measurement in the laboratory.

Causes

See Table 28.6.

Table 28.6 Causes of neonatal/childhood hypoglycaemia

Transient neonatal:	
↓ Substrate/enzyme function	Premature/SGA*
	RDS**
↑ Glucose utilisation	Sepsis hyperinsulinism
	(Beckwith-Wiedemann
	IDM***
	Rhesus disease)
Persistent neonatal	
Recurrent childhood:	
↑ *Glucose utilisation*	Hyperinsulinism
Ketone –ve	Salicylates
	Sepsis
↓ *Hepatic glucose production*	Glycogen storage disease
Ketone +ve	Gluconeogenic defect
+/–↑ Lactate	Galactosaemia
	Fructose intolerance
	Inborn errors of amino acid metabolism (MSUD)
	Severe liver disease (Reye Syndrome)
↓ *Production of alternative fuels*	Fatty acid oxidation defects (MCAD)
Ketone –ve	Ketogenesis defects
Hormonal deficiency	Cortisol (primary or secondary ACTH deficiency)
Ketone +ve	Growth Hormone
Drugs	Alcohol
Ketone +ve/–ve	Salicylates
	Propranolol
	Valproate
	Oral hypoglycaemics

* SGA, small for gestational age.
** RDS, respiratory distress syndrome.
*** IDM, infant of a diabetic mother.
MSUD, Maple syrup urine disease.
MCAD, Medium chain acyl coA dehydrogenase deficency.

The two most common causes of hypoglycaemia by age (beyond the neonatal period) are:

- **Hyperinsulinism** (in the first 2 years). This usually results in persistent, severe hypoglycaemia and may lead to permanent brain damage, as the brain exclusively depends on glucose in the first 2–3 years of life. Treatment is urgent.

- **Ketotic hypoglycaemia** or 'accelerated starvation' (after the first 2 years, but may also occur prior to 2 years). These children are often small for age and were small for gestational age. Poor oral intake or vomiting in the 24 h before the hypoglycaemic episode is common. An early morning seizure in a child should suggest the diagnosis. The cause is unclear and this entity may be one end of the normal spectrum or reaction to fasting. The natural history is for spontaneous remission by 8–10 years.

Signs and symptoms

Neonatal/infantile

- Apnoea, tachypnoea, cyanotic spell.
- Hypotonia, poor cry and feeding.
- Irritability, jitteriness and seizures.

Childhood

- *Catecholamine mediated*: hunger, pallor, sweating, tremor and tachycardia.
- *Neuroglycopaenic effects*: altered conscious state, abnormal behaviour and seizure.

Relevant history

- Gestational duration and birthweight.
- Previous episodes.
- Relationship to meals/feeds and duration of fasting.
- Age at onset of hypoglycaemia.
- Family history of neonatal deaths and affected relatives.
- Drugs – alcohol and insulin.
- Intercurrent illness.

Specific examination features

- Growth parameters (height, weight and head circumference). Overgrowth may suggest hyperinsulinism; underweight, ketotic hypoglycaemia.
- Midline defects (e.g. cleft lip, central incisor and micropenis) may suggest hypopituitarism.
- Muscle bulk, power and tone (glycogen storage disease).
- Hepatomegaly (glycogen storage disease and galactosaemia).
- Jaundice (galactosaemia).
- Cataracts (galactosaemia).

- Unusual odours (e.g. ketones, maple syrup) suggesting metabolic disease.
- Ambiguous genitalia (congenital adrenal hyperplasia with adrenal crisis).

Investigation

Before i.v. glucose is given (and usually before the true blood glucose is available), **obtain blood samples at the time of hypoglycaemia** and send the first urine specimen, as these are essential for diagnosis. Consider performing a catheter urine specimen if patient is stable.

Ketonuria generally excludes hyperinsulinism

See Table 28.3 for first-line investigations.

Specimens should be taken and returned on wet ice as soon as possible to the laboratory.

Do not discard any blood or urine taken at time of hypoglycaemia – send any excess to the laboratory marked 'excess – store'.

Management

- Neonate: 200–300 mg/kg dextrose i.v. (2–3 mL/kg of 10% dextrose) over 5 min, then 5–10 mg/kg per min. *Note*: **10% dextrose solution at 0.1 mL/kg per min will supply 10 mg/kg per min**.
- Older children: 200 mg/kg dextrose i.v. (1 mL/kg of 20% dextrose) over 5 min, then 3–5 mg/kg per min until stable.
- Record the rate of glucose infusion required to maintain euglycaemia (in mg/kg/min).

Note: **Hyperinsulinism is associated with rates over 10 mg/kg/min**

URGENT AUTOPSY FOR SUSPECTED METABOLIC DISEASE

On occasions, a child will die without a formal diagnosis. To diagnose a metabolic disorder post mortem, urgent samples need to be collected prior to the formal autopsy. Fully informed parental consent must be obtained prior to the collection of any samples (see also The death of a child, chapter 15).

- Collect samples as soon as possible after death, preferably within 2 h.

- Note the time between death and the attainment and freezing of all samples.
- Obtain blood, urine, CSF and bile samples, if possible (see Table 28.3), for further metabolic analysis. A vitreous humor specimen should be obtained if urine is unavailable.
- Obtain a skin biopsy for fibroblast culture. One piece full-thickness (2–3 mm surface diameter) in a tissue culture medium bottle, or a viral medium bottle or sterile normal saline without preservatives. Store in a refrigerator at 4°C. **Do not freeze this sample**.
- Obtain skeletal muscle biopsies for light microscopy (LM) and electron microscopy (EM). Muscle samples are preferably from the quadriceps.
  - Two 0.5cm cubes – wrap in aluminium foil, place in a small screw cap tube and completely cover with dry ice. **Store in a freezer at –70°C.**
  - One piece in a glutaraldehyde bottle for EM. Store in a refrigerator at 4°C. **Do not freeze this sample.**
- Obtain liver biopsies for LM and EM. If the parents object to two incisions (muscle and liver), suggest a right upper quadrant incision to take samples from the liver, rectus muscle and skin biopsy.
  - Two cores from a 14-French-gauge cannula or, if open biopsy, two 0.5 cm-cubes – wrap in aluminium foil, place in a small screw-cap tube and completely cover with dry ice. **Store in a freezer at –70°C.**
  - One piece in a glutaraldehyde bottle for EM. Store in a refrigerator at 4°C. **Do not freeze this sample.**
- Blood for DNA tests: 10 mL of heparinised blood (no mixing beads or separating gel) can be sent at room temperature if expected in the laboratory within 24 h, or otherwise frozen.

Note: To avoid mistakes in obtaining and handling of samples, consult with a metabolic specialist.

CHAPTER 29
NEONATAL CONDITIONS

Colin Morley
Peter McDougall
Lex Doyle

ROUTINE CARE

Most aspects of routine care vary with the age of the baby. The vast majority of deliveries are uncomplicated and do not require medical intervention. The baby will start breathing spontaneously and will be kept adequately warm by being swaddled and cuddled by the mother. Early contact helps with establishing bonding and breast-feeding.

The first minutes

Establishing breathing

The baby must start breathing soon after birth. The major stimuli, to start breathing include cooling of the face and physical stimuli as well as hypoxia and acidosis. Normal babies usually start breathing within seconds of birth. If the baby is not breathing, drying it with a towel is a very effective stimulus.

Heat loss after birth

Evaporative cooling occurs very quickly after birth. It is minimised by drying and wrapping the baby in warm towels. A well, term infant will be kept warm by being swaddled and cuddled by the mother. The baby's rectal temperature should stabilise around 37°C (+/– 0.3°C) by an hour of age. If a baby becomes cold it may need controlled warming under a radiant heater or in an incubator and it should always be assessed for illness. Hypothermia and hyperthermia are both bad for babies.

The umbilical cord

This is clamped and cut cleanly close to the skin just after birth. The cut end and the base of the cord must be kept clean and dry. Antiseptic solution, such as chlorhexidine in alcohol, may be applied daily until the cord stump drops off. Omphalitis may occur if this is not done. The plastic clamp can be removed after 2 days.

The first hours

After the infant's temperature is stable, they can be washed with soap and water. There is no hurry to do this. Record the heart rate, colour, respiratory rate and effort, at frequent intervals, depending on the infant's condition.

Often the baby will be very alert and breast feeds should be started at these times.

Vitamin K

All infants, regardless of size, maturity, or ill health, should receive vitamin K mixed micelles 0.1 mL i.m.. This eradicates haemorrhagic disease of the newborn. Claims associating i.m. vitamin K and childhood cancer have not been substantiated.

An increased incidence of both early and late haemorrhagic disease of the newborn occurs in breast-fed infants who received either an oral or inadequate i.m. dose, or no prophylactic vitamin K. Parents who insist on their infant having oral vitamin K must be given instructions that it must be given for 3 doses at 2-weekly intervals from birth.

The first day

After an initial period of alertness the infant will sleep for long periods and may not be too demanding with feeds. However, the infant must:

- *Suck and swallow easily*: if they do not, consider unrecognised prematurity, an abnormality, hypoglycaemia or infection.
- *Pass urine*: many babies pass urine at birth and it is missed. If a boy does not pass urine in the first 24 h, consider urethral valves. This needs careful urological investigation. A reasonable screening test is to ultrasound the bladder and see if it empties completely with micturition.
- *Pass meconium within the first 48 h*: if not, consider low bowel obstruction.

The first examination

The purpose of this examination is to detect congenital abnormalities, reassure the parents and to discuss their concerns. Many major abnormalities will have been seen on antenatal ultrasound, but not all.

- *Observation*: before disturbing the baby observe the posture, behaviour, general appearance, colour and well-being.

- *Chest*: while the baby is quiet examine the heart sounds and rate, pulse characteristics and presence of femoral pulses. Many babies have a very soft murmur in the first few days. If it sounds pathological, there are other signs or it persists, then refer for a cardiac ultrasound examination. Normal babies breathe so shallowly when they are sleeping that it can be difficult to see. Recession and laboured breathing are the most important signs of respiratory difficulty. In babies the rate and depth of each breath can be very variable.
- *Head and neck*: look for scalp defects; fractures; haematomas; lacerations; eye size, anatomy and red reflex; neck cysts, lumps or fistulae; cleft palate; tongue size and shape; ear position, shape, size and tags or fistulae and facial symmetry when crying. A cephalohaematoma is a soft boggy swelling over one bone, usually the parietal, due to blood under the periosteum. It needs no treatment. **Beware of a generalised boggy swelling all over the scalp in a shocked baby**. It may be a subgaleal haemorrhage. Babies can bleed profusely into these and they are a neonatal emergency.
- *Abdomen*: feel for masses (liver, spleen, kidneys, bladder and ovaries), distension and tenderness and examine the genitalia, hernial areas and anus. The liver is often just palpable or percussable in normal babies. The umbilicus should be clean and dry.
- *Limbs*: examine for abnormal fingers, hands, toes and feet; posture of the hands and feet; and the flexibility of the joints.
- *Hips*: carefully examine for congenital dislocation by observation and specific palpation. (See Orthopaedic conditions Chapter 31).
- *Measurement*: naked weight, length and head circumference should be measured, recorded and plotted on the growth chart in the baby's record book.

The first week

- *Feeding*: will be established during this time. After an initial phase of waking frequently until lactation is established, the breast-fed baby should establish a regular cycle of waking for feeds, followed mostly by sleeping. However, some babies will stay awake after some feeds, even in the first week of life. Some babies will sleep for 4 h; others will wake frequently for small feeds. After an initial weight loss of up to 10%, over the first few days, the baby's weight should stabilise and then increase towards the end of the first week.

- *Stools*: change over the first 4–5 days from black sticky meconium, to dark-green, yellow-green and finally loose yellow once full breast-feeding is established. The frequency of bowel actions can vary, but will usually be about once per feed after feeding is established.
- *Urine*: production is usually low in the first few days, but increases after feeding has been established, with a urinary frequency of usually at least once per feed.
- *Jaundice*: occurs in more than 50% of babies after the first 24 h of age, see p. 490.
- *Screening*: is performed on the third day for metabolic conditions, hypothyroidism and cystic fibrosis from a heel prick. Results are available approximately one week after sampling. Negative (normal) results are not notified, but the laboratory will contact the baby's doctor regarding the management of children with positive (abnormal) results and advise on appropriate management. This usually involves an immediate referral to a tertiary paediatric hospital for further testing and treatment.

Behaviour

In the first days, babies mostly sleep and eat; they spend little time awake when not feeding. Their sleep can be quiet or active. In quiet sleep they appear to sleep deeply, breathe quietly and regularly and do not move much. In active sleep (rapid eye movement (REM) sleep), they breathe erratically, make various noises (including crying, vocalising and yawning), have many body movements and may seem to be waking up. Babies may switch from one type of sleep to the other every 5–10 min or so. This behaviour can be confusing to inexperienced parents.

The first month

The baby should be weighed and measured weekly to ensure nutrition is adequate. The results must be written down and plotted on the charts in the baby's book. Weight gain for term babies varies from 150–250 g per week.

Maternal concerns about the baby usually relate to crying, not sleeping enough, not gaining weight, rashes or poor feeding. (See Nutrition, chapter 6 and Behavioural, developmental and sleep problems, chapter 10).

NEONATAL RESUSCITATION

When assessing an apnoeic baby at birth do the following:

- Place the baby on a resuscitation trolley under a radiant heater.
- Stimulate the baby by rubbing with a towel.
- If there is any chance the baby might have aspirated meconium or blood, suction the pharynx.
- Next, count the heart rate. This is the most important parameter to determine how to proceed.
- If it is >100 beats per min (bpm), the baby should respond to stimulation and inflating the lungs with a bag and mask.
- If the heart rate is <100 bpm and the baby does not respond quickly to stimulation or bag and mask ventilation, the baby should be intubated and ventilated. See Table 29.1 for endotracheal tube sizes.
- Ventilate the baby with sufficient pressure (about 30 cm H_2O) to make the lungs expand and therefore the chest and upper abdomen move with each inflation. This should cause a rapid improvement in heart rate followed quickly by the baby becoming pink and starting to breathe.
- The commonest cause for failure of resuscitation is inadequate ventilation. This can be due to a poor seal at the facemask or inadequate pressure. Sometimes pressures up to 50 cm H_2O are required for the first few breaths.
- A baby who does not respond and has a slow heart rate (<60 bpm) needs cardiac massage and may need infusions of bicarbonate, blood or adrenaline to improve cardiac output depending on the underlying problem.
- Admission to a neonatal intensive care unit is mandatory if spontaneous ventilation is not established by 5 min of age.

Table 29.1 Endotracheal tubes

Weight	*ETT size*	*T/e at lips*
<1000 g	2.5 mm	5–5.5 cm
1000–2500 g	3.0 mm	6–7 cm
Term	3.5 mm	9 cm
Large term	Consider 4.0 mm	9 cm

Table 29.2 The Apgar score

Sign	*0 (absent)*	*1 (present but depressed)*	*2 (normal)*
Heart rate	Absent	<100	>100
Respiratory effort	Absent	Slow, irregular	Good, crying
Muscle tone	Limp	Some flexion	Active
Response to stimulation	No response	Grimace	Cry
Colour	Pale, blue	Centrally pink, blue periphery	Pink

Reproduced with permission of *Pediatrics* 94: 558–565, Oct 1994, available at http://rwh.org.au/nets/handbook/index.cfm?doc_id=447.

- The Apgar score is used to assess the condition of the baby at 1, 5 and occasionally 10 min of age. See Table 29.2. The total score ranges from 0–10. A score between 7 and 10 indicates the infant is well. A score between 4 and 7 indicates the baby needs assistance. A score between 0 and 3 indicates severe cardio-respiratory depression. In practice it is best to describe exactly what was happening to the infant.
- Naloxone is rarely required. It should only be given if a mother has received narcotics within 2 h of delivery. When using Naloxone, be aware that the effect can wear off quickly and the baby may then develop apnoea, the most serious sign of narcotic overdose. Do not use Naxolone if there is a possibility of maternal narcotic abuse (risk of fulminant withdrawal in the baby).

VARIATIONS FROM NORMAL

When the baby is fully examined, many normal variants or minor problems will be obvious. If they are obvious to the doctor, most will be obvious to the parents. The parents' anxiety is usually related to what is obvious to them, rather than to its medical importance.

Skin

- *Naevus flammeus* (*'stork-bite'*): dilated capillaries, on the nape of the neck and on the bridge of the nose, eyelids and adjacent forehead. They fade over 6–12 months.

- *Milia*: small white blocked sebaceous glands on the nose. They disappear over the first month.
- *Miliaria*: there are two types – 'crystallina' and 'rubra'. Miliaria crystallina are beads of sweat trapped under the epidermis and are most prominent on the forehead in babies who are overheated. Miliaria rubra, also called 'heat rash', usually appear after a few weeks of age, fluctuate over 2–3 weeks and then disappear. They are related to an increasing activity of the sweat glands. They are prominent on the face, in babies who are overheated.
- *Erythema toxicum ('toxic erythema' or 'urticaria of the newborn')*: this is rash of red 'urticarial' spots over the baby's trunk that peaks at 2–3 days of age and is rarely present after the first week of life. It is harmless and of unknown cause. New lesions have a broad erythematous base up to 2–3 cm diameter with a 1–2 mm papule. Lesions come and go over a few hours during the first few days. The diagnosis can be made with confidence on clinical appearance alone. The differential diagnosis is staphylococcal skin infection, which is persistent and purulent. An examination of the fluid reveals neutrophils and Gram-positive cocci in infection, or eosinophils and no organisms in erythema toxicum.
- *'Mongolian' blue spot*: this condition results in areas of increased melanin deposition over the lower back and sacrum; however, it can be more extensive. Sometimes this is mistaken for bruising. It is present in most babies born to dark-skinned parents. It gradually lightens over a few years, as the rest of the skin becomes more pigmented.
- *Dry skin*: babies who are post mature have a thicker epidermis and hence drier-looking skin after birth. This dry skin may occasionally crack and sometimes bleed around the hands and feet during the first few days. Emollients will help. Otherwise the dry skin should be allowed to peel off naturally, which may take up to 1–2 months.

Deformities

- *Molding*: the skull molds to enable the head to be delivered. This changes to a normal shape over the first few days. In addition there may be postural deformities of the face, skull and limbs that are related to the baby's position in the uterus. These gradually improve after birth, but sometimes they do not disappear completely – very few people are symmetrical, especially in their face.

- *Positional talipes*: is quite common. The foot is deformed from being squashed in the uterus. To determine whether this is pathological test the range of movements of the foot. A normal foot can be flexed and extended so that the angle with the shin is less than or more than 90°. The forefoot should be mobile. A fixed deformity should be referred to a paediatric orthopaedic surgeon for management.

Other

- *Puffy eyelids/scalp oedema*: the newborn infant has excess body fluid at birth. Fluid accumulates easily in the eyelids and, after lying on one side, the lower eye may be more swollen. Scalp oedema is common in the first few hours after a normal birth, but can persist for several days. If it persists, or is generalised, this needs investigating.
- *Bruising/petechiae/subconjunctival haemorrhages*: the part of the baby that was presenting during delivery is commonly bruised. If the cord was wrapped tightly around the neck, the baby may have petechial haemorrhages on the face and head (traumatic cyanosis). Subconjunctival haemorrhages occur in up to 25% of babies delivered normally and do not adversely affect vision. They may persist for up to 2 weeks and must not be confused with postnatal trauma. Bruising is common after forceps deliveries, particularly over bony prominences, but disappears over the first week of life. Less commonly after forceps deliveries, firm nodules may be noted in the subcutaneous tissue at the same sites. This is subcutaneous fat necrosis. It resolves spontaneously over the first month of life.
- *Sucking blisters*: these are common on the lips, particularly the upper lip and need no treatment.
- *Epstein's pearls*: these are small white cysts on the hard palate in the midline. They are benign and disappear in the first weeks after birth.
- *Breast hyperplasia*: a breast bud is palpable in most term babies, regardless of gender. The breasts may become enlarged during the first week and milk may be observed. They should be left alone and the swelling will subside over several months. However, a breast that is swollen, hot, red and tender may be infected.

COMMON MINOR PROBLEMS

- *Hiccups*: these occur frequently after a feed. They are not caused by inadequate burping and are harmless.
- *Snuffles*: these occur in about 1/3 of normal babies in the few weeks after birth. Despite the noise, the baby is otherwise quite well and is able to feed normally. The problem diminishes with time as the baby's feeding becomes more efficient and the nasal passages enlarge. It is only important if it interferes with the baby's ability to suck.
- *Vomiting*: small vomits are harmless. The serious signs are vomit that is bile stained (grass green), blood-stained, projectile, persistent or associated with frequent choking or failure to thrive.
- *Bleeding umbilical cord*: small amounts of bleeding occur rarely as the cord is separating and require no treatment. More profuse bleeding may indicate a bleeding disorder. It may also indicate infection.
- *Umbilical hernia*: this is present in approximately 25% of babies and resolves in almost all. Consider surgical referral if present beyond 2 years.
- *Vaginal skin tag*: a small tag of vaginal skin commonly protrudes between the labia in newborn girls. It is benign and disappears as the labia enlarge.
- *Vaginal discharge*: a small amount of vaginal mucus is universal. In some it can be bloodstained during the first week as the endometrium involutes.
- *Red urine*: a red-orange discoloration of the napkin when the urine is concentrated (common in the first few days of life) may be mistaken for blood, but is usually due to urates.
- *Clicky hips*: some ligamentous clicking is common in all large joints, including the hips. It can be considered normal in the absence of any abnormal movement of the femoral head, restriction of hip movement, strong family history, or breech presentation. However, if there is any doubt, hip ultrasound is indicated.

JAUNDICE

Jaundice is common in the newborn period and is almost always caused by unconjugated hyperbilirubinaemia. The clinical importance of jaundice depends on the time at which it is observed and the gestational age of the baby. Jaundice needs to be taken seriously; if the bilirubin level is too high (>340 μmol/L) brain damage (kernicterus) may occur.

The first 24 hours

- Jaundice in the first 24 h is abnormal. The infant must be admitted to a special care nursery and investigated urgently.
- It is mostly caused by haemolysis, usually ABO or Rhesus incompatibility between mother and fetus. Severe haemolysis leads to a rapid rise in serum bilirubin over a few hours.
- The following investigations are required urgently: the mother and baby's blood group, and the baby's serum bilirubin (total and unconjugated), direct Coombs' test, haemoglobin, white cell count, and platelets. The mother's red cell antibodies may need to be measured.
- Further investigations are needed if there is no haemolysis, or conjugated hyperbilirubinaemia is present.
- Phototherapy should be commenced if the bilirubin level is >150 μmol/L in the first 24 h in a term infant.
- An immediate exchange transfusion may be required if the jaundice is due to rhesus incompatibility and the infant is anaemic (Hb <110 g/L). This primarily corrects the anaemia and removes antibodies. Further exchange transfusions may be required to control the jaundice.
- Frequent monitoring of bilirubin levels is essential as rapid changes may occur. The results should be plotted on a chart and an 'action level' for exchange transfusion established so that mistakes are not made.

Days 2–7

Jaundice is considered to be 'physiological' if the following criteria are satisfied:

- The jaundice appeared on day 2–4.
- The baby is not premature.
- The baby is well (afebrile, feeding well and alert).
- The baby is passing normal-coloured stools and urine.
- There are no other abnormalities.
- Bilirubin levels are not above treatment threshold.

About a 1/3 of term babies become visibly jaundiced by 2–4 days of age. Jaundice is visible once serum bilirubin is above 85–120 μmol/L. Serum bilirubin rarely exceeds 220 μmol/L. If the unconjugated bilirubin is >220 μmol/L, other causes, including infection, should be considered.

A well, term infant, with no haemolysis, is at minimal risk of kernicterus. Ill, term infants, in particular those exposed to hypoxic insults or infants with evidence of haemolysis, are at a higher risk of kernicterus and treatment should be started at lower bilirubin levels. Preterm infants are at increased risk of kernicterus at lower bilirubin levels. For guidelines in the management of jaundice see Tables 29.3, 29.4 and 29.5.

Table 29.3 Management of non-pathologic jaundice in healthy term infants

Age (h)	*Serum bilirubin (μmol)*			
	Consider Phototherapy	*Phototherapy*	*Exchange transfusion if intensive phototherapy fails*	*Exchange transfusion and intensive phototherapy*
<24	–	–	–	–
25–48	>170	>260	>340	>430
49–72	>260	>310	>430	>510
>72	>290	>340	>430	>510

For healthy term babies, phototherapy and exchange transfusion can be provided as recommended in the American Academy of Pediatrics Guidelines (reproduced by permission of *Pediatrics* 94: 558–565, Oct 1994).

In cases of pathologic jaundice, these guidelines are modified and treatment is typically more aggressive. Pathologic jaundice is clinical jaundice at less than 24 h of age, and/or bilirubin rising at greater than 8.5 μmol/L/hr, and/or true haemolysis.

Table 29.4 Management of jaundice in preterm infants: guidelines for phototherapy

Age (h)	*Serum bilirubin (μmol)*		
		Weight (g)	
	<1500	*1500–2000*	*>2000*
<24	>70	>70	>85
24–48	>85	>120	>140
49–72	>120	>155	>200
>72	>140	>170	? 240

Reproduced by permission of *Pediatrics* 94: 558–565, Oct 1994, available from http://rwh.org.au/nets/handbook/index.cfm?doc_id=447.

Table 29.5 Management of jaundice in preterm infants: guidelines for exchange transfusion

Age (h)	*Serum bilirubin (μmol)*		
		Weight (g)	
	<1500	*1500–2000*	*>2000*
<24	>170–255	>255	>270–310
24–48	>170–255	>270	>290–320
49–72	>255	>290	>310–340

For high-risk premature infants: use lower end of range and weight, next lower weight category, and next lower age category in that order. Premature LGA infants: use average birthweight for gestational age, available from http://rwh.org.au/nets/handbook/index.cfm?doc_id=447.

Prolonged jaundice (>14 days)

In a well infant prolonged neonatal jaundice is usually secondary to breast-feeding and is benign. A serum bilirubin should be checked to determine whether the hyperbilirubinaemia is conjugated or unconjugated.

- *Unconjugated bilirubinaemia*: hypothyroidism, infection or red cell enzyme abnormalities should be considered.
  - A sudden onset of jaundice at this age is suggestive of haemolysis caused by a red blood cell enzyme abnormality, most frequently glucose-6-phosphate dehydrogenase (G6PD) deficiency. Urgent admission to hospital is indicated.
- *Conjugated bilirubinaemia*: is uncommon and always pathological. Consider biliary atresia (the stools are white), neonatal hepatitis, a choledochal cyst obstructing the bile duct, galactosaemia or parenteral nutrition.

If the above are excluded and the baby is well and breast-feeding, the likely diagnosis is breast milk jaundice. This occurs in 2–4% of breast-feeding infants, is not associated with kernicterus and does not need any treatment. Reassurance that breast-feeding should continue is very important.

Prolonged jaundice (after the first few days of life) can usually be managed as an outpatient, but may require readmission for investigation or treatment.

RESPIRATORY DISTRESS

Most major causes of respiratory distress will present within the first hours of life. The signs are:

- Increased work of breathing (recession of the lower chest wall and upper abdomen).
- Rapid breathing (>60 breaths per min).
- Expiratory grunt.
- Central cyanosis.

Babies need to be considered for level 3 neonatal intensive care if they require more than 40% oxygen.

Common pulmonary diseases

Respiratory distress syndrome or hyaline membrane disease

- Respiratory distress syndrome (RDS) is primarily caused by immaturity. The incidence increases with decreasing gestation. It affects most babies born at <30 weeks' gestation, but it can occur in term babies, especially those delivered by elective Caesarian section. Due to immaturity of the surfactant, lung structure and fluid clearance, the lungs do not expand easily or evenly. This causes damage to the epithelium and protein exudes on to the surface, forming hyaline membranes.
- Respiratory distress (O_2 requirement, work of breathing) typically increases over 12–24 h before improvement is seen. Rapid deterioration may occur leading to respiratory failure (rising arterial CO_2 level).
- The diagnosis is by clinical features and chest X-ray, which has a generalised fine reticulogranular ('ground glass') appearance with air bronchograms.

- Respiratory support with oxygen, assisted ventilation (CPAP, IPPV) and surfactant therapy may be required.

Transient tachypnoea of the newborn or 'wet lung syndrome'

- This is caused by delayed clearance of foetal lung fluid and commonly occurs in babies born near term by elective Caesarean section. It presents as mild respiratory distress and lasts for up to 1 or 2 days.
- It is diagnosed by chest X-ray, which has coarse streaking of lung fields with fluid in the fissures. Usually the baby is not very ill, needing less than 30% oxygen.

Bacterial infections

- Group B β-haemolytic streptococcus (GBS) is the commonest and most serious cause of pneumonia and septicaemia in the newborn. It is acquired around the time of birth from a colonised mother. Other organisms, including *E. coli*, can also cause pneumonia.
- Pneumonia presents early with severe and progressive respiratory failure. If not treated immediately there is rapid progression to collapse and death.
- Later infections can present with lethargy, temperature instability, poor feeding, respiratory difficulty, apnoea or poor perfusion.
- The chest X-ray of GBS infection is similar to severe RDS and is not diagnostic.
- Because of the rapid and severe nature of GBS septicaemia, all babies with early onset respiratory failure must be treated with penicillin and gentamicin until the cause of the disease is confirmed.

Meconium aspiration syndrome

- Hypoxia before delivery may cause the baby to gasp in-utero and inhale meconium. This causes respiratory difficulty. It is associated with pulmonary hypertension and right to left shunting.
- The chest X-ray shows hyperinflation and patchy consolidation (pneumothorax and pneumomediastinum may follow) or a diffuse hazy appearance.
- Oxygen is the mainstay of therapy, but other respiratory support (CPAP or ventilation) may be required. Antibiotics are given to counter infection.

Pneumothorax

- May occur spontaneously at birth, or secondary to other lung disease. It is a serious cause of respiratory distress that may get worse if it is not recognised and treated.
- The diagnosis is by chest X-ray. Transillumination can be useful.
- The main treatment is an intercostal catheter with an underwater drain at low negative pressure.

Upper airway obstruction

- *Nasal*: may be due to an upper respiratory tract infection, choanal atresia (obstruction to the back of the nose) or traumatic deviated nasal septum. It presents with difficulty in breathing or feeding. Suspect choanal atresia/stenosis if a large-gauge suction tube cannot be passed.
- *Oral*: macroglossia may be associated with Beckwith–Wiedemann syndrome or hypothyroidism. Micrognathia may result in a tongue that obstructs the pharynx.
- *Larynx*: laryngomalacia, subglottic stenosis, laryngeal inflammation or occasionally vocal cord palsy, present with inspiratory stridor and suprasternal and lower chest indrawing.
- *Trachea*: tracheal obstruction presents with an inspiratory and expiratory wheeze and lower chest indrawing. It may be due tracheomalacia or a vascular ring.

Non-pulmonary causes of respiratory difficulty

Cardiac

- Left to right shunts or left sided obstructions cause increased fluid in the lungs making them stiff.

Pulmonary hypertension

- Presents with an increased oxygen requirement and little respiratory difficulty. The lungs on the chest X-ray may look very clear.

Management of respiratory diseases

Before birth

- If possible, anticipate high-risk babies and transfer to a hospital with a level 3 nursery for delivery and neonatal care.
- Betamethasone given to mothers with threatened preterm labour reduces the severity of HMD, halves the mortality and incidence of brain haemorrhages and improves long-term outcome.

General care

- Observation, usually in an incubator.
- Temperature control is essential – aim for a rectal temperature of 37°C (+/– 0.3°C) or axillary temperature range 36.8°C (+/– 0.3°C).
- Avoid enteral feeds initially because they make any respiratory difficulty worse.
- Give intravenous fluids.
- Measure blood glucose, electrolytes, full blood count and CRP.
- Take a blood culture (but not an LP in the acute stage).
- Treat with benzylpenicillin and gentamicin until the blood cultures are known to be clear.

Respiratory care

- A chest X-ray provides the diagnosis in most cases of respiratory difficulty in neonates.
- Monitor cardiorespiratory and blood gas measurements.
  - *Arterial pH* should be maintained at 7.35–7.45. A level of 7.25 or just under may be acceptable, depending on the circumstances.
  - *Arterial* P_aco_2 should be 40–60 mmHg.
  - *Arterial* P_ao_2 A low P_aO_2 means the baby is hypoxic. If the pH is also low, the baby may have a metabolic acidosis and a higher level of inspired oxygen is required. If this does not improve oxygenation, suspect cyanotic heart disease as a cause (see Cardiovascular Conditions, chapter 16).
  - *Arterial bicarbonate* should be 22–26 mmol/L. A low level is due to a metabolic acidosis. The pH will also be low unless the baby has compensated by blowing off CO_2.
  - *Base excess* should be between +3 and –3. If low it indicates a metabolic acidosis. A level of –5 is usually tolerated in small babies without out a significant change in pH.
- In ventilated babies with RDS, especially those <30 weeks' gestation, surfactant should be given down the endotracheal tube as early as possible.
- The inspired oxygen requirement is initially determined using a pulse oximeter. Aim for an oxygen saturation of 90–95%.
- Arterial blood gases should be measured in babies needing >30% oxygen. Aim for a P_aO_2 level between 50–80 mmHg.

- Nasal continuous positive airway pressure (CPAP) is effective for treating RDS or apnoea. It should be used early for any baby who is grunting or showing increased respiratory effort (starting at 7 cm H_2O).
- The decision to ventilate a baby is made on the following criteria:
  - Apnoea not responding to simple treatment.
  - Unsatisfactory arterial blood gases: pH <7.25 with a P_aCO_2 >60 mmHg, or inspired oxygen >60%.

HYPOGLYCAEMIA

- This is defined as a true blood glucose of <2.5 mmol/L. 'Dextrostix' or 'BM stix' are only useful for screening purposes. If these suggest hypoglycaemia, a true blood glucose must be measured.
- Blood glucose should be measured before 1 h of age for infants with the following conditions: infants of diabetic mothers, infants weighing <10th centile, prematurity, large for gestational age, shocked, seizures and infants receiving intravenous infusions.

Clinical features

There are no specific clinical features of hypoglycaemia. The infant may be asymptomatic, or may have apathy, hypotonia, poor feeding, temperature instability, apnoea, jitteriness or convulsions.

Management

- Asymptomatic infants with a true blood glucose of 1.5–2.5 mmol/L: give early, frequent small milk feeds at 90 mL/kg/day. If no response occurs within 2 h, give intravenous dextrose.
- If the blood glucose is <1.5 mmol/L intravenous dextrose should be given. A bolus of 10% dextrose, 2 mL/kg, should be followed by an infusion providing 5–10 mg/kg per min of glucose. The response to therapy should be monitored by frequent blood glucose measurements.
- If the blood glucose is <1 mmol/L and it is difficult to insert an intravenous line, give 0.3 units/kg of glucagon i.m. pending successful insertion of the line, or transfer to a higher level of care.
- Further investigation and treatment is necessary if the glucose requirement is 10 mg/kg per min or greater (see Metabolic conditions, chapter 28).

NEONATAL INFECTION

Infection is one of the commonest preventable causes of neonatal mortality and morbidity. Infection may be acquired from the mother before or at birth (early onset) or postnatally from the environment by droplet spread or handling (late onset). The most frequently encountered bacteria are:

Early onset: Group B β-haemolytic streptococcus, *Escherichia coli* and *Listeria monocytogenes.*

Late onset: Coagulase-negative staphylococci, *Staphylococcus aureus*, Group B β-haemolytic streptococcus, *Klebsiella* spp. and *Pseudomonas* spp.

The most serious viral infection is herpes simplex virus (HSV), but other viruses, especially respiratory syncytial virus (RSV), can cause problems in neonatal nurseries, or soon after discharge home in expremature infants.

Clinical features

The early symptoms and signs may be minimal, but if ignored, rapid progression to overwhelming sepsis may occur.

The following are important warning signs of infection: respiratory difficulty, poor feeding, vomiting, abdominal distension and tenderness, drowsiness, floppiness, pallor, apnoea, seizures, temperature instability, tender limb.

Investigations

If one or more of the warning signs are present it is important to investigate infection. This includes:

- *Blood culture*: arterial or venous – at least 2–4 mL.
- *Urine*: suprapubic aspiration (SPA) under ultrasound imaging if possible.
- Throat and rectal swabs and swabs of any obviously infected lesion.
- Cultures or specific PCR for viral infections.
- Lumbar puncture if meningitis is suspected.

Management

Any ill neonate should be investigated and treated in hospital.

- Start with i.v. benzylpenicillin and gentamicin.
- Add cefotaxime i.v. if meningitis is suspected (see Antimicrobial guidelines) and metronidazole i.v. if abdominal sepsis is suspected.
- If there is any possibility that the baby may have HSV (i.e. the mother has active genital herpes) give aciclovir.
- The antibiotics may need to be changed when cultures are available (see Antimicrobial guidelines).

Careful attention to temperature stability, respiratory status, fluid and electrolytes, blood pressure, blood glucose and haematology is essential.

NEONATAL SEIZURES

Clinical features

- *Subtle*: deviation of the eyes, staring, abnormal sucking or lip smacking, or cycling movements of the limbs.
- *Tonic*: limbs go stiff, frequently associated with apnoea and eye deviation.
- *Clonic*: movement of one or all limbs not stopped by holding the limb.
- These can be distinguished from 'jitteriness' or tremulousness, which have no ocular phenomena, are stimulus sensitive and can be stopped by gentle passive flexion of the limbs.
- *Benign sleep myoclonus*: occurs in a neurologically normal infant only during sleep. The electroencephalogram (EEG) is normal and no treatment is necessary.

Aetiology

The aetiology can usually be determined for neonatal seizures. Causes include:

- Hypoxic ischaemic encephalopathy: the seizures occur within 24 h of the hypoxic episode, often within the first 4–6 h.
- Intracranial haemorrhage.
- Infection: bacterial or viral meningitis.

- Metabolic:
  - Hypoglycaemia.
  - Hypocalcaemia/hypomagnesaemia.
  - Hypo- or hypernatraemia.
  - Kernicterus.
  - Alkalosis.
  - Local anaesthetic intoxication.
  - Inborn errors of metabolism (characterised by intractable seizures, with progressive loss of consciousness, or metabolic acidosis), including:
    - Pyridoxine dependency.
    - Urea cycle disorders.
    - Non-ketotic hyperglycinaemia.
    - Fatty acid oxidation defects.
    - Amino acid/organic acid/hyperammonaemia.
- Drug withdrawal.
- Developmental brain abnormalities.
- Autosomal dominant neonatal seizures.

Investigations

- Blood glucose (must be done immediately).
- Electrolytes, calcium and magnesium.
- Blood gases.
- Cranial ultrasound.
- Urine analysis including ketones and reducing substances.
- Lumbar puncture, blood cultures and viral investigations.
- Metabolic screen: blood ammonia, plasma lactate, urinary organic acids, plasma amino acids and plasma carnitine.
- Cranial CT scan: if focal seizures, birth trauma or uncertain aetiology.
- MRI brain scan: for suspected developmental brain abnormality or ischaemia.
- EEG: to detect seizure activity and to aid prognosis.

Management

Admission to a neonatal intensive care unit is mandatory for all neonates with seizures. Attention to normoglycaemia, optimal ventilation, blood pressure control, fluid and electrolyte balance is essential.

Anticonvulsants

- Phenobarbitone: 20 mg/kg i.v. over 30 min (beware this dose may cause apnoea in a non-ventilated baby). A further 10 mg/kg may be given for refractory seizures followed by 5 mg/kg per day.
- Phenytoin: 20 mg/kg, i.v. over 1 h.
- Clonazepam: up to 0.25 mg. This may cause apnoea. Careful monitoring and the availability of mechanical ventilation are essential.
- Pyridoxine: 50–100 mg i.v. or p.o. should be considered for intractable seizures.

Most infants can be weaned from anticonvulsant therapy within a few days of their last seizure. Some infants who have residual seizures or abnormal neurological signs with an abnormal EEG will require ongoing treatment and specialist referral.

NEONATAL ABSTINENCE SYNDROME

Neonatal abstinence syndrome occurs in babies born to women who are chemically dependent and who may use multiple substances. The babies exhibit signs of withdrawal and may require treatment. The features of withdrawal are assessed using a standardised scoring system.

Do not use Naloxone at delivery in these babies, it may precipitate acute withdrawal associated with seizures.

The onset of withdrawal is variable:

- Heroin: 48–72 h.
- Methadone: may be delayed for up to 1–2 weeks.

Withdrawal may be less evident in premature infants.

Clinical features

Neurological signs:

- Hypertonia, tremors, hyperreflexia.
- Myoclonic jerks, seizures (1–2% heroin, 7% methadone).
- Irritability, restlessness, high-pitched cry.
- Sleep disturbance.

Autonomic system dysfunction:

- Nasal stuffiness, sneezing, yawning.
- Low grade fever, sweating.
- Skin mottling.

Gastrointestinal abnormalities:

- Regurgitation, vomiting, diarrhoea.
- Poor feeding, dysmature swallowing.
- Failure to thrive.

Respiratory symptoms:

- Tachypnoea.
- Increased apnoea.

Skin

- Excoriations (especially around the anus).

Management may involve morphine to assist gradual withdrawal.

POSTNATAL DEPRESSION

Mild to moderate postnatal depression occurs in about 1 in 6 women – a much higher incidence than previously recognised. If severe it may be a risk to the life of both the mother and baby. Postnatal depression can have profound effects on a family and on the child's development. The diagnosis may not always be obvious, so a high level of awareness is required when assessing any baby in the first months of life. Infants of mothers with postnatal depression may present with feeding problems, failure to thrive or excessive crying.

Clinical features

Clinical features in the mother may include:

- Lowered mood/fearfulness.
- Anxiety.
- Disorganisation.
- Inattentiveness to the baby.
- Recurrent presentations to health care professionals.

Management

- Recognise and acknowledge the problem.
- Arrange or refer to appropriate counselling.

- Medication is often necessary.
- Referral to a mother-baby unit or a psychiatric hospital facility may be needed and is often of benefit.

MATERNAL MASTITIS

Mastitis is common in breast-feeding women.

- It presents with aches and pains and fever, women often think they have the 'flu'.
- An examination reveals a tender engorged segment in one or both breasts.
- The organism is usually *Staphylococcus aureus.*

Management

- Prompt treatment is important to prevent abscess formation.
- Oral antibiotics – flucloxacillin 500 mg p.o., 6-hourly.
- Paracetamol and increased fluids.
- Breast-feeding should continue.
- Thorough emptying of the affected breast (the baby is more efficient at this than expression).

PROBLEMS OF THE EX-VERY LOW BIRTHWEIGHT INFANT

While it is not the intention of this chapter to discuss the problems of managing very low birth weight (VLBW) infants (birthweight <1500 g), it is important to be aware of some of the problems that occur after discharge from the neonatal unit.

Bronchopulmonary dysplasia

This is a common chronic lung disease occurring for a few months in very premature infants after RDS. It is characterised by an abnormal chest X-ray and oxygen dependency after 36 weeks' gestation. The majority of infants with bronchopulmonary dysplasia (BPD) can be weaned from oxygen treatment within 4 weeks of the expected date of delivery. A small number require oxygen therapy for months and some are managed at home in oxygen.

These babies are particularly susceptible to respiratory infections in the first 18 months of life and may deteriorate rapidly and need to be readmitted to hospital. If a baby is feeding poorly because of dyspnoea, has retractions of the lower sternum and ribs, apnoeic episodes or is drowsy, urgent admission to hospital is indicated.

In the absence of these signs the infant may be managed at home, but the parents need to be informed of the warning signs and the child reviewed frequently.

Necrotising enterocolitis

This is due to inflammation of the intestine in the early neonatal period. While many babies recover with conservative management (nil orally, intravenous alimentation and antibiotics), some develop necrosis that necessitates bowel resection. The risks to these babies after discharge from hospital are:

- *Stricture formation*: this can present weeks or months after the initial episode. The presenting features of obstruction include: bile-stained vomiting, distension, constipation and failure to thrive.
- *Gastroenteritis*: this can produce severe dehydration very rapidly in a baby who has had a bowel resection. Admission to hospital for intravenous fluids is mandatory.

Hearing deficits

Hearing deficits are common in these babies and hearing must be carefully assessed soon after discharge from hospital.

Visual defects

Visual problems are common and must be screened for soon after discharge from hospital.

Further common problems

- *Inguinal hernias*: require prompt surgical referral as they frequently strangulate.
- *Immunisation*: (see Immunisation, chapter 8) hepatitis B vaccination is recommended just after birth or at 32 weeks' if born prematurely. Immunisation is given at the appropriate postnatal age as per the immunisation schedule. It should not be delayed or the dose reduced because of size or prematurity.

- *Apnoea*: this is a common problem until about 34 weeks' gestation. However, ex-VLBW infants are at increased risk of apnoea until the age of 3 months past their due date after general anaesthesia, or with respiratory infections. Close monitoring is advised at these times.
- *Capillary haemangiomas (strawberry naevus)*: these appear after birth as small raised, red, lobulated and compressible lesions that increase in size over a few months. Most involute during the first two years. Failure to involute or difficult locations may be indications for a referral to a dermatologist for laser or intralesional steroid therapy (see Dermatologic conditions, chapter 20).

CHAPTER 30
NEUROLOGIC CONDITIONS

Andrew Kornberg
Simon Harvey
Wirginia Maixner
Margot Nash

FEBRILE CONVULSIONS

- Febrile convulsions (FC) are usually brief, generalised seizures associated with a febrile illness, in the absence of any central nervous system (CNS) infection or past history of afebrile seizures.
- Febrile convulsions are a genetically determined, age-dependent seizure disorder in which the child has a tendency to have seizures with fever.
- Simple FC refer to seizures that are brief, generalised, self-limited and single.
- Complex FC refer to seizures that are either focal, >15 min, or multiple in a 24 h period.
- They occur in 3–4% of children aged 6 months to 5 years and are recurrent in 25–50%. The most important factor for recurrence is the age of onset of the first febrile seizure; the younger the age, the greater the recurrence risk.
- In otherwise healthy children they are not accompanied by an increased risk of intellectual disability, cerebral palsy, other neurological disorders or death.

Management

- Stop a continuing convulsion (>10 min duration) with i.v. or rectal diazepam 0.2–0.4 mg/kg (max 10 mg).
- General temperature-lowering measures such as removing clothing and administering paracetamol 15 mg/kg may help reduce symptoms of fever.
- A careful search for the cause of fever is required. Most will be due to viral respiratory infections.

- A lumbar puncture need not be performed routinely following a simple FC, but meningitis should be considered in any unwell child, especially when there is a persistently depressed conscious state and in children with multiple or prolonged convulsions. The younger the child the higher the index of suspicion of meningitis.

Recurrence of FC is more likely if the seizure occurs in early infancy and if there is a family history of FC. As FC are usually benign and as anticonvulsants may have significant side effects and do not alter long-term prognosis, these drugs are not routinely recommended for children with recurrent FC. In some circumstances (e.g. children with a history of prolonged FC) parents may be taught to administer rectal diazepam.

About 3% of children with FC subsequently develop afebrile seizures (epilepsy). Predictors include:

- Previous abnormal neurological development.
- A history of epilepsy in first-degree relatives.
- Prolonged (>10 min) FC.
- Focal features present during, or after, the FC.
- Multiple convulsions during a single febrile episode.

When counselling parents, remember that many will have felt that their child nearly died. The excellent long-term prognosis and a 30–50% risk of FC recurrence but low risk of epilepsy needs to be emphasised. Advice on the management of future febrile illnesses and FC is required. A follow-up visit is recommended to review FC and minimise the development of fever phobia in the parents. An electro-encephalogram (EEG) is of little value in single or recurrent, simple or complex FC.

EPILEPSY

Epilepsy (defined notionally as 2 unprovoked seizures) occurs in approximately 5% of children. Seizures may be focal (partial) and/or generalised and the aetiology may be idiopathic (genetic) or symptomatic (malformation, tumour, scar, degenerative).

Electro-encephalogram aids in the characterisation of seizures and epilepsies, but should not be used to distinguish seizures from non-epileptic events unless concurrent video-EEG recording of frequent events is possible.

Brain imaging with CT or MRI is reserved for those in whom there is suspicion from history, examination or EEG that there may be an underlying cerebral lesion. Magnetic resonce imaging is more sensitive in identifying cerebral lesions, particularly subtle abnormalities of the cerebral cortex.

Idiopathic generalised epilepsy

- This term describes the group of childhood epilepsies characterised by recurrent generalised tonic-clonic (GTCS), absence or myoclonic seizures of presumed genetic cause.
- The first seizure usually occurs at 4–16 years of age, in an otherwise normal child.
- The EEG invariably shows generalised spike wave patterns.
- The prognosis is generally good for seizure control and remission in later childhood or adulthood.
- Idiopathic generalised epilepsy syndromes include childhood absence epilepsy, juvenile myoclonic epilepsy, and epilepsy with isolated GTCS.

Partial (focal) seizures

Partial seizures arise from a localised area of cortex in one or both cerebral hemispheres and may be idiopathic, or due to underlying structural pathology. Metabolic disturbances (e.g. hypoglycaemia and hypocalcaemia) may also produce partial seizures.

Two common but distinct forms of partial epilepsy are temporal lobe epilepsy and the benign focal epilepsies of childhood. Partial seizures can arise from anywhere in the brain. Other types of childhood partial epilepsy include frontal lobe epilepsies and occipital lobe epilepsies.

Temporal lobe epilepsy

- Complex partial seizures are the main seizure type and usually manifest by the arrest of activity, staring, autonomic features, mouthing movements, semi-purposeful motor activity and an altered conscious state, sometimes preceded by epigastric or olfactory auras. Seizures may secondarily generalise.
- Seizures typically occur in clusters and are often difficult to treat.
- These children frequently have learning and behavioural problems.
- An EEG may show localised temporal epileptic activity. Structural pathology should be sought using MRI.

Benign focal (partial) epilepsies of childhood

- Onset is typically in mid-childhood (peak 7 years).
- Seizures are commonly nocturnal or early morning. In the centro-temporal (Rolandic) variety, they are usually focal motor or sensory phenomena related to the face, mouth or jaw. The occipital variety may have visual manifestations. Secondarily generalised tonic-clonic seizures may also occur.
- On EEG spike discharges typically occur in the centrotemporal region or occipital region.
- The prognosis is excellent as the seizures are usually infrequent and readily controlled on carbamazepine or valproate if treatment is required. They usually remit before the teenage years.
- Imaging is normally only necessary if clinical or EEG features are atypical or if seizure control is difficult.

Status epilepticus

See Medical emergencies, chapter 1.

ANTICONVULSANT THERAPY

Indications for commencing anticonvulsants

The decision to investigate and treat a child following a seizure depends on many factors. Consideration should be given to a routine EEG in any child with non-febrile, generalised or partial seizures. Brain imaging with CT or MRI is reserved for those in whom there is suspicion from history, examination or EEG that there may be an underlying cerebral lesion. Many children have only a single convulsion and treatment would not normally be commenced unless there are clinical features to suggest an increased risk of recurrence. Epileptic syndrome characterisation from history, EEG and sometimes imaging generally dictates prognosis and the need for long-term therapy.

Antiepileptic medication is only indicated in children at high risk of recurrent epileptic seizures (see Table 30.1).

Principles of anticonvulsant therapy

- Most patients can be controlled well with one anticonvulsant; polypharmacy should be avoided if possible.

Table 30.1 Guidelines for the use of common anticonvulsants

Drug	*Status epilepticus*	*Generalized tonic–clonic seizures*	*Partial: simple, complex or 2° generalised*	*Typical absence (petit mal)*	*Myoclonic/ tonic/atypical absence*	*More common or severe side effects*
Carbamazepine (Tegretol, Tegretol CR)	–	++	+++	–	–	Drowsiness, irritability, GIT, rash
Clobazam (Frisium)	–	+	++	+	++	Drowsiness, irritability
Clonazepam (Rivotril)	+++	+	++	+	+++	Irritability and behaviour disorder, increased secretions
Diazepam (Valium)	+++	–	–	–	+++ (i.v. only)	Drowsiness, respiratory depression
Ethosuximide (Zarontin)	–	–	–	+++	+	Gastrointestinal disturbance, thrombocytopenia
Gabapentin (Neurontin)	–	–	++	–	–	Drowsiness, dizziness, ataxia, fatigue
Lamotrigine (Lamictal)	–	++	++	++	++	Skin rash in 3%: may be severe. Increased risk if rapid introduction or on sodium valproate
Nitrazepam (Mogadon)	–	–	–	–	++	Drowsiness, increased bronchial secretions

Table 30.1 *continued*

Drug	*Status epilepticus*	*Generalized tonic–clonic seizures*	*Partial: simple, complex or 2° generalised*	*Typical absence (petit mal)*	*Myoclonic/ tonic/atypical absence*	*More common or severe side effects*
Phenobarbitone	++	++	+	–	–	Cognitive, irritability, overactivity or drowsiness
Phenytoin sodium (Dilantin)	++	++	++	–	–	Gum hyperplasia, ataxia, nystagmus, serum sickness-like illness, cognitive, rash
Sodium valproate (Epilim)	–	+++	++	+++	+++	Nausea, anorexia vomiting. Rarely severe hepatotoxicity weight gain
Tiagabine (Gabitril)	–	–	+	–	–	Headache, dizziness
Topiramate (Topamax)	–	+	+	–	+	Weight loss, sedation, cognitive nephrolithiasis, paraesthesia
Vigabatrin (Sabril)	–	–	++	–	++ (Infantile spasms)	Excitation, agitation, drowsiness, dizziness, headache, weight gain, constriction of visual fields

* This table shows the relative effectiveness of each drug against each of the major seizure types. It does not represent a comparison of one drug against another. Sodium valproate should be used with caution in children under 3 years, particularly if multiple anticonvulsants are being used and underlying cerebral pathology is present. Cognitive side effects may be seen with all anticonvulsants, particularly benzodiazepines and barbiturates.

The above represents suggestions only. The final decision regarding the most appropriate choice of anticonvulsant can only be made by a physician in possession of details such as age of patient, neurological status, comorbidities, epilepsy syndromes, EEG, patient and parent attitudes and after discussion of potential side effects.

Table 30.2 Non-epileptic paroxysmal events

	Breath-holding attacks	*Shuddering*	*Benign paroxysmal vertigo*	*Infantile self stimulation*	*'Day dreams'*	*Night terrors*	*Nightmares*	*Syncope*
Age	Infancy	Infancy	Preschool	Preschool	School	Preschool/ school age	All ages	All ages
Circumstances	Always upset or a trigger is needed	Anytime/ anywhere	Anytime/ anywhere	Anytime/ anywhere	Commonly school, watching TV, times of inactivity	First third of sleep (non-REM)	Second half of sleep (REM)	Always triggering factor or situational
Frequency	Varies greatly	Sometimes many per day	1 month or less	Daily or less	Varies but not large numbers per day	Nightly or less. Rarely more than one per night	Nightly or less	Occasional
Onset	Sudden, with or without crying	Sudden	Sudden	Sudden	Vague	Sudden	Sudden	Gradual or sudden
Recovery	Slow if hypoxic seizure occurs	Rapid	Rapid	Rapid	Vague. May be 'snapped out'	Returns to sleep	Remains asleep	Gradual
Duration	Seconds to minutes	Seconds	1–5 min	Minutes to hours	Seconds to minutes	Minutes	Minutes	Seconds to minutes

Table 30.2 *continued*

	Breath-holding attacks	*Shuddering*	*Benign paroxysmal vertigo*	*Infantile self stimulation*	*'Day dreams'*	*Night terrors*	*Nightmares*	*Syncope*
Impairment of consciousness	Usually	No	No	No	Apparent but not real	Apparently awake but does not respond	Asleep	Yes
Observations	Cyanotic or pale, limp, may develop opisthotonos/ seizure	Rapid shivering movements maximal in head, trunk and arms	Frightened, pale, holds onto objects to maintain balance or falls	Posturing with stiffening and while lying on side or supine, leaning against firm edge. Irregular breathing, flushing, sweating	Blank staring but no motor automatisms or blinking despite long episodes. Not precipitated by hyperventilation	Screaming, crying inconsolably, may get out of bed. Appears terrified	Nil	May describe light headedness, dizziness or loss of vision. Tonic or tonic/clonic seizure may occur at end
Post-event impairment	Mild unless hypoxic seizure occurs	No	No	No	No	No recollection of event	Good recall of events	Minimal
Main differential	Epilepsy	Epilepsy	Epilepsy	Seizures/ abdominal pain, movement disorder	Absence seizures	Frontal lobe epilepsy	Night terrors	Epilepsy/Cardiac

- Most antiepileptic medications are commenced at a low dose and titrated up to the maintenance dose, to avoid side effects during their introduction ('start low and go slow').
- Individuals vary greatly in dosage requirements and tolerance. Young children and infants typically require relatively large doses.
- Give anticonvulsants an adequate trial before withdrawal.
- If seizure control is inadequate, or non-compliance or clinical toxicity is suspected, anticonvulsant blood levels may be measured for drugs such as phenytoin, phenobarbitone, carbamazepine and valproate. 'Routine' monitoring of phenytoin, phenobarbitone or carbamazepine levels is indicated in young infants or developmentally impaired older children in whom even severe side effects may not be evident.
- Introduce or change one anticonvulsant at a time, except in emergency situations.

Depending on the type of epilepsy, several years free of seizures are generally required before anticonvulsants are withdrawn. This is done gradually over several months.

NON-EPILEPTIC PAROXYSMAL EVENTS

- Many children referred for assessment of epilepsy do not have epilepsy, but some other non-epileptic paroxysmal disorder.
- In differentiating epileptic from non-epileptic events the description of the event is important, but equally important is a description of the circumstances in which the event occurred and the details of what the child was doing immediately before the event.
- Many non-epileptic paroxysmal disorders can be diagnosed positively on history alone, although in some special circumstances more detailed investigations such as video-EEG monitoring may be required.
- The long Q–T syndrome should be considered in any episode of fainting or seizure that is not clearly due to typical breath-holding, vasovagal syncope or a definable epilepsy syndrome.

Table 30.2 lists some of these events and their salient features.

Breath-holding attacks

See Table 30.2 and Behavioural, developmental and sleep problems, chapter 10. In children with severe, recurrent breath-holding attacks, consider iron deficiency.

WEAKNESS OF ACUTE ONSET

The acute onset of symmetrical limb weakness usually has a peripheral neuromuscular or spinal cord origin. Toxins (e.g. snake or tick bite), metabolic disturbance, systemic illness and psychogenic causes need to be considered under appropriate circumstances. Oral polio vaccine is a rare cause of acute flaccid paralysis.

Two key questions require urgent consideration:

- Is there a treatable cause?
- Is there respiratory or pharyngeal dysfunction of sufficient degree to warrant management in an intensive care unit?

Myasthenia gravis

- This diagnosis should be considered in any child with relatively acute onset limb weakness, particularly if accompanied by ptosis, eye movement disorder, pharyngeal or respiratory insufficiency.
- A diagnostic/therapeutic trial of parenteral anticholinesterase is warranted if myasthenia is a possibility.

Guillain-Barré syndrome

- This condition is often not recognised in its early stages when there may only be an 'ataxic' gait.
- The child should be transferred to a tertiary referral centre at the time of diagnosis, as respiratory weakness may occur rapidly and gamma globulin or plasma exchange need to be commenced early if they are to be effective.

Infant botulism

- Suspect in children 2–9 months of age with constipation and rapid onset of weakness, particularly with ophthalmoplegia and bulbar/respiratory weakness.
- A child with suspected infant botulism should be transferred urgently to a centre capable of undertaking long-term ventilation.

Spinal cord compression

- Persistant or severe back pain and stiffness are ominous symptoms requiring prompt attention.
- Myelopathy should always be considered when there is paraparesis or quadriparesis without neurological dysfunction at higher levels.
- Brisk deep tendon reflexes or extensor plantar responses may not be prominent early and a sensory level is often the most important clue to a myelopathy.
- The confirmation or exclusion of trauma, tumour, abscess, haematoma or skeletal anomaly is an urgent priority.
- Spinal imaging is required even when acute 'transverse' myelopathy is suspected.
- Steroid therapy is important in spinal cord compression prior to decompression.

ENCEPHALOPATHIES

Characterised predominantly (but not exclusively) by cerebral hemispheric dysfunction producing at least two of the following;

- Altered conscious state.
- Altered cognitive state/personality.
- Seizures.

The onset can be acute, sub-acute or chronic.

Causes can be grouped into infective (or post-infective), hypoxic, traumatic, epileptic, metabolic, migrainous, raised intracranial pressure and drug or toxin exposure. The primary cause may be systemic or originate in the CNS (see also Encephalitis, Infectious diseases, chapter 27).

Examination

- Often widespread upper motor neurone signs. Meningism may or may not be present.

Investigations

Investigations are guided by history and examination. Consider the following:

- Electrolytes.
- Toxin and metabolic screen.

- Cerebrospinal fluid (microscopy and culture; viral and mycoplasma PCR). *Note*: Contraindications to lumbar puncture (see Procedures, chapter 4).
- EEG.
- Neuroimaging: CT can exclude a mass lesion or acute bleed, but MRI is preferable in most circumstances. Magnetic resonance imaging of the brain and spinal cord may show multifocal demyelination as is seen in Acute Disseminated Encephalomyelitis (ADEM).

Management

- Early specialist referral.
- Identify and treat the primary cause.
- Remember:
  - Adequate seizure control.
  - Consider empiric antimicrobials e.g. cefotaxime and aciclovir (see Infectious diseases, chapter 27).
  - If ADEM is suspected consider high dose i.v. corticosteroids.
  - Early neurosurgical referral if raised intracranial pressure is suspected.

Acute disseminated encephalomyelitis

Acute disseminated encephalomyelitis (ADEM) is a monophasic inflammatory condition of the central nervous system that most commonly affects children and young adults. The usual presentation is with altered conscious state and multifocal neurological disturbance. It typically occurs following a viral prodrome and has been described following a variety of infections including measles, varicella, EBV, *Mycoplasma pneumoniae* and non-specific febrile illnesses.

Clinical

- A prodrome of ataxia prior to onset is typical.
- Encephalopathy: may vary in severity from irritability to coma.
- Multifocal neurological abnormalities such as ataxia, hemiparesis, optic neuritis and cranial nerve palsies.
- A characteristic feature of ADEM is the evolution of symptoms and signs over time: new neurological symptoms and signs appear over the first few days (whereas in encephalitis, the onset is usually explosive without new manifestations after 24–48 h).

Investigation

- Magnetic resonance imaging is the investigation of choice and usually demonstrates white matter changes (gray matter involvement is not uncommon).

Management

General principles as above. Steroids are used in the treatment of ADEM despite the lack of case-controlled studies to prove their efficacy. Anecdotal evidence of their benefit is now strong. Steroid therapy may improve the patient's condition but withdrawal of treatment while the disease is still active may result in the return of original symptoms, or the development of new ones.

Early studies found a mortality rate of up to 20% with a high incidence of neurological sequelae in those who survived. Recent case reports and small series suggest a more favourable prognosis with most individuals recovering fully.

CHRONIC AND RECURRENT HEADACHE

- Migraine is the most common identifiable cause of recurrent or chronic headache in childhood.
- In adolescence, muscle contraction (tension-type) headache is also important.
- Although rare, raised intracranial pressure and systemic illness must also be considered.
- A careful history, examination and follow up will usually yield the correct diagnosis.

History

- Determine the location of the headache and its quality, duration, frequency and time of onset.
- Identify trigger factors (food, sleep deprivation), associated symptoms (e.g. nausea or vomiting, visual disturbance and localising or focal symptoms) and the disruption to normal activities.
- Inquire whether the symptoms are progressive and if there is a family history of migraine or cerebral tumours; recent head

injury; development of visual, gait or coordination difficulties; or changes in personality or intellectual functioning.

- Take a detailed social history.

Distinguishing features

- Migraine without aura is usually a frontotemporal or bilateral headache and in older children it is frequently accompanied by nausea and vomiting, followed by lethargy or sleep. Marked pallor is common and there is commonly a positive family history.
- Migraine headaches with aura or prolonged neurological symptoms are uncommon in young children.
- Migraine has a fluctuating temporal pattern, while tension-type headache tends to be persistent but usually does not interfere with sleep.
- Recurrent morning headaches; headaches that are intense, prolonged and incapacitating or that show a progressive change in character over time suggest intracranial pathology. Such patients, or those with abnormal examination findings, the rarer variants of migraine or those who do not respond to simple treatment measures, require specialist referral.

Examination

- Measure head circumference and blood pressure.
- Auscultate the skull for intracranial bruits; palpate over the sinuses, cervical spine and teeth.
- Perform a thorough neurological examination, including examination of visual acuity and fields, eye movements, optic fundi, coordination and gait.
- Assess the child's growth and pubertal status; inspect the skin for neurocutaneous stigmata.

Management of migraine

- Reassuring the child and parents that migraine is not usually a serious condition is an important part of its management.
- In migraine, trigger avoidance, stress management and the early use of paracetamol 15 mg/kg per dose orally, 4-hourly (max 90 mg/kg per 24 h) during an acute attack is frequently all that is required. Non-steroidal anti-inflammatory medications (e.g.

ibuprofen 2.5–10 mg/kg per dose (max 600 mg) orally, 6–8-hourly) can be useful in the acute attack. The role of sumatriptan in childhood is not yet clear.
- Prophylactic therapy for those with severe or frequent attacks is best used in consultation with a specialist. Propranolol or pizotifen are commonly used. Sodium valproate is also effective in some children with recurrent or chronic migraine syndromes. Other prophylactic agents that can be used include cyproheptadine and amitriptyline.
- Two-thirds of children cease having attacks but 50% of these have recurrences in adult life.

ABNORMAL HEAD SHAPE

Craniosynostosis is an uncommon disorder of childhood affecting 4/10,000 children. It is a condition of premature fusion of the cranial sutures resulting in an abnormal head shape.

The resulting head shape depends on which suture fuses. The common shapes are:
- Scaphocephaly (sagittal suture).
- Brachycephaly (coronal suture).
- Plagiocephaly (lambdoid suture).

The main problem is cosmetic with a small proportion also having intracranial hypertension.

Management

Frank sutural synostosis requires surgical correction.

Postural lambdoid plagiocephaly is not associated with sutural fusion in most cases and as such, may correct spontaneously with changes in sleeping position.

HEAD INJURIES

Assessment

It is essential to determine the nature of the injury, its severity, the time of occurrence and the clinical course prior to the consultation.

Table 30.3 Level of consciousness – Glasgow coma scale

Eye opening		*Verbal Response (modifications for small children in italics)*		*Motor Response*	
Spontaneous	4	Orientated *Appropriate words or social smile, fixes, follows*	5	Obeys commands	6
To speech	3	Confused *Cries but consolable*	4	Localises to stimuli	5
To pain	2	Inappropriate words *Persistently irritable*	3	Withdraws to stimuli	4
Nil	1	Incomprehensible words *Restless & agitated*	2	Abnormal flexion	3
		Nil	1	Extensor responses	2
				Nil	1

- General and neurological examination findings will provide a baseline for further assessment and must be carefully recorded. In the unconscious patient the presence of brain stem signs must be assessed.
- Assessment using the Glasgow coma chart is essential (see Table 30.3).
- Cervical spine injury must also be diagnosed or excluded as it may occur in association with head injury.

Radiological examination

- A skull X-ray is not performed routinely in patients presenting with a non-localised head injury and is not used to determine whether a child requires admission. If a child is assessed as being clinically unwell after a head injury, they should be transferred immediately to a centre with paediatric neurosurgical expertise; the transfer should not be delayed by the taking of a skull X-ray.
- If the child is unwell enough to warrant a skull X-ray, they should be in hospital under observation. There is no place for a skull X-ray 'just in case'. The only exception is the child with a large scalp haematoma who is otherwise perfectly well, where a depressed skull fracture cannot be excluded clinically.
- A cervical spine X-ray is necessary when there is a suggestion that the spine may have been injured and in all patients with severe head injuries.

- A CT scan is indicated in all patients with significant head injury, particularly if there is the possibility of an intracranial haematoma, as suggested by severe headache and vomiting, a depressed conscious state or focal neurological signs.
- An MRI is indicated in those children in whom there is suspicion of a spinal cord injury or a vascular injury or anomaly.

Blunt head injury

This form of injury is due to an impact on a flat surface that produces an acceleration-deceleration type of injury.

Effects

- *Scalp haematomas*: are common in the infant or young child, they may be responsible for a significant reduction in the circulating blood volume.
- *Skull fracture*: significant injuries may not necessarily have a skull fracture, but the majority do. Conversely, a skull fracture may not be associated with significant brain injury. The fracture is usually linear and it may extend to the skull base. The involvement of the nasal, paranasal or middle ear spaces implies that the injury is compound, with a risk of infection. Check for CSF rhinorrhoea or otorrhoea.
- *Concussion*: the duration of unconsciousness is an indicator of the severity of the concussion.
- *Localised brain damage*: this is due to either local deformity at impact (which is not generally an important factor except for some injuries in infancy), or surface laceration of the brain due to brain movement within the skull.
- *Intracranial haemorrhage*: subarachnoid and subdural haemorrhages are usually due to a surface laceration of the brain. In extradural haemorrhage, a dural vessel is torn by distortion at or near the point of impact, especially if on the lateral aspect of the head.
- Intracerebral haemorrhage may result from local damage or a shearing injury within the brain.

Clinical course

Most patients rapidly recover from the effects of concussion in 12–24 h. A delay or reversal of recovery suggests haemorrhage, brain swelling, infection or an extracranial complication – most commonly an impairment of ventilation (hypercarbia → brain swelling).

Management

Mild

- A brief loss of consciousness (<5 min) without other neurological symptoms or signs suggests a mild injury and these patients can be sent home after an initial 4 h observation in emergency.
- An adequate explanation and written information must be given to the parents regarding signs suggesting deterioration and indications for re-presentation (see below).
- The patient should be reviewed the following day, either by the local medical officer or in emergency.

Blows to the side of the head are potentially serious and these patients should be admitted.

Serious

A more serious head injury is indicated by:

- A longer period of unconsciousness.
- Increasingly severe headache with or without vomiting.
- A deterioration in the conscious state, behaviour or vital signs.
- Neurological defects.
- Bleeding or CSF leak from the nose or ear.
- Severe bleeding from a scalp wound.
- A superficial haematoma on the side of the head may be associated with an extradural haematoma, even if no fracture is seen on the X-ray.

Children with these signs will require admission and must be observed carefully for at least 48 h.

Delayed presentation

These can be grouped into four categories:

- Symptoms and signs as described for potentially serious head injuries – admit.
- Patients with a wide linear fracture and a large scalp haematoma – admit.
- Patients with a skull X-ray showing a narrow linear fracture, but who do not require admission on clinical grounds – discuss with a neurosurgeon.
- Apparently well patients – send home after appropriate advice, with instructions to return immediately if there is any deterioration.

Localised head injury

In these injuries the damage is predominantly confined to a focal area of the head. Injuries of this type are relatively more common in children than in adults.

Effects

- Simple or compound depressed fractures are common.
- Infection may occur with compound injuries.
- Focal contusion or laceration of the brain may be present to a varying size or depth, and may produce neurological signs or seizures.
- Concussion may be absent.

Management

- X-rays are always required and should be performed as part of the admission including, where indicated, tangential views. Computed tomography (CT) is indicated in focal injuries.
- Admission for neurosurgical assessment is required in most cases.
- To prevent wound infection all patients with external compound head injuries should receive antibiotics (flucloxacillin i.v., with contamination add gentamicin i.v. and metronidazole i.v.) and the wound covered by a head dressing. Prophylactic antibiotics are not indicated, however, for patients with internal compound fractures (base of skull) with CSF leaks. These patients should be observed closely and, if they develop a fever with no obvious focus, given empiric antibiotics (e.g. flucloxacillin 50 mg/kg (max 2 g) i.v. 4–6-hourly and cefotaxime 50 mg/kg (max 2 g) i.v. 6-hourly).

Head injury instructions to parents

For the next 24 h keep a careful watch over the patient who should be roused at least every 2 h. The child must be reassessed immediately if the parent notices any of the following:

- The child becomes unconscious or more difficult to rouse.
- The child becomes confused, irrational or delirious.
- There are convulsions or spasms of the face and limbs.
- The child complains of persistent headache or has neck stiffness.
- Repeated vomiting.
- Bleeding from the ear or recurrent watery discharge from the ear or nose.

CARE OF THE UNCONSCIOUS PATIENT

- Maintain the airway.
- Observe for vital and basal neurological signs.
- Protect the cervical spine.
- Ensure temperature regulation.
- Fluid and electrolyte balance.
- Nasogastric aspiration to avoid the inhalation of gastric contents (orogastric if the base of the skull is fractured).

Anticipate complications

Early evaluation is essential to assess the development of complications, such as compression and infection. Observing for complications associated with extracranial injury is also important. The patient who is not improving should be referred to a neurosurgeon.

CEREBROSPINAL FLUID SHUNT PROBLEMS

Subacute shunt obstruction

Cause

- *Upper end block*. The tube is too long or blocked by the choroid plexus.
- *Lower end block*. The tube is too short or blocked by abdominal tissues.
- *Fracture/disconnection.*

Symptoms

- Headache.
- Drowsiness.
- Vomiting.
- Fits.
- The same as a previous episode.

Signs

- Fontanelle tension.
- Abnormal cranial percussion note.
- Focal neurological signs.

- Change in vital signs.
- Deterioration in the conscious state.
- Recent increase in head circumference in infants.

Specific signs

- *Upper end block.* The pump depresses but it does not refill.
- *Lower end block.* The pump is difficult to depress. An X-ray of the chest or abdomen will give an indication of the length of the tube.
- *Fracture/disconnection.* The signs depend on the site of the disconnection. Ventricular tube disconnection is unusual and has the same signs as upper end block. Pump disconnection produces local swelling. Fracture along the course of the tubing may produce local swelling. X-rays may demonstrate a disconnection.

Assessment

The neurosurgeon will want to know the:

- Symptoms and signs, including the state of the pump and shunt tubing.
- Findings on plain X-ray, CT head or ultrasound.
- Type of shunt: atrial or peritoneal.

Shunt infection

These infections are often indolent and should be suspected in any child with a shunt who is constitutionally unwell with fevers. There may be associated obstruction, with symptoms and signs as above.

CHAPTER 31
ORTHOPAEDIC CONDITIONS

Kerr Graham
Peter Barnett

NEONATAL ORTHOPAEDIC CONDITIONS

Developmental dysplasia of the hip

This condition was previously known as congenital dislocation of the hip; however, not all cases are present at birth and the hips are not necessarily dislocated. Risk factors are breech delivery, caesarean section, family history, congenital foot abnormality, other congenital anomalies, being the first-born and being female.

Diagnosis

General screening

All neonates should have a clinical examination for hip joint instability: the Ortolani and Barlow tests. The baby should be relaxed. With the knee flexed, the thumb is placed over the lesser trochanter and the middle finger over the greater trochanter. The pelvis is steadied with the other hand and the flexed thigh is abducted and adducted. Any clunk or jerk where a dislocation reduces allowing the hip to abduct fully, is a positive Ortolani's sign. The demonstration of acetabular dislocation by levering the femoral head in and out of the acetabulum is a positive Barlow's sign (see Figure 31.1).

Selective screening

Infants in high-risk groups and those with an abnormal routine clinical screening examination should have an ultrasound examination of their hips.

- As clinical diagnosis can be difficult and ultrasound has diagnostic limitations, the repeated examination of children during the first year of life is important.
- X-rays are helpful after 3 months.

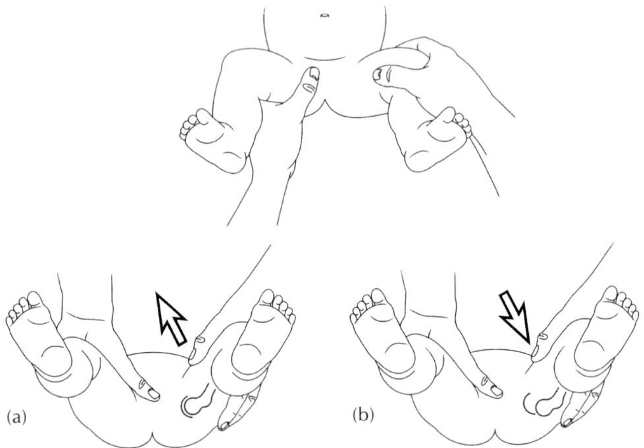

Fig. 31.1 Screening for developmental dysplasia of the hip. (a) Ortolani's sign, (b) Barlow's sign.

Management

The earlier the diagnosis, the easier the management.

- Most neonates can be successfully treated by abduction bracing with a Pavlik harness.
- Operative treatments, including open reduction, may be required with later diagnosis.

Club foot (congenital talipes equinovarus)

Most infants with abnormal-looking feet are said to have 'talipes'. However, the majority have postural problems such as talipes calcaneovalgus (excessive dorsiflexion and eversion), metatarsus varus (adduction of the forefoot) or postural talipes equinovarus (see Figure 31.2). These deformities are usually mild and mobile; that is, they correct easily and fully with the pressure of one finger. They resolve spontaneously with no treatment.

The true club foot deformity is more severe and is often stiff. The foot is in equinus, with the hind foot in varus and the forefoot supinated.

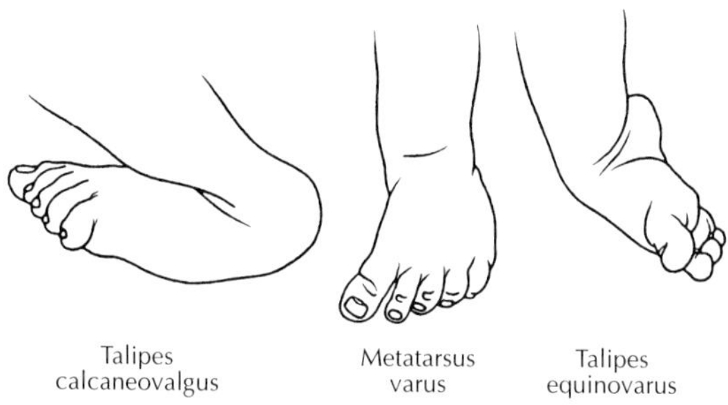

Fig. 31.2 Congenital foot deformities

Management

- All require manipulation and casting.
- Soft tissue surgery is required for many.
- Bone surgery is required for a few.

TORSIONAL AND ANGULAR DEFORMITIES IN CHILDREN

Many children are seen with normal angular or torsional variants. It can be difficult to distinguish physiological variation from pathological conditions. The range of 'normality' is very wide, but what parents accept is much narrower. The physiological variations in normal children can result in as much anxiety as the pathological disorders.

Intoeing

Intoeing in childhood can be due to metatarsus varus, internal tibial torsion or medial femoral torsion.

See Table 31.1, Figures 31.3 and 31.4.

Out-toeing

Infants and toddlers have restricted internal rotation at the hip because of an external rotation soft tissue contracture, not retroversion of the femur.

Table 31.1 Intoeing in childhood

	Metatarsus varus	*Internal tibial torsion*	*Medial femoral torsion*
Synonyms	Metatarsus adductus		Inset hips
Age at presentation	Birth	Toddler	Child
Site of problem	Foot	Tibia	Femur
Examination	Sole of foot bean shaped	Thigh–foot angle is inwards	Arc of hip rotation favours internal rotation
Management	Observe or cast	Observe and reassure	Observe, rarely surgery
When to refer if not resolved	3 months after presentation	6 months after presentation	8 years after presentation

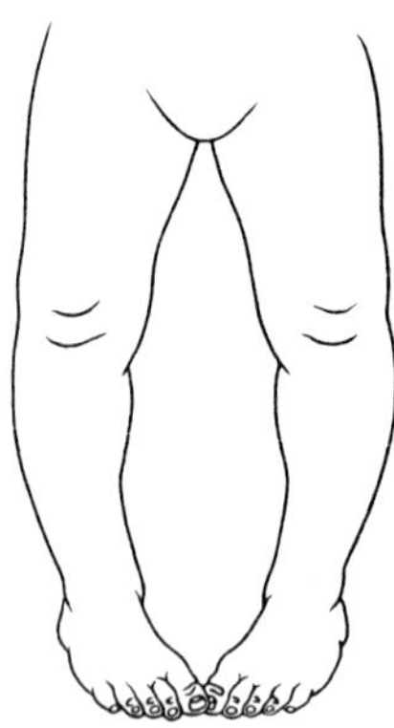

Fig. 31.3 Internal tibial torsion

Infants

- Present with a 'Charlie Chaplin' posture between 3–12 months.
- The child weight bears and walks normally.
- Resolution occurs with no treatment.

Children

- May be due to neurologic disorder.
- Surgery may be necessary.

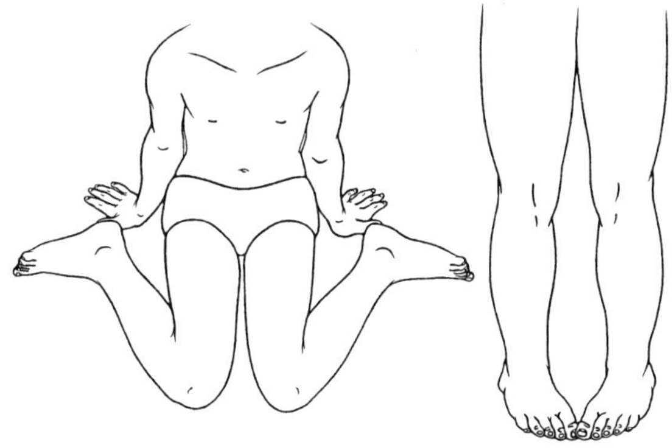

Fig. 31.4 Medial femoral torsion

Bow-legs (genu varum)

The vast majority are physiological. Rare causes include skeletal dysplasias, rickets and Blount's disease (tibia vara).

Presentation

- Toddlers are usually bowed until 3 years of age.
- Physiological bowing is symmetrical, not excessive and improves with time.

Management

Monitor intercondylar separation (ICS; see Figure 31.5). Refer when ICS is greater than 6 cm, is not improving or when it is asymmetric.

Knock-knees (genu valgum)

Again, the vast majority are physiological. Rare causes are rickets and trauma.

Presentation

- Children are usually knock-kneed from 3–8 years.
- Physiological knock-knee is symmetrical, not excessive and improves with time.

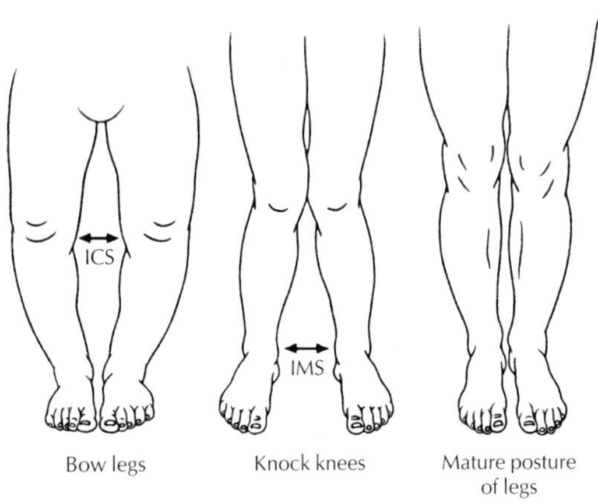

Fig. 31.5 Postural variants in the lower limbs

Management

- Monitor the intermalleolar separation (IMS; see Figure 31.5).
- Refer if IMS greater than 8 cm.

Note: Most children with bow-legs or knock-knees are normal with <1% having an underlying problem.

Flat feet (pes plano valgus)

This condition is painless and asymptomatic. *Note*: If painful or stiff, referral is needed.

Causes

- Physiological (in the vast majority): all newborns have flat feet due to fat that fills the medial longitudinal arch; 80% of children develop a medial arch by their sixth birthday.
- Tarsal coalition (in older children and adolescents only).

Management

- No treatment is required unless the condition is painful or stiff.
- The condition is unaffected by orthotics or exercises.
- The majority of cases resolve spontaneously.

TRAUMA

The management of fractures and dislocations is an integral part of the overall management of the trauma patient. Common fractures in children involve the wrist, elbow, clavicle, distal tibia, fibula and femur. Each has distinct management strategies but there are common themes.

Assessment

Patients presenting with a suspected fracture or dislocation require a full evaluation of the fracture and exclusion of damage to other structures.

An accurate history of the mechanism of injury will determine which structures may potentially be damaged.

Note: Consider child abuse in infants with fractures (see Child abuse, chapter 14).

Examination

- Closed or open fracture (the latter will require operative intervention).
- Deformity or swelling. *Note*: acute swelling in children usually indicates a fracture.
- Neurological status distal to the injury.
- Peripheral pulses – if the blood flow to the limb is compromised, emergency orthopaedic consultation is necessary.

Management

- The affected limb should be splinted by a board or plaster slab prior to an X-ray.
- Analgesia (usually parenteral) is required (e.g. morphine 0.05–0.1 mg/kg dose i.v.).
- An X-ray should be obtained of the suspected fracture site, with additional views to include the joints above and below the suspected fracture site. An anteroposterior and lateral view should be obtained.
- If the angle between the shaft of the bone and the fractured fragment is greater than 15–20°, manipulation of the fracture needs to occur prior to the placement of a plaster. Forearm fractures in children 6 years or older can usually be manipulated using a local anaesthetic block (e.g. Bier's block, see Procedures, chapter 4).

- If the fracture involves both cortices of the bone, plaster the joints above and below (e.g. above the elbow for a forearm fracture).
- A simple undisplaced greenstick or buckle fracture can be treated in a short cast/backslab.

Home treatment after a full plaster

- Elevate the limb above the heart level for the next 24–48 h.
- A sling should only be worn after this period and the hand should not be below the elbow while in the sling.
- Crutches should only be used by children over 6–7 years of age.
- Written plaster instructions should be explained and given to parents.

Follow up

For patients who have had a manipulation of fracture or a fracture involving both cortices of the bone, a repeat X-ray should be obtained in 1 week to ensure the correct position is maintained. Plaster should remain in place for 3–6 weeks, depending on the degree of injury. Following the removal of the cast, the bone is still at risk of re-fracture for the next 8–12 weeks; therefore, contact sports are not recommended during this period.

Description of fractures

It can be useful to use a specific, technical vocabulary to describe fractures for the purposes of documentation, or discussion with a colleague. The issues to be considered are:

- The anatomical site of the fracture – which bone? Which side? For example, right humerus or left tibia. In most long bones it is helpful to specify whether the fracture is in the upper, middle or distal third of the bone.
- The fracture type should be specified i.e. open or closed. An open fracture has a wound which communicates with the exterior, a closed fracture has an intact soft tissue envelope.
- Further description of the actual appearance of the fracture line, e.g. transverse, oblique, spiral or comminuted (more than one fragment).
- The displacement of the fracture should be described e.g. undisplaced, angulated or displaced. Angulation is described by drawing a line along both major fragments and measuring the angle of intersection. Displacement is best described by comparing the

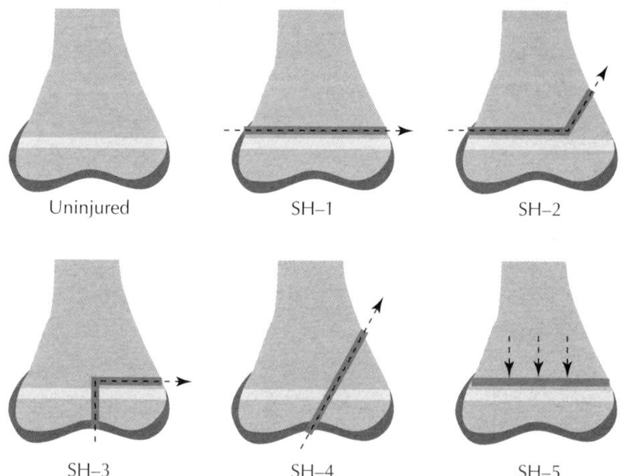

Fig. 31.6 Salter Harris (SH) classification of growth plate injuries.

displacement of the bone ends with the width of the bone at that point e.g. half a diameter displaced or completely displaced.

- Fractures in the expanded ends of long bones are usually described as metaphyseal and injuries to the growth plate are described according to the Salter Harris classification (see Figure 31.6).

From these terms, a complete description of any fracture can be given that should be meaningful to a colleague who cannot see the X-rays. For example, a femoral shaft fracture might be described as a closed, displaced, midshaft fracture of the left femur with 30° of angulation and one complete diameter of displacement.

SPECIFIC MANAGEMENT OF SOME COMMON FRACTURES

Clavicle

- Sling for 2–3 weeks.
- Inform the parents of the lump that will develop at the fracture site and that may be visible for up to 1 year.
- No contact sports for 6 weeks.
- No follow-up X-ray is necessary in children, but it is required in adolescents.

Humerus

Surgical neck

- *Undisplaced*: sling for 3 weeks.
- *Displaced*: frequently treated with a collar and cuff – refer for follow up.

Shaft

- Check the integrity of the radial nerve.
- *Undisplaced*: collar and cuff. A U-shaped plaster slab may be applied to the humerus to reduce movement and minimise knocks.
- *Transverse, displaced or comminuted*: refer for an immediate orthopaedic consultation.

Supracondylar

- Check the integrity of the radial artery, radial nerve, median nerve and ulnar nerve.
- If there is vascular compromise, extend the elbow until perfusion returns.
- *Undisplaced*: collar and cuff (under clothing) with the elbow flexed for 3–4 weeks.
- *Angulated, displaced or comminuted*: refer for an immediate orthopaedic consultation.

Epiphyseal and intra-articular

- Refer for an immediate orthopaedic consultation.

Radius and ulna

Shaft

- *Undisplaced*: above elbow plaster, follow up with an orthopaedic opinion.
- *Displaced*: refer for an immediate orthopaedic consultation.

Distal end

- *Undisplaced and non-deformed clinically*:
  - If a single cortex only is involved, use a short arm cast/backslab for 3–4 weeks.
  - If both cortices are involved, plaster above the elbow – refer for an orthopaedic opinion within a week with repeat X-ray.

- *Displaced and clinically deformed*: use local anaesthesia manipulation plaster (LAMP) in the emergency department.
- *Totally displaced* with fracture ends not touching: use general anaesthesia manipulation plaster (GAMP) in theatre.

Metacarpals

- Check carefully for rotation at the fracture site.
- *Undisplaced*: volar slab; follow up with an orthopaedic opinion.
- *Displaced*: refer for an immediate orthopaedic consultation.

Phalanges (hand)

- Check carefully for rotation at the fracture site.
- Intra-articular fractures require anatomical reduction.
- *Undisplaced*: strap to the adjacent finger for 3–4 weeks.
- *Displaced*: refer for an immediate orthopaedic or plastic surgical consultation; some may be reduced under regional nerve block (see Procedures, chapter 4).

Femur

- Isolated femur fractures in young children rarely cause hypotension; however, in adolescents and patients with multi-trauma an intravenous line should be inserted.
- Ensure adequate analgesia with nitrous oxide, opioids and a femoral nerve block (see Procedures, chapter 4).
- Apply simple skin traction, refer for an immediate orthopaedic consultation.

Tibia

- *Undisplaced proximal or midshaft*: above-knee plaster, follow up with an orthopaedic opinion within 1 week (there is a risk of valgus deformity).
- *Undisplaced distal*: below-knee plaster, follow up with an orthopaedic opinion.
- *Displaced*: will need manipulation, refer for an immediate orthopaedic consultation.

Toddlers' fracture

- This is a clinical diagnosis in a young child where a fractured tibia is suspected on clinical grounds (i.e. non-weight bearing after a fall or tender tibia/fibula on palpation), but no abnormality is detected on X-ray.

- Exclude septic arthritis/osteomyelitis.
- Apply an above-knee plaster for pain relief, or allow weight bearing as the child desires if the pain is minimal.
- Limping will continue for 6 weeks.

Ankle

- *Undisplaced*: below-knee plaster, follow up with an orthopaedic opinion.
- *Displaced*: will need manipulation, refer for an immediate orthopaedic consultation.

Metatarsals

- *Undisplaced*: lower leg plaster slab, followed by elevation, follow up with an orthopaedic opinion within 1 week.

ANKLE INJURY

True sprains or soft tissue injuries are more common in adolescents. Younger children with open growth plates are more likely to sustain a growth plate injury or fracture and should be treated in a plaster cast.

Clinical assessment

- Mechanism of injury – it is usually caused by an inversion injury to the ankle.
- Was the patient able to bear weight immediately after the injury?
- Where is the swelling most prominent?
- What is the point of maximal tenderness?

Investigation

X-rays are required if:

- Deformity is present.
- Maximal tenderness occurs over the tibia or fibula.
- The patient is unable to weight bear.

Note: If the patient is tender over the growth plate of the tibia or fibula and the X-rays are normal, the patient has a Salter-Harris 1 epiphyseal injury and it should be treated in a below-knee plaster. However, if there is a large amount of swelling use a plaster slab.

If none of the above conditions apply, the treatment will depend on the severity of symptoms.

Management: mild–moderate sprain

Remember the RICE acronym:

- *Rest*: weight bearing should not occur for a few days to a period of 2–3 weeks.
- *Ice*: should be applied every 2–3 h for 15 min during the first 48 h; then heat can be applied.
- *Compression*: should be accomplished either with a firm bandage or a plaster slab.
- *Elevation*: the limb should be elevated on a few pillows whenever possible to allow the swelling to subside.

Management: severe sprain

Treat like a fracture:

- Use below-knee plaster (or if the swelling is severe, a plaster slab followed by a full plaster) for 2–4 weeks.
- No weight bearing for the first week.
- Gradual rehabilitation should occur after several days of rest. This includes gentle weight bearing and ankle exercises to strengthen the damaged ankle ligaments (initially plantar- and dorsiflexion exercises as soon as possible; later toe raises and inversion/eversion exercises when the pain has subsided).

PULLED ELBOW

Clinical features

- This injury usually occurs at the age of 1–3 years.
- The cause of injury is usually another person pulling the child's arm forcefully. There may be a crack or popping sound at the time. Occasionally, it may occur after a fall.
- The arm is held pronated and slightly flexed (i.e. limp by their side as if they are ignoring it).
- The child is not distressed and is not using the apparently lifeless limb.
- Palpation from the clavicle to the wrist does not demonstrate any swelling or tenderness.
- Supination of the arm causes pain.

Investigations

If the symptoms are typical of a pulled elbow, no investigations are necessary.

Management

- Hold the child's hand as if to shake it and with your other hand encircle the elbow with the thumb over the annular ligament of the radius.
- Gently apply traction and supinate the hand. Flex the forearm at the elbow all the way to the shoulder. You should feel a pop as the radial head is relocated.
- The child should be moving the arm normally within 10–15 min.

Note: If the history is not typical, there is swelling or your attempts at reduction fail, an X-ray of the elbow should be obtained to exclude a radial head fracture.

LIMP IN CHILDHOOD

Limp is a common presenting complaint in childhood (see Table 31.2).

Clinical assessment

- Is the limp acute, subacute or chronic?
- Is there associated pain or fever or both?
- Are there other constitutional symptoms?
- Have there been previous episodes of pain or limp?
- What position is the leg held in (e.g. flexed and externally rotated)?
- Does joint movement or bony pressure cause pain?
- Is there limitation of movement?

Table 31.2 Differential diagnosis of limp in childhood

Acute	*Subacute*	*Chronic*
Fracture	Juvenile rheumatoid arthritis	Cerebral palsy
Irritable hip	Tumour/leukaemia	Developmental dysplasia of the hips
Septic arthritis	Acute on chronic SCFE	Perthes' disease
Osteomyelitis		Chronic SCFE

SCFE, slipped capital femoral epiphysis.

Investigations

- Full blood examination (FBE), differential, erythrocyte sedimentation rate (ESR) and C-reactive protein (CRP).
- Plain X-ray of the joint or affected limb.
- Ultrasound of hip if it is painful (looking for fluid in the joint).
- Bone scan (after orthopaedic consultation).

Management

This will depend on the underlying problem:

- Slipped capital femoral epiphysis (SCFE), tumours, Perthes' disease or developmental dysplasia of the hip should be referred immediately to an orthopaedic surgeon.
- Toddlers' fractures may be occult and not seen on an X-ray. If the child is afebrile then observation is appropriate.
- A bone scan should be arranged for worsening or changing symptoms.

Irritable hip (transient synovitis)

The usual presentation is a child who is constitutionally well with a partial limp and difficulty walking. This is a common condition. A child who is constitutionally well presents with a painful hip and difficulty walking. This condition needs to be distinguished from the others listed in Table 31.2. Although it is the commonest reason for limp in the preschooler, irritable hip is a diagnosis of exclusion.

Usual clinical features

- Occurs in 3–8 year olds.
- History of a recent viral illness (which lasts 1–2 weeks).
- Absence of trauma.
- Children are able to walk, but with pain.
- Severity of the symptoms may vary with time.
- Child is afebrile and appears well.
- There is a mild to moderate decrease in the range of motion due to pain, particularly internal rotation.

Note: The less movement in the joint, the more likely the cause is infective.

Investigations

- These are the same as for limp (see previous; ultrasound usually demonstrates an effusion).
- X-rays and FBE are normal with an ESR of <20.

Note: The history, symptoms and signs of an irritable hip overlap with septic arthritis, which is a serious condition requiring urgent treatment. If there is any suspicion of bone or joint sepsis, paediatric orthopaedic consultation is required and admission to hospital should be arranged.

Management

Rest in bed and simple analgesics are the treatment of choice. The more the child can rest, the quicker the recovery. Patients may have a relapse if they increase their activity too quickly. Occasionally, these patients need to be admitted to hospital for bed rest and observation.

Acute bone and joint sepsis: septic arthritis and osteomyelitis

Septic arthritis (SA) and osteomyelitis (OM) can affect any joint or bone, but most commonly involve the lower limbs. **Septic arthritis is an orthopaedic emergency. Drainage and antibiotics are essential to prevent long-term morbidity**.

Clinical features

- Acute onset of limp/non-weight bearing/non-movement of the limb (may be delayed in OM).
- Pain is localised to the joint or the metaphysis of the bone. Hip pain may be referred to knee.
- Irritability and poor feeding in infants.
- Temperature is usually >38.5°C.
- Joint is held in a mid-range position.
- Pain on all movements with a decreased range of movement (severe in SA).

Investigations

(As for limp – see previous).

- ESR is usually >20–30.
- White cell count (WCC) is raised in SA and is usually raised in OM.
- A bone scan may be indicated if the diagnosis is not clear.

Management

- Admit to hospital; keep nil orally.
- Collect all possible specimens for culture **before** starting antibiotics, including blood culture (all patients) and fluid from the involved joint (consult with the orthopaedic team before starting antibiotics).
- Intravenous antibiotics to cover *Staphylococcus aureus*. Cover should be broadened in neonates and children who have not had Hib vaccine to include *Haemophilus influenzae* and other Gram-negative organisms. See Antimicrobial guidelines.
- Duration of antibiotics: for uncomplicated, acute haematogenous septic arthritis and osteomyelitis, intravenous antibiotics are required until defervescence, improvement in symptoms and signs and evidence of reduced inflammatory markers (CRP falls before ESR). This is often 3–5 days. Oral antibiotics are then administered to complete a minimum 3-week course. For disease with any evidence of complication (duration of symptoms ≥ 14 days, changes of chronicity on plain X-ray, any underlying disease, penetrating injury or delayed response to treatment) intravenous treatment should be prolonged for at least 7–14 days and the total duration of treatment should be at least 4–6 weeks.

Urgent paediatric orthopaedic consultation and possibly surgery is required.

Perthes' disease

This is a specific hip disease of childhood. Affected children have a generalised disorder of growth with a tendency to low birthweight and delayed bone age. The pathology is avascular necrosis of the capital femoral epiphysis followed by a sequence of changes including resorption of necrotic bone, reossification and remodelling. This sequence of events is seen radiologically as density of the capital epiphysis, patchy osteolysis, new bone formation and remodelling with a variable degree of femoral head deformity.

Clinical features

- Age range: 2–12 years, but the majority present between 4 and 8 years.
- Sex ratio: 5 males to 1 female, 20% bilateral.
- Symptoms: pain and limp, usually for at least 1 week.
- Signs: restriction of hip motion.

Investigations

- X-ray.
- A bone scan is useful in the early stages before the signs are clear on X-ray.

Management principles

- Resting the hip in the early irritable phase.
- Regaining motion if the hip is stiff.
- Containing the hip by bracing or surgery in selected patients.

Slipped capital femoral epiphysis

Can occur acutely or chronically. Early detection will prevent later morbidity.

Clinical features

- Age: this occurs in late childhood to early adolescence. Maximum incidence in girls aged 10–12 years and boys 12–14 years.
- Weight is usually >90th percentile.
- Pain in the hip or knee (often pain only in the knee).
- Limp.
- The hip appears externally rotated and shortened.
- Decreased hip movement, particularly internal rotation.
- The condition can be bilateral.

Investigation

Take an X-ray of the pelvis and a frog leg lateral of the affected hip.

Management

- The patient should not weight bear if this diagnosis is considered.
- Urgent orthopaedic referral and surgery to prevent further slipping is required.

SCOLIOSIS

Definitions

- Scoliosis is a curvature in the spine when viewed from the frontal (coronal) plane.
- A structural scoliosis occurs when the curvature has an element of rotation and may progress with growth.
- A non-structural scoliosis may be secondary to a problem outside the spine, such as unequal leg lengths.

Detection

The most common type of scoliosis is adolescent scoliosis, affecting girls in 90% of cases. Because abnormal spinal curvatures start small and may progress with time and growth, efforts have been made to detect the condition at an early stage by school screening programs. This is usually done by the forward bend test, in which the examiner observes the spine from behind as the subject bends forwards. Flexion of the spine usually demonstrates the deformity much more clearly because of the asymmetry of the ribs and chest wall. Very small curves are relatively common and it can be difficult to decide when an X-ray is required, which curves are likely to progress and which require brace treatment or surgery. The risk of curve progression is related to the age at presentation and the size and cause of the curve.

Ten per cent of normal adolescents have a curve of 5° or more, but only 2% have curves of >10°.

Management

All children with scoliosis should be referred to a paediatric orthopaedic surgeon.

- If the curvature <20° – observe.
- If the curvature is 20–40° – a brace is recommended.
- If the curvature is >40° – surgery is required.

CHAPTER 32
RENAL CONDITIONS AND ENURESIS

Colin Jones
Annie Moulden

Significant renal disease in childhood usually presents in one of the following ways:

- Antenatal ultrasound abnormality of the urinary tract.
- Urinary tract infection (UTI).
- Functional voiding disorder.
- Proteinuria (including nephrotic syndrome).
- Haematuria.
- Hypertension.
- Acute renal failure.
- Chronic renal failure.

ANTENATAL ABNORMALITIES

See Figure 32.1. Antenatal abnormalities.

URINARY TRACT INFECTIONS

All children with a first UTI need investigation.

Diagnosis

Urine infections are diagnosed by bacterial growth on midstream urine (MSU), catheter (CSU) or suprapubic aspirate (SPA) specimens of urine. A clean catch specimen is prone to contamination.

Bag urine specimen collection

- Do not send for culture.
- Use for initial screening only.
- In sick infants or those where the suspicion of UTI is high (e.g. renal tract anomaly or previous UTI), a bag specimen **should not**

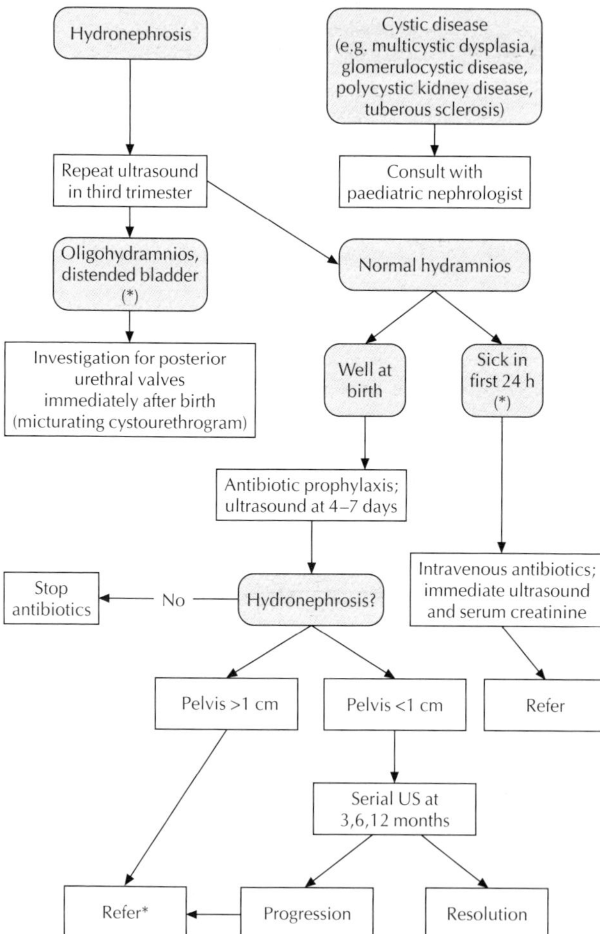

* Consult a paediatric nephrologist or urologist early in all cases

Fig. 32.1 Antenatal abnormalities

be taken, as it only delays the diagnosis. A SPA (preferred) or CSU sample should be obtained as part of the septic workup (see Infectious diseases, chapter 27).

Urine 'ward test' strips

Are useful as a screening test in a child with a low suspicion of a UTI, not as a diagnostic test in a child with a high chance of a UTI. The ward test strips for leucocytes or nitrites are negative in up to 15% of UTI in infants when organism counts are high and are negative in 50% or more of cases with low counts of organisms.

Midstream urine specimen collection

This can be obtained from children who are able to void on request (usually by 3–4 years of age). The child's genitalia are first washed with warm water. In girls the labia should be separated. The child is asked to void. After passing the first few millilitres, a specimen is collected.

- A pure growth of 10^8 c.f.u./L in a MSU is proof of a UTI.
- A pure growth of $>10^5$–10^8 c.f.u./L in a MSU is suggestive of a UTI (correlate with clinical setting).
- Up to 50% of urine specimens from patients with symptomatic UTI have no pyuria or nitrituria.

Suprapubic aspirate collection

(See Procedures, chapter 4)

- Aspirated urine should be sterile, hence any pure growth of bacteria indicates infection.

Catheter specimen collection

(See Procedures, chapter 4)

- These are useful in infants after a failed SPA or in older children who are unable to void on request. A pure growth of $>10^5$ c.f.u./L indicates infection.

Management

- Blood culture and electrolytes.
- Do not omit an LP in a sick child just because UTI has been diagnosed. All infants <3 months should have a lumbar puncture. Consider a lumbar puncture in all infants aged 3 months–2 years.

- Most infants <12 months of age with a UTI and older children with acute pyelonephritis (fever, vomiting and loin/abdominal pain) require benzyl penicillin 60 mg/kg i.v. (max 2 g) 6-hourly and gentamicin 7.5 mg/kg i.v. (<10 yr) or 6.0 mg/kg i.v. (>10 yr) (max 240 mg) daily.
- In older children without pyelonephritis, a 5-day course of oral antibiotics is usually sufficient (see Antimicrobial guidelines). Antibiotic sensitivity should be checked when available (usually at 48 h).
- In children at high risk of recurrent UTI (<12 months old, strong family history of vesico-ureteric reflux or recurrent UTI) prophylactic antibiotics should be commenced immediately after the treatment antibiotic course has finished.
- Prophylactic antibiotics should be continued until the minimal initial investigations have been performed and a decision is then made on the basis of the anatomy of the urinary tract and other clinical indicators (see Figure 32.2). See also Antimicrobial guidelines.
- For neonates <1 month old or preterm infants, discuss with a specialist.

Minimal initial follow-up investigations

Forty per cent of children with UTI have renal tract abnormalities, including vesico-ureteric reflux (VUR; 35%), reflux nephropathy (renal scarring; 12%), pelvi-ureteric junction (PUJ) or vesico-ureteric junction (VUJ) obstruction (together 4–6%), and other congenital abnormalities.

The following can be helpful:

- Renal ultrasound (U/S). Early renal U/S is required if infant <12 months old or obstruction suspected.
- A DMSA scan performed 2–4 years after the last UTI to indicate whether the renal injury requires further follow up.
- Micturating cystourethrogram (MCU) is recommended in children under 1 year of age where there is clinical evidence of bladder dysfunction (palpable bladder that does not empty, poor urinary stream), increased serum creatinine or the U/S shows hydroureter, hydronephrosis or renal abnormality. In the child with recurrent UTI the demonstration of VUR may lead to the use of prophylactic antibiotics until the child is able to perform a midstream urine sample.

Investigation of siblings of a child with vesico-ureteric reflux

- Fifty per cent of siblings of a child will all have or have had VUR. An U/S should be performed.

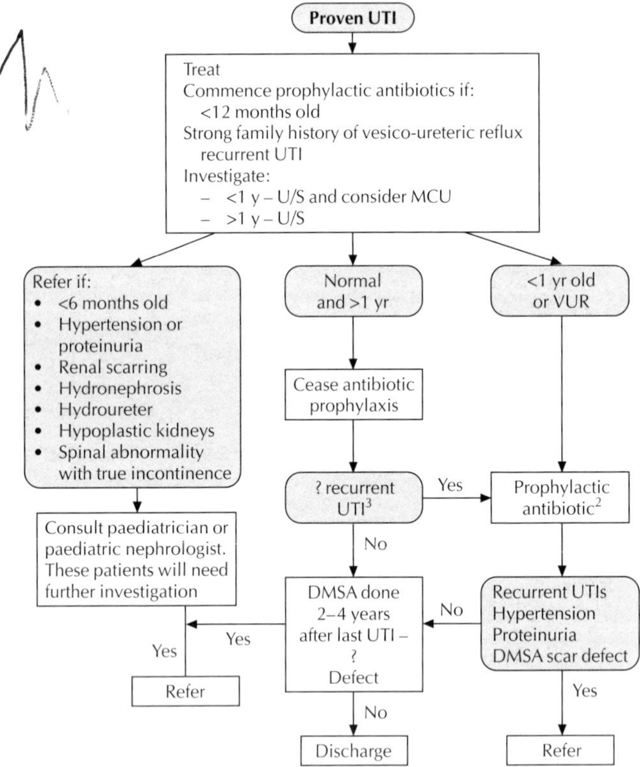

U/S, ultrasound
MCU, micturating cystourethrogram
VUR, vesicoureteric reflux

[1] A normal U/S does not exclude scarring/dysplasia.

[2] The duration of prophylactic antibiotic usage varies with common practice patterns being: (a) until age 1 in patient <1 yr without VUR: (b) until out of nappies (when an MSU can be performed approximately 3–4 yr of age) in patients with VUR

[3] Risk factors in recurrent febrile UTI are VUR, female sex, functional voiding disorders (daytime wetting) and young age. Constipation is associated with bladder dysfunction. Hygeine is rarely a factor

Fig. 32.2 An outline of the management of a proven urinary tract infection

PROTEINURIA

Isolated proteinuria

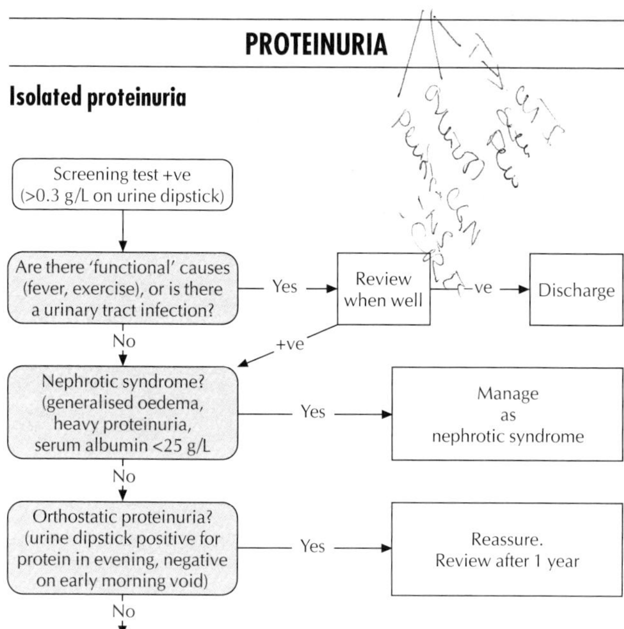

Work-up in consultation with paediatrician/paediatric nephrologist:

History

- Family history of renal disease, deafness
- Medications (e.g. gold, penicillamine, probenecid, amphotericin)
- Other symptoms related to urinary tract or systemic disease

Examination

- Height, weight, blood pressure

Urinalysis (including specific gravity), *microscopy and culture*

Renal function

- Serum creatinine, electrolytes
- 24 h urine collection for protein

Further investigations may be indicated
(e.g. renal ultrasound, protein electrophoresis, C3, serum lipids, renal biopsy)

Fig. 32.3 Isolated proteinuria

Nephrotic syndrome

Diagnosis

The diagnosis of nephrotic syndrome is made on the basis of proteinuria (>40 mg/m^2 per h on a recumbent urine, usually >3 g/1.73 m^2/day; usually 3+ to 4+ on dipstick testing), generalised oedema, hypoalbuminaemia (<25 g/L) and hypercholesterolaemia (>4.5 mmol/L).

Management

Exclude life-threatening complications

- Sepsis (e.g. peritonitis).
- Symptomatic hypovolaemia (e.g. cool extremities and postural hypotension).
- Symptomatic thromboembolism (e.g. venous sinus thrombosis: convulsions and a reduced conscious state; deep venous thrombosis and pulmonary embolism).
- Symptomatic oedema (e.g. marked ascites, respiratory distress with pleural effusions and skin breakdown).

Admit to hospital: for initial assessment and patient and family education.

Medication

(*Note*: Minor variations in protocol may exist between different centres.)

- Administer prednisolone according to the following dosage schedule: prednislone 60 mg/m^2 per day as a single dose up to (max 80 mg/day) for 4 weeks. Then:
  - 40 mg/m^2 alternate day for 4 weeks.
  - 20 mg/m^2 per alternate day for 4 weeks.
  - 15 mg/m^2 per alternate day for 4 weeks.
  - 10 mg/m^2 per alternate day for 4 weeks.
  - 5 mg/ m^2 per alternate day for 4 weeks.
- Phenoxymethylpenicillin: 12.5 mg/kg (max 1 g) oral twice daily to prevent pneumococcal sepsis while oedematous.
- Aspirin: 10 mg/kg per alternate day (to reduce the incidence of arterial thromboses) until oedema clears.

Note: The long-term prognosis of nephrotic syndrome is dependent on the response to prednisolone.

For m^2 formulae, see Appendix 4.

Treatment of complications

- *Symptomatic oedema*: concentrated albumin (i.e. 20%) 1 g/kg (5 mL/kg), i.v. over 4 h with frusemide 1 mg/kg at 2 and 4 h after the start of the infusion.
- *Circulatory insufficiency*: concentrated albumin 1 g/kg, i.v. over 4 h. (Administer frusemide only if the circulation is markedly improved at the end of the infusion – it is dangerous in hypovolaemic patients.)
- *Thromboembolism*: systemic anticoagulation with heparin, followed by warfarin for 3–6 months.
- *Sepsis*: high-dose antibiotic therapy to cover *Streptococcus pneumoniae, Haemophilus influenzae* and *Escherichia coli* (e.g. cefotaxime 50 mg/kg (max 2 g) i.v. 6-hourly).
- *Suspected primary peritonitis*:
  - Use a peritoneal tap to establish diagnosis.
  - If early diagnosis and minimal symptoms, antibiotic therapy alone may be sufficient.
  - Usually requires laparotomy for a peritoneal lavage.

Additional treatments

If the patient does not respond to steroids, refer to a specialist for consideration of cyclophosphamide or cyclosporin A treatment.

Indications for renal biopsy

- Age: <1 year of age.
- Failure to respond to prednisolone within 3–4 weeks of treatment using 60 mg/m^2 per day, either at diagnosis or with relapse.
- Nephritic/nephrotic syndrome (increased blood pressure, moderate haematuria and renal impairment without evidence of peripheral circulatory insufficiency).
- Low complement (C3).

Relapse

Most (75%) patients relapse.

- This is usually precipitated by a febrile illness or an allergic reaction.
- Four days of heavy proteinuria (>100 mg/dL; i.e. 3+ to 4+ on urine dipstick) distinguishes relapse from transient proteinuria associated with a febrile illness.

- Treat with: prednisolone 60 mg/m² per day till proteinuria dip test result in 0, trace or +. Then:
  - 40 mg/m² alternate day for 2 weeks.
  - 20 mg/m² alternate day for 2 weeks.
  - 15 mg/m² alternate day for 2 weeks.
  - 10 mg/m² alternate day for 2 weeks.
  - 5 mg/m² alternate day for 2 weeks.

Use penicillin and aspirin if the patient becomes oedematous (see previous).

Indications for referral

Refer to a specialist in cases of:

- Nephritic/nephrotic syndrome.
- Complications.
- Failure to respond to steroids in 2–3 weeks.
- Frequent relapsing nephrotic syndrome or steroid dependence.

HAEMATURIA

See Figure 32.4: Haematuria assessment.

HYPERTENSION

Measurement of blood pressure

- Use a cuff with a bladder that covers at least 75% of the arm's length.
- Take in the right arm, with the patient sitting; if initially increased, retake after resting quietly.

Definition

The 95th percentiles for blood pressure (BP) at different ages in childhood are as follows:

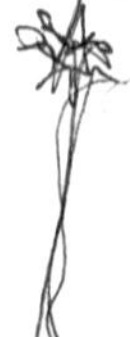

Newborn: 95/70
0–6 years: 115/75
6–13 years: 120/80
13–16 years: 135/85
16–18 years: 140/90

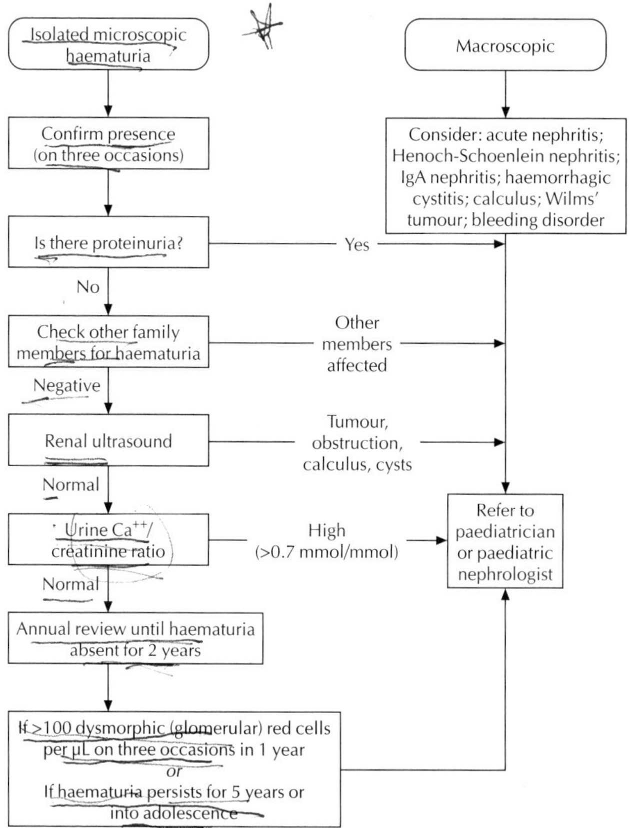

Fig. 32.4 Haematuria assessment

Causes

See Table 32.1.

Cautions

- As in adults, treatment of the asymptomatic child should not be based on a single BP measurement. Blood pressure should be repeated on three occasions to confirm sustained elevation. Twenty-four-hour ambulatory BP monitoring is suitable for most children >5 years of age.

Table 32.1 Causes of secondary hypertension in childhood

Secondary causes	
Renal (75%)	Post-infectious glomerulonephritis Chronic glomerulonephritis Obstructive uropathy Polycystic kidney disease Autosomal recessive Autosomal dominant Reflux nephropathy Renovascular Haemolytic uraemic syndrome
Cardiovascular (15%)	Coarctation of the aorta
Endocrine (5%)	Phaeochromocytoma Hyperthyroidism Congenital adrenal hyperplasia Primary hyperaldosteronism Cushing's syndrome
Other (5%)	Neuroblastoma Neurofibromatosis Glucocorticoids Increased intracranial pressure

- Blood pressure 'tracks' poorly (i.e. only 20–40% of children with BP higher than the 80th percentile still remain in that group 10 years later). Children placed on medication for essential hypertension should undergo a trial of no treatment after their BP has been controlled for 9 months.
- There are no proven advantages of lowering asymptomatic blood pressure in normal children in terms of modifying adult cardiovascular risk.
- Blood pressure reduction slows the progression of renal impairment in people with renal disease. Children with renal impairment should have their BP target range set at less than the mean BP for their age.
- Hypertensive children should be referred to a specialist for investigation for causes outlined in Tables 32.1 and 32.2.
- In asymptomatic hypertension, the BP should be lowered slowly.
- Angiotensin-converting enzyme inhibitors are the usual drug of choice for chronic treatment and should be started in low doses then increased, with monitoring of potassium and creatinine.

Table 32.2 Initial investigation of established hypertension

Urine	MSU, careful urinalysis (dipstick)
	Microscopy
	Urinary catecholamines
Blood	Creatinine
	Potassium
	Bicarbonate
Imaging	Renal ultrasound
	DMSA scan

Management

Asymptomatic hypertension

Refer to a specialist.

Symptomatic hypertension

This requires immediate treatment:

- In a conscious child, who is not vomiting, give a crushed nifedipine tablet by nasogastric tube or swallowed with water. The dose is nifedipine 5 mg oral (<2 years of age); nifedipine 10 mg oral (>2 years of age). Repeat 20 minutely, titrating to BP control.
- In a child with impaired consciousness or vomiting either:
  - Labetalol 0.2 mg/kg i.v. push over 2 min. If no response in 5–10 min, increase to 0.4 mg/kg (max 60 mg) *or*
  - Nitroprusside 0.3–8.0 mcg/kg per min constant infusion (need ICU monitoring), *or*
  - Diazoxide 1 mg/kg i.v. push repeated 5–10 minutely to 5 mg/kg.
- Hypertension due to catecholamine production: phentolamine 0.1 mg/kg i.v. bolus (to 5 mg).
- Head trauma/increased intracranial pressure: labetalol or nitroprusside. *Note*: Nifedipine/diazoxide contraindicated.

GLOMERULONEPHRITIS

Glomerulonephritis presents as either proteinuria, haematuria, hypertension, acute renal failure or chronic renal failure (see appropriate sections). See Table 32.3.

Table 32.3 Types of Glomerulonephritis

Type of Glomerulonephritis (GN)	*Clinical Features*
Thin membrane nephropathy	Microscopic haematuria
Minimal lesion GN	Nephrotic syndrome (oedema, proteinuria, hypoalbuminemia)
Post infectious GN	Nephritic syndrome – microscopic haematuria (often macroscopic), hypertension, oliguria, renal impairment 2–3 weeks following infection
IgA nephropathy	Microscopic haematuria and episodes of haematuria coincident with mucosal infection and loin pain
HSP nephritis	Haematuria, +/– nephrotic/nephritic features
Chronic GN (focal segmental glomerulosclerosis membrano-proliferative GN, membranous GN)	Chronic nephritic – nephrotic syndrome usually with nephrotic features dominating
Acute severe nephritis (SLE nephritis, crescentic GN, ANCA +ve GN, some HSP GN)	Acute nephritic-nephrotic syndrome usually with nephritic features dominating

GN Glomerulonephritis
ANCA Anti neutrophil cytoplasmic antibody
HSP Henoch Schoenlein Purpura

ACUTE RENAL FAILURE

Definition

Acute renal failure is the change in glomerular filtration such that the renal solute load (electrolytes, other ions and nitrogenous wastes) cannot be excreted. There are two main forms:

- *Oliguric*: acute reduction in urine output to <0.5 mL/kg per h. This form is more complex to manage (see Figure 32.5).
- *Polyuric*: often subacute and clinically unapparent, until the fluid intake is reduced and the patient becomes dehydrated due to an inappropriately high urine output.

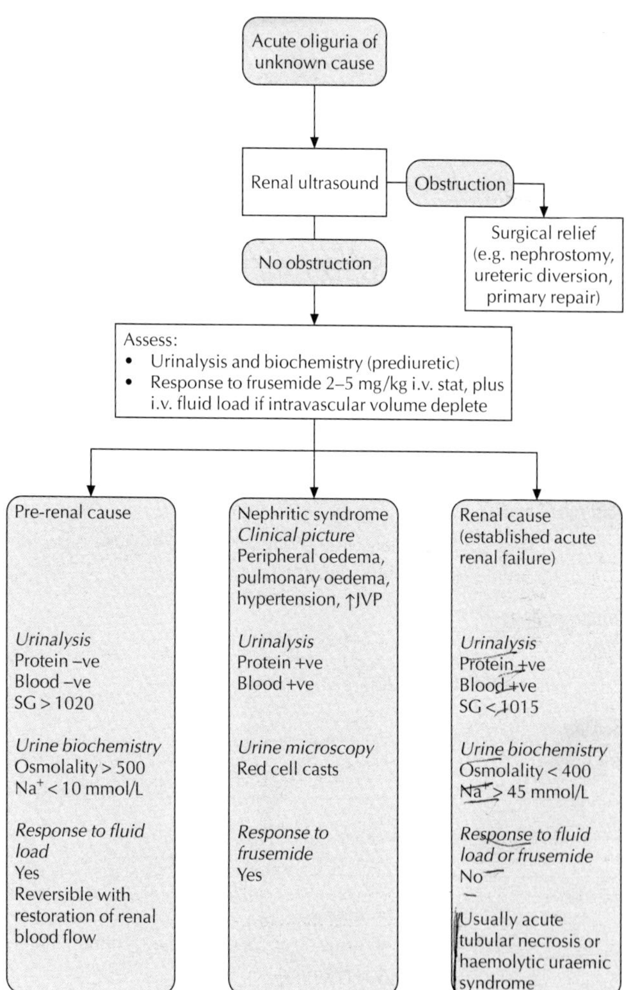

Fig. 32.5 Differentiation of types of oliguria

Causes

Pre-renal

- Dehydration (e.g. gastroenteritis).
- Shock.
- Sepsis.
- Nephrotic syndrome.

Renal

- Crescentic glomerulonephritis: acute post-infectious glomerulonephritis, membranoproliferative glomerulonephritis, Henoch-Schonlein purpura, and antineutrophil cytoplasmic antibody-associated haemolytic uraemic syndrome.
- Acute tubular necrosis.
- Crush injury (myoglobinuria).
- Urinary tract infection with septicaemia.
- Nephrotoxin (e.g. gentamicin).

Post-renal

- Obstruction, especially to a single kidney. The cause is usually apparent from the clinical context of the illness.

Management

Water

Limit to insensible losses (300 mL/m^2) plus urine output.

Sodium

Principle:

Intake = urine sodium + other sodium losses.

- *Oliguric*: minimal Na^+ intake.
- *Polyuric*: measure the urine $[Na]^+$ and volume of urine. Generally, about 75 mmol/L is required.

Potassium

There should be no intravenous or oral intake until losses of K^+ are established.

Hyperkalaemia

- Repeat venous or arterial serum K^+ urgently. Arrange haemofiltration or dialysis in the patient who has renal failure.
- ECG: peaked T waves, wide QRS, increased PR interval, decreased P and R waves, ST segment depression and a prolonged QT interval.
- *If K^+ >7 mmol/L with ECG changes*:
  - 10% calcium gluconate 0.5 mL/kg i.v. over 3–5 min (do not mix with bicarbonate). Works in seconds.
  - Insulin plus concurrent glucose infusion: 0.1 U/kg rapid-acting insulin and 2 mL/kg 50% dextrose. Works in minutes.
  - Arrange dialysis urgently.
- *If K^+ >7 mmol/L, no ECG changes*:
  - $NaHCO_3$ 1–3 mmol/kg (shifts K^+ intracellularly); however, there is the risk of hypocalcaemic tetany with decreased pH. Works within the hour.
  - Dextrose 0.5 g/kg per h (10% dextrose at 5 mL/kg/h) until blood glucose reaches 14 mmol/L (shifts K^+ intracellularly). Works within the hour.
  - Arrange dialysis urgently.
- *If K^+ >6mmol/L*:
  - Na^+ – K^+ exchange resin; e.g. Resonium A, 1 g/kg p.o. (action within 6–12 h) or p.r. (action within 30 min; may repeat in 1–2 h).
  - Arrange dialysis.

Acidosis

Correct with bicarbonate **(mmol = base deficit × weight × 0.3)** over 4 h as long as:

- The patient is not severely hypocalcaemic (HCO_3 may lower Ca and cause convulsions).
- The accompanying Na load does not cause fluid overload (e.g. hypertension and pulmonary oedema).

Hypocalcaemia

This is usually due to increased serum phosphate.

- A low phosphate diet.
- Calcium carbonate (phosphate binder).
- Symptomatic hypocalcaemia may require i.v. calcium gluconate.

- There is a danger of metastatic calcification if the $Ca^{2+} \times PO_4^{3-}$ product is >5–6.
- If there is increased phosphate, consider dialysis.

Uraemia

- An acute rise in serum urea to more than 30 mmol/L may cause CNS symptoms.
- Protein restriction and high-quality protein food are required.
- High carbohydrate diet.

Indications for dialysis/haemofiltration

- Fluid overload (hypertension or pulmonary oedema) not responding to frusemide.
- Hyperkalaemia.
- Severe metabolic acidosis.
- Progressive uraemia.
- Dialysable nephrotoxin.
- Hyperammonaemia.
- The reduction of intravascular volume to facilitate total parenteral nutrition or blood transfusion.

CHRONIC RENAL FAILURE

Presentation

- Known renal disease.
- Growth failure.
- Rickets.
- Anaemia: normochromic, normocytic.
- Laboratory test: increased serum creatinine, increased urea, increased phosphate and metabolic acidosis.
- Radiological studies: small kidney, with other renal disease; e.g. obstruction uropathy.
- Proteinuria.
- Urinary tract infection.

Management

Investigation of the cause and treatment of chronic renal failure should be performed in conjunction with a specialist.

NOCTURNAL ENURESIS

Nocturnal enuresis is defined as bed-wetting in a child 5 years of age or older. It is the second commonest paediatric condition affecting 20% of 5 year olds, 5% of 10 year olds and up to 1% of adults.

Cause

- Enuresis is due to a genetically based arousal disorder (autosomal dominant with variable penetrance) and in some cases an associated nocturnal anti-diuretic hormone (ADH) insufficiency. It is essential to discuss family history, as enuretics are often very relieved to know other family members were affected.
- Enuresis occurs if the bladder becomes full and the child does not wake from sleep.
- All children with enuresis have an arousal disorder that interferes with their ability to wake to bladder distension.
- Nocturnal polyuria due to overnight ADH insufficiency may compound the problem (up to 60% of children with nocturnal enuresis have failed to develop the normal circadian rhythm of ADH secretion).
- Psychological issues are often present but are predominantly due to the enuresis, not the cause of it, and improve with resolution of the wetting.

Management

See Figure 32.6

- The spontaneous remission rate is only 15% per year.
- All children 6 years and over, for whom wetting has become a problem, should be offered treatment.
- Initial measures should include cessation of fluid restriction, treatment of constipation if present and the keeping of charts to document progress. First-line treatment is an alarm; either a bed alarm or a personal alarm. Through a combination of conditioning and other factors this treatment will cure about 60% of children.
- Alarm treatment is most effective when everyone involved is motivated and regular practitioner support is provided during the treatment period.

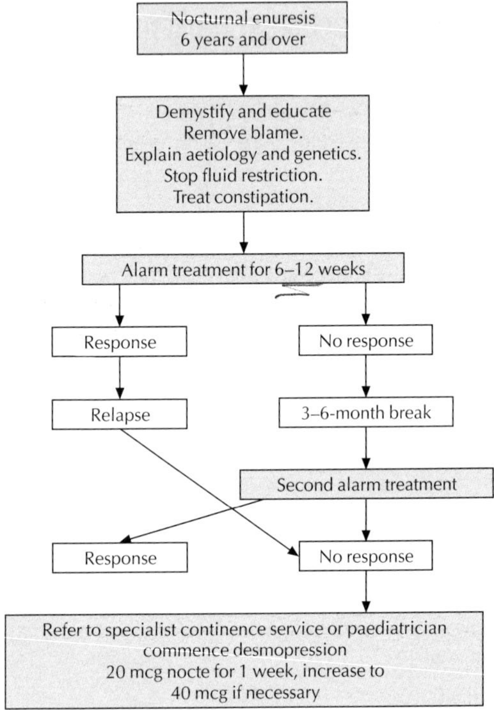

Fig. 32.6 Management of nocturnal enuresis

- In Australia alarms can be hired through hospitals or pharmacies or continence services in the community.
- Relapse after successful therapy can be minimised using a fluid load (before bed) for a week at the end of the treatment period.
- Failure to respond to an alarm warrants a trial of desmopressin (Minirin), 20–40 mcg, intranasal at night.
- The response rate to desmopressin is about 60% and it is palliative rather than curative. Desmopressin can be used temporarily as a stop-gap (e.g. school camps), for long periods and is safe provided an excessive fluid load is not ingested after a dose is given.

- The alarm may be retried each year, as the response improves with increasing age.
- There is no indication for the use of imipramine (Tofranil) now that desmopressin is available as a safer alternative.
- Fluid restriction, star charts, hypnosis, chiropractic treatments and other remedies have not been shown to be effective.

DAY-WETTING (FUNCTIONAL VOIDING DISORDER)

Daytime wetting is a distressing and embarrassing symptom with a significant impact on self-esteem. It affects about 5% of Australian children between 5–12 years of age, girls more often than boys. It is difficult to treat and should be managed in consultation with a specialist.

There are a number of different causes of day-wetting. The following classification is useful in determining appropriate investigations and management.

Urge incontinence

- Symptoms are urgency, frequency, posturing (squatting) and wetting.
- The condition is caused by detrusor (bladder) instability; i.e. dysfunctional overactivity in the detrusor muscle during bladder filling.
- More girls are affected than boys.
- There is an association with recurrent UTI, vulvovaginitis and constipation.
- The condition often coexists with vesico-ureteric reflux and reflux nephropathy.
- Management includes treating any coexistent UTI and constipation, regular voiding, bladder training with the aim of increasing bladder capacity and anticholinergic medication to reduce detrusor spasm.

Dysfunctional voiding

- There is a lack of coordination between detrusor and bladder neck activity with poor relaxation of the external sphincter during voiding.

- The condition is associated with increased intravesical pressure, high residual urine volumes and at times upper tract dilatation.
- Management relies on teaching sphincter relaxation (i.e. pelvic floor relaxation) and ensuring optimal voiding techniques.

Diurnal enuresis

- This condition is characterised by complete bladder emptying of reasonably large volumes of urine in children who appear to be unaware of the need to void, especially when distracted by other activities (typically when watching TV or on the computer).
- It is likely to be due to a combination of developmental and personality factors with some of these children being inattentive and unaware of their bodily needs.
- Management is dependent on increasing the child's awareness of bladder sensation using behaviour modification techniques (e.g. star charts).

Neurological and urological pathology

- Exclude ectopic ureter and fistulae (history of constant dribbling) urethral obstruction neurogenic bladder. Examine the external genitalia and directly visualise of the urethra.
- Examining the back and assessing the lower limb neurological function should highlight spinal cord anomalies, especially a tethered cord.

Investigation

- All children with day-wetting should have a urine microscopy, culture and a renal and bladder ultrasound, including an assessment of residual urine volume.
- Ultrasound should be repeated 2-yearly in children refractory to treatment.

CHAPTER 33
RESPIRATORY CONDITIONS

John Massie
Michael Marks

ASTHMA

Establishing the diagnosis and pattern of asthma

The two main components of asthma pathology include:

- Airway inflammation.
- Reactive airways (bronchoconstriction).

The important clinical features are:

- Wheeze.
- Shortness of breath.
- Chest tightness.
- Cough.
- Response of symptoms to bronchodilators.
- Ask also for interval symptoms, for example: symptoms at night (waking the patient), early in the morning, at rest during the day, during physical activity/sport.

Note: Cough alone, in the absence of wheeze, is rarely asthma.

Common triggers of asthma are:

- Upper respiratory tract infections (URTI).
- Exercise.
- Exposure to cold air.
- Allergen exposure.

The important clinical settings where asthma is more common

- Individuals with allergic disease (perennial rhinitis, hay fever, eczema).
- First-degree relatives with asthma.
- First-degree relatives with atopic disease.

There may be very few physical findings between acute attacks. Look for:

- Hyperinflation.
- Pectus carinatum.
- Expiratory wheeze (generalised).
- Growth parameters
- Side effects of medication (e.g. oral candidiasis in those taking inhaled steroids).

Keep in mind other diagnoses if there are atypical findings, such as digital clubbing (suppurative lung disease), tracheal shift (mediastinal mass) or localised wheeze (inhaled foreign body).

In most cases the diagnosis of asthma in children is a clinical diagnosis.

- While wheezing is a cardinal feature of asthma there are a number of other causes for wheeze. In particular, wheeze is common in young children and may be due to small airway calibre rather than asthma.
- The natural history for most children with episodic (infrequent or frequent) asthma is that it will improve over time.
- The diagnosis of asthma is not always straightforward and a therapeutic trial of asthma treatment is sometimes required. In this circumstance it is important that the treating doctor, the referring doctor and the patient/parents realise that the treatment is a trial and that a label of asthma is not applied inappropriately. Remember that an apparent response to therapy may in fact be the natural history of the underlying disease improving. Reconsider the diagnosis if there is a significant escalation in treatment.

Investigations

Usually investigations are not required, however, tests that may help with the diagnosis and management of asthma are:

Spirometry

- Children over the age of 6 years can learn to perform spirometry accurately.
- Peak flow measurements are unreliable in children. They are inadequate for establishing the diagnosis and monitoring the progress of asthma.
- Airway obstruction is defined as FEV1 < 80% (predicted), FEV1/FVC <75%, MMEF25–75 <67% (predicted).

- If there is evidence of airway obstruction assess bronchodilator reversibility (an improvement of FEV1 of 12% in absolute values).
- In most cases spirometry is unhelpful during an acute admission unless there is a difference between the perceived symptoms and objective clinical measures.

Exercise challenge

- May be performed in children able to do accurate spirometry.
- Seventy per cent of asthmatic children have exercise-induced bronchoconstriction.
- Fifteen per cent reduction in FEV1 following exercise is considered significant.

Chest X-rays

- Chest X-rays are not routinely required in either the acute or interval management of asthma.
- Chest X-rays may be required if there is evidence of a complication (e.g. mucous plugging). Note that pneumothorax is very uncommon complication of acute asthma in children.
- Chest X-rays are helpful if symptoms are not explained by asthma and may be caused by another diseases (e.g. mediastinal mass, suppurative lung disease or foreign body).

Management of acute asthma

See also Medical emergencies, chapter 1 for the management of critical asthma.

Assessment of the severity of an attack

The severity of acute asthma can be classified as mild, moderate, severe or critical. The most reliable indicators are mental state and work of breathing (comprising accessory muscle use and recessions) (see Table 33.1).

- The initial arterial O_2 saturation (SaO_2) in air, heart rate and ability to talk should be used as additional features in assessing the severity of acute asthma.
- Wheeze intensity, central cyanosis, pulsus paradoxus or peak expiratory flow are not reliable for the assessment of the severity of acute asthma.
- Arterial blood gases, chest X-ray and spirometry should not be routinely used in assessing the severity of acute asthma.

Treatment of an acute attack

See Table 33.2.

Table 33.1 Assessment of the severity of an acute asthma attack

Sign	*Mild*	*Moderate*	*Severe*	*Critical*
Mental State	Normal	Normal	Agitated	Confused/drowsy
Work of breathing	Normal	Mildly increased	Moderately/ markedly increased	Maximally increased or exhausted

Hospital discharge and home treatment

Patients should be discharged from medical care when they are stable and can be cared for at home. Education of caregivers is an important component of this process.

Writing an individual asthma action plan assists caregivers in treating asthma in the current and subsequent episodes. The key elements are in the plan are:

- Daily treatment.
- Treatment of minor symptoms.
- Treatment of acute exacerbation.
- Emergency plan.

Drug delivery

Ensure that delivery devices are appropriate to the patient's age (see Table 33.3).

- Inhalations are given with a spacer with a mask firmly applied to the face (in younger children) and with the lips around a mouthpiece for older children.
- Shake the puffer initially and then after every 3 puffs.
- Load with 1 puff at a time (and repeat).
- If the child uses tidal breathing, allow 5–6 breaths. If the child is able to take larger breaths (this is best), wait until they take 1–2 breaths.
- Frequency – in hospital, doses may be given frequently as indicated by severity and response. The use of oxygen between treatments does not preclude using a spacer.
- Spacers should be washed in household detergent weekly to reduce static and then air-dried (spacers should not be rinsed, rubbed or towel dried).
- Selection of appropriate delivery system is crucial for good asthma management. Older children and adolescents should help choose their preferred delivery device to facilitate adherence.

Table 33.2 Treatment of an acute asthma attack

	Mild	*Moderate*	*Severe*	*Critical*
Oxygen	No	No	If SaO_2 <92%	Yes
Inhaled ß$_2$-agonist salbutamol)	6–12 puffs pMDI/spacer[1] once review after 20 min	6–12 puffs pMDI/spacer[1] 3 times in 1st h (every 20 min) review 10 min after 3rd dose	6–12 puffs pMDI/spacer[1] 3 times in 1st h (every 20 min) review 10 min after 3rd dose	Nebulised continuous (e.g. salbutamol[2]
Ipratropium	No	No	2 or 4 puffs pMDI/spacer[3] 3 times in 1st hour only (every 20 min)	Nebulised (250 mcg) –3 times in 1st hour only (every 20 min; add to salbutamol)
Corticosteroids	Usually no	Oral prednisolone 1 mg/kg/dose –once daily for up to 3 days	Oral prednisolone 1 mg/kg/dose –once daily for up to 3 days –IV if vomiting	IV methyl prednisolone 1 mg/kg/dose –6 hourly on day one
IV ß$_2$-agonist (e.g. salbutamol)	No	No	No	Consider if poor response to initial therapy[4]
Aminophylline	No	No	No	Consider if poor response to initial therapy[5]
Observation/admission	Usually discharge home after initial observation	Observe for at least 1 hour the decide need for hospital admission	Admit to hospital Frequent review	Arrange admission to ICU

[1] salbutamol (100 mcg/puff) delivered by pMDI and spacer – 6 puffs if <6 yo, 12 puffs if ≥6 yo
[2] salbutamol 0.5% solution delivered by nebuliser
[3] ipratropium (40 mcg/puff) delivered by pMDI and spacer – 2 puffs if <6 yo, 4 puffs if ≥6 yo
[4] salbutamol 5 mcg/kg/min for 1 hour IV (load), then 1 mcg/kg/minute infusion
[5] aminophylline loading dose 10 mg/kg (maximum 250 mg) over 1 hour (if patient previously taking theophylline, measure serum level to decide need for loading dose; then infusion 1.1 mg/kg/hour if age 1–9 years, 0.7 mg/kg/hour if 10+ years. Aminophylline and salbutamol must be given by separate IV lines
[6] Reduce frequency of ß$_2$-agonist if improving. If no change, continue 20 minutely ß$_2$-agonist. If deteriorating, treat as critical.

Table 33.3 Drug delivery devices

Delivery System	*Age*
Pressurised metered dose inhaler (pMDI)	>8 (reliever only, mild symptoms)
pMDI + Small volume spacer	
• Mask	0–3 years
• No mask	3–5 years
pMDI + large volume spacer	>5 years
Turbuhaler	>8 years
Accuhaler	>8 years
Autohaler	>8 years

All asthma preventers and symptom controllers, prescribed as pMDI, should be delivered through a spacer regardless of the age of the patient.

Principles of interval asthma management

After establishing the diagnosis it is important to determine the pattern of asthma in order to prescribe the appropriate treatment. (See Tables 33.4 and 33.5 respectively)

Table 33.4 Pattern of asthma

Classification of Pattern	*Common Features*
Infrequent Episodic	Episodes 6–8 weeks apart or more Attacks usually not severe Symptoms rare between attacks Normal examination and lung function between episodes
Frequent Episodic	Attacks <6 weeks apart Attacks more troublesome Increasing symptoms between attacks Normal examination and lung function between episodes
Persistent	Daytime symptoms >2 days/week Nocturnal symptoms >1 night/week Attacks <6 weeks apart May have abnormal lung function Multiple Emergency Department visits or hospital admissions

Table 33.5 Interval treatment

	Preventer	*Symptom controller*	*Reliever*
Infrequent episodic	Nil	Nil	Short-acting $ß_2$-agonist as needed*
Frequent episodic	Inhaled corticosteroids (most patients will be well controlled on 100–200 mcg/day fluticasone (or equivalent)	Nil	$ß_2$-agonist as needed*
Persistent	Inhaled corticosteroids (most patients will be well controlled on 100–200 mcg/day fluticasone (or equivalent)	If on $\geq$ 250 mcg/day fluticasone and poorly controlled: add a long acting $ß_2$-agonist (maximum effective dose of fluticasone is 500 mcg/day) If symptoms poorly controlled on maximum inhaled therapy consider oral corticosteroids, theophyllines, or leukotriene receptor antagonists.	Short-acting $ß_2$-agonist as needed*

* For children who experience exercise induced symptoms – consider pre-treatment with prior to exercise (e.g. Salbutamol 2×100 mcg puffs)

A number of issues should be attended to at subsequent check-ups, including:

- Symptom review – in particular nocturnal and exercise symptoms.
- Review of asthma action plan and medication regime.
- Adherence with medication.
- Avoiding precipitants (e.g. allergens).
- Avoidance of cigarette smoking (personal and environmental).
- Monitoring of growth and development.

ACUTE VIRAL BRONCHIOLITIS

See Figure 33.1 Assessment and management of acute viral bronchiolitis.

PNEUMONIA

Clinical features

- Tachypnoea, fever and cough. There may be signs of respiratory distress.
- Focal signs in the chest may be difficult to detect in young infants.
- A diagnosis of pneumonia, especially in younger children, can often only be made with radiological confirmation.

Cause

- *Respiratory viruses* are the most common cause of pneumonia in young infants in developed countries. There is generally only mild to moderate constitutional disturbance. There may be scattered inspiratory crackles on auscultation.
- *Mycoplasma pneumoniae* is the commonest pathogen in children over 5 years old, but is a less common cause of pneumonia in younger children. Typically symptoms develop over several days before the cough, often with a systemic illness. Cough is prominent and crackles may be focal or widespread. Children are usually unwell and focal signs are present in the chest.
- *Streptococcus pneumoniae* is the most common bacterial pathogen in all age groups followed by non-typeable *Haemophilus influenzae* and *Staphylococcus aureus*. Group A β haemolytic streptococcus is less common but may cause severe pneumonia. Many older children can be managed at home, but most under the age of 24 months should be admitted to hospital.

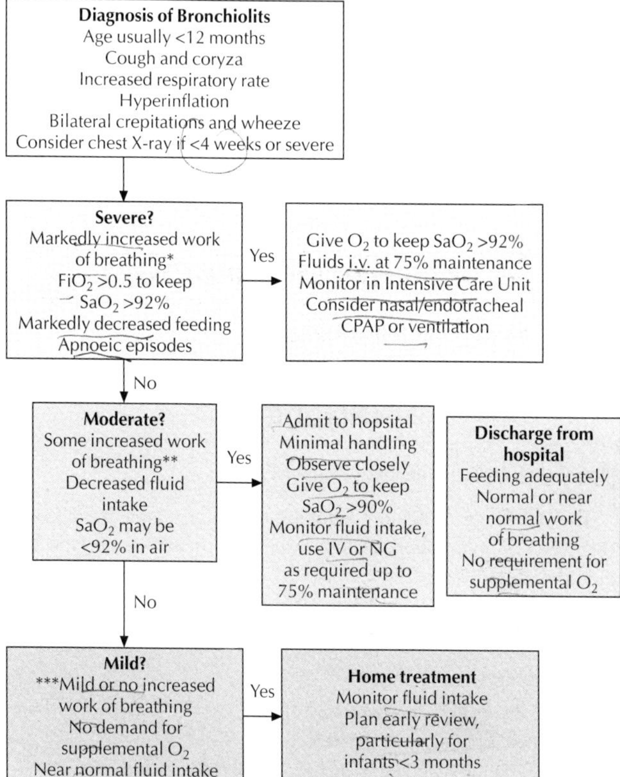

Diagnosis of Bronchiolits
Age usually <12 months
Cough and coryza
Increased respiratory rate
Hyperinflation
Bilateral crepitations and wheeze
Consider chest X-ray if <4 weeks or severe
Severe?
Markedly increased work of breathing*
FiO2 >0.5 to keep SaO2 >92%
Markedly decreased feeding
Apnoeic episodes
Yes
Give O2 to keep SaO2 >92%
Fluids i.v. at 75% maintenance
Monitor in Intensive Care Unit
Consider nasal/endotracheal CPAP or ventilation
No
Moderate?
Some increased work of breathing**
Decreased fluid intake
SaO2 may be <92% in air
Yes
Admit to hopsital
Minimal handling
Observe closely
Give O2 to keep SaO2 >90%
Monitor fluid intake, use IV or NG as required up to 75% maintenance
Discharge from hospital
Feeding adequately
Normal or near normal work of breathing
No requirement for supplemental O2
No
Mild?
***Mild or no increased work of breathing
No demand for supplemental O2
Near normal fluid intake
Yes
Home treatment
Monitor fluid intake
Plan early review, particularly for infants <3 months

Notes:
* Routine CXR is not required for children with typical clinical features.
** Use the respiratory rate, accessory muscle use and recessions to judge the work of breathing.
*** Very young infants and infants with a comorbidity (e.g. cardiac disease, Down syndrome, chronic lung disease etc) are at greatest risk of severe disease. These infants may need admission for observation if they have mild bronchiolitis. Administration of β2 agonists may be distressing for young infants and is of no proven value.

Fig. 33.1 Assessment and management of acute viral bronchiolitis

Management

See Figure 33.2 Management of pneumonia.

PHARYNGITIS/TONSILLITIS, ACUTE OTITIS MEDIA AND URTI

See Ear, nose and throat conditions, chapter 21.

LARYNGOTRACHEOBRONCHITIS (CROUP)

See Figure 33.3 Management of croup.

EPIGLOTTITIS

See also Medical emergencies, chapter 1.

The incidence of acute epiglottitis has fallen markedly in countries where immunisation against *Haemophilus influenzae* type b is widespread. However, it continues to occur (child not immunised, immunisation failure, other bacteria) and if the diagnosis is not made promptly, a child with epiglottitis is likely to die.

Clinical features

Epiglottitis differs from laryngotracheobronchitis in the following ways:

- Cough is not a prominent feature.
- Most children appear toxic because of associated sepsis.
- The onset is with fever and lethargy. Symptoms of respiratory obstruction develop after 2–6 h. There may be a history of a preceding upper respiratory tract infection.
- The stridor is soft and the expiratory element is often dominant with a snoring or gurgling quality.
- Difficulty in swallowing with drooling of saliva is common.

Management

See Medical emergencies, chapter 1.

Treatment of contacts

- Rifampicin prophylaxis 20 mg/kg (max 600 mg) p.o. daily for 4 days (<1 month 10 mg/kg p.o. for 4 days).

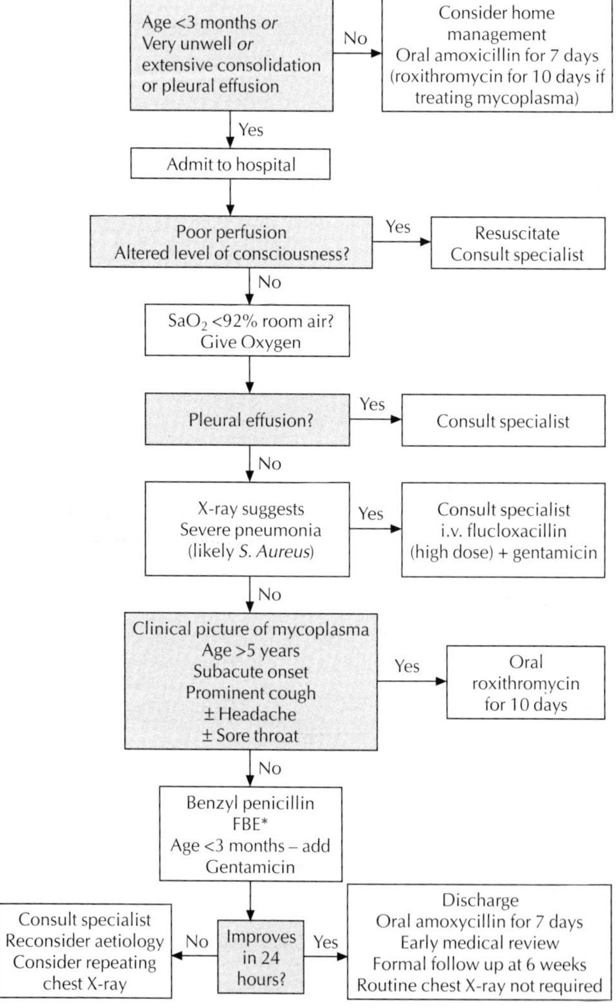

* Other investigations as indicated. Blood culture positive in less than 5% of cases; Nasopharyngeal aspirate for viral identification not usually helpful; Mycoplasma serology may be helpful if diagnosis in doubt.

Fig. 33.2 Management of pneumonia (previously well patient >1 month old)

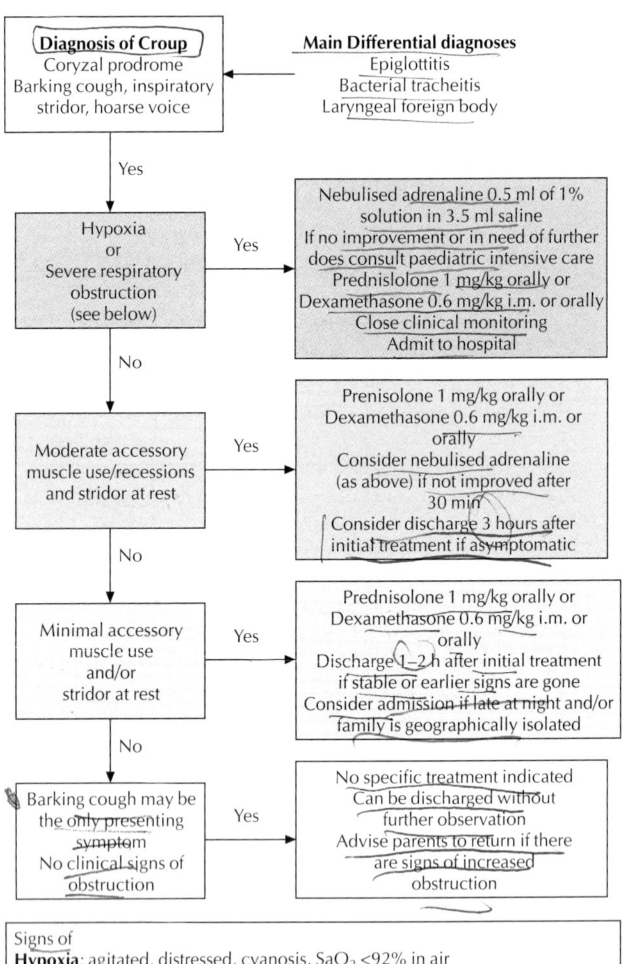
Diagnosis of Croup
Coryzal prodrome
Barking cough, inspiratory stridor, hoarse voice
Main Differential diagnoses
Epiglottitis
Bacterial tracheitis
Laryngeal foreign body
Yes
Hypoxia or Severe respiratory obstruction (see below)
Yes
Nebulised adrenaline 0.5 ml of 1% solution in 3.5 ml saline
If no improvement or in need of further does consult paediatric intensive care
Prednislolone 1 mg/kg orally or
Dexamethasone 0.6 mg/kg i.m. or orally
Close clinical monitoring
Admit to hospital
No
Moderate accessory muscle use/recessions and stridor at rest
Yes
Prenisolone 1 mg/kg orally or
Dexamethasone 0.6 mg/kg i.m. or orally
Consider nebulised adrenaline (as above) if not improved after 30 min
Consider discharge 3 hours after initial treatment if asymptomatic
No
Minimal accessory muscle use and/or stridor at rest
Yes
Prednisolone 1 mg/kg orally or
Dexamethasone 0.6 mg/kg i.m. or orally
Discharge 1–2 h after initial treatment if stable or earlier signs are gone
Consider admission if late at night and/or family is geographically isolated
No
Barking cough may be the only presenting symptom
No clinical signs of obstruction
Yes
No specific treatment indicated
Can be discharged without further observation
Advise parents to return if there are signs of increased obstruction
Signs of
Hypoxia: agitated, distressed, cyanosis, SaO2 <92% in air
Severe Obstruction: marked accessory muscle use/recessions
Note: Risk Factors for severe disease: subglottic stenosis (either congenital or prolonged intubation), age <6 months, Down syndrome (or other neurological abnormalities). Consider admission for such children even with mild symptoms

Fig. 33.3 Management of croup

WHOOPING COUGH (PERTUSSIS)

Whooping cough continues to be widespread in many communities because of sub-optimal uptake of childhood immunisation and waning immunity in adolescents and adults immunised as children (the current vaccines give protection for only 5–10 years).

Clinical features

- Starts with a coryzal illness that resembles an URTI (infectious period).
- The cough continues for many weeks to months, is paroxysmal and may be associated with facial suffusion and vomiting. In some children the paroxysm is terminated by an inspiratory whoop. The cough is often only recognised as pertussis at this stage (paroxysmal phase).
- The child appears well between coughing paroxysms.
- In small infants pertussis can present with apnoea alone.

Diagnosis

- Diagnosis can be made on clinical grounds.
- Lymphocyte count may be elevated ($>20 \times 10^9$/L)
- In the acute phase the diagnosis can be confirmed by identifying *Bordetella pertussis* from a nasopharyngeal aspirate (culture, immunofluorescence, PCR).
- Pertussis serum IgA is specific (but not sensitive) for past infection. It may be elevated after 3 weeks and persist for 2 years.

Management

- No pharmacological agents improve the clinical course of whooping cough.
- Clearance of nasal carriage of *B. pertussis* has been best studied with erythromycin estolate for 14 days but the estolate preparation is no longer available in Australia. Comparative studies suggest that a shorter course of clarithromycin is as effective and possibly more effective than erythromycin. The current recommendation is clarithromycin 7.5 mg/kg (max 500 mg) oral twice daily for 7 days.
- Treat household and other close contacts with clarithromycin (same dosage) for 7 days.

- Infants >3 months of age with culture proven pertussis do not need to receive pertussis vaccine, although vaccination of previously infected children is safe.
- Admission: infants <6 months, apnoea, cyanosis, not coping with the cough, poor feeding, systemically unwell.
- In hospital: careful observation, including the use of an apnoea monitor. If paroxysms occur frequently and are associated with marked cyanosis, nursing in oxygen may be of some help.

COUGH

Cough is a common symptom in children. The degree to which a family becomes concerned about the frequency and severity of a child's cough seems to be extremely variable. There is often a poor correlation between a parental report of cough and objective measures.

Cough is best thought of in the following diagnostic groups:

Recurrent cough

These are episodes of cough lasting a few days to a few weeks with completely asymptomatic periods between. There are two common causes: viral respiratory tract infection and asthma.

Viral respiratory tract infection

Cough with a viral respiratory infection, although typically lasting 7–10 days, may persist for 4–8 weeks or even longer. Initially it may be loose but later in the course it may become dry. It may be perceived by the family to be worse at night.

Asthma

While cough can be a troublesome symptom of asthma, it rarely occurs without some evidence of airways obstruction (e.g. wheeze). There is considerable doubt as to whether the entity of 'cough variant asthma' (in which cough is the only symptom of asthma) exists in children. Be very reluctant to diagnose asthma in the absence of evidence of airways obstruction. The management of asthma is based on the severity and duration of the airways obstruction, not on the cough.

Subacute cough

There are a number of entities in addition to post-viral infection in which cough can last some weeks to 2 or 3 months. They include:

- Whooping cough.
- An inhaled foreign body.
- *Mycoplasma pneumoniae* infection.
- Segmental or lobar collapse following an acute respiratory infection.
- Tuberculosis.
- Psychogenic.

Whooping cough and psychogenic cough should be diagnosed on the pattern of the cough. The others may be diagnosable by a chest X-ray.

Persistent cough

This is a cough of many months or even years. Ask carefully about a wet or productive cough. In suppurative lung disease the cough is often worse on waking in the morning and there may be a history of response to antibiotics.

The likely causes of a persistent cough are:

- Cystic fibrosis.
- Other causes of bronchiectasis – primary cilia dyskinesia, agammaglobulinaemia and other immune-deficient states.
- Recurrent aspiration (upper airway incoordination, gastro-oesophageal reflux).
- Insidious onset bronchiectasis without an apparent cause.
- Smoker's cough in adolescents.

Bronchiectasis probably commences with suppurative bronchitis. If this has been present for < 6–12 months, it may be completely reversible without permanent lung damage, following a prolonged course of antibiotics (weeks to months) and physiotherapy.

Management

- The single most important aspect of management is to make a diagnosis and explain its nature to the parents. The effects of passive smoking should be discussed.
- Most cough suppressants provide only partial relief.
- Specific therapy is indicated for asthma, tuberculosis and segmental or lobar collapse. A foreign body must be removed bronchoscopically.
- It is often much more difficult to control the cough of asthma than the wheeze.

FOREIGN BODY IN THE BRONCHIAL TREE

Clinical features

Symptoms

- Coughing or choking episodes while eating solid foods (classically nuts) or while sucking a small plastic toy or similar object. This history should never be dismissed.
- Persistent coughing and wheezing.
- Beware of the sudden onset of a first wheezing episode in a toddler in whom there is no history of allergy, especially if it follows a choking episode.
- Parents may not volunteer the history of possible inhalation (many foreign body aspirations are not witnessed).

Signs

- There may be no physical signs or alternatively reduced breath sounds over the whole or part of one lung.
- Wheeze.

Investigations

Chest X-ray in full inspiration and full expiration to exclude obstructive hyperinflation or an area of collapse. The X-ray should include the nasopharynx to the chest. Normal X-rays do not exclude a foreign body.

Management

Bronchoscopy is indicated for all patients with a suspected inhaled foreign body.

- Bronchoscopy in children is difficult and it requires an expert paediatric endoscopist teamed with an experienced paediatric anaesthetist. It should only be done in a tertiary paediatric centre. Rigid bronchoscopy is preferred.
- In most cases the removal of the foreign body improves symptoms and corticosteroids or antibiotics are rarely indicated.

CHAPTER 34
RHEUMATOLOGIC CONDITIONS

Roger Allen
Jane Munro

Musculoskeletal symptoms and signs are common in children and adolescents and may be the presenting feature of a broad spectrum of conditions. Clinical features and laboratory findings may be relatively non-specific in rheumatological conditions and it is important to look for disease patterns when evaluating the presenting complaint and conducting a systems review.

EVALUATION OF ARTHRITIS/ARTHRALGIA

History

- Check the nature of onset – is it acute or insidious?
- **Acute onset monoarticular arthritis associated with fever is septic until proven otherwise.**
- Check the timing of symptoms during the day – as a general guide:
  - Early morning stiffness = inflammatory.
  - Post-activity pain = mechanical.
- Check duration of illness – if >6 weeks it is less likely to be reactive/post-viral arthritis.
- Are there any intercurrent infections (respiratory, enteric or skin)? Post-viral infections are probably the commonest cause of transient arthritis.
- Has the child been taking any medications (e.g. cefaclor)?
- What does the child, or parent, consider to be the most symptomatic site – is it in the joint, muscle, adjacent bone or a more diffuse area?
- Check for extra-articular symptoms – ensure a thorough systems review and keep the three following diagnoses in mind:
  - Systemic lupus erythematosus (SLE).
  - Acute lymphoblastic leukaemia (ALL).
  - Inflammatory bowel disease (IBD).

- Assess whether the normal physical activities or interests have been interrupted.
- Assess the functional milieu of the patient (e.g. school progress, family and peer relationships and stress experiences).
- Check the family history for other types of inflammatory arthritis, particularly the spondyloarthropathies, autoimmune disorders and pain syndromes (e.g. fibromyalgia or other models for pain behaviour).

Examination

Observe the patient as they move about the room, watch them undress and be opportunistic when examining them.

- Examine all joints, not only the site of the presenting complaint. There may be inflammation without symptoms in juvenile chronic arthritis (JCA).
- Aim to localise the site of maximal discomfort (e.g. is it the joint capsule, adjacent bone or muscle belly, tendon or ligament attachments?).
- Examine for signs of systemic diseases with an articular component, extra-articular features of JCA or both. In particular examine the skin, eyes, abdomen, nails and lymph nodes.

A musculoskeletal assessment should include:

- Joints – signs of inflammation such as swelling or tenderness, the range of movement and deformity.
- Entheses – bone attachment sites of ligaments/tendons (e.g. Achilles tendon).
- Tendon sheaths of fingers and toes (e.g. dactylitis in psoriasis).
- Gait – antalgic (pain) or limp, Trendelenburg's sign.
- Muscle tenderness, muscle wasting or weakness (e.g. inability to toe or crouch walk).
- Patellar tracking pattern – does the patella move vertically on walking?
- Shoe sole and heel-wearing pattern.
- Leg length measurement.
- Spinal flexion, including Schober's test (the measurement of the lumbosacral range should increase by at least 6 cm on maximal flexion; the starting range is between the lumbosacral junction and a point 10 cm above).
- Assessment of growth parameters.

Investigations

There is no one diagnostic test for JCA.

Often useful

- Full blood examination (FBE), erythrocyte sedimentation rate (ESR) and C-reactive protein (CRP). Normal inflammatory markers do not exclude the diagnosis.
- Synovial fluid culture – if sepsis is considered.
- Antinuclear antibody (ANA) – beware of over-interpretation as up to 20% of normal children may have a low positive ANA.

Occasionally useful

- Specific bacterial/viral studies if the clinical picture is suggestive (e.g. ASOT, antiDNase B, Yersinia and parvovirus serology).
- Rheumatoid factor – in polyarticular patients, older children or if the pattern of disease appears unusual.
- Human leucocyte antigen (HLA) B27 – if spondyloarthropathy is suspected (remember almost 9% of the Caucasian population are positive).
- Imaging – plain X-ray, bone scan and ultrasound. In early arthritis, plain films usually give no more information than a careful examination. They may be useful for difficult sites such as the hip, or if there is a long history of arthritis.
- Diagnostic aspirate – worthwhile if sepsis or haemarthrosis is considered, but will not necessarily differentiate between other inflammatory arthritides.

Not useful

- Serum uric acid.

CAUSES OF ARTHRITIS/ARTHRALGIA IN CHILDHOOD

Juvenile chronic (rheumatoid) arthritis

Assessment

- Age of onset <16 years of age.
- Minimum duration of arthritis – 6 weeks (some criteria suggest 3 months).
- **Most acute non-septic arthritis is not JCA.**

Disease subtypes

- *Pauciarticular*: affects 4 or fewer joints:
  - Young, often ANA-positive females (can get asymptomatic severe uveitis that does not correlate with activity of arthritis – screen 3 monthly).
  - Older, often B27-positive males (who may have an evolving spondyloarthropathy).
- *Polyarticular*: affects 5 or more joints; sero- (rheumatoid factor) positive or negative.
- *Systemic*: joint involvement plus fever, rash and lymphadenopathy.

It is useful to look for:

- Features suggestive of a spondyloarthropathy: enthesitis, sacro-ileitis or acute uveitis.
- Nail pits/scalp rash (indicative of psoriasis).
- Rash of Still's disease (faint urticarial-like erythema) – mostly when febrile.
- Uveitis (especially pauci-JCA patient) by slit-lamp.
- Inflammatory features, including subtle behavioural features such as withdrawal/excessive irritability.

Management

Depends on the clinical picture of disease severity and subtype.

Principles:

1. Preserve joint function.
2. Control pain.
3. Manage complications.

Multidisciplinary approach – including psychosocial support

Physical therapy is essential to maintain joint range and function. Splinting should be considered where appropriate.

Medication

- Initially non-steroidal anti-inflammatory drugs (NSAIDs): e.g. naproxen, indomethacin, diclofenac or ibuprofen.
- Then usually low dose methotrexate to minimise joint destruction.
- Other options include corticosteroids in systemic JCA and intra-articular injections (used early in mono or pauciarticular arthritis).

Spondyloarthropathies

- Uncommon (more frequent in males) with onset >10 years of age.
- HLA B27 positive (80%), often raised inflammatory markers.
- Intermittent episodes of enthesitis (tender at tendon insertions) and low back pain/sacroiliitis.
- Acute uveitis (usually clinically evident).
- Management: NSAIDs such as naproxen; sulfasalazine in refractory cases.

Henoch-Schonlein purpura (HSP)

A small vessel vasculitis.

Clinical features

- Most common age of onset 2–8 years.
- Evolving crops of palpable purpura – predominantly buttocks and legs.
- Abdominal pain (occasionally melaena) may precede rash.
- Large joint migratory arthritis of variable duration and severity.
- Nephritis.
- Other (e.g. oedema dorsum of the feet and hands, acute scrotal swelling and 'bruising', fever and fatigue).
- Exclude other causes of purpura (see Dermatologic conditions, chapter 20).

Investigations

- Full blood examination (to exclude thrombocytopenia).
- Urinalysis – haematuria/proteinuria.
- Renal function – urea/creatinine and urinary protein estimation.

Management

- Supportive – bed rest and analgesia.
- Corticosteroids – may reduce the duration of abdominal pain, but it is uncertain if they significantly affect other features.
- Refer to a specialist if renal dysfunction, hypertension or surgical complications develop.

Irritable hip (transient synovitis)

See Orthopaedic conditions, chapter 31.

Septic arthritis

See Orthopaedic conditions, chapter 31.

Kawasaki Disease

See Infectious diseases, chapter 27.

POSTINFECTIOUS ARTHRITIS

Acute rheumatic fever

See Infectious diseases, chapter 27.

Post-streptococcal reactive arthritis

- Afebrile symmetrical non-migratory poly- or pauciarticular arthritis.
- Arthritis responds slowly to anti-inflammatories.
- Carditis may occur and form part of a spectrum with acute rheumatic fever.
- Consider penicillin prophylaxis if carditis is present.

Post-enteric reactive arthritis

- Mainly *Salmonella, Shigella* and *Yersinia* (also reported with *Campylobacter* and *Giardia*).
- It is clinically similar to the spondyloarthropathies; i.e., predominantly lower limb (including sacroiliitis), enthesitis is common and positive family history (especially if HLA B27 positive). However, it may not present with all the classic clinical features.
- Consider Crohn's disease or ulcerative colitis.
- Associated features – acute anterior uveitis and sterile pyuria.
- Treatment – NSAIDs: indomethacin 0.5–1.0 mg/kg (max 75 mg) p.o. 8-hourly is often the most effective.

Post-viral arthritis

- Many viral illnesses are associated with arthritis
- It is uncertain in most situations whether it is the primary (infective) or secondary (reactive) event; e.g., Epstein-Barr virus, rubella, adenovirus, varicella (beware septic arthritis secondary to infected skin lesion), parvovirus B19 and hepatitis B.
- A transient arthritis often follows a non-specific 'viral' illness, the confirmation of which may be difficult and unnecessary.
- Treatment – NSAIDs probably shorten the duration.

NON-INFLAMMATORY CAUSES OF JOINT PAIN

Benign nocturnal limb pain ('growing pains')

- Onset at 3–7 years, often occurs in the evenings and at night.
- Well between attacks.
- Recurrent pain mainly involving the knee, calf and shin.
- No symptoms or signs of inflammation either on history or examination.
- Investigations (if carried out) are normal.
- Management involves analgesia (usually paracetamol) and reassurance; heat and massage/rubbing often help.

Benign hypermobility

- Common, particularly in the older child/adolescent (≤7, all the features are normal variants)
- Typical sites:
  - Hyperextension of the fingers parallel to the forearm.
  - Apposition of the thumb to the anterior forearm.
  - Hyperextension of the elbows, knees, or both more than 10°.
  - Excessive dorsiflexion of the ankles.
  - Hip flexion allowing the palms to be placed flat on ground.
- Pain occurs typically in the afternoon or after exercise and occurs mostly in the lower limbs.
- The child may have features of patello-femoral dysfunction.
- The child may have transient joint effusions.
- Management: symptomatic treatment and reassurance.

Complex regional pain syndrome

See Pain management, chapter 3.

OTHER RHEUMATOLOGICAL DISORDERS

Maintain an index of suspicion regarding other rheumatological disorders (e.g. SLE, dermatomyositis connective tissue disorders). Enquire about the following symptoms:

- Lethargy, weight loss, mouth ulcers, alopecia or frontal hair breaking.
- Recurrent fevers.

- Raynaud's phenomenon, rashes or photosensitivity.
- Ophthalmological symptoms: red sore eyes, change in vision or dry eyes.
- Weakness.
- Consider investigating with: C3, C4, ANA, dsDNA, ENA, CK, LDH or LFT.

CHAPTER 35
SURGICAL CONDITIONS

John Hutson
Chris Kimber

INGUINOSCROTAL CONDITIONS

The underlying pathological basis of an inguinal hernia, an encysted hydrocele of the cord and a scrotal hydrocele is the persistence of a patent processus vaginalis after the completion of testicular descent.

The causes of groin lumps in neonates are:

- Undescended testes.
- Inguinal hernia – if irreducible, irritable baby, tender lump in the groin.
- Encysted hydrocele of the cord, unable to be reduced – e.g., well baby, mobile lump, unable to get above it.
- Lymphadenitis with abscess formation – rare condition, often not diagnosed until operation.

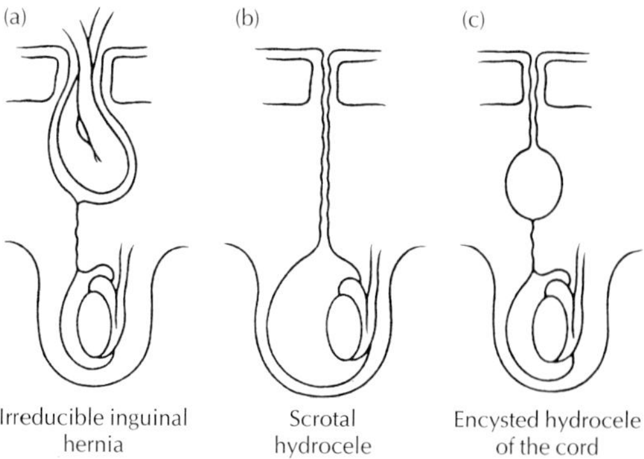

Fig. 35.1 Inguinoscrotal conditions

Inguinal hernia

An inguinal hernia occurs when the patent processus vaginalis is large enough to allow bowel, omentum or ovary to protrude through the inguinal canal and sometimes, in males, down to the scrotum. The younger the child, the greater the risk of bowel or ovary becoming strangulated. Bowel strangulation in boys compresses the testicular vessels and may result in testicular ischaemia. Surgery is always required and this is performed as a day case, except when the baby is less than 4 weeks of age.

Reducible inguinal hernia

Table 35.1 Reducible inguinal hernia

Age at presentation	*Timing of surgical consultation*	*Appropriate operating time*
Birth–6 weeks	Day of diagnosis	Next available list
6 weeks–6 months	Within few days	Within 2 weeks
6 months–6 years	Within 2 weeks	Within 2 months

Irreducible inguinal hernia

Urgent surgical referral is indicated. The majority of irreducible inguinal hernias can be manually reduced by a surgical specialist and surgery is performed within 48 h. Pain relief is appropriate to aid with reduction. The use of ice packs or traction is inappropriate.

Scrotal hydrocele, encysted hydrocele of the cord

In these conditions, the patent processus vaginalis is narrow and enables peritoneal fluid, but not abdominal contents, into the cord structures. A patent processus vaginalis often closes of its own accord in the first 18 months of life (see Figure 35.1b and c).

The important clinical signs are:

- Brilliantly transilluminable swelling.
- Narrow cord above the swelling.
- Swelling does not empty on squeezing and a normal testicle is felt in it.
- Non-tender.

If a hydrocele persists beyond 2 years of age, surgery is recommended and an inguinal herniotomy (i.e. division of patent processus vaginalis) is performed as a day case.

Undescended testes

When the testis cannot be brought to the bottom of the scrotum, it is 'undescended'. An assessment should be made by a paediatric surgeon between 3–6 months of life and an orchidopexy performed at 6–12 months of age as a day case.

Some children present with undescended testis later in childhood (4–10 years). This is probably an acquired condition secondary to failure of elongation of the spermatic cord with age. Surgery is recommended, if the testis does not remain in the bottom of the scrotum to optimise fertility and reduce the risk of malignancy and torsion.

The acute scrotum

A child with a painful, tender or red scrotum should be seen by a surgeon as a matter of urgency. Without surgical exploration, it is usually impossible to differentiate between the two common causes:

- Torsion of the testicular appendage
- Torsion of the testis.

Torsion of the testis can occur at any age. In older children it is characterised by more severe pain and vomiting. A testis lying horizontally in the scrotum indicates an anatomical predisposition to torsion and may cause intermittent testicular pain.

Ultrasound is unreliable in distinguishing between torsion of the testis and torsion of the testicular appendage and often delays critical operative treatment. Epididymo-orchitis is a rare disease in pre-pubertal boys who do not have urinary tract infections and should not be considered part of the initial differential diagnosis. Mumps orchitis is not seen before puberty.

THE PENIS

The foreskin/prepuce

The foreskin is normally adherent to the glans at birth and remains so for a variable period of time. It is usually fully retractable by 4 years of age,

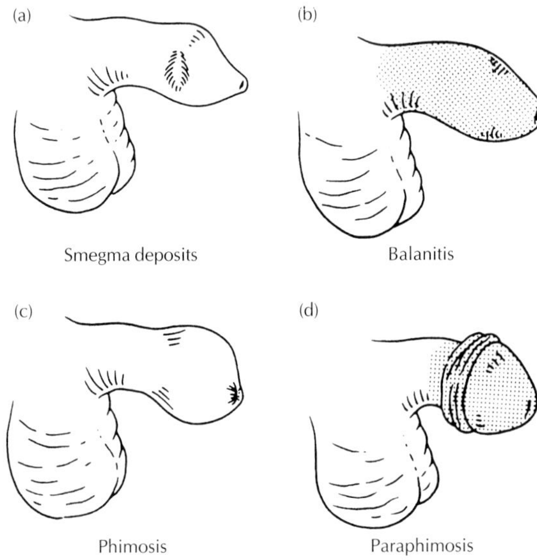

Fig. 35.2 Conditions of the penis

but partial adherence is still normal up to 10 years of age. There is no need to retract the foreskin in preschool children.

Smegma deposits

These present as firm yellow-white masses beneath the prepuce in non-retractile foreskins (see Figure 35.2a). They are often confused with tumours or cysts of the penis, but are a normal variant and require no treatment.

Balanitis

This is an infection under the foreskin with redness, inflammation, swelling and sometimes a white exudate (see Figure 35.2b). Immediate treatment with local penile toilet, i.e., soaking in an antiseptic solution, local antiseptic ointment (e.g. neomycin eye ointment) beneath the foreskin and oral antibiotics (e.g. cotrimoxazole) are usually sufficient. If the whole penile shaft skin is red and swollen to the pubis, intravenous antibiotics may be required.

Phimosis

This is scarring of the preputial opening, which causes:

- Urinary obstruction.
- Ballooning of the foreskin on micturition.

It is often the end result of recurrent episodes of balanitis (see Figure 35.2c). It usually requires circumcision if severe, although mild cases respond to topical 0.5% betamethasone valerate cream applied 4 times daily for 14 days.

Paraphimosis

This acutely painful condition results from a retracted foreskin trapped behind the glans and forming an oedematous ring constricting the exposed and swollen glans penis (see Figure 35.2d). Manual reduction should be attempted in all cases. **Ice should not be applied**. The use of topical local anaesthetic cream, such as EMLA cream (do not use adrenaline-containing creams) 5 min prior to reduction, facilitates this procedure. Failure to reduce the paraphimosis requires urgent surgical consultation.

Circumcision

There is no indication for neonatal circumcision. The indications for circumcision are phimosis and recurrent balanitis. Hypospadias is an absolute contraindication, as the foreskin may be required for penile reconstruction. **Circumcision is not required for cleanliness** and less than 10% of Australian male children are currently being circumcised. It is an unnecessary operation with complications of surgery and anaesthesia.

UMBILICAL HERNIA

Umbilical hernia – the protrusion of the umbilicus – is a common finding in newborn children and usually resolves in the first 12 months of life. If it persists, operation as a day case is recommended prior to commencing school. The operation is primarily cosmetic, although strangulation during adult life – particularly during pregnancy – can occur.

ACUTE ABDOMINAL PAIN

Abdominal pain is a common symptom in children. Acute appendicitis must be distinguished from common causes of abdominal pain, including gastrointestinal and urinary tract infection and constipation.

Appendicitis

The symptoms and signs of appendicitis are related to the degree of peritoneal irritation and the position of the appendix. Diagnosis is straightforward if there is localised peritonitis with guarding in the right iliac fossa, however, peritonitis may not occur in retrocaecal appendicitis and in pelvic appendicitis there may be only vague suprapubic tenderness. Repeated clinical examination and abdominal ultrasound may help identify these difficult cases. Rectal examination is very rarely required in children.

Urinary tract infection may be excluded by urine testing (see Renal conditions and enuresis, chapter 32). Blood, protein and white cells may all be present in the urine in acute appendicitis. Nitrites are more specific for urinary tract infections. Gastrointestinal infections often produce a local ileus but no peritonitis and are frequently distinguished by 'squelchiness' in the right iliac fossa on examination; from air and fluid in the ileum.

Diagnosing appendicitis in the young child (<4 years of age) is difficult. It is important to refer a child who complains of persistent abdominal pain, even if this is associated with vomiting or diarrhoea. In particular, suspect significant peritonitis if the child does not allow abdominal examination.

Intussusception

Consider intussception in infants aged 3-months to 2-years presenting with vomiting, intermittent abdominal pain and lethargy/pallor. These early symptoms should be acted on, rather than awaiting the classic 'red currant jelly stool', which is a feature of advanced disease. The abdominal mass is central, beneath the rectus abdominis on the right side and is often difficult to feel. Contrast enema should not be performed in the presence of peritonitis, significant dehydration or established bowel obstruction.

An infant with suspected intussusception requires urgent surgical assessment and radiological investigations for diagnosis and treatment. While an ultrasound may aid in the diagnosis, a contrast air or barium enema is required in order to reduce the intussusception. These procedures should only be undertaken by an experienced radiologist with a surgical team immediately available.

VOMITING IN INFANCY

Table 35.2 Vomiting in infancy

Green vomit	*Curdled milk*
Differential Diagnosis: • Malrotation • Infection (gastroenteritis / meningitis / UTI) • Small bowel obstruction (rare)	Differential Diagnosis: • Pyloric stenosis • Gastro-oesophageal reflux • Infection (UTI/gastroenteritis/ meningitis)
Management: (*after exclusion of major sepsis*): URGENT SURGICAL REFERRAL.	Projectile vomiting ± weight loss/gastric peristalsis: URGENT SURGICAL REFERRAL.

Malrotation and volvulus

Green vomiting without an obvious septic cause is an indication for urgent surgical consultation, to exclude intestinal malrotation and its associated lethal complication of midgut volvulus. Initially, there are usually no other symptoms or signs of abdominal disease. Abdominal distension is not usually seen; do not wait for distension to develop.

This condition requires urgent referral.

Pyloric stenosis

Pyloric stenosis with vomiting of gastric contents is a significant metabolic condition. It may be difficult to diagnose. It should be suspected when vomiting is projectile, particularly if associated with failure to thrive.

Gastric peristalsis occurs due to the pyloric obstruction. This is clearly visible on the baby's abdominal wall and if the stomach is not grossly distended with fluid and/or air, the pyloric tumour is readily palpable. Ultrasound is only required if the diagnosis is unclear and the pyloric tumour cannot be felt.

Management

Vomiting in these infants results in loss of gastric fluid (water and HCl). The kidneys can initially conserve H^+, but once the baby becomes dehydrated, water and Na^+ are conserved in exchange for K^+ and H^+. The resulting condition is hypovolaemia with alkalosis, low chloride and potassium. Even if serum K^+ is normal, there is a total body potassium deficiency.

Metabolic complications

A significant metabolic alkalosis (chloride <100 mmol/L; pH <7.45 and sodium <130 mmol/L) is present only in significant cases. Inappropriate rehydration with low-sodium-containing fluids can result in cerebral oedema.

An appropriate fluid for resuscitation is 1/2 normal saline with 5% dextrose. Potassium should be added once the baby is passing urine (refer to Table 35.3).

If the baby's weight prior to the onset of symptoms is known, fluid deficit is easily calculated. Maintenance requirements may be calculated at 100 ml/kg/24 hours.

For example; a baby normally weighing 3 kg now weighs 2.7 kg

- Deficit 300 gram (10% dehydration) – Replacement required 300 ml
- Maintenance required – 300 mL/24 hours
- For resuscitation over 12 hours, 450 mL is required in this period, i.e. 38 mL/hour

For a simple guideline to facilitate fluid calculations if the baby's weight is not known see Table 35.3.

Table 35.3 Fluid calculations in pyloric stenosis

Clinical state	*Fluids preoperative period/first 12–16 h*	*Monitoring*
Mildly dehydrated <5% Clinically well, reduced urine output Electrolytes usually normal	No bolus required 1/2 normal saline & 5% Dextrose with 20 mmol/l KCL in each litre Rate = 1.5 × maintenance for 12 h	Check O_2 saturations Monitor Pulse, Urine output Glucose, U & E, creatinine 12-hourly
Moderately dehydrated 5–10% Mildly lethargic, pale, dry mouth Poor urine output Low chloride +/– sodium	Bolus normal saline 20 ml / kg in 30 min Then 1/2 normal saline & 5% Dextrose with 30 mmol/l KCL in each litre Rate = 2 × maintenance for 12 h	Monitor O_2 saturations, pulse, BP and urine output. Glucose, U & E, creatinine 12-hourly
Severely dehydrated 10% Lethargic, pale, mottled, dry mouth, no urine, tachycardia & may have low BP Low chloride & sodium +/– Low potassium	Bolus normal saline 20 ml / kg in 30 min Then 1/2 normal saline & 5% Dextrose with 30 mmol KCL in each litre Rate = 2 × maintenance Continue up to 16 h or further if clinically indicated	Monitor O_2 saturations, pulse, BP and urine output. Glucose, U & E, creatinine 12-hourly

RECTAL BLEEDING

See Table 35.4. See also Gastrointestinal conditions, chapter 24.

Table 35.4 Rectal bleeding

Sick neonate	Necrotising enterocolitis (NEC) Malrotation Severe enteritis
Well neonate	Ingested maternal blood Bleeding disorder Anal fissure
Well child: Bright red blood	Anal fissure Polyp (with mucus)
Well child: Dark blood	Meckel's diverticulum Peptic ulcer/varices Inflammatory bowel disease

NECK LUMPS

The enlargement of cervical lymph nodes is common with upper respiratory infections. Consider bacterial infection with abscess formation in infants and children with large (2–4 cm) tender masses. There is often no underlying redness in cervical abscesses because the lymph nodes are beneath the deep fascia. Skin involvement occurs late in the disease. Fluctuance is the indication for surgical referral for incision and drainage.

The development of indolent, non-tender, persistent lymphadenopathy in infants 1–3 years of age is often due to mycobacterial lymph node infection, e.g. mycobacterium avium complex (MAC). Purple discolouration in the overlying skin indicates an underlying abscess, which requires surgical treatment. Large (>3–4 cm) or suspicious lymph nodes need a biopsy to exclude malignancy.

Table 35.5 Urgent neonatal conditions

Symptom	*Diagnosis*	*Investigation*	*Management*
Excessive drooling Feed intolerance	Oesophageal atresia	Passage of 10 F catheter by mouth, stops at ~10 cm	Oropharyngeal suction
Respiratory distress with scaphoid abdomen	Diaphragmatic hernia	Abdominal and chest X-rays – bowel loops in chest	O_2 No bag and masking Nasogastric tube
Intestinal contents in a sac	Exomphalos (consider Beckwith-Weidemann syndrome, especially if infant is large)	Blood glucose	10% IV dextrose Temperature control Nasogastric tube
Prolapsed intestinal contents	Gastroschisis	–	Cover with kitchen wrap Temperature control Nasogastric tube
Green vomiting	Malrotation Bowel obstruction	Abdominal X-ray U & Es (Barium study only after surgical referral)	Nasogastric drainage

URGENT NEONATAL SURGICAL CONDITIONS

Important warning signs

- Excessive drooling of frothy secretions from the mouth may suggest oesophageal atresia.
- Bile-stained vomiting is always abnormal (malrotation may be present and requires urgent treatment)
- Delayed passage of meconium (beyond 24 h) is abnormal and may indicate Hirschsprung's disease.
- Inguinoscrotal hernias need urgent attention to avoid strangulation.

All the conditions following require urgent paediatric surgical consultation and transfer to a tertiary centre.

Oesophageal atresia

Excessive drooling or frothy, mucousy secretions from the mouth in a newborn suggests an inability to swallow. The test for oesophageal atresia is to pass a 10-French gauge catheter (which will not curl up) gently through the mouth.

- In the baby with oesophageal atresia, the catheter stops at 10 cm from the gums.
- In a normal baby, it passes to 20–25 cm and returns acid on litmus testing.

First aid includes:

- Nil orally.
- Intravenous fluids.
- Frequent oropharyngeal suction (every 10–15 min), to prevent aspiration.

Urgent transfer is required.

Diaphragmatic hernia

Respiratory distress in a newborn with a scaphoid abdomen suggests diaphragmatic hernia. Cardiac displacement and a chest X-ray showing bowel loops in the chest (left side more commonly) confirms the diagnosis. First aid is described in Table 35.5. If a baby with suspected or diagnosed diaphragmatic hernia needs mechanical ventilation, intubate the trachea; bag and mask ventilation may exacerbate respiratory distress by distending the bowel.

Exomphalos/gastroschisis

These anterior abdominal wall defects place the child at risk of heat and water loss from the exposed surface of the sac (exomphalos) or bowel (gastroschisis). First and is described in Table 35.5.

Sacrococcygeal teratoma

Any lump over the coccyx of the baby should be assumed to be a teratoma until proven otherwise and needs immediate referral at birth.

Ambiguous genitalia

Genitalia that are frankly ambiguous need urgent consultation with an experienced paediatric endocrinologist or surgeon on the first day of life (see Endocrine conditions, chapter 21).

An enlarged clitoris in an apparent female is also abnormal and needs immediate referral.

Hypospadias may overlap with ambiguous genitalia. This needs a careful initial assessment, if the diagosis of hypospadias has been made, someone has already assumed the gender is male. If one or both testes are undescended, or the scrotum is bifid, or both, the baby should be treated as having ambiguous genitalia until proven otherwise with immediate referral for further investigation.

CHAPTER 36
PRESCRIBING FOR CHILDREN

Noel Cranswick
Yashwant Sinha

Knowledge of drug administration in children and infants is essential to the practice of paediatrics. The majority of registered medicines do not have indications or dosing for children.

There are many issues unique to paediatrics that influence drug choice and dose (e.g. virtually all pharmacokinetic parameters change with age). Dosage regimens need to take into account factors such as growth, organ development and sexual maturation.

Both unlicensed and off-label use are commonplace in paediatric practice as a result of inadequate paediatric data.

Unlicensed drug use is the use of an unapproved drug, an untested formulation of an approved drug or a non-pharmacopoeial substance as a medicine.

Off-label prescribing is the use of a drug in a manner other than that recommended in the manufacturer's product information.

Dosing considerations

- Most medicines in children are dosed by weight.
- A few medications, especially cytotoxic drugs, may only have dosing information by surface area (see Appendix 4).
- Always attempt to obtain accurate weight and height data prior to calculating the appropriate initial dose.

Table 36.1 Guidelines for best prescribing practice

- Dose by weight (use a calculator)
- Check the dose
- Do not exceed the maximum adult dose
- Check for allergies and contraindications
- Write legible prescriptions

- In emergencies standard nomograms for weight and height may be utilised for these calculations.

Adverse drug reactions

- Are common but under-recognised in children.
- All suspected and proven adverse drug reactions (ADR) no matter how trivial, should be reported.
- Suspected allergic reactions should be confirmed and follow-up provided. Potentially avoidable ADR should be identified and patients should be given a permanent record (e.g. card or medical alert bracelet) as appropriate.

There are two main types:

Type A adverse drug reaction

- These are predictable from the known pharmacology of the drug and are dose dependent.
- Examples include opiate sedation and tachycardia with β-2-agonists.

Type B adverse drug reaction

- These are less common, unpredictable and dose-independent.
- They are often serious and usually require ceasing the drug e.g. Steven-Johnson syndrome (most commonly associated with anticonvulsants).

Therapeutic drug monitoring

- Relatively few drugs need therapeutic drug monitoring.
- Drugs where it is beneficial usually either have a narrow therapeutic index or serum levels are well correlated with efficacy or safety.
- Serum levels may be important to determine toxicity in overdose (e.g. paracetamol and iron).
- Timing of samples for monitoring will vary depending upon the actual drug but accurate recording of the drug dose, administration time and sample time is essential.

Drug errors

- Paediatric patients are at high risk of drug errors.
- Certain drugs are commonly associated with medication errors in children (e.g. opiates, paracetamol, antibiotics, 50% dextrose and electrolytes such as i.v. Ca^{2+} and Mg^{2+}).

- Extra care should be taken when prescribing or administering these medicines.
- When prescribing for children, the following factors should be taken into consideration:
  - Children's doses vary widely and so there is no standard dose (as there is with adults).
  - Some drugs are documented as total daily dose while others are per dose – this can cause confusion.
  - Calculations are required for most childhood dosing and so errors may occur during this step.
  - Some paediatric preparations may cause confusion in those unfamiliar with their use.
  - The small doses used in children may cause measuring and administration errors.
  - Misplacement or misreading of decimal points can lead to error.

Drug interactions

- Drug interactions are always possible when using more than one medicine, however, relatively few drug combinations result in clinically significant sequelae.
- The potential increases with number of drugs prescribed.
- Are more common in sick patients, especially with multiple organ pathologies.
- Drugs with a narrow therapeutic window are more likely to be involved in significant interactions.

Complementary medicines

- Many patients take alternative or complementary products, often these are available 'over the counter'.
- Families may not mention these when asked about medication use and a specific history should be sought.
- Such products can cause adverse drug reactions and be involved in drug interactions.

APPENDIX 1
GROWTH CHARTS AND PUBERTAL STAGING

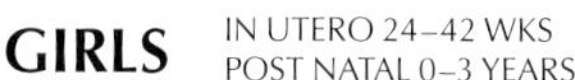

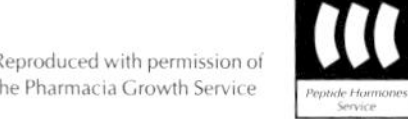

INTRAUTERINE GROWTH CURVES (COMPOSITE MALE/FEMALE)

Measuring techniques: (as for ages 0–36 months—see over page)

Additional Notes: Gestational ages are recorded in completed weeks from the first day of the mother's last menstrual period. Foetal growth is influenced by many factors including age, body weight, height, parity, ethnic origin of the mother and sex of the foetus. Corrections for some of these factors are found in the quoted reference.

Data Source: W.H. Kitchen et al *Revised intrauterine growth curves for an Australian hospital population.* Aust. Paediatr. J. *(1983) 19:157–161.*

BIRTH LENGTH
HEAD CIRCUMFERENCE
WEEKS OF GESTATION

BIRTH WEIGHT
WEEKS OF GESTATION

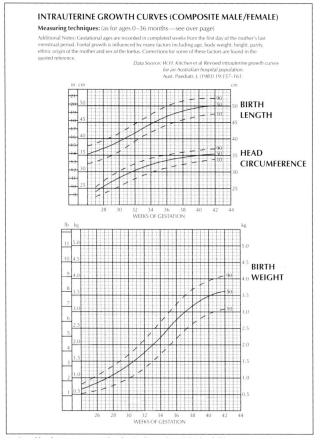

Designed by the Department of Endocrinology, The Adelaide Children's Hospital, 1989.

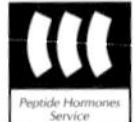

GIRLS 0–3 YEARS
LENGTH PERCENTILE CHART

cm MOTHER'S HEIGHT_______________ FATHER'S HEIGHT_______________ cm in

Supine length (recommended up to the age of 3 so that there is overlap with standing height at 2 to 3) is taken on a flat surface, with the child lying on her back. One observer holds her head in contact with a board at the top of the table and another straightens the legs and turns the feet upward to be at right angles to the legs and brings a sliding board in contact with the child's heels.

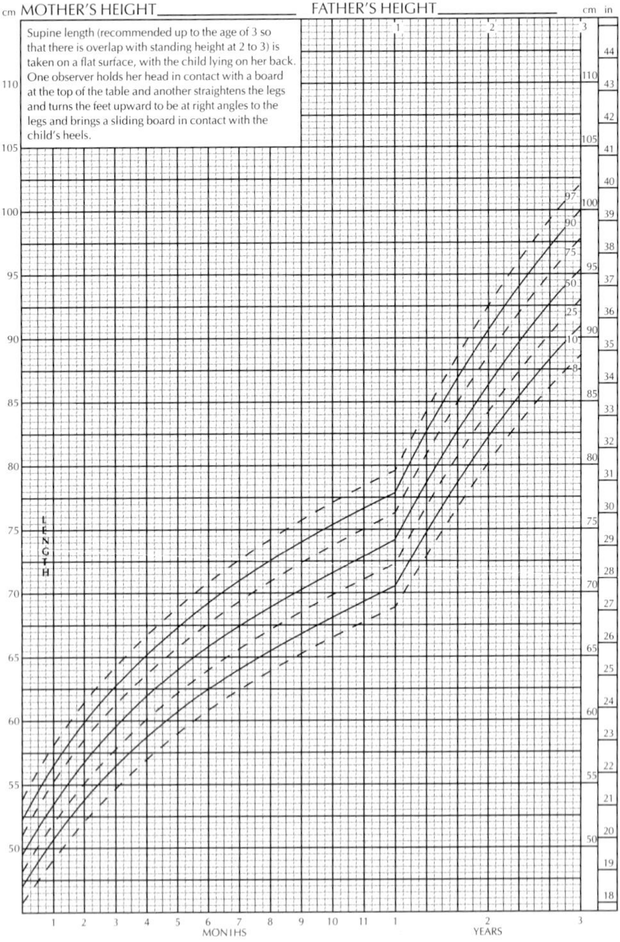

Data Source: Hamill P.V.V.: NCHS growth curves for children. DHEW publication (PHS) 78–1650

GIRLS 0–3 YEARS WEIGHT PERCENTILE CHART

Reproduced with permission of the Pharmacia Growth Service

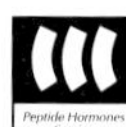

Weight should be taken in the nude, or as near thereto as possible. If a surgical gown or minimum underclothing (vest and pants) is worn, then its estimated weight (about 0.1 kg) must be subtracted before weight is recorded. Weights are conveniently recorded to the last completed 0.1 kg above the age of six months. The bladder should be empty.

DATE	AGE	LENGTH	WEIGHT	HEAD CIRCUM.

SIMPLIFIED CALCULATION OF BODY SURFACE AREA (BSA)

$$BSA\ (m^2) = \sqrt{\frac{Ht\ (cm) \times Wt\ (kg)}{3600}}$$

Ref: Mosteller R.D.
Simplified calculation of body surface area
N.Engl. J.Med. 1987; 317:1098.

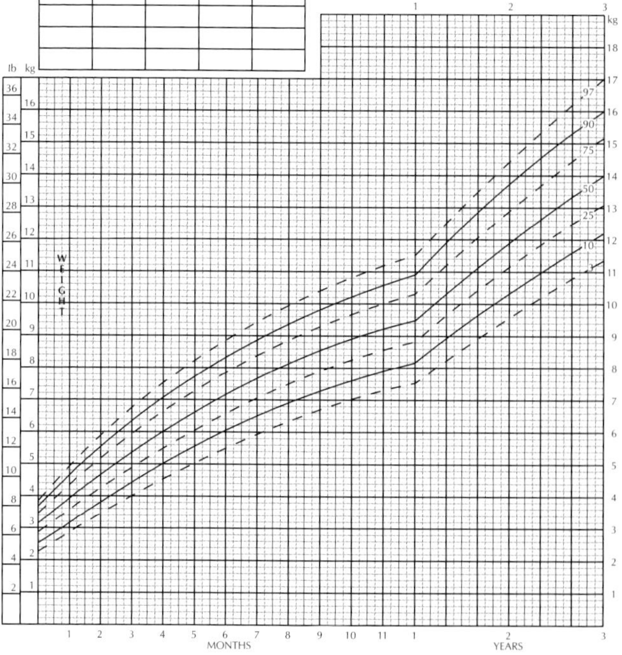

Data Source: Hamill P.V.V.: NCHS growth curves for children. DHEW publication (PHS) 78–1650

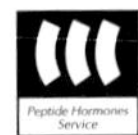

Reproduced with permission of the Pharmacia Growth Service

HEAD CIRCUMFERENCE GIRLS

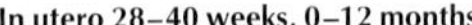

In utero 28–40 weeks, 0–12 months

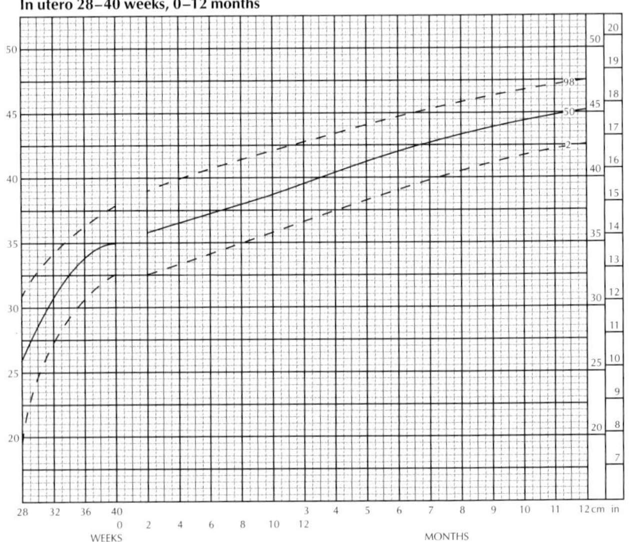

1–3 years

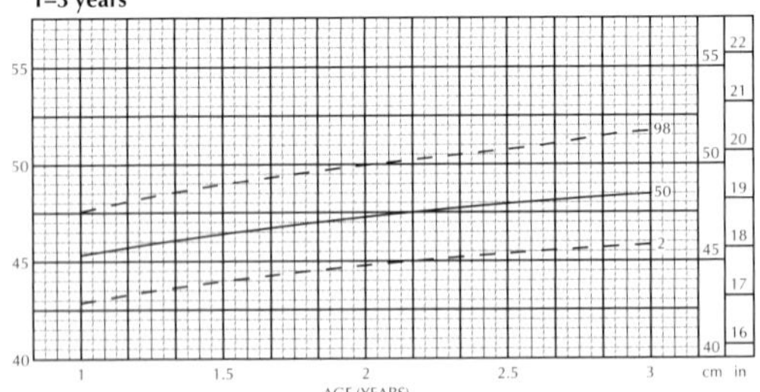

MEASURING TECHNIQUE HEAD CIRCUMFERENCE

The tape should be placed over the eyebrows, above the ears and over the most prominent part of the occiput taking a direct route. A paper tape is preferable to plastic which stretches unacceptably. Record to nearest 0.1 cm.

SOURCES

Head circumference 0–3 years from NSW Health Commission Publication (Jones DL and Hemphill W, 1974).

Head circumference 28–40 weeks gestation from Kitchen WH Aust. Paediatr. J. *(1983) 19:157–161.*

BOYS

IN UTERO 24–42 WKS
POST NATAL 0–3 YEARS

Reproduced with permission of the Pharmacia Growth Service

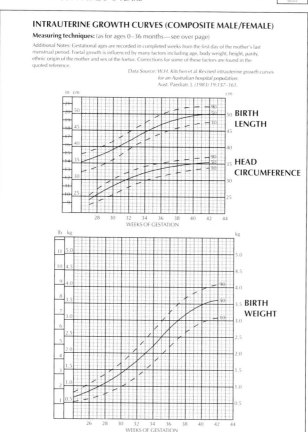

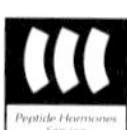

INTRAUTERINE GROWTH CURVES (COMPOSITE MALE/FEMALE)

Measuring techniques: (as for ages 0–36 months—see over page)

Additional Notes: Gestational ages are recorded in completed weeks from the first day of the mother's last menstrual period. Foetal growth is influenced by many factors including age, body weight, height, parity, ethnic origin of the mother and sex of the foetus. Corrections for some of these factors are found in the quoted reference.

Data Source: W.H. Kitchen et al *Revised intrauterine growth curves for an Australian hospital population.* Aust. Paediatr. J. *(1983) 19:157–161.*

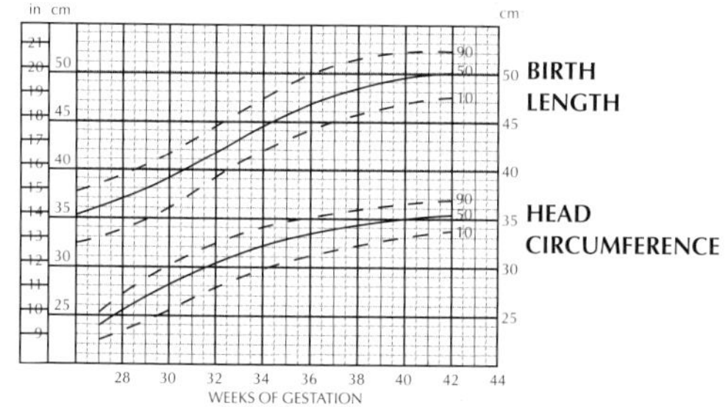

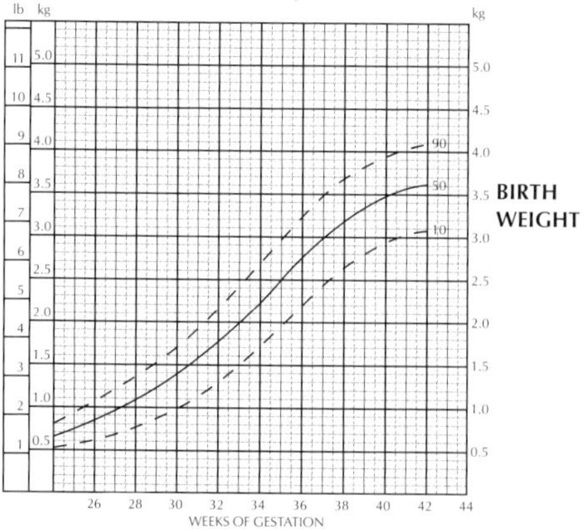

Designed by the Department of Endocrinology, The Adelaide Children's Hospital, 1989.

BOYS 0–3 YEARS
LENGTH PERCENTILE CHART

Reproduced with permission of the Pharmacia Growth Service

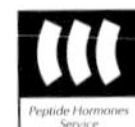

MOTHER'S HEIGHT________ FATHER'S HEIGHT________

Supine length (recommended up to the age of 3 so that there is overlap with standing height at 2 to 3) is taken on a flat surface, with the child lying on his back. One observer holds his head in contact with a board at the top of the table and another straightens the legs and turns the feet upward to be at right angles to the legs and brings a sliding board in contact with the child's heels.

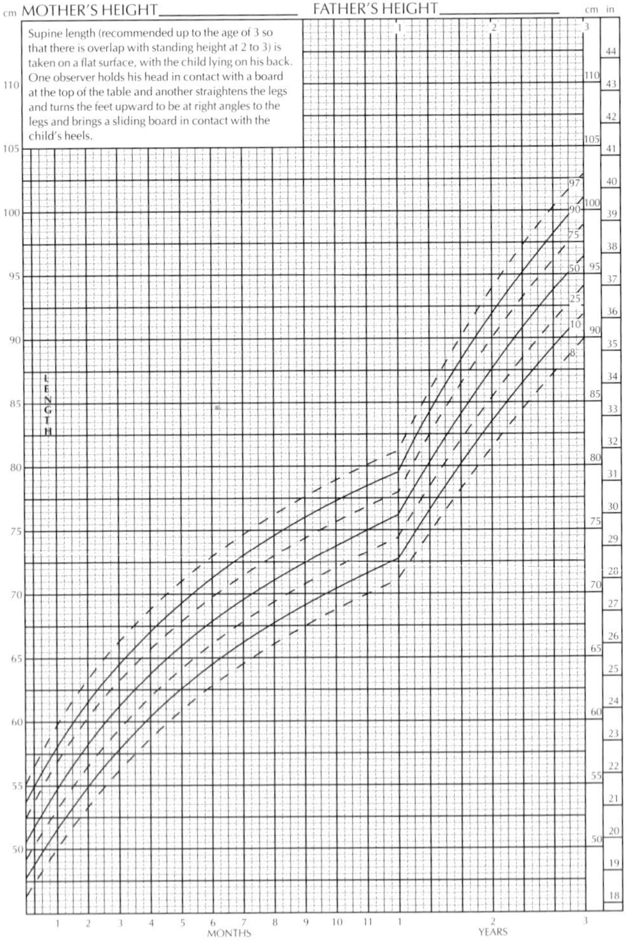

Data Source: Hamill P.V.V.: NCHS growth curves for children. DHEW publication (PHS) 78–1650

BOYS 0–3 YEARS
WEIGHT PERCENTILE CHART

Reproduced with permission of the Pharmacia Growth Service

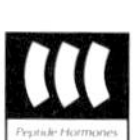

Weight should be taken in the nude, or as near thereto as possible. If a surgical gown or minimum underclothing (vest and pants) is worn, then its estimated weight (about 0.1 kg) must be subtracted before weight is recorded. Weights are conveniently recorded to the last completed 0.1 kg above the age of six months. The bladder should be empty.

DATE	AGE	LENGTH	WEIGHT	HEAD CIRCUM.

SIMPLIFIED CALCULATION OF BODY SURFACE AREA (BSA)

$$\text{BSA (m}^2\text{)} = \sqrt{\frac{\text{Ht (cm)} \times \text{Wt (kg)}}{3600}}$$

Ref: Mosteller R.D.
Simplified calculation of body surface area
N.Engl. J.Med. 1987; 317:1098.

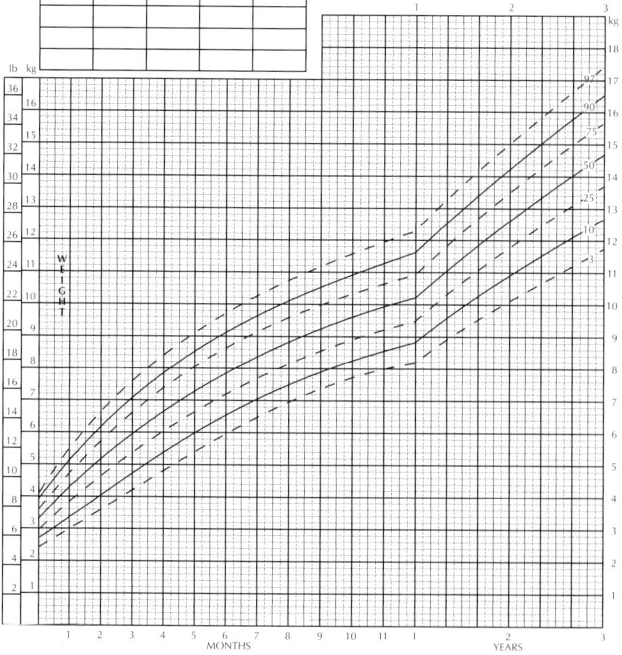

lb kg

WEIGHT

97 90 75 50 25 10 3

MONTHS

YEARS

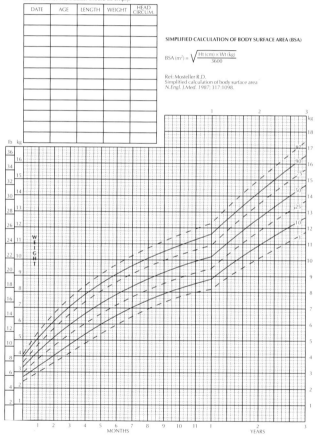

Data Source: Hamill P.V.V.: NCHS growth curves for children. DHEW publication (PHS) 78–1650

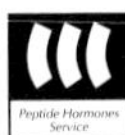

HEAD CIRCUMFERENCE BOYS

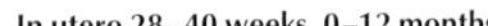

In utero 28–40 weeks, 0–12 months

Reproduced with permission of the Pharmacia Growth Service

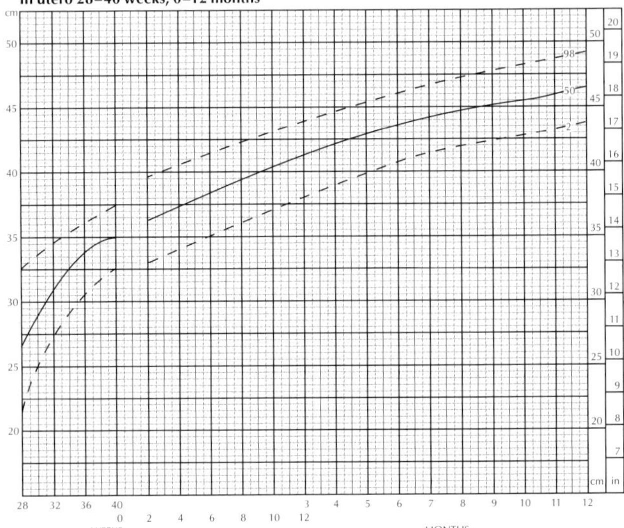

1–3 years

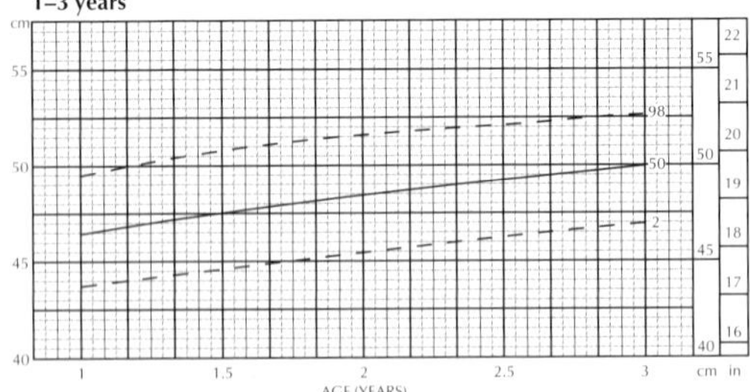

MEASURING TECHNIQUE HEAD CIRCUMFERENCE

The tape should be placed over the eyebrows, above the ears and over the most prominent part of the occiput taking a direct route. A paper tape is preferable to plastic which stretches unacceptably. Record to nearest 0.1 cm.

SOURCES

Head circumference 0–3 years from NSW Health Commission Publication (Jones DL and Hemphill W, 1974).

Head circumference 28–40 weeks gestation from Kitchen WH Aust. Paediatr. J. *(1983) 19:157–161.*

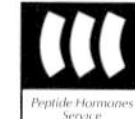

GIRLS: 2 TO 18 YEARS HEIGHT PERCENTILE

Reproduced with permission of the Pharmacia Growth Service

MOTHER'S HEIGHT________________ FATHER'S HEIGHT________________

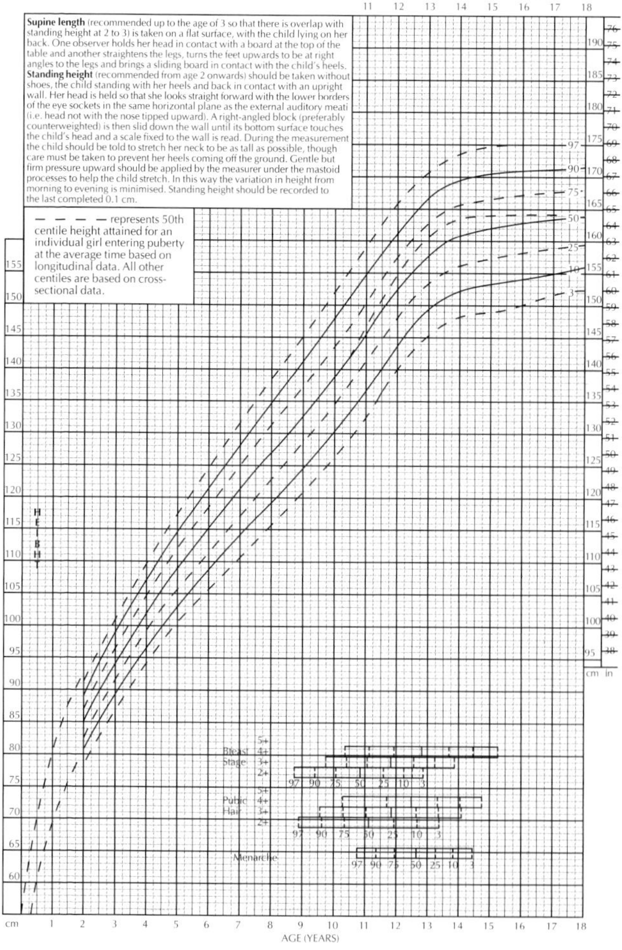

Supine length (recommended up to the age of 3 so that there is overlap with standing height at 2 to 3) is taken on a flat surface, with the child lying on her back. One observer holds her head in contact with a board at the top of the table and another straightens the legs, turns the feet upwards to be at right angles to the legs and brings a sliding board in contact with the child's heels. **Standing height** (recommended from age 2 onwards) should be taken without shoes, the child standing with her heels and back in contact with an upright wall. Her head is held so that she looks straight forward with the lower borders of the eye sockets in the same horizontal plane as the external auditory meati (i.e. head not with the nose tipped upward). A right-angled block (preferably counterweighted) is then slid down the wall until its bottom surface touches the child's head and a scale fixed to the wall is read. During the measurement the child should be told to stretch her neck to be as tall as possible, though care must be taken to prevent her heels coming off the ground. Gentle but firm pressure upward should be applied by the measurer under the mastoid processes to help the child stretch. In this way the variation in height from morning to evening is minimised. Standing height should be recorded to the last completed 0.1 cm.

— — — — represents 50th centile height attained for an individual girl entering puberty at the average time based on longitudinal data. All other centiles are based on cross-sectional data.

Source: Adapted from Hamill P.V.V.: NCHS growth curves for children. DHEW publication (PHS) 78–1650

GIRLS: 2 TO 18 YEARS
WEIGHT PERCENTILE

Weight should be taken in the nude, or as near thereto as possible. If a surgical gown or minimum underclothing (vest and pants) is worn, then its estimated weight (about 0.1 kg) must be subtracted before weight is recorded. Weights are conventionally recorded to the last completed 0.1 kg above the age of six months. The bladder should be empty.

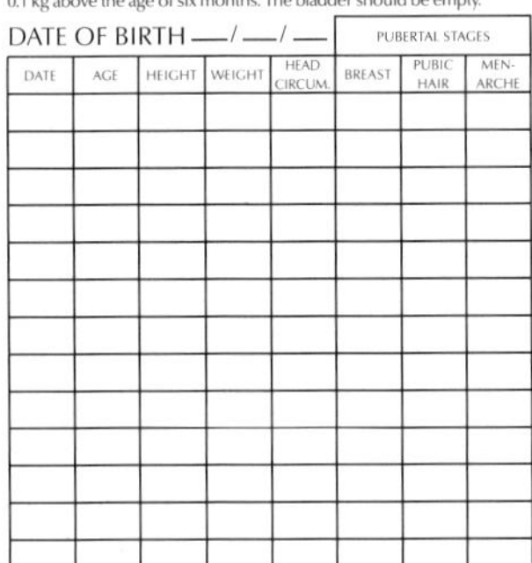

DATE OF BIRTH —/—/—

DATE	AGE	HEIGHT	WEIGHT	HEAD CIRCUM.	PUBERTAL STAGES: BREAST	PUBERTAL STAGES: PUBIC HAIR	PUBERTAL STAGES: MEN-ARCHE

BODY-MASS INDEX

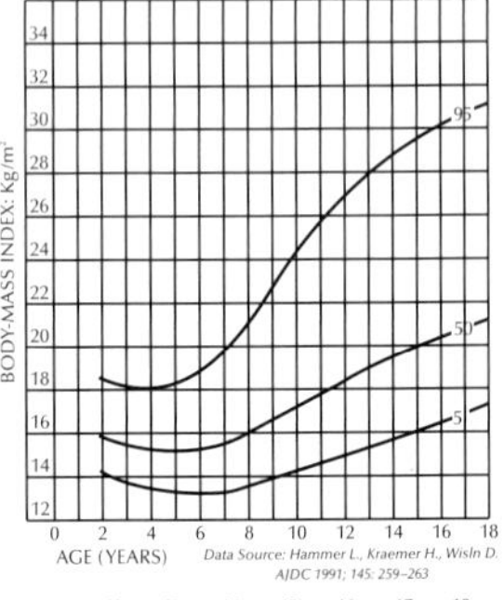

Data Source: Hammer L., Kraemer H., Wisln D. AJDC 1991; 145: 259–263

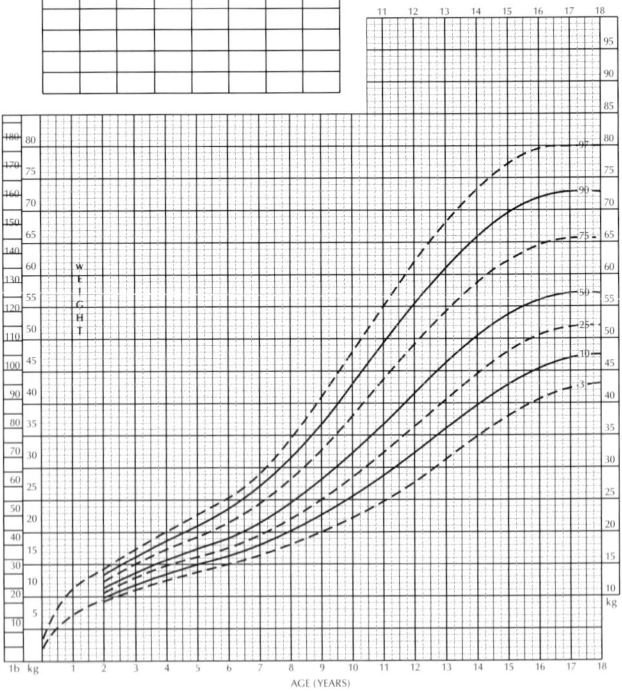

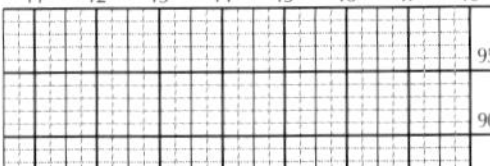

Source: Adapted from Hamill P.V.V.: NCHS growth curves for children. DHEW publication (PHS) 78–1650

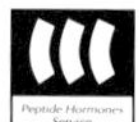

Reproduced with permission of the Pharmacia Growth Service

HEAD CIRCUMFERENCE, GIRLS

Head Circumference: The tape should be placed over the eyebrows, above the ears and over the most prominent part of the occiput taking a direct route. A paper tape is preferable to plastic, which stretches unacceptably under tension. The maximum measurement should be recorded to the nearest 0.1 cm.

Data Source: 2–5 yr. Jones DL (1973) NSW Health Comm. Publ. 5–18 yr Nellhaus G. Pediatrics (1968) 41:106–114

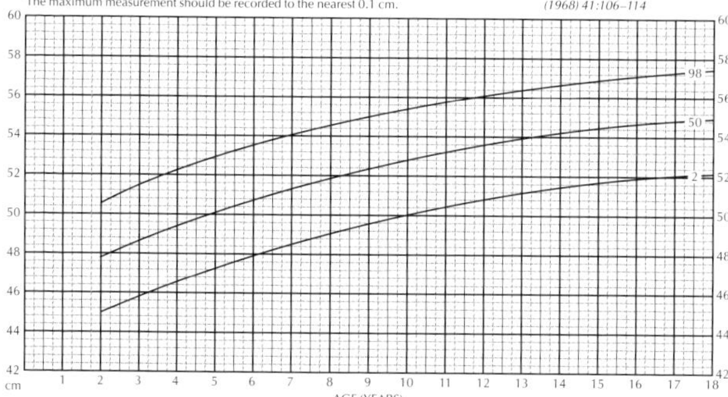

HEIGHT VELOCITY, GIRLS

The standards are appropriate for velocity calculated over a whole year period, not less, since a smaller period requires wider limits (the 3rd and 97th centiles for whole year being roughly appropriate for the 10th and 90th centiles over six months). The yearly velocity should be plotted at the mid-point of a year. The centiles given in black are appropriate to children of average maturational tempo, who have their peak velocity at the average age for this event. The red line is the 50th centile line for the child who is two years early in maturity and age at peak height velocity, and the blue line refers to a child who is 50th centile in velocity but two years late. The arrows mark the 3rd and 97th centiles at peak velocity for early and late maturers.

Centiles for girls maturing at average time — 97, 50, 3

97 and 3 centiles at peak height velocity for ^ v

Early (+2SD) maturers

Late (–2SD) maturers

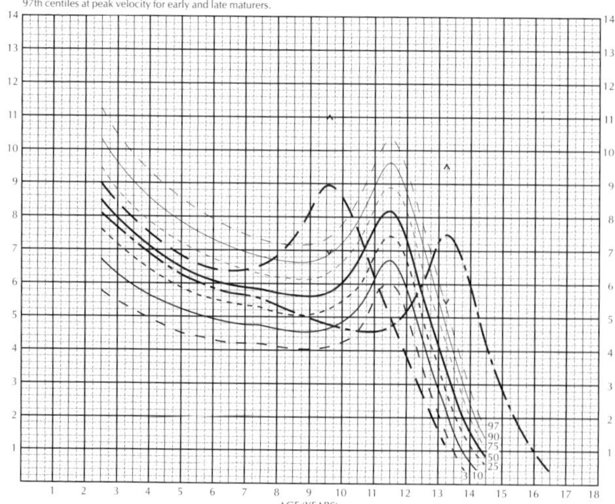

Reproduced by permission of © Castlemead Publications

Data Source: Tanner J, Davis PSW, *Journal of Pediatrics* 1985:107

BOYS: 2 TO 18 YEARS
HEIGHT PERCENTILE

Reproduced with permission of the Pharmacia Growth Service

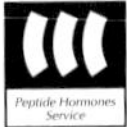

MOTHER'S HEIGHT________________ FATHER'S HEIGHT________________

Supine length (recommended up to the age of 3 so that there is overlap with standing height at 2 to 3) is taken on a flat surface, with the child lying on his back. One observer holds his head in contact with a board at the top of the table and another straightens the legs, turns the feet upwards to be at right angles to the legs and brings a sliding board in contact with the child's heels. **Standing height** (recommended from age 2 onwards) should be taken without shoes, the child standing with his heels and back in contact with an upright wall. His head is held so that he looks straight forward with the lower borders of the eye sockets in the same horizontal plane as the external auditory meati (i.e. head not with the nose tipped upward). A right-angled block (preferably counterweighted) is then slid down the wall until its bottom surface touches the child's head and a scale fixed to the wall is read. During the measurement the child should be told to stretch his neck to be as tall as possible, though care must be taken to prevent his heels coming off the ground. Gentle but firm pressure upward should be applied by the measurer under the mastoid processes to help the child stretch. In this way the variation in height from morning to evening is minimised. Standing height should be recorded to the last completed 0.1 cm.

— — — — represents 50th centile height attained for an individual boy entering puberty at the average time based on longitudinal data. All other centiles are based on cross-sectional data.

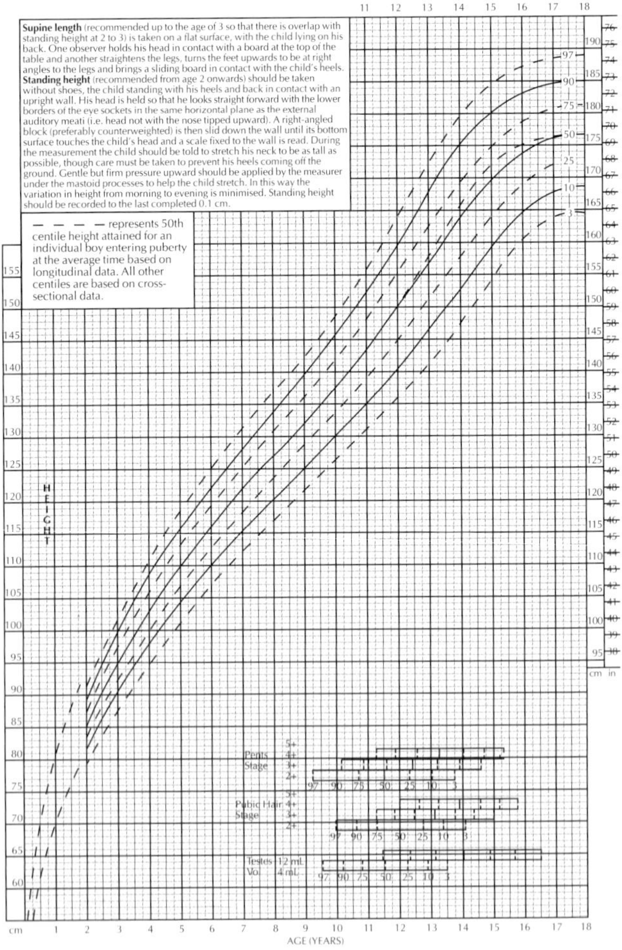

HEIGHT

Centiles: 97, 90, 75, 50, 25, 10, 3

Pents Stage 2+ 3+ 4+ 5+ — 97 90 75 50 25 10 3

Pubic Hair Stage 2+ 3+ 4+ 5+ — 97 90 75 50 25 10 3

Testes Vol 4 mL 12 mL — 97 90 75 50 25 10 3

cm: 60 65 70 75 80 85 90 95 100 105 110 115 120 125 130 135 140 145 150 155 160 165 170 175 180 185 190

in: 38 39 40 41 42 43 44 45 46 47 48 49 50 51 52 53 54 55 56 57 58 59 60 61 62 63 64 65 66 67 68 69 70 71 72 73 74 75 76

AGE (YEARS) 1 2 3 4 5 6 7 8 9 10 11 12 13 14 15 16 17 18

Source: Adapted from Hamill P.V.V.: NCHS growth curves for children. DHEW publication (PHS) 78–1650

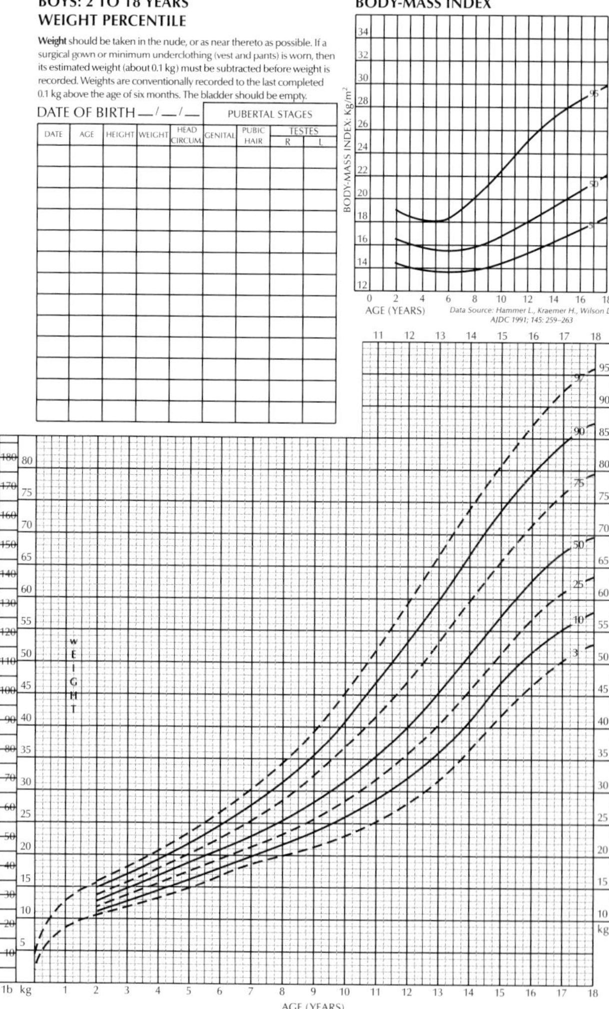

BOYS: 2 TO 18 YEARS WEIGHT PERCENTILE

Weight should be taken in the nude, or as near thereto as possible. If a surgical gown or minimum underclothing (vest and pants) is worn, then its estimated weight (about 0.1 kg) must be subtracted before weight is recorded. Weights are conventionally recorded to the last completed 0.1 kg above the age of six months. The bladder should be empty.

DATE OF BIRTH __/__/__

DATE	AGE	HEIGHT	WEIGHT	HEAD CIRCUM.	PUBERTAL STAGES: GENITAL	PUBIC HAIR	TESTES R	TESTES L

Source: Adapted from Hamill P.V.V.: NCHS growth curves for children. DHEW publication (PHS) 78–1650

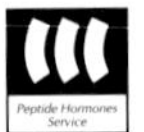

Reproduced with permission of the Pharmacia Growth Service

HEAD CIRCUMFERENCE, BOYS

Head Circumference: The tape should be placed over the eyebrows, above the ears and over the most prominent part of the occiput taking a direct route. A paper tape is preferable to plastic, which stretches unacceptably under tension. The maximum measurement should be recorded to the nearest 0.1 cm.

Data Source: 2–5 yr. Jones DL (1973) NSW Health Comm. Publ. 5–18 yr Nellhaus G. Pediatrics (1968) 41:106–114

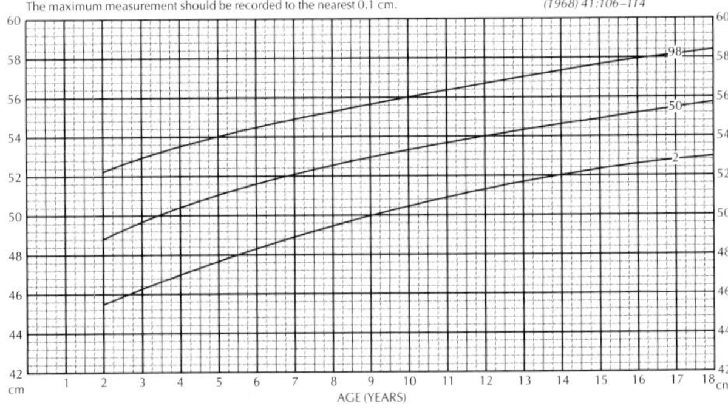

HEIGHT VELOCITY, BOYS

The standards are appropriate for velocity calculated over a whole year period, not less, since a small period requires wider limits (the 3rd and 97th centiles for whole year being roughly appropriate for the 10th and 90th centiles over six months). The yearly velocity should be plotted at the mid-point of a year. The centiles given in black are appropriate to children of average maturational tempo, who have their peak velocity at the average age for this event. The red line is the 50th centile line for the child who is two years early in maturity and age at peak height velocity, and the green line refers to a child who is 50th centile in velocity but two years late. The arrows mark the 3rd and 97th centiles at peak velocity for early and late maturers.

Centiles of whole-year velocity for maturers at average time — 97, 50, 3

97 and 3 centile at peak height velocity for
Early (+2SD) maturers
Late (–2SD) maturers

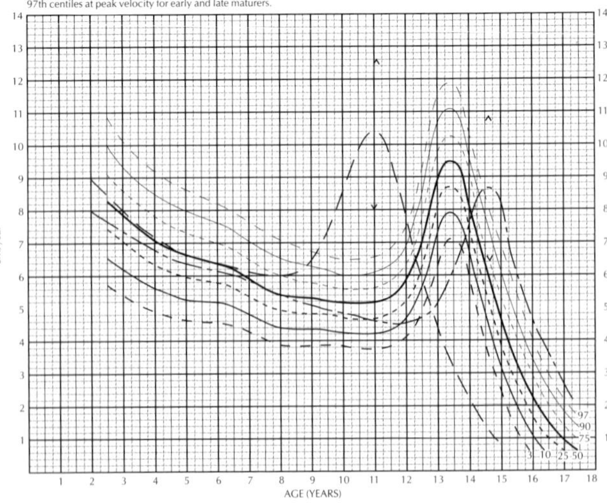

Data Source: Tanner J, Davis PSW, *Journal of Pediatrics* 1985:107

GIRLS 2–18

Reproduced with permission of the Pharmacia Growth Service

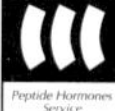

Breast Development

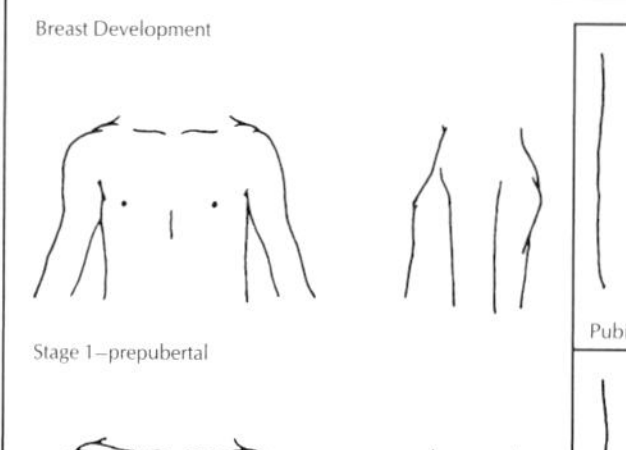

Stage 1–prepubertal

Stage 2–elevation of breasts and papilla

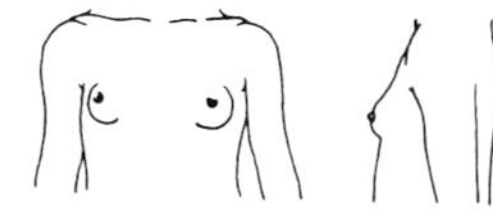

Stage 3–further elevation and areola but no separation of contours

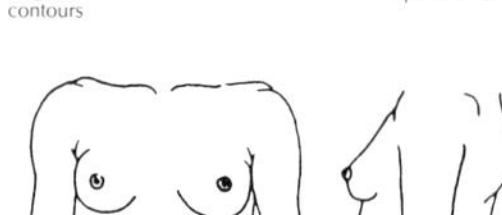

Stage 4–areola and papilla form a secondary mound above level of the breast

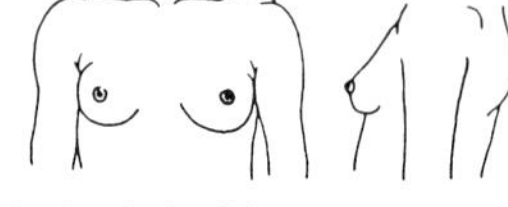

Stage 5–areola recesses to the general contour of the breast

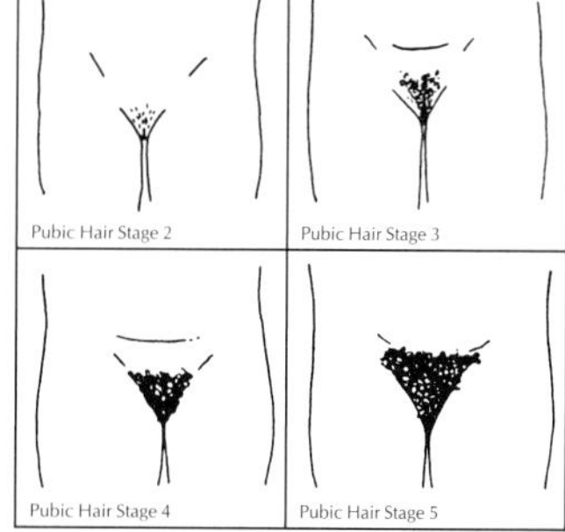

STAGES OF PUBERTY

Ages of attainment of successive stages of pubertal sexual development are given in the height centile chart overpage. The stage Pubic Hair 2+ represents the state of a child who shows the pubic hair appearance stage 2 but not stage 3 (see below). The centiles for age at which this state is normally seen are given, the 97th centile being considered as the early limit, the 3rd centile as the late limit. The child's puberty stages may be plotted at successive ages (Tanner, *Growth at Adolescence*, 2nd Ed., 1962).

Pubic hair:

Stage 1. Pre-adolescent. The vellus over the pubes is not further developed than that over the abdominal wall, i.e. no pubic hair.

Stage 2. Sparse growth of long, slightly pigmented downy hair, straight or slightly curled, chiefly along labia.

Stage 3. Considerably darker, coarser and more curled. The hair spreads sparsely over the junction of the pubes.

Stage 4. Hair now adult in type, but area covered is still considerably smaller than in the adult. No spread to the medial surface of thighs.

Stage 5. Adult in quantity and type with distribution of the horizontal (or classically 'feminine') pattern. Spread to medial surface of thighs but not up linea alba or elsewhere above the base of the inverse triangle (spread up linea alba occurs late and is rated stage 6).

Designed by the Department of Endocrinology, The Adelaide Children's Hospital, 1989.

BOYS 2–18

Reproduced with permission of the Pharmacia Growth Service

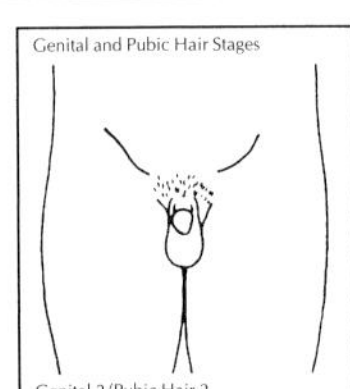

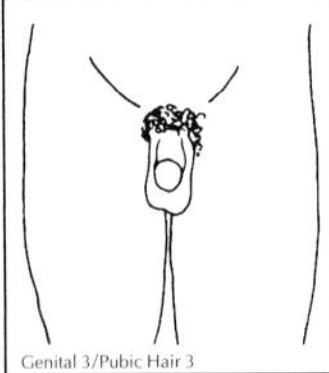

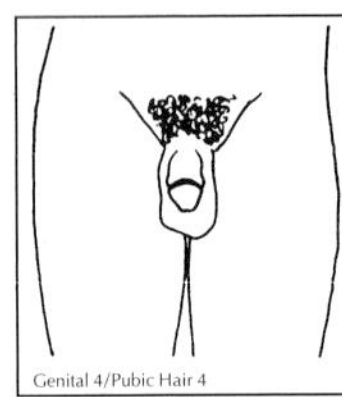

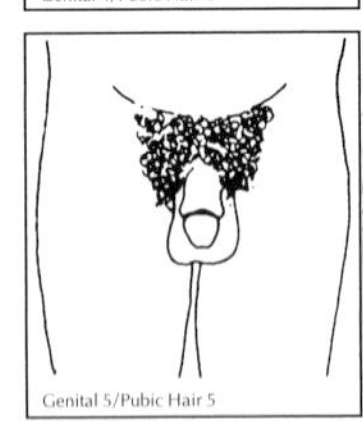

STAGES OF PUBERTY

Ages of attainment of successive stages of pubertal sexual development are given in the height centile chart overpage. The stage Pubic Hair 2+ represents the state of a child who shows the pubic hair appearance stage 2 but not stage 3 (see below). The centiles for age at which this state is normally seen are given, the 97th centile being considered as the early limit, the 3rd centile as the late limit. The child's puberty stages may be plotted at successive ages (Tanner, *Growth at Adolescence*, 2nd Ed., 1962). Testis sizes are judged by comparison with the Prader orchidometer (Zachmann, Prader, Kind, Haflinger and Budliger, *Helv. Paed. Acta.* 29, 61–72, 1974).

Genital (penis) development:

Stage 1. Pre-adolescent, testes, scrotum and penis are of about the same size and proportion as in early childhood.
Stage 2. Enlargement of scrotum and testes. Skin of scrotum reddens and changes in texture. Little or no enlargement of penis at this stage.
Stage 3. Enlargement of the penis which occurs at first mainly in length. Further growth of the testes and scrotum.
Stage 4. Increased size of penis with growth in breadth and development of glans. Testes and scrotum larger; scrotal skin darkened.
Stage 5. Genitalia adult in size and shape.

Pubic hair:

Stage 1. Pre-adolescent. The vellus over the pubes is not further developed than that over the abdominal wall, i.e. no pubic hair.
Stage 2. Sparse growth of long, slightly pigmented downy hair, straight or slightly curled at the base of the penis.
Stage 3. Considerably darker, coarser and more curled. The hair spreads sparsely over the junction of the pubes.
Stage 4. Hair now adult in type, but area covered is still considerably smaller than in the adult. No spread to the medial surface of thighs.
Stage 5. Adult in quantity and type with distribution of the horizontal (or classically 'feminine') pattern. Spread to medial surface of thighs but not up linea alba or elsewhere above the base of the inverse triangle (spread up linea alba occurs late and is rated stage 6).

Stretched Penile Length

Measured from the pubo-penile skin junction to the tip of the glans (Schonfeld and Beebe, *J. of Urology* 48, 759–777, 1942).

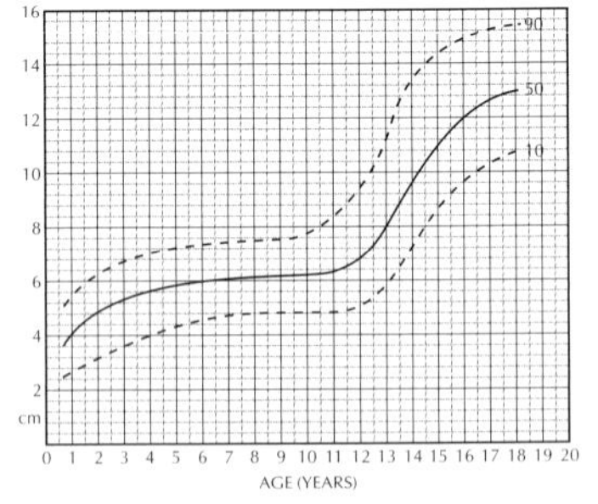

Designed by the Department of Endocrinology, The Adelaide Children's Hospital, 1989.

APPENDIX 2
PHARMACOPOEIA

This pharmacopoeia is reproduced directly from 'Drug doses', 12th edition, published in 2001 by the Royal Children's Hospital, Melbourne, with permission from Frank Shann. Considerable care has been taken to see that the information in this pharmacopoeia is accurate, but the user is advised to check the doses carefully. The authors shall not be responsible for any errors in this publication.

Acetazolamide 5–10 mg/kg/dose (adult 100–250 mg) 6–8 H (daily for epilepsy) oral.

Acetylcholine chloride Adult (NOT/kg): 1% instil 0.5–2 mL into anterior chamber of the eye.

Acetylcysteine Paracetamol poisoning (regardless of delay): 150 mg/kg in 5%D IV over 1 hr; then 10 mg/kg/hr for 20 hr (delay <10 hr), 32 hr (delay 10–16 hr), 72 hr (delay >16 hr) and longer if still encephalopathic; oral 140 mg/kg stat, then 70 mg/kg/dose 4 H for 72 hr. Monitor serum K^+. Give if paracetamol >1000 μmol/L (150 mg/L) at 4 hr, >500 μmol/L 8 hr, >250 μmol/L 12 hr. Lung disease: 10% soltn 0.1 mL/kg/dose (adult 5 mL) 6–12 H nebulised or intratracheal. Meconium ileus equivalent: 5 mL/dose (NOT/kg) of 20% soltn 8 H oral; 60–100 mL of 50 mg/mL for 45 min PR. CF: 4–8 mg/kg/dose 8 H oral. Eye drops 5% + hypromellose 0.35%: 1–2 drops/eye 6–8 H.

Aciclovir Neonate to 12 wk: 20 mg/kg/dose IV over 1 hr daily (<30 wk gest), 18 H (30–32 wk), 12 H (1st wk life), 8 H (2–12 wk) for 2 wk (3 wk for encephalitis). EB virus, herpes encephalitis, immunocompromised, or varicella (>12 wk old): 500 mg/m^2/dose (adult 10 mg/kg) 8 H IV over 1 hr. Cutaneous herpes (>12 wk old): 250 mg/m^2/dose (12 wk–12 yr), 5 mg/kg/dose (adult) 8 H IV over 1 hr. Genital herpes (NOT/kg): 200 mg/dose oral × 5/day for 10 days, then 200 mg/dose × 2–3/day for 6 mo if reqd. Zoster (NOT/kg): 400 mg/dose (<2 yr) or 800 mg/dose (≥2 yr) oral × 5/day for 7 days. Cold sores: apply 5% cream × 5/day. Eye: apply 3% oint × 5/day.

Activated charcoal See charcoal, activated.

Adenosine 0.1 mg/kg (adult 3 mg) stat rapid IV push, incr by 0.05 mg/kg (adult 3 mg) every 2 min to max 0.35 mg/kg (adult 18 mg).

Adrenaline Croup: 1% (L isomer) or 2.25% (racemic) 0.05 mL/kg/dose diluted to 4 mL by inhaltn; or 1/1000 0.5 mL/kg/dose (max 6 mL) by inhaltn. Cardiac arrest (repeat if reqd): 0.1 mL/kg of 1/10,000 IV or intracardiac; via ETT 0.1 mL/kg of 1/1000. Anaphylaxis: 0.05–0.1 mL/kg/dose of 1/10,000 IV, repeat if reqd. SC: 0.01 mg/kg (0.01 mL/kg of 1/1000) up to 0.1 mg/kg, × 3 doses 20 min apart if reqd. IV infsn 0.05–2 mcg/kg/min: child; for 65 kg adult 5 mg in 50 mL at 2 mL/hr is 0.05 mcg/kg/min.

Albendazole Pinworm, threadworm, roundworm, hookworm, whipworm: 20 mg/kg (adult 400 mg) oral once (may repeat after 2 wk). *Strongyloides*, cutaneous larva migrans, *Taenia, H. nana, O. viverrini, C. sinesis*: 20 mg/kg (adult 400 mg) daily for 3 days, repeated in 3 wk. 7.5 mg/kg/dose (adult 400 mg) 12 H for 8–30 days (neurocysticercosis); 12 H for three 28 day courses 14 days apart (hydatid).

Albumin 20%: 2–5 mL/kg IV. 4%: 10–20 mL/kg. If no loss from plasma: dose (mL/kg) = 5 × (increase g/L)/(% albumin).

Alendronate Adults (NOT/kg), oral. Osteoporosis 10 mg daily; slow release 35 mg weekly (prevention), 70 mg weekly (treatment). Paget's 40 mg daily.

Alginic acid (Gaviscon single strength) <1 yr: liquid 2 mL with feed 4 H. 1–12 yr: liquid 5–10 mL, or 1 tab after meals. >12 yr: liquid 10–20 mL, or 1–2 tab after meals.

Allopurinol 10 mg/kg/dose (adult 300 mg) 12–24 H oral, or (chemotherapy) 50–100 mg/m^2/dose 6 H IV, oral.

Alpha tocopheryl acetate One alpha-tocopheryl (at) equivalent = 1 mg d-at = 1.1 mg d-at acetate = 1.5 mg dl-at acetate = 1.5 u vit E. Abetalipoproteinaemia: 100 mg/kg (max 4 g) daily oral. Cystic fibrosis: 45–200 mg (NOT/kg) daily oral. Newborn (high dose, toxicity reported): 10–25 mg/kg daily IM or IV, 10–100 mg/kg daily oral.

Alprostadil (prostaglandin E1, PGE1) To maintain PDA: 0.01–0.1 mcg/kg/min (10–100 ng/kg/min); for 0.01 mcg/kg/min (10 ng/kg/min), put 60 mcg/kg in 50 mL saline, run at 0.5 mL/hr. Pul vasodil with 0.1 mcg/kg/min (100 ng/kg/min), put 500 mcg in 83/Wt mL saline and run at 1 mL/hr (5.0 mcg/kg/min nitroglyc = 2.0 mcg/kg/min nitropr = 0.1 mcg/kg/min PGE1 approx). Erectile dysfunction (adult NOT/kg): 2.5 mcg intracavernous inj, incr in 2.5 mcg increments if reqrd to max 60 mcg (max of 3 doses/wk).

Alteplase (tissue plasminogen activator) 0.1–0.6 mg/kg/hr IV for 6–12 hr (longer if no response); keep fibrinogen >100 mg/dL (give cryoprecipitate 1 bag/5 kg), give heparin 10 u/kg/hr IV, give fresh frozen plasma (FFP) 10 mL/kg IV daily in infants. Local IA infsn: 0.05 mg/kg/hr, give FFP 10 mL/kg IV daily. Blocked central line: 0.5 mg/2 mL (<10 kg) 2 mg/2 mL (>10 kg) per lumen left for 2–4 hr, withdraw drug, flush with saline; repeat once in 24 hr if reqd.

Aluminium acetate 13% soltn (Burrow's lotion): for wet compresses, or daily to molluscum contagiosum.

Aluminium hydroxide 25 mg/kg/dose (adult 0.5–1 g) 4–6 H oral. Gel (64 mg/mL) 0.1 mL/kg/dose 6 H oral.

Aluminium hydroxide 40 mg/mL, magnesium hydroxide 40 mg/mL, simethicone 4 mg/mL (Mylanta, Gelusil) 0.5–1 mL/kg/dose (adult 10–20 mL) 6–8 H oral. ICU: 0.5 mL/kg/dose 3 H oral if gastric pH <5.

Amethocaine Gel 4% in methylcellulose (RCH AnGel): 0.5 g to skin, apply occlusive dressing, wait 30–60 min, remove gel. 0.5%, 1%: 1–2 drops/eye.

Amikacin Single daily dose IV or IM. Neonate: 15 mg/kg stat, then 7.5 mg/kg (<30 wk) 10 mg/kg (30–35 wk) 15 mg/kg (term <1 wk) daily. 1 wk–10 yr: 25 mg/kg day 1, then 18 mg/kg daily. >10 yr: 20 mg/kg day 1, then 15 mg/kg (max 1.5 g) daily. Trough level <5.0 mg/L (RCH sent to St.V's).

Amiloride 0.2 mg/kg/dose (adult 5 mg) 12–24 H oral.

Aminocaproic acid 3 g/m^2 (adult 5 g) over 1 hr IV, then 1 g/m^2/hr (adult 1–1.25 g/hr). Prophylaxis: 70 mg/kg/dose 6 H IV, oral.

Aminophylline (100 mg aminophylline = 80 mg theophylline) Load: 10 mg/kg (max 500 mg) IV over 1 hr. Maintenance: 1st wk life 2.5 mg/kg/dose 12 H; 2nd wk life 3 mg/kg/dose 12 H; 3 wk–12 mo ((0.12 × age in wk) + 3) mg/kg/dose 8 H; 1–9 yr 1.1 mg/kg/hr (55 mg/kg in 50 mL at 1 mL/hr), or 6 mg/kg/dose IV over 1 hr 6 H; 10–16 yr or adult smoker 0.7 mg/kg/hr (<35 kg 35 mg/kg in 50 mL at 1 mL/hr; >35 kg 25 mg/mL at 0.028 mL/kg/hr), or 4 mg/kg/dose IV over 1 hr 6 H; adult non-smoker 0.5 mg/kg/hr (25 mg/mL at 0.02 mL/kg/hr), or 3 mg/kg/dose IV over 1 hr 6 H; elderly 0.3 mg/kg/hr (15 mg/kg in 50 mL at 1 mL/hr), or 2 mg/kg/dose IV over 1 hr 6 H. Monitor theophylline level: 60–80 μmol/L (neonate), 60–110 (asthma) (× 0.18 = mcg/mL).

Amiodarone IV: 25 mcg/kg/min for 4 hr, then 5–15 mcg/kg/min (max 1.2 g/24 hr). Oral: 4 mg/kg/dose (adult 200 mg) 8 H 1 wk, 12 H 1 wk, then 12–24 H. After starting tablets, taper IV infsn over 5 days. Reduce dose of digoxin and warfarin. Pulseless VF or VT: 5 mg/kg IV.

Amitriptyline hydrochloride Usually 0.5–1 mg/kg/dose (adult 25–50 mg) 8 H oral. Enuresis: 1–1.5 mg/kg nocte.

Amoxicillin 10–25 mg/kg/dose (adult 0.25–1 g) 8 H IV, IM or oral; or 20 mg/kg/dose 12 H oral. Severe inftn: 50 mg/kg/dose (adult 2 g) IV 12 H (1st wk life), 6 H (2–4 wk), 4–6 H or constant infsn (4+ wk).

Amoxicillin and clavulanic acid Dose as for amoxicillin. 4:1 (non-Duo products) given 8 H, 7:1 (Duo) 12 H oral.

Amoxycillin See amoxicillin.

Amphotericin B 0.5–1.5 mg/kg/day by continuous infusion IV; total dose 30–35 mg/kg over 4–8 wk. Oral (NOT/kg): 100 mg 6 H treatment, 50 mg 6 H prophylaxis. Bladder washout: 25 mcg/mL. Cream or ointment 3%: apply 6–12 H.

Amphotericin, lipid complex or liposomal 2–3 mg/kg daily over 1 hr IV. Total dose typically 20–60 mg/kg over 2–4 wk.

Ampicillin 10–25 mg/kg/dose (adult 0.25–1 g) 6 H IV, IM or oral. Severe inftn: 50 mg/kg/dose (max 2 g) IV 12 H (1st wk life), 6 H (2–4 wk), 3–6 H or constant infsn (4+ wk).

Ampicillin 1 g + sulbactam 0.5 g 25–50 mg/kg/dose (adult 1–2 g) of ampicillin 6 H IM or IV over 30 min.

Amrinone <4 wk old: 4 mg/kg IV over 1 hr, then 3–5 mcg/kg/min. >4 wk: 1–3 mg/kg IV over 1 hr, then 5–15 mcg/kg/min.

Antivenom to Australian box jellyfish, snakes (black, brown, death adder, sea, taipan, tiger), spiders (funnel-web) and ticks Dose depends on amount of venom injected, not size of patient. Higher doses needed for multiple bites, severe symptoms or delayed administration. Give adrenaline 0.005 mg/kg (0.005 mL/kg of 1 in 1000) SC. Initial dose antivenom usually 1–2 amp diluted 1/10 in Hartmann's soltn IV over 30 min. Monitor PT, PTT, fibrinogen, platelets. Give repeatedly if symptoms or coagulopathy persist.

Antivenom to black widow spider (USA), red back spider (Australia) 1 amp IM, may repeat in 2 hr. Severe envenomation: 2 amp diluted 1/10 in Hartmann's soltn IV over 30 min.

Aprotinin (1 kIU = 140 ng = 0.00056 epu, 1 mg = 7143 kIU) 1,200,000 kIU/m^2 IV over 1 hr (plus 1,200,000 kIU/m^2 in prime), then 300,000 kIU/m^2/hr; half for "low dose". Adult (NOT/kg): 2,000,000 kIU IV over 1 hr (plus 2,000,000 kIU in prime), then 500,000 kIU/hr; half for "low dose". Prophylaxis: 4000 kIU/kg, then 2000 kIU/kg/dose 6 H IV.

Arginine hydrochloride Dose (mg) = BE × Wt (kg) × 70 (give half this) IV over 2 hr.

Ascorbic acid Burn (NOT/kg): 200–500 mg daily IV, IM, SC, oral. Metabolic dis (NOT/kg): 250 mg (<7 yr) 500 mg (>7 yr) daily oral. Scurvy (NOT/kg): 100 mg/dose 8 H oral for 10 days. Urine acidification: 10–30 mg/kg/dose 6 H.

Aspirin 10–15 mg/kg/dose (adult 300–600 mg) 4–6 H oral. Antiplatelet: 3–5 mg/kg (max 100 mg) daily. Kawasaki: 10 mg/kg/dose 6 H (low dose) or 25 mg/kg/dose 6 H (high dose) for 2 wk, then 3–5 mg/kg daily. Arthritis: 25 mg/kg/dose (max 2 g) 6 H for 3 days, then 15–20 mg/kg/dose 6 H. Salicylate level (arthritis) midway between doses 0.7–2.0 mmol/L (× 13.81 = mg/100 mL).

Aspirin 25 mg + dipyridamole 200 mg Adult (NOT/kg) 1 sustained release cap 12 H oral.

Atenolol Oral: 1–2 mg/kg/dose (adult 50–100 mg) 12–24 H. IV: 0.05 mg/kg (adult 2.5 mg) every 5 min until response (max 4 doses), then 0.1–0.2 mg/kg/dose (adult 5–10 mg) over 10 min 12–24 H.

Atracurium besylate 0.3–0.6 mg/kg stat, then 0.1–0.2 mg/kg when reqd or 5–10 mcg/kg/min IV.

Atropine sulphate 0.02 mg/kg (max 0.6 mg) IV or IM, then 0.01 mg/kg/dose 4–6 H. Organophosphate poisoning: 0.05 mg/kg (adult 2 mg) IV, then 0.02–0.05 mg/kg/dose (adult 2 mg) every 15–60 min until atropinised (continue 12–24 hr). Colic: see phenobarbitone.

Azathioprine 25–75 mg/m^2 (approx 1–3 mg/kg) daily oral, IV.

Azithromycin 15 mg/kg (adult 500 mg) day 1, then 7.5 mg/kg (adult 250 mg) days 2–5 oral. Trachoma: 20 mg/kg (adult 1 g) wkly × 3. MAC prophylaxis (adult): 1.2 g wkly. Gp A strep: 20 mg/kg daily × 3.

Aztreonam 30 mg/kg/dose (adult 1 g) 8 H IV. Severe inftn: 50 mg/kg/dose (adult 2 g) 12 H (1st wk life), 8 H (2–4 wk), 6 H or constant infsn (4+ wk).

Bacillus Calmette-Guérin (BCG) vaccine (CSL) Live. Intradermal (1 mg/mL): 0.075 mL (<3 mo) or 0.1 mL (>3 mo) once. Percutaneous (60 mg/mL suspension): 1 drop on skin, inoculated with Heaf apparatus, once.

Bacillus Calmette-Guérin (BCG) suspension, about 5 × 10^8 cfu/vial Adult: 1 vial (OncoTICE) or 3 vials (ImmuCyst) left in bladder for 2 hr each wk for 6 wks, then at 3, 6, 12, 18 and 24 mo.

Bacitracin 400 u/g + neomycin 5 mg/g + polymyxin B 5000 u/g (Neosporin) Ointment or eye ointment: apply × 2–5/day. Powder:

apply 6–12 H (skin inftn), every few days (burns). Eye drops: see gramicidin.

Baclofen 0.2 mg/kg/dose (adult 5 mg) 8 H oral, incr every 3 days to 1 mg/kg/dose (adult 25 mg, max 50 mg) 8 H. Intrathecal infsn: 2–20 mcg/kg (max 1000 mcg) per 24 hr.

Beclomethasone dipropionate Rotacap or aerosol (NOT/kg): 100–200 mcg (<8 yr), 150–400 mcg (>8 yr) × 2/day (rarely × 4/day). Nasal (NOT/kg): aerosol or pump (50 mcg/spray): 1 spray 12 H (<12 yr), 2 spray 12 H (>12 yr).

Benzhexol >3 yr: 0.02 mg/kg/dose (adult 1 mg) 8 H, incr to 0.1–0.3 mg/kg/dose (adult 1.5–5 mg) 8 H oral.

Benzocaine 1%–20% topical: usually applied 4–6 H.

Benztropine >3 yr: 0.02 mg/kg (adult 1 mg) stat IM or IV, may repeat in 15 min. 0.02–0.06 mg/kg/dose (adult 1–3 mg) 12–24 H oral.

Benzyl benzoate 25% lotion. Scabies: apply from neck down after a hot bath, remove in bath after 24 hr; repeat after 5 days. Lice: apply to infected region, wash off after 24 hr; repeat after 7 days.

Benzylpenicillin See penicillin G.

Beractant (bovine surfactant, Survanta) 25 mg/mL soltn. 4 mL/kg intratracheal 2–4 doses in 48 hr, each dose in 4 parts: body inclined down with head to right, body down head left, body up head right, body up head left.

Beta carotene Porphyria: 1–5 mg/kg (adult 30–300 mg) daily oral.

Betamethasone 0.01–0.2 mg/kg daily oral. Betamethasone has no mineralocorticoid action, 1 mg = 25 mg hydrocortisone in glucocorticoid action. Gel 0.05%; cream, lotion or ointment, 0.02%, 0.05%, 0.1%: apply sparingly 8–24 H.

Betamethasone acetate 3 mg/mL with betamethasone sodium phosphate 3.9 mg/mL (Celestone Chronodose) Adult: 0.25–2 mL (NOT/kg) IM, IA or intralesional injection.

Bethanecol Oral: 0.2–1 mg/kg/dose (adult 10–50 mg) 6–8 H. SC: 0.05–0.1 mg/kg/dose (adult 2.5–5 mg) 6–8 H.

Bicarbonate Slow IV: dose (mmol) = BE × Wt/4 (<5 kg), BE × Wt/6 (child), BE × Wt/10 (adult). These doses correct half the base deficit. Alkalinise urine: 0.25 mmol/kg 6–12 H oral.

Bisacodyl NOT/kg: <12 mo 2.5 mg PR, 1–5 yr 5 mg PR or 5–10 mg oral, >5 yr 10 mg PR or 10–20 mg oral. Enema: half daily (6 mo–3 yr), 1 enema daily (>3 yr).

Bismuth subcitrate (colloidal) 5 mg/kg/dose (adult 240 mg) 12 H oral 30 min before meal. *H. pylori* (adult, NOT/kg): 107.7 mg/dose × 4/day with meals and nocte for 2 wk + tetracycline 500 mg/dose × 4/day + metronidazole 200 mg with meals and 400 mg nocte; see also omeprazole.

Bismuth subsalicylate See bismuth subcitrate.

Blood 4 mL/kg packed cells raises Hb 1 g%. 1 bag = 300 mL.

Botulinum toxin type A NOT/kg: 1.25–2.5 u/site (max 5 u/site) IM, max total 200 u in 30 days. Oesoph achalasia: 100 u per session divided between 4–6 sites.

Botulinum toxin type B NOT/kg: usual total dose 2500–10,000 u, repeated every 3–4 mo if reqd.

Bretylium tosylate 5–10 mg/kg IV over 1 hr, then 5–30 mcg/kg/min.

Bromocriptine mesylate 0.025 mg/kg/dose (adult 1.25 mg) 8–12 H, incr wkly to 0.05–0.2 mg/kg/dose (adult 2.5–10 mg) 6–12 H oral. Inhibit lactn, NOT/kg: 2.5 mg/dose 12 H for 2 wk.

Budesonide Metered dose inhaler (NOT/kg): <12 yr 50–200 mcg 6–12 H, reducing to 100–200 mcg 12 H; >12 yr 100–600 mcg 6–12 H, reducing to 100–400 mcg 12 H. Nebuliser (NOT/kg): <12 yr 0.5–1 mg 12 H, reducing to 0.25–0.5 mg 12 H; >12 yr 1–2 mg 12 H, reducing to 0.5–1 mg 12 H. Croup: 2 mg (NOT/kg) by nebuliser. Nasal spray or aerosol (NOT/kg): 64–128 mcg/nostril 12–24 H. Crohn's dis, adult (NOT/kg): 9 mg daily for 8 wk, then reduce over 4 wk.

Bupivacaine Max dose: 2–3 mg/kg (0.4–0.6 mL/kg of 0.5%). With adrenaline: max dose: 3–4 mg/kg (0.6–0.8 mL/kg of 0.5%). Epidural: 2 mg/kg (0.4 mL/kg 0.5%) stat intraop, then 0.25 mg/kg/hr (0.2 mL/kg/hr 0.125%) postop. Epidural in ICU: 25 mL 0.5% + 1000 mcg (20 mL) fentanyl + saline to 100 mL at 2–8 mL/hr in adult.

Caffeine citrate 2 mg citrate = 1 mg base. 1–5 mg/kg/dose (adult 50–250 mg) of citrate 4–8 H oral, PR. Neonate: 20 mg/kg stat of citrate, then 5 mg/kg daily oral or IV over 30 min; weekly level 5–30 mg/L midway between doses.

Calamine Lotion: usually applied 6–8 H.

Calcifediol (25-OH D3) Deficiency: 1–2 mcg/kg daily oral.

Calciferol (ergocalciferol) See vitamin D2.

Calcipotriol 50 mcg/g ointment: apply 12–24 H.

Calcitonin Hypercalcaemia: 4 u/kg/dose 12–24 H IM or SC, may incr up to 8 u/kg/dose 6–12 H. Paget's: 1.5–3 u/kg (max 160 u) × 3/wk IM or SC.

Calcitriol (1,25-OH vitamin D3) Renal failure, vit D-resistant rickets: 0.02 mcg/kg daily oral, incr by 0.02 mcg/kg every 4–8 wk according to serum calcium.

Calcium (as carbonate, lactate or phosphate) NOT/kg: Neonate: 50 mg × 4–6/day; 1 mo 3 yr: 100 mg × 2–5/day oral; 4–12 yr: 300 mg × 2–3/day; >12 yr: 1000 mg × 1–2/day.

Calcium carbonate Adult NOT/kg: 840 mg 8–12 H oral.

Calcium chloride 10% soltn (0.7 mmol/mL Ca): 0.2 mL/kg (max 10 mL) slow IV stat. Requirement <16 yr 2 mL/kg/day IV. Inotrope: 0.5–2 mmol/kg/day (0.03–0.12 mL/kg/hr).

Calcium gluconate 10% soltn (0.22 mmol/mL Ca): 0.5 mL/kg (max 20 mL) slow IV stat. Requirement <16 yr 5 mL/kg/day IV. Inotrope: 0.5–2 mmol/kg/day (0.1–0.4 mL/kg/hr).

Calcium polystyrene sulfonate (Calcium Resonium) 0.3–0.6 g/kg/dose (adult 15–30 g) 6 H NG (+ lactulose), PR.

Canrenoate potassium 3–8 mg/kg (adult 150–400 mg) daily IV.

Captopril Beware hypotension. 0.1 mg/kg/dose (adult 5 mg) 8 H oral, incr if reqd to max 2 mg/kg/dose (adult 50 mg) 8 H.

Carbamazepine 2 mg/kg/dose (adult 100 mg) 8 H oral, may incr over 2–4 wk to 5–10 mg/kg/dose (adult 250–500 mg) 8 H. Level 20–40 μmol/L (× 0.24 = mg/L), done Mo-Fri 1100 RCH.

Carbenicillin 382 mg tab, adult (NOT/kg): 1–2 tab 4 H oral.

Carbenoxolone sodium Adult (NOT/kg): 20–50 mg 6 H oral. Mouth gel 2%, or 2 g granules in 40 mL water, apply 6 H.

Carbimazole 0.4 mg/kg/dose (adult 20 mg) 8–12 H oral for 2 wk, then 0.1 mg/kg/dose (adult 5–10 mg) 8–24 H.

Carnitine, L form IV: 5–15 mg/kg/dose (max 1 g) 6 H. Oral: 25 mg/kg/dose 6–12 H (max 3 g/day).

Carob bean gum (Carobel Instant) NOT/kg: 1 scoop (1.8 g) in 100 mL water, give 10–20 mL by spoon; or add half a scoop to every 100–200 mL of milk.

Cefaclor monohydrate 10–15 mg/kg/dose (adult 250–500 mg) 8 H oral. Slow release tab 375 mg (adult, NOT/kg): 1–2 tab 12 H oral.

Cefdinir 14 mg/kg (adult 600 mg) daily (or in two divided doses) oral.

Cefditoren 4–8 mg/kg/dose (adult 200–400 mg) 12 H oral.

Cefepime hydrochloride 25 mg/kg/dose (adult 1 g) 12 H IM or IV over 5 min. Severe inftn: 50 mg/kg/dose (adult 2 g) IV 8–12 H or constant infsn.

Cefixime 5 mg/kg/dose (adult 200 mg) 12–24 H oral.

Cefodizime 25 mg/kg/dose (max 1 g) 12 H IV or IM.

Cefonicid 15–50 mg/kg (adult 0.5–2 g) IV or IM daily.

Cefoperazone 25–60 mg/kg/dose (adult 1–3 g) 6–12 H IV over 1 hr or IM.

Cefotaxime 25 mg/kg/dose (adult 1 g) 12 H (<4 wk), 8 H (4+ wk) IV. Severe inftn: 50 mg/kg/dose (adult 2–3 g) IV 12 H (preterm), 8 H (1st wk life), 6 H (2–4 wk), 4–6 H or constant infsn (4+ wk).

Cefotetan 25 mg/kg/dose (adult 1 g) 12 H IM, IV. Severe inftn: 50 mg/kg/dose (max 2–3 g) 12 H or constant infsn.

Cefoxitin 25–60 mg/kg/dose (adult 1–3 g) 12 H (1st wk life), 8 H (1–4 wk), 6–8 H (>4 wk) IV.

Cefpirome 25–50 mg/kg/dose (adult 1–2 g) 12 H IV.

Cefpodoxime 5 mg/kg/dose (adult 100–200 mg) 12 H oral.

Cefprozil 15 mg/kg/dose (adult 500 mg) 12–24 H oral.

Ceftazidime 15–25 mg/kg/dose (adult 0.5–1 g) 8 H IV or IM. Severe inftn, CF: 50 mg/kg/dose (max 2 g) 12 H (1st wk life), 8 H (2–4 wk), 6 H or constant infsn (4+ wk).

Ceftibuten 10 mg/kg (adult 400 mg) daily oral.

Ceftizoxime 25–60 mg/kg/dose (adult 1–3 g) 6–8 H IV.

Ceftriaxone sodium 25 mg/kg/dose (adult 1 g) 12–24 H IV, or IM (in 1% lignocaine). Severe inftn: 50 mg/kg/dose (max 2 g) daily (1st wk life), 12 H (2+ wk). Epiglottitis: 100 mg/kg (max 2 g) stat, then 50 mg/kg (max 2 g) after 24 hr. Meningococcus prophylaxis (NOT/kg): child 125 mg, >12 yr 250 mg IM in 1% lignocaine once.

Cefuroxime Oral: 10–15 mg/kg/dose (adult 250–500 mg) 12 H. IV: 25 mg/kg/dose (adult 1 g) 8 H. Severe inftn: 50 mg/kg/dose (max 2 g) IV 12 H (1st wk life), 8 H (2nd wk), 6 H or constant infsn (>2 wk).

Celecoxib Usually 2 mg/kg/dose (adult 100 mg) 12 H, max 4 mg/kg/dose (adult 200 mg) 12 H oral.

Cephalexin 7.5 mg/kg/dose (adult 250 mg) 6 H, or 15 mg/kg/dose (adult 500 mg) 12 H oral.

Cephalothin 15–25 mg/kg/dose (adult 0.5–1 g) 6 H IV or IM. Severe inftn: 50 mg/kg/dose (max 2 g) IV 4 H or constant infsn. Irrigation fluid: 2 g/L (2 mg/mL).

Cephamandole 15–25 mg/kg/dose (adult 0.5–1 g) 6–8 H IV over 10 min or IM. Severe inftn: 40 mg/kg/dose (adult 2 g) IV over 20 min 4–6 H or constant infsn.

Cephazolin 10–15 mg/kg/dose (adult 0.5 g) 6 H IV or IM. Severe inftn: 50 mg/kg/dose (adult 2 g) IV 4–6 H or constant infsn. Surgical proph: 50 mg/kg IV at induction.

Cetirizine 0.25 mg/kg/dose (adult 10 mg) 12–24 H oral.

Cetylpyridinium + benzocaine Mouthwash (Cepacaine): apply 3 H prn. Do not swallow.

Chloral hydrate Hypnotic: 50 mg/kg (max 2 g) stat (up to 100 mg/kg, max 5 g, in ICU). Sedative: 8 mg/kg/dose 6–8 H oral or PR.

Chloramphenicol Severe inftn: 40 mg/kg (max 2 g) stat, then 25 mg/kg/dose (max 1 g) IV, IM or oral. 1st wk life daily; 2–4 wk 12 H; >4 wk 8 H for 5 days, then 6 H. Eye drops, oint: apply 2–6 H. Ear: 4 drops 6 H. Serum level 20–30 mg/L at 2 hr, <15 mg/L trough.

Chloroquine, base Oral: 10 mg/kg (max 600 mg) daily × 3 days. IM: 4 mg/kg/dose (max 300 mg) 12 H for 3 days. Prophylaxis: 5 mg/kg (adult 300 mg) oral × 1/wk. Lupus, rheu arthritis: 12 mg/kg (max 600 mg) daily, reduce to 4–8 mg/kg (max 400 mg) daily oral.

Chlorothiazide 5–20 mg/kg/dose (adult 0.25–1 g) 12–24 H oral, IV.

Chlorpheniramine maleate 0.1 mg/kg/dose (adult 4 mg) 6–8 H oral.

Chlorpheniramine maleate 1.25 mg + phenylephrine 2.5 mg in 5 mL Syrup (NOT/kg): 1.25–2.5 mL (0–1 yr), 2.5–5 mL (2–5 yr), 5–10 mL (6–12 yr), 10–15 mL (>12 yr) 6–8 H oral.

Chlorpromazine Oral or PR: 0.5–2 mg/kg/dose (max 100 mg) 6–8 H; up to 20 mg/kg/dose 8 H for psychosis. IM (painful) or slow IV (beware hypotension): 0.25–1 mg/kg/dose (usual max 50 mg) 6–8 H.

Chlorpropamide Adult: initially 125–250 mg (NOT/kg) daily oral, max 500 mg daily.

Chlortetracycline 3% cream or ointment: apply 8–24 H.

Cholera vaccine, parenteral (CSL) Inactivated. 2 doses SC 7–28 days apart: 0.1 mL then 0.3 mL (<5 yr), 0.3 mL then 0.5 mL (5–9 yr), 0.5 mL then 1 mL (>9 yr). Boost every 6 mo (use 1st dose).

Cholera vaccine, oral (Orochol) Live. >2 yr: 1 sachet + 100 mL water. Boost every 6 mo.

Cholestyramine NOT/kg: 1 g/dose (<6 yr), 2–4 g/dose (6–12 yr), 4 g/dose (>12 yr) 4–12 H oral with feeds. 16% paste: apply 8–12 H.

Cimetidine Oral: 5–10 mg/kg/dose (adult 300–400 mg) 6 H, or 20 mg/kg (adult 800 mg) nocte. IV: 10–15 mg/kg/dose (adult 200 mg) 12 H (newborn), 6 H (>4 wk).

Ciprofloxacin 5–10 mg/kg/dose (adult 250–500 mg) 12 H oral, 4–7 mg/kg/dose (adult 200–300 mg) 12 H IV. Severe inftn, or cystic fibrosis: 20 mg/kg/dose (max 750 mg) 12 H oral, 10 mg/kg/dose (max 400 mg) 8 H IV; higher doses used occasionally. Meningococcus proph: 15 mg/kg (max 500 mg) once oral. Reduce dose of theophylline.

Ciprofloxacin, eye drops 0.3%. Corneal ulcer: 2 drops/15 min for 6 hr then 2 drops/30 min for 18 hr (day 1), 2 drops 1 H (day 2), 2 drops 4 H (day 3–14). Conjunctivitis: 1–2 drops 4 H; if severe 1–2 drops 2 H when awake for 2 days, then 6 H.

Cisapride 0.2 mg/kg/dose (adult 5–15 mg) 6–8 H oral.

Cisplatin 60–100 mg/m^2 IV over 6 hr every 3–4 wk × 6 cycles.

Clarithromycin 7.5–15 mg/kg/dose (adult 250–500 mg) 12 H oral. Slow release tab, adult (NOT/kg): 0.5 g or 1 g daily.

Clindamycin 6 mg/kg/dose (adult 150–450 mg) 6 H oral. IV or IM >28 days: 10 mg/kg/dose (adult 600 mg) 8 H (IV over 30 min). Neonate: 5 mg/kg/dose 12 H (preterm <1 wk old), 5 mg/kg/dose 8 H (preterm >1 wk, term <1 wk), 7.5 mg/kg/dose 8 H (term >1 wk) IV over 30 min. Severe inftn (>28 days): 15–20 mg/kg/dose (adult 900 mg) 8 H IV over 1 hr. Acne soltn 1%: apply 12 H.

Clioquinol 10 mg/g cream, 100% powder: apply 6–12 H.

Clobazam 0.1 mg/kg (adult 10 mg) daily oral, incr if reqd to max 0.4 mg/kg/dose (adult 20 mg) 8–12 H oral.

Clomiphene Adult: 50 mg (NOT/kg) daily for 5 days oral, incr to 100 mg daily for 5 days if no ovulation.

Clomipramine 0.5–1 mg/kg/dose (adult 25–50 mg) 12 H oral, incr if reqd to max 2 mg/kg/dose (adult 100 mg) 8 H.

Clonazepam 1 drop = 0.1 mg. 0.01 mg/kg/dose (max 0.5 mg) 12 H oral, slowly incr to 0.05 mg/kg/dose (max 2 mg) 6–12 H oral. Status (may be repeated), NOT/kg: neonate 0.25 mg (if ventilated), child 0.5 mg, adult 1 mg IV.

Clonidine 3–5 mcg/kg slow IV, 1–6 mcg/kg/dose (adult 50–300 mcg) 8–12 H oral. Migraine: start with 0.5 mcg/kg/dose 12 H oral. Analgesia: 2.5 mcg/kg premed oral, 0.3 mcg/kg/hr IV, 1–2 mcg/kg local block; ventilated 0.5–2 mcg/kg/hr (1 mcg/kg/hr is 50 mcg/kg in 50 mL at 1 mL/hr (<12 kg), or 25 mcg/kg in 50 mL at 2 mL/hr (>12 kg)) + midazolam 1 mcg/kg/min (3 mg/kg in 50 mL at 1 mL/hr).

Clotrimazole Topical: 1% cream or solution 8–12 H. Vaginal (NOT/kg): 1% cream or 100 mg tab daily for 6 days, or 2% cream or 500 mg tab daily for 3 days.

Cloxacillin 15 mg/kg/dose (adult 500 mg) 6 H oral, IM or IV. Severe inftn: 25–50 mg/kg/dose (adult 1–2 g) IV 12 H (1st wk life), 8 H (2–4 wk), 4–6 H (>4 wk) or constant infsn (>4 wk).

Coal tar, topical 0.5% incr to max 10%, applied 6–8 H.

Cocaine Topical: 1–3 mg/kg.

Codeine phosphate Analgesic: 0.5–1 mg/kg/dose (adult 15–60 mg) 4 H oral, IM, SC. Antitussive: 0.25–0.5 mg/kg/dose (adult 15–30 mg) 6 H.

Co-dergocrine mesylate Adult: usually 3.0–4.5 mg (NOT/kg) daily before meal oral or sublingual. 300 mcg (NOT/kg) daily IM, SC or IV infsn.

Colchicine Acute gout: 0.02 mg/kg/dose (adult 1 mg) 2 H oral (max 3 doses/day). Chronic use (gout, FMF): 0.01–0.04 mg/kg (adult 0.5–2 mg) daily oral.

Colfosceril palmitate (Exosurf Neonatal) Soltn 13.5 mg/mL. Prophylaxis: 5 mL/kg intratracheal over 5 min immediately after birth and at 12 hr and 24 hr if still ventilated. Rescue: 5 mL/kg intratracheal over 5 min, repeat in 12 hr if still ventilated.

Colistin sulphomethate sodium 2.6 mg = 1 mg colistin base = 30,000 u. IM, or IV over 5 min: 40,000 u/kg/dose (adult 2 million u) 8 H, or 1.25–2.5 mg/kg/dose of colistin base 12 H. Oral or inhaled: 30,000–60,000 u/kg/dose (adult 1.5–3 million u) 8 H.

Colistin 3 mg/mL + neomycin 3.3 mg/mL Otic: 4 drops 8 H.

Colonic lavage (macrogol) soltns Poisoning, severe constipation: if bowel sounds present, 30 mL/kg/hr oral or NG for 4–8 hr (until rectal effluent clear). Before colonoscopy: 1 L (<1 yr), 1.5–1.75 L (1–10 yr), 2–3 L (>10 yr) oral, NG.

Corticotrophin releasing factor or hormone (CRF, CRH) See corticorelin.

Cortisone acetate 1–2.5 mg/kg/dose 6–8 H oral. Physiological: 7.5 mg/m^2/dose 8 H. Cortisone acetate 1 mg = hydrocortisone 1.25 mg in mineralo- and gluco-corticoid action.

Cotrimoxazole (trimethoprim 1 mg + sulphamethoxazole 5 mg) TMP 1.5–3 mg/kg/dose (adult 80–160 mg) 12 H IV over 1 hr or oral. Renal prophylaxis: TMP 2 mg/kg (max 80 mg) daily oral. Pneumocystis: TMP 250 mg/m^2 stat, then 150 mg/m^2 8 H (<11 yr) or 12 H (>10 yr) IV over 1 hr; in renal failure dose interval (hr) = serum creatinine (mmol/L) × 135 (max 48 hr); 1 hr post-infsn serum TMP 5–10 mcg/mL, SMX 100–200 mcg/mL. IV infsn: TMP max 1.6 mg/mL in 5% dext.

Coumarin Oral: 1–8 mg/kg (adult 50–400 mg) daily. Cream 100 mg/g: apply 8–12 H.

Cromoglycate See sodium cromoglycate.

Crotamiton 10% cream or lotion: apply × 2–3/day.

Cryoprecipitate Low factor 8: 1 u/kg incr activity 2% (half-life 12 hr); usual dose 5 mL/kg or 1 bag/4 kg 12 H IV for 1–2 infns (muscle, joint), 3–6 infns (hip, forearm, retroperitoneal, oropharynx), 7–14 infns (intracranial). Low fibrinogen: usual dose 5 mL/kg or 1 bag/4 kg IV. A bag is usually 20–30 mL: factor 8 about 5 u/mL and 100 u/bag, fibrinogen about 10 mg/mL and 200 mg/bag.

Cyanocobalamin (Vit B12) 20 mcg/kg/dose (adult 1000 mcg) IM daily for 7 days then wkly (treatment), monthly (prophylaxis). IV dangerous in megaloblastic anaemia.

Cyclopentolate hydrochloride 0.5%, 1%: 1 drop/eye, repeat after 5 min. Pilocarpine 1% speeds recovery.

Cyclophosphamide A typical regimen is 600 mg/m^2 IV over 30 min daily for 3 days, then 600 mg/m^2 IV wkly or 10 mg/kg twice wkly (if leucocytes >3000/mm^3).

Cyclosporin 1–3 mcg/kg/min IV for 24–48 hr, then 5–8 mg/kg/dose 12 H reducing by 1 mg/kg/dose each month to 3–4 mg/kg/dose oral. Eczema, juv arth, nephrotic, psoriasis: 1.5–2.5 mg/kg/dose 12 H. Trough level by Abbott TDx monoclonal specific assay (× 2.5 = non-specific assay level) on whole blood (done Tu, Fri 1400 at RCH): 100–250 ng/mL (marrow), 300–400 ng/mL first 3 mo then 100–300 ng/mL (kidney), 200–250 first 3 mo then 100–125 (liver), 100–400 ng/mL (heart, lung).

Cyproheptadine 0.1 mg/kg/dose (adult 4 mg) 8–12 H oral. Migraine: 0.1 mg/kg (adult 4 mg), repeated in 30 min if reqd.

Cyproterone acetate 1 mg/kg/dose (adult 50 mg) 12 H oral. Prec puberty: 25–50 mg/m^2/dose 8–12 H oral. Hyperandrogenism: 50–100 mg daily days 5–14, with oestradiol valerate 1 mg daily days 5–25.

Cysteamine bitartrate 0.05 mg/m^2/dose 6 H oral, incr over 6 wk to 0.33 mg/m^2/dose (<50 kg) or 0.5 mg/kg/dose (>50 kg) 6 H.

Dalteparin sodium Proph (adult): 2500–5000 u SC 1–2 hr preop, then daily. Venous thrombosis (adult): 100 u/kg/dose 12 H SC, or infuse 200 u/kg/day IV (anti-Xa 0.5–1 u/mL 4 hr post dose). Haemodialysis: 5–10 u/kg stat, then 4–5 u/kg/hr IV (acute renal failure, anti-Xa 0.2–0.4 u/mL); 30–40 u/kg stat, then 10–15 u/kg/hr (chronic renal failure, anti-Xa 0.5–1 u/mL).

Danazol 2–4 mg/kg/dose (adult 100–200 mg) 6–12 H oral.

Dantrolene Hyperpyrexia: 1 mg/kg/min until improves (max 10 mg/kg), then 1–2 mg/kg/dose 6 H for 1–3 days IV or oral. Spasticity: 0.5 mg/kg/dose (adult 25 mg) 6 H, incr over 2 wk if reqd to 3 mg/kg/dose (adult 50–100 mg) 6 H oral.

Dapsone 1–2 mg/kg (adult 50–100 mg) daily oral. Derm herpet: 1–6 mg/kg (adult 50–300 mg) daily oral. See also pyrimethamine.

DDAVP See desmopressin.

Desferrioxamine Antidote: 10–15 mg/kg/hr IV for 12–24 hr (max 6 g/24 hr) if Fe >60–90 μmol/L at 4 hr or 8 hr; some also give 5–10 g (NOT/kg) once oral. Thalassaemia (NOT/kg): 500 mg per unit blood; and 5–6 nights/wk 1–3 g in 5 mL water SC over 10 hr, 0.5–1.5 g in 10 mL water SC over 5 min.

Desipramine 1–5 mg/kg/dose (adult 25–50 mg) 8–12 H oral.

Desmopressin (DDAVP) 1 u = 1 mcg. Nasal: 5–10 mcg (0.05–0.1 mL) per dose (NOT/kg) 12–24 H; enuresis 10–40 mcg nocte. IV: 2 mcg in 1 L fluid, and replace urine output + 10% H. Haemophilia, von Wille: 0.3 mcg/kg (adult 20 mcg) IV over 1 hr 12–24 H.

Dexamethasone 0.1–0.25 mg/kg/dose 6 H oral or IV. BPD: 0.1 mg/kg/dose 6 H for 3 days, then 8 H 3 days, 12 H 3 days, 24 H 3 days, 48 H 7 days. Cerebral oedema: 1.5 mg/kg (adult 10 mg) stat, then 0.25 mg/kg 4–6 H (adult 4 mg) IV. Congenital adrenal hypoplasia: 0.27 mg/m^2 daily oral. Croup, severe: 0.6 mg/kg (max 12 mg) IM stat, then prednisolone 1 mg/kg/dose 8–12 H oral. Eye drops 0.1%: 1–2 drops per eye 3–8 H. Dexamethasone has no mineralocorticoid action, but 1 mg = 25 mg hydrocortisone in glucocorticoid action.

Dexamphetamine 0.2 mg/kg (max 10 mg) daily oral, incr if reqd to max 0.6 mg/kg/dose (max 40 mg) 12 H.

Dexchlorpheniramine maleate 0.05 mg/kg/dose (adult 2 mg) 6–8 H oral. Repetab (adult NOT/kg): 6 mg 12 H oral.

Diazepam 0.1–0.4 mg/kg (adult 10–20 mg) IV or PR. 0.04–0.2 mg/kg/dose (adult 2–10 mg) 8–12 H oral. Do not give by IV infsn (binds to PVC). Premed: 0.2–0.4 mg/kg oral, PR.

Diazoxide Hypertension: 1–3 mg/kg (max 150 mg) stat by rapid IV injection (severe hypotension may occur) repeat once if reqd, then 2–5 mg/kg/dose IV 6 H. Hyperinsulinism: <12 mo 5 mg/kg/dose 8–12 H oral; >12 mo 30–100 mg/m^2 per dose 8 H oral.

Diclofenac 1 mg/kg/dose (adult 50 mg) 8–12 H oral, PR. Eye drops 0.1%: preop 1–5 drops over 3 hr, postop 3 drops stat, then 1 drop 4–8 H. Topical gel: apply 2–4 g 6–8 H.

Dicloxacillin 15–25 mg/kg/dose (adult 250–500 mg) 6 H oral, IM or IV. Severe inftn: 25–50 mg/kg/dose (max 2 g) IV 12 H (1st wk life), 8 H (2–4 wk), 4–6 H or constant infsn (>4 wk).

Digitoxin 4 mcg/kg/dose (max 0.2 mg) 12 H oral for 4 days, then 1–6 mcg/kg (adult usually 0.15 mg, max 0.3 mg) daily.

Digoxin 15 mcg/kg stat and 5 mcg/kg after 6 H, then 3–5 mcg/kg/dose (usual max 200 mcg IV, 250 mcg oral) 12 H slow IV or oral. Level 6 hr or more after dose: 1.0–2.5 nmol/L (× 0.78 = ng/mL), done Mo-Sat 1400 at RCH.

Digoxin immune FAB (antibodies) IV over 30 min. Dose (to nearest 40 mg) = serum digoxin (nmol/L) × Wt (kg) × 0.3, or mg ingested × 55. Give if >0.3 mg/kg ingested, or level >6.4 nmol/L or 5.0 ng/mL.

Dihydrocodeine 0.5–1 mg/kg/dose 4–6 H oral.

Dihydroergotamine mesylate Adult (NOT/kg): 1 mg IM, SC or IV, repeat hourly × 2 if needed. Max 6 mg/wk.

Diltiazem 1 mg/kg/dose (adult 60 mg) 8 H, incr if reqd to max 3 mg/kg/dose (adult 180 mg) 8 H oral. Slow release (adult, NOT/kg): 120–240 mg daily, or 90–180 mg 8–12 H oral.

Diphenhydramine hydrochloride 1–2 mg/kg/dose (adult 50–100 mg) 6–8 H oral.

Diphenoxylate 2.5 mg and atropine 25 mcg tab (Lomotil) Adult (NOT/kg): 1–2 tab 6–8 H oral.

Diphtheria vaccine, adult (CSL) Inactivated. 0.5 mL IM stat, 6 wk later, and 6 mo later (3 doses). Boost every 10 yr.

Diphtheria vaccine, child <8 yr (CSL) Inactivated. 0.5 mL IM stat, 6 wk later, and 6 mo later (3 doses). Boost with adult vaccine.

Diphtheria + pertussis (whole cell) + tetanus vaccine (Triple Antigen) Inactivated. 0.5 mL IM at 2 mo, 4 mo, 6 mo, 18 mo and 4–5 yr of age (5 doses).

Diphtheria + pertussis (acellular) + tetanus vaccine (Infanrix, Tripacel) Inactivated. 0.5 mL IM at 2 mo, 4 mo, 6 mo, 18 mo and 4–5 yr of age (5 doses).

Diphtheria + pertussis (acellular) + tetanus + hepatitis B vaccine (Infanrix Hep B) Inactivated. 0.5 mL at 2 mo, 4 mo, 6 mo (3 doses), and (without hep B) 18 mo.

Diphtheria + tetanus vaccine, adult (ADT) Inactivated. 0.5 mL IM stat, 6 wk later, and 6 mo later (3 doses). Boost every 10 yr.

Diphtheria + tetanus vaccine, child <8 yr (CDT) Inactivated. 0.5 mL IM stat, 6 wk later, 6 mo later (3 doses). Boost with ADT.

Dipyridamole 1–2 mg/kg/dose (adult 50–100 mg) 6–8 H oral. See also aspirin + dipyridamole.

Disopyramide Oral: 1.5–4 mg/kg/dose (adult 75–200 mg) 6 H. IV: 2 mg/kg (max 150 mg) over 5 min, then 0.4 mg/kg/hr (max 800 mg/day). Level 9–15 μmol/L (× 0.3395 = mcg/mL).

Disulfiram Adult (NOT/kg): 500 mg oral daily for 1–2 wk, then 125–500 mg daily.

Dobutamine IV infsn 1–20 mcg/kg/min: for 65 kg adult 250 mg in 50 mL at 2 mL/hr is 2.5 mcg/kg/min.

Docusate sodium NOT/kg: 100 mg (3–10 yr), 120–240 mg (>10 yr) daily oral. Enema (5 mL 18% + 155 mL water): 30 mL (newborn), 60 mL (1–12 mo), 60–120 mL (>12 mo) PR.

Docusate sodium 100 mg + bisacodyl 10 mg <2 yr half suppos, 1–11 yr half to 1 suppos, >11 yr 1 suppos daily.

Docusate sodium 50 mg + sennoside 8 mg, tab >12 yr: 1–4 tabs at night oral.

Domperidone Oral: 0.2–0.4 mg/kg/dose (adult 10–20 mg) 4–8 H. Rectal suppos: adult (NOT/kg) 30–60 mg 4–8 H.

Dopamine IV infsn 1–20 mcg/kg/min: for 65 kg adult 200 mg in 50 mL at 2 mL/hr is 2 mcg/kg/min.

Dopexamine IV infsn 0.5–6 mcg/kg/min: for 65 kg adult 50 mg in 50 mL at 2 mL/hr is 0.5 mcg/kg/min.

Dornase alpha (deoxyribonuclease I) NOT/kg: usually 2.5 mg (max 10 mg) inhaled daily (5–21 yr), 12–24 H (>21 yr).

Dothiepin 0.5–1 mg/kg/dose (adult 25–50 mg) 8–12 H oral.

Doxapram 5 mg/kg IV over 1 hr, then 0.5–1 mg/kg/hr for 1 hr (max total dose 400 mg).

Doxycycline Over 8 yr: 2 mg/kg/dose (adult 100 mg) 12 H for 2 doses, then daily oral. Severe: 2 mg/kg/dose 12 H. Malaria proph: 2 mg/kg (adult 100 mg) daily oral.

Droperidol Antiemetic: postop 0.02–0.05 mg/kg/dose (adult 1.25 mg) 4–6 H IM or slow IV, chemother 0.02–0.1 (adult 1–5 mg) 1–6 H. Psychiatry, neuroleptanalgesia, IM or slow IV: 0.1 mg/kg (adult 2.5 mg) stat, incr if reqd to max 0.3 mg/kg/dose (adult 15 mg) 4–6 H. Psychiatry, oral: 0.1–0.4 mg/kg/dose (adult 5–20 mg) 4–8 H.

Econazole nitrate Topical: 1% cream, powder or lotion 8–12 H. Vaginal: 75 mg cream or 150 mg ovule twice daily.

Eformoterol Caps 12 mg (NOT/kg): 1 cap (5–12 yr) or 1–2 caps (adult) inhaled 12 H.

Enalapril 0.1 mg/kg (adult 2.5 mg) daily oral, incr over 2 wk if reqd to max 0.5 mg/kg/dose (adult 5–20 mg) 12 H.

Enoximone IV: 5–20 mcg/kg/min. Oral: 1–3 mg/kg/dose (adult 50–150 mg) 8 H.

Ephedrine 0.25–1 mg/kg/dose (adult 12.5–60 mg) 4–8 H oral, IM, SC or IV. Nasal (0.25%–1%): 1 drop each nostril 6–8 H, max 4 days.

Epoetin alpha, beta 20–50 u/kg × 3/wk, incr to max 240 u/kg × 1–3/wk SC, IV. When Hb >10 g%: 20–100 u/kg × 23/wk.

Epoprostenol (prostacyclin, PGI2) 0.01 mcg/kg/min IV. Chronic pul ht: 2 ng/kg/min IV, incr to 20–40 ng/kg/min. Pul vasodil: 0.01 mcg/kg/min epoprost = 5 mcg/kg/min nitroglyc = 2 mcg/kg/min nitropr = 0.1 mcg/kg/min PGE1.

Ergometrine maleate Adult (NOT/kg): 250–500 mcg IM or IV; 500 mcg 8 H oral, sublingual or PR.

Ergonovine maleate See ergometrine maleate.

Ergotamine tartrate >10 yr (NOT/kg): 2 mg sublingual stat, then 1 mg/hr (max 6 mg/episode, 10 mg/wk). Suppos (1–2 mg): 1 stat, may repeat once after 1 hr.

Erythromycin Oral or slow IV (max 5 mg/kg/hr): usually 10 mg/kg/dose (adult 250–500 mg) 6 H; severe inftn 15–25 mg/kg/dose (adult 0.75–1 g) 6 H. 2% gel: apply 12 H.

Esmolol 0.5 mg/kg (500 mcg/kg) IV over 1 min, then 50 mcg/kg/min for 4 min; if poor response repeat 0.5 mg/kg and give 50–200 mcg/kg/min; rarely given for >48 hr.

Etanercept 0.4 mg/kg (max 25 mg) twice wkly deep SC.

Ethacrynic acid IV: 0.5–1 mg/kg/dose (adult 25–50 mg) 12–24 H. Oral: 1–4 mg/kg/dose (adult 50–200 mg) 12–24 H.

Ethambutol hydrochloride 25 mg/kg once daily for 8 wk, then 15 mg/kg daily oral. Intermittent: 35 mg/kg × 3/wk. IV: 80% oral dose.

Ethamsylate 12.5 mg/kg/dose (max 500 mg) 6 H oral, IM, IV.

Ethanol, dehydrated (100%) Vessel sclerosis: inject max of 1 mL/kg.

Ethanolamine oleate 5% soltn, adult (NOT/kg): 1.5–5 mL per varix (max 20 mL per treatment).

Ethionamide TB: 15–20 mg/kg (max 1 g) at night oral. Leprosy: 5–8 mg/kg (max 375 mg) daily.

Ethosuximide 10 mg/kg (adult 500 mg) daily oral, incr by 50% each wk to max 40 mg/kg (adult 2 g) daily. Trough level 0.3–0.7 mmol/L.

Etidocaine 0.5%–1.5% soltn: max 6 mg/kg (0.6 mL/kg of 1%) parenteral, or 8 mg/kg (0.8 mL/kg of 1%) with adrenaline.

Etidronate 5–20 mg/kg daily oral (no food for 2 hr before and after dose) for max 6 mo. IV: 7.5 mg/kg daily for 3–7 days.

Etomidate 0.3 mg/kg slow IV.

Factor 8 concentrate (vial 200–250 u), recombinant antihaemophilic factor (rAHF) Joint 20 u/kg, psoas 30 u/kg, cerebral 50 u/kg. 2 × dose (u/kg) = % normal activity, e.g. 35 u/kg gives peak level of 70% normal.

Factor 8 inhibitor bypassing fraction IV infsn max 2 u/kg/min: joint 50 u/kg/dose 12 H, mucous mem 50 u/kg/dose 6 H, soft tissue 100 u/kg/dose 12 H, cerebral 100 u/kg/dose 6–12 H.

Famciclovir Zoster, varicella: 5 mg/kg/dose (adult 250 mg) 8 H oral for 7 days; immunocompromised 10 mg/kg/dose (adult 500 mg) 8 H for 10 days. Genital herpes (adult, NOT/kg): 125 mg 12 H oral for 5 days (treat), 250 mg (suppress) 12 H; immunocompromised 500 mg 12 H for 7 days (treat), 500 mg daily (suppress).

Famotidine 0.5–1 mg/kg/dose (adult 20–40 mg) 12–24 H oral. 0.5 mg/kg/dose (max 20 mg) 12 H slow IV.

Fat emulsion 20% See lipid emulsion.

Felodipine 0.1 mg/kg (adult 2.5 mg) daily, incr if reqd to 0.5 mg/kg (adult 10 mg) daily oral.

Fenoterol Oral: 0.1 mg/kg/dose 6 H. Resp soltn 1 mg/mL: 0.5 mL/dose diluted to 2 mL 3–6 H (mild), 1 mL/dose diluted to 2 mL 1–2 H (moderate), undiluted continuous (severe, in ICU). Aerosol (200 mcg/puff): 1–2 puffs 4–8 H.

Fentanyl 1–2 mcg/kg/dose (adult 50–100 mcg) IM or IV; infuse 2–4 mcg/kg/hr (<25 kg: 100 mcg/kg in 50 mL at 1–2 mL/hr, >25 kg: amp 50 mcg/mL at 0.04–0.08 mL/kg/hr). Ventltd: 5–10 mcg/kg stat or 50 mcg/kg IV over 1 hr; infuse 5–10 mcg/kg/hr (amp 50 mcg/mL at 0.1–0.2 mL/kg/hr). Patch (lasts 72 hr) in adult (NOT/kg): 25 mcg/hr, incr if reqd by 25 mcg/hr every 3 days. Epidural: 0.5 mcg/kg stat, or 0.4 mcg/kg/hr.

Ferrous salts Prophylaxis 2 mg/kg/day elemental iron oral, treatment 6 mg/kg/day elemental iron oral. Fumarate 1 mg = 0.33 mg iron. Gluconate 1 mg = 0.12 mg iron; so Fergon (60 mg/mL gluconate) prophylaxis 0.3 mL/kg daily, treatment 1 mL/kg daily oral. Sulphate (dried) 1 mg = 0.3 mg iron; so Ferro-Gradumet (350 mg dried sulphate) prophylaxis 7 mg/kg (adult 350 mg) daily, treatment 20 mg/kg (adult 1050 mg) daily oral.

Filgrastim (granulocyte CSF) Idiopathic or cyclic neutropenia: 5 mcg/kg daily SC or IV over 30 min. Congenital neutropenia: 12 mcg/kg daily

SC or IV over 1 hr. Marrow transplant: 20–30 mcg/kg daily IV over 4–24 hr, reducing if neutrophils >1 × 109/L.

Flecainide 2–3 mg/kg/dose (max 100 mg) 12 H oral, may incr over 2 wk to 7 mg/kg/dose (max 200 mg) 8–12 H. IV over 30 min: 0.5–2 mg/kg/dose (max 150 mg) 12 H.

Flucloxacillin Oral: 12.5–25 mg/kg/dose (adult 250–500 mg) 6 H. IM or IV: 25 mg/kg/dose (adult 1 g) 6 H. Severe inftn: 50 mg/kg/dose (adult 2 g) IV 12 H (1st wk life), 8 H (2–4 wk), 6 H or constant infsn (>4 wk).

Fluconazole 6 mg/kg (adult 200 mg) stat, then 3 mg/kg (adult 100 mg) daily oral or IV. Severe inftn: 12 mg/kg (adult 400 mg) stat, then 6–12 mg/kg (adult 200–400 mg) daily IV.

Flucytosine (5-fluorocytosine) 400–1200 mg/m^2/dose (max 2 g) 6 H IV over 30 min, or oral. Peak level 50–100 mcg/mL, trough 25–50 mcg/mL (× 7.75 = μmol/L).

Fludrocortisone acetate 150 mcg/m^2 daily oral. Fludrocortisone 1 mg = hydrocortisone 125 mg in mineralocorticoid activity, 10 mg in glucocorticoid.

Flumazenil 5 mcg/kg every 60 sec to max total 40 mcg/kg (adult 2 mg), then 2–10 mcg/kg/hr IV.

Flunitrazepam Adult (NOT/kg): 0.5–2 mg at night, oral.

Fluoxetine 0.5 mg/kg (max 20 mg) daily, incr to max 1 mg/kg /dose (max 40 mg) 12 H oral. Weekly 90 mg cap: 1 per wk.

Fluticasone Inhaled (NOT/kg): 50–100 mcg/dose (child), 100–500 mcg/dose (adult) 12 H. 0.05% soltn: 1–4 sprays/nostril daily. 0.05% cream: apply sparingly daily.

Fluvastatin 0.4 mg/kg (adult 20 mg) nocte oral, incr to 0.8 mg/kg (adult 40 mg) nocte if required.

Fluvoxamine 2 mg/kg/dose (adult 100 mg) 8–24 H oral.

Folic acid NOT/kg. Deficiency: 50 mcg (neonate), 0.1–0.25 mg (<4 yr), 0.5–1 mg (>4 yr) daily IV, IM, SC or oral. Metabolic disease: 5 mg/day oral. Pregnancy: 0.5 mg (high risk 4 mg) daily oral.

Folinic acid See calcium folinate.

Follicle stimulating hormone (FSH) Adult (NOT/kg), monitor urinary oestrogen. Anovulation: usually 50–150 IU SC daily for 9–12 days. Superovulation (2 wk after starting GnRH agonist): 100–225 IU/kg daily starting day 3 of cycle.

Foscarnet 20 mg/kg IV over 30 min, then 200 mg/kg/day by constant IV infsn (less if creatinine >0.11 mmol/L) or 60 mg/kg/dose 8 H IV over 2 hr. Chronic use: 90–120 mg/kg IV over 2 hr daily.

Framycetin sulfate (Soframycin) Subconjunctival: 500 mg in 1 mL water daily × 3 days. Bladder: 500 mg in 50 mL saline 8 H × 10 days. Eye/ear 0.5%: 23 drops 8 H, ointment 8 H.

Framycetin sulfate 15 mg/g + gramicidin 0.05 mg/g Cream or ointment (Soframycin topical): apply 8–12 H.

Framycetin sulfate 5 mg + gramicidin 0.05 mg + dexamethasone 0.5 mg/mL (Sofradex) Eye/ear: 2–3 drops 6–8 H, ointment 8–12 H.

Fresh frozen plasma Contains all clotting factors. 10–20 mL/kg IV. 1 bag is about 230 mL.

Frusemide Usually 0.5–1 mg/kg/dose (adult 20–40 mg) 6–24 H (daily if preterm) oral, IM, or IV over 20 min (no faster than 0.05 mg/kg/min IV). IV infsn: 0.1–1 mg/kg/hr.

Fusidic acid Fusidic acid (susp) absorption only 70% that of sodium fusidate (tabs). Suspension: 15–20 mg/kg (adult 750 mg) 8 H oral. For tablets and IV, see sodium fusidate.

Gabapentin 10 mg/kg (adult 300 mg) once day 1, oral, 12 H day 2, 8 H day 3, then adjusted to 10–20 mg/kg/dose (adult 300–1200 mg) 8 H.

Ganciclovir 5 mg/kg/dose 12 H IV over 1 hr for 2–3 wk; then 5 mg/kg IV daily, or 6 mg/kg IV on 6 days every wk, or 20 mg/kg/dose (adult 1 g) 8 H oral. Congenital CMV: 7.5 mg/kg/dose 12 H IV over 2 hr.

Gentamicin Single daily dose IV or IM. Neonate: 5 mg/kg stat, then 2.5 mg/kg (<30 wk) 3.5 mg/kg (30–35 wk) 5 mg/kg (term <1 wk) daily. 1 wk–10 yr: 8 mg/kg day 1, then 6 mg/kg daily. >10 yr: 7 mg/kg day 1, then 5 mg/kg daily (max 240–360 mg) daily. Trough level <1.0 mg/L, done daily 1000, 1600, 2200 at RCH.

Glibenclamide Adult (NOT/kg): initially 2.5 mg daily oral, max 20 mg daily.

Glucagon 1 u = 1 mg. 0.04 mg/kg (adult 1–2 mg) IV or IM stat, then 10–50 mcg/kg/hr (0.5 mg/kg in 50 mL at 1–5 mL/hr) IV. Beta-blocker overdose: 0.1 mg/kg IV stat, then 0.3–2 mcg/kg/min.

Glucose See dextrose.

Glucose electrolyte solution Not dehydrated: 1 heaped teaspoon sucrose in a large cup of water (4% sucrose = 2% glucose); do NOT add salt. Dehydrated: 1 sachet of Gastrolyte in 200 mL water; give frequent small sips, or infuse through a nasogastric tube.

Glutamic acid 10–20 mg/kg (adult 0.5–1 g) oral with meals.

Glyceryl trinitrate Adult (NOT/kg): sublingual tab 0.3–0.9 mg/dose (lasts 30–60 min); sublingual aerosol 0.4–0.8 mg/dose; slow-release buccal tab 1–10 mg 8–12 H; transdermal 0.5–5 cm of 2% ointment, or 5–15 mg patch 8–12 H. IV infsn 1–10 mcg/kg/min: adult 50 mg in 50 mL at 0.8 mL/hr is 0.2 mcg/kg/min; use polyethylene-lined syringe and tubing (not PVC). Pul vasodil: 5 mcg/kg/min nitroglyc = 2 mcg/kg/min nitropr = 0.1 mcg/kg/min PGE1.

Glycopyrronium bromide Dose as for glycopyrrolate.

Gramicidin 25 mcg/mL + neomycin 2.5 mg/mL + polymyxin B 5000 u/mL (Neosporin) Eye drops: 1–2 drops/eye every 15–30 min, reducing to 6–12 H.

Griseofulvin (Grisovin, Fulcin) 10–20 mg/kg (adult 0.5–1 g) daily oral.

Griseofulvin, ultramicrosize (Griseostatin) 5.5–7 mg/kg (adult 330–660 mg) daily oral.

***Haemophilus influenzae* type b, vaccines** Inactivated. <12 mo: give diphtheria protein conjugate (HibTITER, ProHIBiT), or tetanus conjugate (Act-HIB, Hiberix) 0.5 mL IM at 2 mo, 4 mo, 6 mo and 15 mo; or meningococcal conjugate (Pedvax HIB) 0.5 mL IM at 2 mo, 4 mo and 15 mo. If 1st dose >18 mo: give 1 dose of HibTITER or Pedvax HIB.

Haloperidol 0.01 mg/kg (max 0.5 mg) daily, incr up to 0.1 mg/kg/dose 12 H IV or oral; up to 2 mg/kg/dose (max 100 mg) 12 H used rarely. Acutely disturbed: 0.1–0.2 mg/kg (adult 5–10 mg) IM. Long-acting decanoate ester: 1–6 mg/kg IM every 4 wk.

Heparin 1 mg = 100 u. Low dose: 75 u/kg stat, then 10–15 u/kg/hr IV (500 u/kg in 50 mL at 1 mL/hr = 10 u/kg/hr). Full dose: 75 u/kg (adult 5000 u) stat, then 30 u/kg/hr (<12 mo), 20 u/kg/hr (child), 15 u/kg/hr (adult) IV adjusted to give APTT 60–85 sec (anti-Xa 0.3–0.7 u/mL). Heparin lock: 100 u/mL.

Heparin calcium Low dose: 75 u/kg/dose SC 12 H.

Hepatitis A vaccine (Havrix) Inactivated. 0.5 mL (child) or 1 mL (adult) IM stat, and after 6–12 mo (2 doses). Boost every 5 yr.

Hepatitis A vaccine (VAQTA) Inactivated. 0.5 mL (child) or 1 mL (>17 yr) IM stat, and after 6–18 mo (2 doses).

Hepatitis A + hepatitis B vaccine (Twinrix) Inactivated. 1–15 yr 0.5 mL, >15 yr 1 mL IM stat, after 1 mo, and after 6 mo (3 doses). Boost every 5 yr.

Hepatitis B vaccine (Engerix-B, HB Vax II) Inactivated. Engerix-B 10 mcg/dose (<10 yr), 20 mcg (>9 yr); HB Vax II 2.5 mcg/dose (<10 yr), 5 mcg (10–19 yr), 10 mcg (>19 yr), 40 mcg (dialysis) IM stat, after 1 mo, and after 6 mo (3 doses). Boost every 5 yr approx. See also diphtheria and *Haemophilus* vaccines.

Homatropine 2%, 5% soltn: 1–2 drops/eye 4 H.

Hydralazine 0.1–0.2 mg/kg (adult 5–10 mg) stat IV or IM, then 4–6 mcg/kg/min (adult 200–300 mcg/min) IV. Oral: 0.4 mg/kg/dose (adult 20 mg) 12 H, slow incr to 1.5 mg/kg/dose (usual max 50 mg) 6–8 H.

Hydrochloric acid Use soltn of 100 mmol/L (0.1 m = 0.1 n = 100 mEq/L); give IV by central line only. Alkalosis: dose (mL) = BE × Wt × 3 (give half this); maximum rate 2 mL/kg/hr. Blocked central line: 1.5 mL/lumen over 24 hr.

Hydrochlorothiazide 1–1.5 mg/kg/dose (adult 25–50 mg) 12–24 H oral.

Hydrochlorothiazide + quinapril 10/12.5, 20/12.5 Adult (NOT/kg): 10/12.5 tab daily oral, incr if reqd to 20/12.5 tab, max two 10/12.5 tab daily.

Hydrocortisone Usually 0.5–2 mg/kg/dose (adult 25–50 mg) 6–8 H oral, reducing as tolerated. 0.5%, 1% cream, ointment: apply 6–12 H. 1% cream + clioquinol: apply 8–24 H. 10% rectal foam: 125 mg/dose.

Hydrocortisone sodium succinate 2–4 mg/kg/dose 3–6 H IM, IV reducing as tolerated. Physiological: 5 mg/m^2/dose 6–8 H oral; 0.2 mg/kg/dose 8 H IM, IV. Physiological, stress: 1 mg/kg/dose 6 H IM, IV.

Hydrogen peroxide 10 volume (3%). Mouthwash 1:2 parts water. Skin or ear disinfectant 1:1 part water.

Hydroxocobalamin (Vit B12) 20 mcg/kg/dose (adult 1000 mcg) IM daily for 7 days then wkly (treatment), then every 2–3 mo (prophyl); IV dangerous in megaloblastic anaemia. Homocystinuria, methylmalonic acidur: 1 mg daily IM.

Hydroxychloroquine sulphate Doses as sulphate. Malaria: 10 mg/kg (max 600 mg) daily for 3 days; prophylaxis 5 mg/kg (max 300 mg) once a wk oral. Arthritis, SLE: 3–6.5 mg/kg (adult 200–600 mg) daily oral.

Hydroxyzine 2 mg/kg/dose (adult 25–100 mg) 6–8 H oral. 0.5–1 mg/kg/dose (adult 25–100 mg) 4–6 H if reqd IM.

Hyoscine 0.01 mg/kg/dose (max 0.6 mg) 6 H, IM or IV. Transdermal patch: 1.5 mg patch: >10 yr 1 every 72 hr.

Hyoscine hydrobromide 6–8 mcg/kg (max 400 mcg) 6–8 H IV, IM, SC. Motion sickness 300 mcg tab (NOT/kg): 0.25 tab (2–7 yr), 0.5 tab (7–12 yr), 1–2 tab (>12 yr) 6–24 H oral 30 min before, may repeat in 4 hr.

Hyoscine *N*-butylbromide 0.5 mg/kg/dose (adult 20–40 mg) 6–8 H IV, IM or oral.

Hyoscyamine (L-atropine) 2–5 mcg/kg/dose (adult 100–300 mcg) 4–6 H oral, sublingual, IM or IV.

Ibuprofen 5–10 mg/kg/dose (adult 200–400 mg) 4–8 H oral. Arthritis: 10 mg/kg/dose (adult 400–800 mg) 6–8 H. Cystic fibrosis: 20–30 mg/kg/dose 12 H. PDA: 10 mg/kg stat, then 5 mg/kg after 24 and 48 hr IV over 15 min.

Imipenem-cilastatin 15 mg/kg/dose (adult 500 mg) 6 H IV over 30 min. Severe inftn: 25 mg/kg/dose IV over 1 hr (adult 1 g) 12 H (1st wk life), 8 H (2–4 wk), 6–8 H or constant infsn (4+ wk).

Imipramine 0.5–1.5 mg/kg/dose (adult 25–75 mg) 8 H oral. Enuresis: 5–6 yr 25 mg, 7–10 yr 50 mg, >10 yr 50–75 mg nocte.

Immunoglobulin, CMV 100–200 mg/kg IV over 2 hr. Transplant: daily for first 3 days, wkly × 6, monthly × 6.

Immunoglobulin, diphtheria 250 u IM once.

Immunoglobulin, hepatitis B 400 u IM within 5 days of needlestick, repeat in 30 days; 100 u IM within 24 hr birth to baby of Hep B carrier.

Immunoglobulin, antilymphocyte (thymocyte) Horse (Atgam): 10–15 mg/kg daily for 3–5 days IV over 4 hr; occasionally up to 30 mg/kg daily. Rabbit (ATG-Fresenius): 2.5–5 mg/kg daily over 4–6 hr IV.

Immunoglobulin, normal, human Hypogammaglobulinaemia: 10–15 mL/kg of 6% soltn (600–900 mg/kg) IV over 5–8 hr, then 5–7.5 mL/kg (300–450 mg/kg) over 3–4 hr monthly; or 0.6 mL/kg of 16% soltn (100 mg/kg) every 2–4 wk IM. Sepsis: 0.5 g/kg IV over 4 hr. Kawasaki, Guillain-Barré, ITP, myasth gravis, Still's dis: 35 mL/kg of 6% soltn (2 g/kg) IV over 16 hr stat, then if required 15 mL/kg (900 mg/kg) IV over 8 hr each month. Prevention hep A: 0.1 mL/kg (16 mg/kg) IM. Prevention measles: 0.2 mL/kg (32 mg/kg) IM (repeat next day if immunocompromised).

Immunoglobulin, rabies (Hyperab, Imogam) 20 IU (0.133 mL)/kg IM once (half infiltrated around wound), with rabies vaccine.

Immunoglobulin, Rh 1 mL (625 IU, 125 mcg) IM within 72 hr of exposure. Large transfusion: 0.16 mL (100 IU, 20 mcg) per mL Rh-positive red cells (maternal serum should be anti-D positive 24–48 hr after injection).

Immunoglobulin, respiratory syncytial virus 750 mg/kg every month IV (50 mg/mL: 1.5 mL/kg/hr for 15 min, 3 mL/kg/hr for 15 min, then 6 mL/kg/hr).

Immunoglobulin, tetanus (TIG) IM preparation: 250–500 IU (1–2 amp). IV preparation: 4000 IU (100 mL) at 0.04 mL/kg/min for 30 min, then 0.075 mL/kg/min.

Immunoglobulin, zoster Prevention of chickenpox in immunocompromised, 0.4–1.2 mL/kg (max 6 mL) IM.

Indomethacin 0.5–1 mg/kg/dose (adult 25–50 mg) 8 H (max 6 H) oral or PR. PDA: 0.1 mg/kg (<1 kg) or 0.2 mg/kg (≥1 kg) day 1, then 0.1 mg/kg daily days 2–7 oral or IV over 1 hr.

Infliximab 3 mg/kg (arthritis, with methotrexate) 5 mg/kg (Crohn's) IV over 2 hr, then (if response) after 2 wk, 6 wk, and then 5–10 mg/kg every 8 wk.

Influenza A and B vaccine (Fluvax, Vaxigrip) Inactivated. 0.125 mL (3 mo–2 yr), 0.25 mL (2–6 yr), 0.5 mL (>6 yr) SC stat and 4 wk later (2 doses). Boost annually (1 dose).

Insulin Regular insulin: 0.05–0.2 u/kg prn, or 0.05–0.1 u/kg/hr (5 u/kg in 50 mL at 0.5–1 mL/hr); later 1 u/10 g dextrose IV. For hyperkalaemia: 0.1 u/kg insulin and 2 mL/kg 50% dextrose IV. In TPN: 5–25 u/250 g dextrose. SC insulin (onset/peak/duration): lispro 10–15 min/1 hr/2–5 hr; aspart 15–20 min/1 hr/3–5 hr; regular 30–60 min/4 hr/6–8 hr; isophane (NPH) 2–4 hr/4–12 hr/18–24 hr; zinc (Lente) 2–3 hr/7–15 hr/24 hr; glargine 1.5 hr/none/24 hr; crystalline zinc (Ultralente) 4–6 hr/10–30 hr/24–36 hr; protamine zinc 4–8 hr/15–20 hr/24–36 hr.

Interferon alfa-2a, recombinant Haemangioma: 1 million u/m^2 daily SC or IM incr over 4 wk to 2–3 million u/m^2 daily for 16–24 wk, then × 3/wk. Hep B, C: 3–6 million u/m^2 × 3/wk SC or IM for 4–6 mo; higher doses may be reqd in hep B.

Interferon alfa-2b, recombinant Condylomata: 1 million u into each lesion (max 5) × 3/wk for 5 wk. Haemangioma: as for interferon alfa-2a. Hepatitis B, C: monotherapy as for interferon alfa-2a; hep C refractory to interferon monotherapy (adult, NOT/kg) 3 million u × 3/wk IM or SC, plus ribavirin oral 400 mg morning and 600 mg evening (<75 kg), or 600 mg morning and evening (>75 kg).

Interferon alfa-n3 Warts (NOT/kg): 250,000 u injected into base of wart (max 10 doses/session) × 2/wk for max 8 wk.

Interferon alfacon-1 Hepatitis C (adult, NOT/kg): usually 9 mcg (7.5 mcg if not tolerated) × 3/wk SC for 24 wk; if relapse 15 mcg × 3/wk SC for 6 mo.

Interferon beta-1a Mult scler (adult, NOT/kg): Avonex 30 mcg (6 million IU) once a wk IM, Rebif 44 mcg × 3/wk SC.

Interferon beta-1b Mult scler (adult, NOT/kg): 250 mcg (8 million IU) SC alternate days.

Interferon gamma-1b Chronic gran dis: 1.5 mcg/kg (body area ≤0.5 m^2) or 50 mcg/m^2 (area >0.5 m^2) × 3/wk SC.

Ipecacuanha syrup (total alkaloids 1.4 mg/mL) 12 mL/kg (adult 30 mL) stat oral, NG. May repeat once in 30 min.

Ipratropium bromide Resp soltn (250 mcg/mL): 0.251 mL diluted to 4 mL 4–8 H; severe attack every 20 min for 3 doses, then 4–6 H. Aerosol 20 mcg/puff: 2–4 puffs 6–8 H. Nasal: 84 mcg/nostril 6–12 H.

Iron See ferrous gluconate, ferrous sulphate.

Iron dextran, iron polymaltose Fe 50 mg/mL: dose (mL) = 0.05 × Wt × (15 – Hb in g%) IM (often in divided doses). IV infsn possible (but dangerous).

Isoconazole Topical: 1% cream 12 H. Vaginal: 600 mg (2 tab) once.

Isoetharine Inhaltn soltn (1%): 0.5 mL diltd to 4 mL 3–6 H (mild), 1 mL diltd to 4 mL 1–2 H (moderate), undiltd constant (severe, in ICU). Aerosol 340 mcg/puff: 1–2 puffs 4–6 H.

Isoniazid 10 mg/kg (max 300 mg) daily oral, IM or IV. TB meningitis: 15–20 mg/kg (max 500 mg) daily.

Isoprenaline Aerosol 80–400 mcg/puff: 1–3 puffs 4–8 H. IV infsn <33 kg: 0.3 mg/kg in 50 mL at 1 mL/hr = 0.1 mcg/kg/min; >33 kg: 0.1 mcg/kg/min using 1/5000 (0.2 mg/mL) soltn = 0.03 × Wt mL/hr; for 65 kg adult 4 mg in 50 mL at 2 mL/hr is 0.05 mcg/kg/min.

Isosorbide dinitrate Sublingual: 0.1–0.2 mg/kg/dose (max 10 mg) 2 H or as needed. Oral: 0.5–1 mg/kg/dose (max 40 mg) 6 H or as needed. Slow release tab, adult (NOT/kg): 20–80 mg/dose 12 H. IV infsn 0.6–2 mcg/kg/min: for 65 kg adult 50 mg in 50 mL at 2.5 mL/hr is 0.5 mcg/kg/min.

Isotretinoin Adult: 0.5–1 mg/kg daily oral for 2–4 wk, reducing if possible to 0.1–0.2 mg/kg daily for 15–20 wk. 0.05% gel: apply sparingly at night.

Ispaghula husk Adult (NOT/kg): 1–2 teaspoonfuls 6–12 H oral. Half this dose 6–12 yr.

Isradipine 0.05 mg/kg/dose 12 H oral, may incr after 2–4 wk gradually to 0.1–0.2 mg/kg/dose (max 10 mg) 12 H.

Itraconazole 2–4 mg/kg/dose (adult 100–200 mg) 12–24 H oral after food. Trough level >0.5 mcg/mL at 10–14 days.

Ivermectin 0.15–0.4 mg/kg (adult 12–24 mg) oral every 6–12 mo.

Kanamycin Single daily dose IV or IM. Neonate: 15 mg/kg stat, then 7.5 mg/kg (<30 wk) 10 mg/kg (30–35 wk) 15 mg/kg (term <1 wk) daily. 1 wk–10 yr: 25 mg/kg day 1, then 18 mg/kg daily. >10 yr: 20 mg/kg day 1, then 15 mg/kg (max 1.5 g) daily. Trough level <5.0 mg/L.

Ketamine Sedation, analgesia: 2–4 mg/kg IM, 4 mcg/kg/min IV. Anaesthesia: 5–10 mg/kg IM, 1–2 mg/kg IV, infsn 10–40 mcg/kg/min. Premed: 5 mg/kg oral.

Ketoconazole Oral: 5 mg/kg/dose (adult 200 mg) 12–24 H. 2% cream: apply 12–24 H. 2% shampoo: wash hair, apply liquid for 5 min, wash off.

Ketoprofen 1–2 mg/kg/dose (adult 50–100 mg) 6–12 H (max 4 mg/kg or 200 mg in 24 hr) oral, IM, PR. Slow release, adults (NOT/kg): 200 mg daily.

Ketorolac Oral: 0.2 mg/kg/dose (max 10 mg) 4–6 H (max 0.8 mg/kg/day or 40 mg/day). IM: 0.6 mg/kg (max 30 mg) stat, then 0.2–0.4 mg/kg/dose (max 20 mg) 4–6 H for 5 days, then 0.2 mg/kg/dose (max 10 mg) 6 H.

Ketotifen Child >2 yr (NOT/kg): 1 mg/dose 12 H oral with food. Adult (NOT/kg): 1–2 mg/dose 12 H oral with food.

Labetalol 1–2 mg/kg/dose (adult 50–100 mg) 12 H oral, may incr wkly to max 10 mg/kg/dose (max 600 mg) 6 H.

Lactulose 3.3 g/5 mL soltn. Laxative: 0.5 mL/kg/dose 12–24 H oral. Hepatic coma: 1 mL/kg/dose hourly until bowel cleared, then 6–8 H.

Lamotrigine 0.2 mg/kg (adult 25 mg) oral daily, incr slowly if reqd to max 1–4 mg/kg/dose (adult 50–200 mg) 12 H. Double dose if taking carbamazepine, phenobarbitone, phenytoin or primidone; halve dose if taking valproate.

Levodopa + benserazide (4:1) Adult (NOT/kg): initially levodopa 100 mg/dose 8 H oral; if not controlled, incr wkly by 100 mg/day to max 250 mg/dose 6 H.

Levodopa + carbidopa 250 mg/25 mg and 100 mg/10 mg tabs. Adult (NOT/kg): initially one 100/10 tab 8 H oral; if not controlled, substitute one 250/25 tab for one 100/25 tab every 2nd day; if not controlled on 250/25 8 H, incr by one 250/25 tab every 2nd day to max 6–8 tab/day.

Lignocaine IV 1 mg/kg (0.1 mL/kg of 1%) over 2 min, then 15–50 mcg/kg/min: for 65 kg adult 1 g in 50 mL at 5 mL/hr is 25 mcg/kg/min. VF: 1 mg/kg (0.1 mL/kg of 1%) IV. Nerve block: without adrenaline max

4 mg/kg (0.4 mL/kg of 1%), with adrenaline 7 mg/kg (0.7 mL/kg of 1%). Topical spray: max 3–4 mg/kg (xylocaine 10% spray pack: about 10 mg/puff). Topical 2% gel, 2.5% compound mouth paint/gel (SM-33), 2% and 4% soltn, 5% ointment, 10% dental ointment: apply 3 H prn.

Lignocaine 2.5% + prilocaine 2.5% Cream (EMLA): 1.5 g/10 cm^2 under occlusive dressing for 1–3 hr.

Lincomycin 10 mg/kg/dose (adult 600 mg) 8 H oral, IM or IV over 1 hr. Severe inftn: 15–20 mg/kg/dose (adult 1.2 g) IV over 2 hr 6 H.

Lindane 1% cream, lotion. Scabies: apply from neck down, wash off after 8–12 hr. Lice: rub into hair for 4 min, then wash off; repeat after 24 hr (max × 2/wk).

Liothyronine sodium (T3) Oral: 0.2 mcg/kg/dose (adult 10 mcg) 8 H, may incr to 0.4 mcg/kg/dose (adult 20 mcg) 8 H. IV: 0.1–0.4 mcg/kg/dose (adult 5–20 mcg) 8–12 H. Septic shock: 0.1–0.2 mcg/kg/hr (adult 100–200 mcg/day) IV infsn.

Lipid 20% emulsion: 1–3 g/kg/day IV (mL/hr = g/kg/day × Wt × 0.21).

Lisinopril 0.1 mg/kg (adult 5 mg) daily oral, may incr over 4–6 wk to 0.2–1 mg/kg (adult 10–20 mg) daily.

Lithium (salts) 5–20 mg/kg/dose 8–24 H oral. Slow release tab 4–50 mg (adult, NOT/kg): 1–2 tab 12 H. Maintain trough level 0.8–1.6 mmol/L (>2 mmol/L toxic).

Loperamide 0.05–0.1 mg/kg/dose (adult 2–4 mg) 8–12 H oral, incr if reqd to max 0.4 mg/kg/dose (max 4 mg) 8 H.

Lorazepam 0.02–0.06 mg/kg/dose (adult 1–3 mg) 8–24 H oral. IV: 0.05–0.2 mg/kg IV over 2 min, then 0.01–0.1 mg/kg/hr.

Magnesium chloride 10% 0.48 g/5 mL = Mg 1 mmol/mL. 0.4 mL/kg/dose 12 H slow IV. Myoc infarct (NOT/kg): 5 mL/hr IV for 6 hr, then 1 mL/hr for 24–48 hr. VF: 0.1–0.2 mL/kg IV.

Magnesium hydroxide Antacid: 10–40 mg/kg/dose (max 2 g) 6 H oral. Laxative: 50–100 mg/kg (max 5 g) oral.

Magnesium sulphate Deficiency: 50% mag sulph (2 mmol/mL) 0.2 mL/kg/dose (max 10 mL) 12 H IM, slow IV. Asthma, digoxin tachycardia, eclampsia, prem labour, pul ht: 50% 0.1 mL/kg (50 mg/kg) IV over 20 min, then 0.06 mL/kg/hr (30 mg/kg/hr); keep serum Mg 1.5–2.5 mmol/L (pul ht 3–4 mmol/L). Myoc infarct (NOT/kg): 50% 2.5 mL/hr (5 mmol/hr) IV for 6 hr, then 0.5 mL/hr (1 mmol/hr) for 24–48 hr. VF: 50% 0.05–0.1 mL/kg (0.1–0.2 mmol/kg) IV. Laxative: 0.5 g/kg/dose (max 15 g) as 10% soltn 8 H for 2 days oral.

Maldison 0.5% liquid: 20 mL to hair, wash off after 12 hr.

Mannitol 0.25–0.5 g/kg/dose IV (2–4 mL/kg of 12.5%, 1.25–2.5 mL/kg of 20%, 1–2 mL/kg of 25%) 2 H prn, provided serum osmolality <320–330 mmol/L.

Measles vaccine (Attenuvax) Live. >12 mo: 0.5 mL SC once.

Measles + mumps vaccine (Rimparix) Live. >12 mo: 0.5 mL SC once.

Measles + mumps + rubella vaccine (MMRII, Priorix) Live. >12 mo: 0.5 mL SC.

Mebendazole NOT/kg: 100 mg/dose 12 H × 3 days. Enterobiasis (NOT/kg): 100 mg once, may repeat after 24 wks.

Mebeverine 135 mg tab: adult (NOT/kg) 13 tab daily oral.

Mefenamic acid 10 mg/kg/dose (adult 500 mg) 8 H oral.

Mefloquine 15 mg/kg (adult 750 mg) stat, then 10 mg/kg (adult 500 mg) after 6–8 hr. Prophylaxis: 5 mg/kg (adult 250 mg) once a wk.

Meningococcus gp A, C, W135 and Y vaccine (Mencevax ACWY, Menomune) Inactivated. >2 yr: 0.5 mL SC. Boost 1–3 yrly.

Meropenem 10–20 mg/kg/dose (adult 0.5–1 g) 8 H IV over 5–30 min. Severe inftn: 20–40 mg/kg/dose (adult 1–2 g) 12 H (1st wk life) 8 H (>1 wk) or constant infsn.

Metaraminol IV: 0.01 mg/kg stat (repeat prn), then 0.1–1 mcg/kg/min and titrate dose against BP. SC: 0.1 mg/kg.

Methadone Usually 0.1–0.2 mg/kg/dose (adult 5–10 mg) 6–12 H oral, SC or IM.

Methionine 50 mg/kg/dose (max 2.5 g) oral 4 H for 4 doses. Prophylaxis: 1 mg to paracetamol 5 mg.

Methotrexate Leukaemia: typically 3.3 mg/m^2 IV daily for 4–6 wk; then 2.5 mg/kg IV every 2 wk, or 30 mg/m^2 oral or IM × 2/wk; higher doses with folinic acid rescue. Intrathecal: 12 mg/m^2 wkly for 2 wk, then monthly. Arthritis: 10–20 mg/m^2 wkly oral, IV, IM or SC. Adult psoriasis: 0.2–0.5 mg/kg wkly oral, IV or IM until response, then reduce.

Methylcellulose Constipation: 30–60 mg/kg/dose (adult 1.5–3 g) with at least 300 mL fluid 12 H oral.

Methylene blue 1–2 mg/kg/dose (G6PD deficiency 0.4 mg/kg) IV, repeated as reqd. Septic shock: 0.5 mg/kg over 15 min IV, then 0.1–0.25 mg/kg/hr.

Methylphenidate 0.1 mg/kg/dose oral 8 am, noon and (occasionally) 4 pm; incr if reqd to max 0.5 mg/kg/dose (adult 20 mg). Long acting: 20–60 mg (18–54 mg in USA) in morning.

Methylprednisolone Asthma: 0.5–1 mg/kg/dose 6 H oral, IV or IM day 1, 12 H day 2, then 1 mg/kg daily, reducing to minimum effective dose. Severe croup: 4 mg/kg IV stat, then 1 mg/kg/dose 8 H. Severe sepsis before antibiotics (or within 4 hr of 1st dose): 30 mg/kg IV once. Spinal cord injury (within 8 hr): 30 mg/kg stat, then 5 mg/kg/hr 2 days. Lotion 0.25%: apply sparingly 12–24 H. Methylpred 1 mg = hydrocortisone 5 mg in glucocorticoid activity, 0.5 mg in mineralocorticoid.

Methylprednisolone aceponate 0.1% cream, ointment: apply 12–24 H.

Methyltestosterone NOT/kg: 2.5–12.5 mg/day buccal.

Methysergide maleate 0.02 mg/kg/dose (adult 1 mg) 12 H oral, incr if reqd to max 0.04 mg/kg/dose (adult 2 mg) 8 H for 3–6 mo.

Metoclopramide 0.15–0.3 mg/kg/dose (adult 10–15 mg) 6 H IV, IM, oral; 0.2–0.4 mg/kg/dose (adult 10–20 mg) 8 H PR. Perioperative: 0.5 mg/kg IV. With chemother: up to 1–2 mg/kg 4 H IV.

Metolazone 0.1–0.2 mg/kg (adult 5–10 mg) daily oral. Up to 0.5 mg/kg (adult 30 mg) daily short term.

Metoprolol IV: 0.1 mg/kg (adult 5 mg) over 5 min, repeat every 5 min to max 3 doses, then 1–5 mcg/kg/min. Oral: 1–2 mg/kg/dose (adult 50–100 mg) 6–12 H.

Metronidazole 15 mg/kg (max 1 g) stat, then 7.5 mg/kg/dose (max 1 g) 12 H in neonate (1st maintenance dose 48 hr after load if <2 kg, 24 hr in term baby), 8 H (4+ wk) IV, PR or oral. Giardiasis: 30 mg/kg (adult 2 g) daily × 3 oral. Amoebiasis: 40 mg/kg/dose (adult 2.4 g) 8 H × 5 days oral. Topical gel 0.5%: apply daily. Level 60–300 μmol/mL (× 0.17 mcg/mL).

Mianserin 0.2–0.5 mg/kg/dose (adult 10–40 mg) 8 H oral.

Miconazole 7.5–15 mg/kg/dose (adult 0.6–1.2 g) 8 H IV over 1 hr. Topical: 2% cream, powder, lotion, tincture or gel 12–24 H. Vaginal: 2% cream or 100 mg ovule daily × 7.

Microlax enema <12 mo 1.25 mL, 12 yr 2.5 mL, >2 yr 5 mL.

Midazolam Sedation: usually 0.1–0.2 mg/kg (adult 5 mg) IV or IM, up to 0.5 mg/kg used safely in children; 0.2 mg/kg (repeated in 10 min if reqd) nasal; 0.5 mg/kg (max 20 mg) oral. Infusion (ventltd): 3 mg/kg in 50 mL at 1–4 mL/hr (1–4 mcg/kg/min); fitting usually 2–4 mL/hr (range 1–18 mL/hr); sedatn 1 mL/hr + clonidine 0.5–2 mcg/kg/hr.

Milrinone 50 mcg/kg IV over 10 min, then 0.25–0.75 mcg/kg/min (max 1.13 mg/kg/day).

Minocycline Over 8 yr: 4 mg/kg (max 200 mg) stat, then 2 mg/kg/dose (max 100 mg) 12 H oral or IV over 1 hr.

Minoxidil 0.1 mg/kg (max 5 mg) daily, incr to max 0.5 mg/kg/dose (max 25 mg) 12–24 H oral. Male baldness: 2% soltn 1 mL 12 H to dry scalp.

Mometasone furoate 0.1% cream or oint: apply daily. 50 mcg spray: adult 2 sprays/nostril daily.

Montelukast NOT/kg: 4 mg (2–5 yr) 5 mg (6–14 yr) 10 mg (>14 yr) daily at bedtime, oral.

Morphine Half life 2–4 hr. IM: neonate 0.1 mg/kg, child 0.2 mg/kg, adult 10–20 mg. IV (ventilated): 0.1–0.2 mg/kg/dose (adult 5–10 mg). Infsn of 1 mg/kg in 50 mL 5% dextrose: ventilated neonate 0.5–1.5 mL/hr (10–30 mcg/kg/hr), child or adult 1–3 mL/hr (20–60 mcg/kg/hr). Patient controlled: 20 mcg/kg boluses (1 mL of 1 mg/kg in 50 mL) with 5 min lockout time + (in child) 5 mcg/kg/hr. Oral: double parenteral dose; slow release, start with 0.6 mg/kg/dose 12 H and incr every 48 hr if reqd.

Mumps vaccine (Mumpsvax) Live. >12 mo: 0.5 mL SC once. See also measles + mumps + rubella vaccine.

Mupirocin 2% ointment: apply 8–12 H.

Nalidixic acid 15 mg/kg/dose (adult 1 g) 6 H oral, reducing to 7.5 mg/kg/dose (adult 500 mg) 6 H after 2 wk.

Naloxone Opiate intoxication (including newborn): 0.1 mg/kg (max 2 mg) stat IV, IM, SC or intratracheal, then 0.01 mg/kg/hr IV. Postop sedatn: 0.002 mg/kg/dose repeat every 2 min, then 0.01 mg/kg/hr (0.2 mcg/kg/min) IV.

Naltrexone 0.5 mg/kg (adult 25 mg) stat, then 1 mg/kg (adult 50 mg) daily oral.

Naproxen 1 mg = 1.1 mg naproxen sodium. >2 yr: 5–10 mg/kg/dose (adult 250–500 mg) 8–12 H oral. Adult (NOT/kg): 500 mg/dose 12 H PR.

Nedocromil Inhltn: 4 mg (2 puffs) 6 H, reducing to 12 H when improved. 2% eye drops: 1 drop/eye 6–24 H.

Neomycin 1 g/m^2/dose 4–6 H oral (max 12 g/day). Bladder washout: 40–2000 mg/L.

Neostigmine Reverse relaxants: 0.05–0.07 mg/kg/dose (adult 0.5–2.5 mg) IV; suggested dilution: neostigmine (2.5 mg/mL) 0.5 mL + atropine (0.6 mg/mL) 0.5 mL + saline 0.5 mL, give 0.1 mL/kg IV. Myasth gravis: 0.2–0.5 mg/kg/dose (adult 1–2.5 mg) 2–4 H IM, SC.

Netilmicin Single daily dose IV or IM. Neonate: 5 mg/kg stat, then 2.5 mg/kg (<30 wk), 3.5 mg/kg (30–35 wk), 5 mg/kg (term <1 wk) daily. 1 wk–10 yr: 8 mg/kg day 1, then 6 mg/kg daily. >10 yr: 7 mg/kg day 1, then 5 mg/kg daily (max 240–360 mg) daily. Trough level <1.0 mg/L.

Nicardipine 0.4–0.8 mg/kg/dose (adult 20–40 mg) 8 H oral. 1–3 mcg/kg/min (max 20 mg/hr) IV.

Nicotine resin chewing gum NOT/kg: 2–4 mg chewed over 30 min when inclined to smoke; usually need 16–24 mg/day, max 60 mg/day.

Nicotine transdermal patches Usually 21 mg, 14 mg, and 7 mg per 24 hr. Adult: if smoked >20 cig/day apply strongest patch daily 3–4 wk, medium patch daily 3–4 wk (initial dose if smoked ≤20 cig/day), then weakest patch daily 3–4 wk.

Nicotinic acid Hypercholesterolaemia and hypertriglyceridaemia: 5 mg/kg/dose (adult 200 mg) 8 H, gradually incr to 20–30 mg/kg/dose (adult 1–2 g) 8 H oral.

Nifedipine Caps 0.25–0.5 mg/kg (adult 10–20 mg) 6–8 H, tabs 0.5–1 mg/kg/dose (adult 20–40 mg) 12 H oral or sublingual.

Nimodipine 10–15 mcg/kg/hr (adult 1 mg/hr) IV for 2 hr, then 10–45 mcg/kg/hr (adult 2 mg/hr). Adult: 60 mg/dose 4 H oral.

Nisoldipine Slow release: 0.2 mg/kg (adult 10 mg) daily oral, incr to 0.4–0.8 mg/kg (adult 20–40 mg) daily.

Nitrazepam Child epilepsy: 0.125–0.5 mg/kg/dose 12 H oral. Hypnotic (NOT/kg): 2.5–5 mg (child) 5–10 mg (adult) nocte.

Nitric oxide 1–40 ppm (up to 80 ppm used occasionally). 0.1 L/min of 1000 ppm added to 10 L/min gas gives 10 ppm. [NO] = Cylinder [NO] × (1 – (Patient FiO_2/Supply FiO_2)). [NO] = Cylinder [NO] × NO flow/Total flow.

Nitrofurantoin 1.5 mg/kg/dose (adult 50–100 mg) 6 H oral. Prophylaxis: 1–2 mg/kg (adult 50–100 mg) at night.

Noradrenaline IV infsn: 0.05–0.5 mcg/kg/min.

Norethisterone Contraception: 350 mcg daily, starting 1st day of menstruation. Menorrhagia: 10 mg 3 H until bleeding stops, then 5 mg 6 H for 1 wk, then 5 mg 8 H for 2 wk.

Norethisterone + ethinyloestradiol (0.5 mg/35 mcg or 1 mg/35 mcg) × 21 tab, + 7 inert tab Contraception: 1 tab daily, starting 1st day of menstruation.

Norethisterone 1 mg + mestranol 50 mcg Contraception: 1 tab daily from 5th to 25th day of menstrual cycle.

Norethisterone 1 mg + oestradiol 2 mg Adult: 1 tab daily.

Norethisterone + oestradiol patches Adult (NOT/kg): 0 mg/4 mg (Estraderm 50) patch × 2/wk for 2 wk, then 30 mg/10 mg (Estragest 250/50) patch × 2/wk for 2 wk.

Norfloxacin 10 mg/kg/dose (adult 400 mg) 12 H oral.

Norgestimate 0.25 mg + ethinyloestradiol 0.035 mg + 7 inert tab Contraception: 1 tab daily, starting 1st day of menstruation.

Norgestrel See levonorgestrel.

Normacol granules 6 mo–5 yr half teasp 12 H, 6–10 yr 1 teasp 12 H, >10 yr 1 teasp 8 H.

Nortriptyline 0.5–1.5 mg/kg/dose (adult 25–75 mg) 8 H oral.

NTBC (nitro-trifluoromethylbenzoyl cyclohexanedione) 0.5 mg/kg/dose 12 H oral.

Nystatin 500,000 u (1 tab) 6–8 H NG or oral. Neonates: 100,000 u (1 mL) 8 H, prophylaxis 50,000 u (0.5 mL) 12 H. Topical: 100,000 u/g gel, cream or ointment 12 H. Vaginal: 100,000 u 12–24 H.

Oestradiol NOT/kg. Menopause: transdermal patch 3.8 mg, 5.7 mg or 7.6 mg (releases 50, 75 or 100 mcg/day) apply every 7 days (add progestogen for 14 days per month if uterus intact). Induction puberty: 0.5 mg alternate days oral, incr over 2–3 yr to 2 mg/day (add progestogen for 14 days per month when dose 1.5 mg/day or when bleeding occurs). Tall stature: 12 mg/day oral until bone age >16 yr (add progestogen for 14 days per cycle). Gonadal failure: 2 mg/day oral (add progestogen for 14 days per cycle).

Oestradiol 2 mg or 4 mg (× 12 tab), oestradiol 1 mg (× 6 tab), oestradiol 2 mg or 4 mg + norethisterone 1 mg (× 10 tab) 1 tab daily, starting 5th day of menstruation. Vaginal tab 25 mcg: 1 tab daily for 2 wk, then 1 tab × 2/wk. See also norethisterone + oestradiol.

Oestradiol 2 mg (× 11 tab), oestradiol 2 mg + cyproterone 1 mg (× 10 tab) 1 tab daily for 21 days (starting 5th day of menstruation), then 7 days with no tablet.

Oestradiol 2 mg + norethisterone 1 mg Adult 1 tab daily.

17-beta-Oestradiol 2 mg vaginal ring, replace every 3 mo.

Oestriol Inductn puberty: 0.25 mg/day incr to 2 mg/day (+ progestogen 12 days/cycle) oral. Epiphyseal maturtn: 10 mg/day (+ progestogen 12 days/cycle). Vaginal: 0.5 mg daily, reducing to × 2/wk. Patch (Menorest) 37.5 (3.28 mg), 50 (4.33 mg), 75 (6.57 mg), 100 (8.66 mg): apply 1 patch × 2/wk (adjust dose monthly), with medroxyprogesterone acetate (if uterus intact) 10 mg × 10 days/month.

Ofloxacin 5 mg/kg/dose (adult 200 mg) 8–12 H, or 10 mg/kg/dose (adult 400 mg) 12 H oral or IV over 1 hr. 0.3%: 1 drop/eye hrly for 2 days (4 H overnight), reducing to 3–6 H.

Omeprazole Usually 0.4–0.8 mg/kg/dose (adult 20–40 mg) 12–24 H oral. ZE synd: 1 mg/kg/dose (adult 60 mg) 12–24 H oral, incr up to 3 mg/kg (adult 120 mg) 8 H if reqd. IV: 2 mg/kg (max 80 mg) stat, then 1 mg/kg (max 40 mg) 8–12 H. *H. pylori*: 0.8 mg/kg/dose (adult 40 mg) daily oral with metronidazole 8 mg/kg/dose (adult 400 mg) 8 H + amoxycillin 10 mg/kg/dose (adult 500 mg) 8 H for 2 wk.

Ondansetron IV: prophylaxis 0.15 mg/kg (adult 4 mg); treatment 0.2 mg/kg (adult 8 mg) over 5 min, or 0.2–0.5 mcg/kg/min. Oral: 0.1–0.2 mg/kg/dose (usual max 8 mg) 6–12 H.

Oxacillin 15–30 mg/kg/dose 6 H oral, IV, IM. Severe inftn: 40 mg/kg/dose (max 2 g) 12 H (1st wk life), 8 H (2nd wk), 6 H or constant infsn (>2 wk).

Oxandrolone 0.1–0.2 mg/kg (adult 2.5–20 mg) daily oral. Turner's synd: 0.05–0.1 mg/kg daily.

Oxazepam 0.2–0.5 mg/kg/dose (adult 10–30 mg) 6–8 H oral.

Oxybutynin <5 yr: 0.2 mg/kg/dose 8–12 H oral. >5 yr (NOT/kg): 2.5–5 mg 8–12 H oral. Slow release: adult 5–30 mg daily oral.

Oxycodone 0.1–0.2 mg/kg/dose (adult 5–10 mg) 4–6 H oral, incr if reqd. Slow release: 0.6–0.9 mg/kg/dose (adult 10 mg) 12 H oral, incr if reqd. Suppos: adult 30 mg 6–8 H PR.

Oxymorphone Usually 0.02–0.03 mg/kg/dose (adult 1–1.5 mg) 4–6 H IM or SC. Slow IV: 0.01 mg/kg/dose (adult 0.5 mg) 4–6 H. PR: 0.1 mg/kg (adult 5 mg) 4–6 H.

Oxytetracycline >8 yr (NOT/kg): 250–500 mg/dose 6 H oral, or 250–500 mg/dose 6–12 H slow IV.

Oxytocin Labour (NOT/kg): 1–4 mU/min IV, may incr to 20 mU/min max. Lactation: 1 spray (4 IU) into each nostril 5 min before infant feeds.

Packed cells 4 mL/kg raises Hb 1 g%. 1 bag is about 300 mL.

Pamidronate Osteoporosis, OI: 3–7 mg/kg daily oral, 1.0 mg/kg/dose (adult 15–90 mg) IV over 4 hr daily × 3 every 4 mo, or once every 3–4 wk. Hypercalcaemia 20–50 mg/m^2 (depending on Ca level) IV over 4 hr every 4 wk.

Pancreatic enzymes With meals (NOT/kg): usually 1–3 Cotazyme-S Forte cap, 1–5 Pancrease cap oral. Max lipase 10,000 u/kg/day.

Pancuronium ICU: 0.1–0.15 mg/kg IV prn. Theatre: 0.1 mg/kg IV, then 0.02 mg/kg prn. Infsn: 0.25–0.75 mcg/kg/min.

Pantoprazole 1.0 mg/kg (adult 40 mg) 12–24 H oral, IV. GI haemorrhage, adult: 80 mg stat, then 8 mg/hr. ZE: 80 mg 8–12 H adjusted to achieve acid <10 mmol/L.

Papaveretum (Omnopon) 0.2 mg/kg/dose IV, 0.4 mg/kg/dose IM (half life 2–4 hr). ICU: 0.3 mg/kg/dose IV, 0.6 mg/kg/dose IM.

Papaveretum (20 mg/mL) + hyoscine (0.4 mg/mL) 0.4 mg/kg (P) + 0.008 mg/kg (H) = 0.02 mL/kg/dose IM.

Paracetamol Oral: 20 mg/kg stat, then 15 mg/kg/dose 4 H (max 4 g/day); child usual daily max 60 mg/kg (90 mg/kg short term). Rectal: 40 mg/kg stat, then 30 mg/kg/dose 6 H (max 5 g/day). Overdose: see acetylcysteine.

Paraffin Liquid: 1 mL/kg (adult 30–45 mL) daily oral. Liquid 50% + white soft 50%, ointment: apply 6–12 H.

Paraffin 65% + agar NOT/kg: 6 mo–2 yr 5 mL, 3–5 yr 5–10 mL, >5 yr 10 mL 8–24 H oral.

Paraffin, phenolphthalein and agar (Agarol) NOT/kg: 6 mo–2 yr 2.5 mL, 3–5 yr 2.5–5 mL, >5 yr 5 mL 8–24 H oral.

Paraldehyde IM: 0.2 mL/kg (adult 10 mL) stat, then 0.1 mL/kg/dose 4–6 H. IV: 0.2 mL/kg (adult 10 mL) over 15 min, then 0.02 mL/kg/hr (max 1.5 mL/hr). Rectal or NG: 0.3 mL/kg/dose (adult 5–10 mL) diluted 1:10.

Penicillamine (D-penicillamine) Arthritis: 1.5 mg/kg/dose (adult 125 mg) 12 H oral, incr over several months to max 3 mg/kg/dose (adult 375 mg) 6–8 H. Wilson's dis, lead poisoning: 5–7.5 mg/kg/dose (adult 250–500 mg) 6 H oral. Cystinuria: 7.5 mg/kg/dose (adult 250–1000 mg) 6 H oral, titrated to urine cystine <100–200 mg/day.

Penicillin, benzathine 1 mg = 1250 u. Usually 25 mg/kg (max 900 mg) IM once. Venereal disease: 40 mg/kg (max 1.8 g) IM once. Strep proph: 25 mg/kg (max 900 mg) IM 3–4 wkly, or 10 mg/kg IM 2 wkly.

Penicillin, benzathine + procaine 900 mg/300 mg in 2 mL: 0–2 yr half vial, 3 yr or more 1 vial IM once.

Penicillin, benzyl (penicillin G, crystalline) 1 mg = 1667 u. 30 mg/kg/dose 6 H. Severe inftn: 50 mg/kg/dose (max 2 g) IV 12 H (1st wk life), 6 H (2–4 wk), 4 H or constant infsn (>4 wk).

Penicillin, procaine 1 mg = 1000 u. 25–50 mg/kg (max 1.2–2.4 g) 12–24 H IM. Single dose: 100 mg/kg (max 4.8 g).

Penicillin V See phenoxymethylpenicillin.

Pentamidine isethionate 3–4 mg/kg (1.7–2.3 mg/kg base) IV over 2 hr or IM daily for 10–14 days (1 mg base = 1.5 mg mesylate = 1.74 mg isethionate). Neb: 600 mg/6 mL daily for 3 wk (treatment), 300 mg/3 mL every 4 wk (prophylaxis).

Pentastarch 10% soltn: 10–40 mg/kg IV.

Pentazocine Oral: 0.5–2.0 mg/kg/dose (adult 25–100 mg) 3–4 H. SC, IM or slow IV: 0.5–1 mg/kg/dose (adult 30–60 mg) 3–4 H. PR: 1 mg/kg/dose (adult 50 mg) 6–12 H.

Pentobarbital See pentobarbitone.

Pentobarbitone 0.5–1 mg/kg/dose (adult 30–60 mg) 6–8 H oral, IM, slow IV. Hypnotic: 2–4 mg/kg (adult 100–200 mg).

Permethrin 1% creme rinse (head lice): wash hair, apply creme for 10 min, wash off; may repeat in 2 wk. 5% cream (scabies): wash body, apply to whole body except face, wash off after 12–24 hr.

Pethidine 0.5–1 mg/kg/dose (adult 25–50 mg) IV, 0.5–2 mg/kg/dose (adult 25–100 mg) IM (half life 2–4 hr). Infsn: 5 mg/kg in 50 mL at 1–4 mL/hr (0.1–0.4 mg/kg/hr). PCA 5 mg/kg in 50 mL: Usually bolus 2 mL with lockout 5 min, optional background 0.5 mL/hr.

Pheniramine 0.5–1 mg/kg/dose (adult 25–50 mg) 6–8 H oral. Slow release tab 75 mg at night.

Phenobarbitone Loading dose in emergency: 20–30 mg/kg IM or IV over 30 min stat. Ventilated: repeat doses of 10–15 mg/kg up to 100 mg/kg per day (beware hypotension). Usual maintenance: 5 mg/kg (adult 300 mg) daily IV, IM or oral. Infant colic: 1 mg/kg/dose 4–8 H oral. Level 80–120 μmol/L (× 0.23 = mcg/mL) done Mo-Fr 1100 at RCH.

Phenoxybenzamine 0.2–0.5 mg/kg (adult 10–40 mg) 8–12 H oral. Cardiac surgery: 1 mg/kg IV over 1–4 hr stat, then 0.5 mg/kg/dose 8–12 H IV over 1 hr or oral.

Phenoxymethylpenicillin (penicillin V) 7.5–15 mg/kg/dose (adult 250–500 mg) 6 H oral. Proph: 12.5 mg/kg/dose (adult 250 mg) 12 H oral.

Phentolamine 0.1 mg/kg stat, then 5–50 mcg/kg/min IV.

Phenylephrine IV: 2–10 mcg/kg stat (adult 500 mcg), then 1–5 mcg/kg/min; for 65 kg adult 25 mg in 50 mL at 8 mL/hr is 1 mcg/kg/min. SC or IM: 0.1–0.2 mg/kg (max 10 mg). Oral: 0.2 mg/kg/dose (max 10 mg) 6–8 H. 0.15%, 10% eye drops: 1–2 drops/eye 6–8 H. 0.25%, 0.5% nose drops: 1–3 drops/sprays per nostril 6–8 H.

Phenyltoloxamine 1 mg/kg/dose (adult 50 mg) 8 H oral.

Phenytoin Loading dose in emergency: 15–20 mg/kg (max 1.5 g) IV over 1 hr. Initial maintenance, oral or IV: 2 mg/kg/dose 12 H (preterm); 3 mg/kg/dose 12 H (1st wk life), 8 H (2 wk–4 yr), 12 H (5–12 yr); 2 mg/kg/dose (usual max 100 mg) 8 H >12 yr. Level 40–80 μmol/L (× 0.25 = mcg/mL), done Mo, We and Fr at RCH.

Pholcodine 0.10.2 mg/kg/dose (adult 5–15 mg) 6–12 H oral.

Phosphate, potassium (1 mmol/mL) 0.1–1.5 mmol/kg/day (max 70 mmol/day) IV infsn.

Phosphate, sodium NOT/kg: 250 mg (<4 yr) 250–500 mg (>4 yr) 6 H oral.

Phosphate, sodium (Fleet enema) Na 1.61 mEq/L + PO_4 4.15 mEq/L + P 1.38 mEq/L: 33 mL (2–5 yr), 66 mL (5–11 yr), 133 mL (adult) rectal.

Physostigmine 0.02 mg/kg (max 1 mg) IV every 5 min until response (max 0.1 mg/kg), then 0.5–2.0 mcg/kg/min.

Phytomenadione (vitamin K1) Deficiency with haemorrhage: FFP 10 mL/kg, then 0.3 mg/kg (max 10 mg), IM or IV over 1 hr. Prophylaxis in neonates (NOT/kg): 1 mg (0.1 mL) IM at birth; or 2 mg (0.2 mL) oral at birth, at 3–5 days, and by 4 wk (give half dose if <1.5 kg). Warfarin reversal: 0.1 mg/kg (max 5 mg) SC or oral (repeat if reqd); if severe haemorrhage 0.3 mg/kg (max 10 mg) with FFP 10 mL/kg. Mitochondrial disease (NOT/kg): 10 mg/dose 6 H oral.

Pilocarpine 0.1 mg/kg/dose (adult 5 mg) 4–8 H oral. 0.5%, 1%, 2%, 3%, 4% eye drops: 1–2 drops 6–12 H.

Pimecrolimus 1% cream: apply 12 H.

Pimozide 0.04 mg/kg (adult 20 mg) daily oral, incr if reqd to max 0.4 mg/kg (adult 20 mg) daily.

Pine tar Gel, solution: 5 mL to baby bath, 15–30 mL to adult bath; soak for 10 min.

Piperacillin 50 mg/kg/dose (adult 2–3 g) 6–8 H IV. Severe inftn: 75 mg/kg/dose (adult 4 g) 8 H (1st wk life) 6 H (2–4 wk) 4–6 H (>4 wk) or constant infsn.

Piperacillin 1 g + tazobactam 125 mg Dose as for piperacillin.

Piperazine 75 mg/kg (max 4 g) oral daily for 2 days (ascaris), 7 days (pinworm).

Piroxicam 0.2–0.4 mg/kg (adult 10–20 mg) daily oral. Gel 5 mg/g: apply 1 g (3 cm) 6–8 H for up to 2 wk.

Pizotifen NOT/kg: 0.5 mg daily oral, incr if reqd to max 0.5 mg morning and 1 mg at night.

Platelets 10 mL/kg IV stat, then as reqd. 1 unit approx 60 mL.

Pneumococcal vaccine, polysaccharide (Pneumovax 23) Inactivtd. >2 yr: 0.5 mL SC or IM once. Boost every 5 yr.

Pneumococcal vaccine, CRM conjugate (Prevenar) Inactivated. 0.5 mL IM. <6 mo: 2 mo, 3 mo, 4 mo, 12–15 mo (4 doses). 6–11 mo: 6 mo, 7 mo, 12–15 mo (3 doses). 12–23 mo: 2 doses 2 mo apart. >23 mo 1 dose.

Podophyllotoxin 0.5% paint: apply 12 H for 3 days, then none for 4 days; 4 wk course.

Poliomyelitis vaccine, oral (Sabin) Live. 2 drops oral at 2 mo, 4 mo and 6 mo (3 doses). Boost at 5 yr, and if going to epidemic area.

Poliomyelitis vaccine, SC (IPOL) Inactivated. 0.5 mL SC stat, 8 wk later, and 8 wk later (3 doses). Boost 12 mo later, and at school entry.

Poloxamer 10% soltn 8 H oral: <6 mo 10 drops/dose, 6–18 mo 15 drops/dose, 18 mo–3 yr 25 drops/dose.

Poractant alfa (porcine surfactant, Curosurf) Intratracheal: 200 mg/kg stat, then up to 4 doses of 100 mg/kg 12 H if required.

Potassium Deficiency: usually 0.3 mmol/kg/hr (max 0.4 mmol/kg/hr) for 4–6 hr IV, then 4 mmol/kg/day. Max oral 1 mmol/kg/dose (<5 yr), 0.5 mmol/kg/dose (>5 yr). Maintenance 2–4 mmol/kg/day. 1 g KCl = 13.3 mmol K, 7.5% KCl = 1 mmol/mL.

Potassium guaiacolsulphonate 1–3 mg/kg/dose (adult 50–160 mg) 4–6 H oral.

Povidone-iodine Cream, oint, paint, soltn: apply 6–12 H.

Praziquantel 20 mg/kg/dose oral once (tapeworm), 4 H × 3 doses (schistosomiasis), 8 H × 6 doses (other flukes), 8 H 14 days (cysticercosis).

Prazosin 5 mcg/kg (max 0.25 mg) test dose, then 0.025–0.1 mg/kg/dose (adult 1–5 mg) 6–12 H oral.

Prednisolone Oral. Alopecia, autoimm liver, Crohn's, epilepsy, SLE, ulcerative col: 2 mg/kg daily, gradually reducing. Asthma: 0.5–1 mg/kg/dose 6 H for 24 hr, 12 H for the next 24 hr, then 1 mg/kg daily. Croup: 1 mg/kg stat and in 12 hr; severe 4 mg/kg stat, then 1 mg/kg/dose 8–12 H. ITP: 4 mg/kg daily. Nephrotic: 60 mg/m^2 (max 80 mg) daily, reducing over several months. Physiological: 4–5 mg/m^2 daily. Prednisolone 1 mg = hydrocortisone 0.8 mg in mineralocorticoid action, 4 mg in glucocorticoid. See also methylprednisolone.

Prednisolone acetate 1% + phenylephrine 0.12% 1–2 drops/eye 6–12 H.

Prednisolone sodium phosphate 0.5% ear/eye drops: 1–3 drops 2–6 H.

Prednisone Action equivalent to prednisolone.

Primaquine Usually 0.3 mg/kg (adult 15 mg) daily for 14–21 days oral. Gameteocyte: 0.7 mg/kg (adult 45 mg) once.

Primidone Initially 2.5 mg/kg (adult 125 mg) at night, incr if reqd to max 15 mg/kg/dose (adult 750 mg) 12 H oral. Trough level (phenobarbitone) 60–120 μmol/L.

Probenicid 25 mg/kg (adult 1 g) stat, then 10 mg/kg/dose (adult 500 mg) 6 H oral.

Probucol 10 mg/kg/dose (adult 500 mg) 12 H oral.

Procainamide IV: 0.4 mg/kg/min (adult 20 mg/min) for max 25 min, then 20–80 mcg/kg/min (max 2 g/day). Oral: 5–8 mg/kg/dose 4 H. Level 3–10 mcg/mL.

Procaine Max dose 20 mg/kg (1 mL/kg of 2%).

Prochlorperazine 1 mg base = approx 1.5 mg edisylate, maleate or mesylate. Only use if >10 kg. Oral (salt): 0.2 mg/kg/dose (adult 5–10 mg) 6–8 H, slow incr if reqd to max 0.6 mg/kg/dose (max 35 mg) 6 H in psychosis. IM, slow IV (salt): 0.2 mg/kg (adult 12.5 mg) 8–12 H. Buccal (salt): 0.05–0.1 mg/kg (max 6 mg) 12–24 H. PR (base): 0.2 mg/kg (adult 25 mg) 8–12 H.

Progesterone Adult (NOT/kg). Premenst syn: 200–400 mg/dose PV or PR 12–24 H (last half of cycle). Dysfunctional uterine haemorrhage: 5–10 mg/day IM for 5–10 days before menses. Prevent abrtn: 25–100 mg IM every 2–4 days.

Promazine Oral: 2–4 mg/kg/dose (adult 100–200 mg) 6 H. IM 0.7 mg/kg/dose (max 50 mg) 6–8 H.

Promethazine Antihist, antiemetic: 0.2–0.5 mg/kg/dose (adult 10–25 mg) 6–8 H IV, IM or oral. Sedative, hypnotic: 0.5–1.5 mg/kg/dose (adult 25–100 mg).

Proxymetacaine 0.5%: 1–2 drops/eye before procedure.

Propafenone Oral: 3–5 mg/kg/dose (adult 150–300 mg) 8 H. IV: 1–2 mg/kg over 15 min, then 10–20 mcg/kg/min.

Propantheline bromide 0.3–0.6 mg/kg/dose (adult 15–30 mg) 6 H oral.

Propiverine 0.3 mg/kg/dose (adult 15 mg) 6–12 H oral.

Propofol Child: 2.5–3.5 mg/kg stat, then 7.5–15 mg/kg/hr IV. Adult: 1–2.5 mg/kg stat, then 3–12 mg/kg/hr IV.

Propoxyphene See dextropropoxyphene.

Propranolol IV: 0.02 mg/kg (adult 1 mg) test dose then 0.1 mg/kg (adult 5 mg) over 10 min (repeat × 13 prn), then 0.1–0.3 mg/kg/dose (adult 5–15 mg) 3 H. Oral: 0.2–0.5 mg/kg/dose (adult 10–25 mg) 6–12 H, slow incr to max 1.5 mg/kg/dose (max 80 mg) 6–12 H if required.

Propylthiouracil 50 mg/m^2/dose 8 H oral, reduce according to response.

Protamine IV 1 mg/100 u heparin (0.5 mg/100 u if >1 hr since heparin dose) slow IV stat; subsequent doses of protamine 1 mg/kg (max 50 mg). 1 mg per 25 mL pump blood. Heparin 1 mg = 100 u (half life 1–2 hr).

Prothrombinex See coagulation factor, human.

Pseudoephedrine 1 mg/kg/dose (adult 60 mg) 6–8 H oral. Slow release: adult (NOT/kg) 120 mg/dose 12 H.

Pumactant (ALEC) Preterm babies (NOT/kg): disconnect ETT, rapidly inject 100 mg in 1 mL saline via catheter at lower end ETT, flush with 2 mL air; repeat after 1 hr and 24 hr. Prophylaxis if unintubated: 100 mg into pharynx.

Pyrantel Threadworm: 10 mg/kg (adult 750 mg) once oral, may repeat 2 wkly × 3 doses. Roundworm, hookworm: 20 mg/kg (adult 1 g) once, may repeat in 7 days. Necator: 20 mg/kg (adult 1 g) daily × 23 doses.

Pyrazinamide 20–35 mg/kg (max 1.5 g) daily oral, or 75 mg/kg (max 3 g) × 2/wk.

Pyridostigmine Myas gravis: 5–7 mg/kg/dose (usual max 200 mg) 4–6 H oral. 180 mg slow release tab (Timespan), adult (NOT/kg): 1–3 tabs 12–24 H. 1 mg IV, IM or SC = 30 mg oral.

Pyridoxine With isoniazid or penicillamine (NOT/kg): 5–10 mg daily IV or oral. Fitting: 10–15 mg/kg daily IV or oral. Siderobl anaem: 2–8 mg/kg (max 400 mg) daily IV or oral.

Pyrimethamine 12.5 mg and dapsone 100 mg (Maloprim) 1–4 yr quarter tab wkly, 5–10 yr half tab, >10 yr 1 tab.

Pyrimethamine 25 mg and sulphadoxine 500 mg (Fansidar) <4 yr half tab once, 4–8 yr 1 tab, 9–14 yr 2 tabs, >14 yr 3 tabs. Prophylaxis: <4 yr quarter tab wkly, 4–8 yr half tab, 9–14 yr three-quarter tab, >14 yr 1 tab.

Quinidine, base 10 mg/kg stat, then 5 mg/kg/dose (max 333 mg) 4–6 H oral. IV: 6.3 mg/kg (10 mg/kg of gluconate) over 2 hr, then 0.0125 mg/kg/min. IM: 15 mg/kg stat, then 7.5 mg/kg/dose (max 400 mg) 8 H. NOTE: 1 mg base = 1.2 mg sulphate = 1.3 mg bisulphate = 1.6 mg gluconate.

Quinine, base Oral: 8.3 mg/kg/dose (max 500 mg) 8 H for 7–10 days. Parenteral: 16.7 mg/kg (20 mg/kg of dihydrochloride) IV over 4 hr or IM, then 8.3 mg/kg/dose 8 H IV over 2 hr or IM for 2–3 days, then 8.3 mg/kg/dose 8 H oral for 5 days. NOTE: 1 mg base = 1.7 mg bisulphate = 1.2 mg dihydrochloride = 1.2 mg ethyl carbonate = 1.3 mg hydrobromide = 1.2 mg hydrochloride = 1.2 mg sulphate.

Ramipril 0.05 mg/kg (adult 2.5 mg) oral daily, may incr over 4–6 wk to 0.1–0.2 mg/kg (adult 5–10 mg) daily.

Ranitidine IV: 1 mg/kg/dose (adult 50 mg) slowly 6–8 H, or 2 mcg/kg/min. Oral: 2–4 mg/kg/dose (adult 150 mg) 8–12 H, or 300 mg (adult) at night.

Ranitidine bismuth citrate 8 mg/kg/dose (adult 400 mg) 12 H oral; to eradicate *H. pylori*, add an antibiotic.

Reserpine 0.005–0.01 mg/kg/dose (adult 0.25–0.5 mg) 12–24 H oral.

Ribavirin Inhltn (Viratek nebulizer): 20 mg/mL at 25 mL/hr (190 mcg/L of gas) for 12–18 hr/day for 3–7 days. Oral: 5–15 mg/kg/dose 8–12 H. Hepatitis C: see interferon alfa-2b.

Riboflavine NOT/kg: 5–10 mg daily oral. Organic acidosis (NOT/kg): 50–200 mg daily oral, IM or IV.

Rifampicin 10–15 mg/kg (max 600 mg) daily oral fasting, or IV over 3 hr (monitor AST). Prophylaxis: *N. meningitidis* 10 mg/kg daily (neonate), 10 mg/kg (max 600 mg) 12 H for 2 days; *H. influenzae* 10 mg/kg daily (neonate), 20 mg/kg (max 600 mg) daily for 4 days.

Risedronate Osteoporosis: 0.1 mg/kg (adult 5 mg) daily oral; slow release 0.7 mg/kg (adult 35 mg) weekly. Paget's: 0.5 mg/kg (adult 30 mg) daily oral.

Risperidone 0.02 mg/kg/dose (adult 1 mg) 12 H, incr if reqd to 0.15 mg/kg/dose (adult 2–4 mg, max 8 mg) 12 H oral.

Rituximab 370 mg/m^2 by IV infsn wkly × 4.

Rofecoxib 0.25–0.5 mg/kg/dose (adult 12.5–25 mg) daily oral.

Ropivacaine 4–5 mg/kg (adult max 200–250 mg). Postop infusion 0.2–0.4 mg/kg/hr (adult 12–20 mg/hr).

Roxithromycin 2.5–4 mg/kg/dose (adult 150 mg) 12 H oral.

Rubella vaccine (Ervevax, Meruvax II) Live >12 mo: 0.5 mL SC once. See also measles + mumps + rubella vaccine.

Salbutamol 0.1–0.15 mg/kg/dose (adult 2–4 mg) 6 H oral. Inhaltn: mild resp soltn (5 mg/mL, 0.5%) 0.5 mL/dose diluted to 4 mL, or nebule 2.5 mg/2.5 mL 3–6 H; moderate 0.5% soltn 1 mL/dose diluted to 4 mL, or nebule 5 mg/2.5 mL 1–2 H; severe (in ICU) 0.5% soltn undiluted continuous. Aerosol 100 mcg/puff: 1–2 puff 4–6 H. Rotahaler: 200–400 mcg 6–8 H. IM or SC: 10–20 mcg/kg/dose (adult 500 mcg) 3–6 H. IV: child 5–10 mcg/kg/min for 1 hr, then 1–2 mcg/kg/min (1 mcg/kg/min using 1 mg/mL soltn = 0.06 × Wt mL/hr).

Salicylic acid Cradle cap: 6% soltn (Egocappol) 12 H 3–5 days. Plantar warts: 15% soltn × 1–2/day, 40% medicated disc 24–48 H.

Salmeterol Aerosol, diskhaler (NOT/kg): 50–100 mcg 12 H. See also fluticasone + salmeterol.

Selenium sulphide 2.5% shampoo × 2/wk for 2 wk.

Sennoside Tab 7.5 mg daily (NOT/kg): 6 mo–2 yr half–1 tab, 3–10 yr 1–2 tabs, >10 yr 2–4 tabs. Granules 2–2.5 mg/teasp, 12–24 H (NOT/kg): <6 mo quarter–half teasp, 6 mo–2 yr half–1 teasp, 3–10 yr 1–2 teasp.

Simvastatin Initially 0.2 mg/kg (adult 10 mg) daily, may incr every 4 wk to max 1 mg/kg (adult 40 mg) daily oral.

Sodium Deficit: to increase serum Na by 0.5 mmol/L/hr (maximum safe rate), infusion rate (mL/hr) = 2 × Wt (kg)/(% saline infused); number of hours of infusion = (140 – serum Na)/8. 4 mL/kg of *x*% saline raises serum Na by *x* mmol/L. Need 2–6 mmol/kg/day. NaCl M.W. = 58.45, 1 g NaCl = 17.1 mmol Na, NaCl 20% = 3.4 mmol/mL.

Sodium cromoglycate Inhalation (Intal): 1 cap (20 mg) 6–8 H, 2 mL soltn (20 mg) 6–8 H, aerosol 1–10 mg 6–8 H. Eye drops (2%): 1–2 drops per eye 4–6 H. Oral: 5–10 mg/kg/dose (max 200 mg) 6 H oral. Nasal (Rynacrom): insufflator 5 mg in each nostril 6 H, spray 1 puff in each nostril 6 H.

Sodium ferric gluconate Fe 12.5 mg/mL. 0.05 mL/kg (adult 2 mL) test dose IV over 1 hr, then 0.25 mL/kg (adult 10 mL) IV over 1 hr with each dialysis (usually for 8 doses).

Sodium nitroprusside IV infsn 0.5–10 mcg/kg/min: for 65 kg adult 50 mg in 50 mL at 2 mL/hr is 0.5 mcg/kg/min. If used for >24 hr, max rate 4 mcg/kg/min. Max total 70 mg/kg with normal renal function (or sodium thiocyanate <1725 μmol/L, × 0.058 = mg/L). Pul vasodil: 2 mcg/kg/min nitropr = 5 mcg/kg/min nitroglyc = 0.1 mcg/kg/min PGE1 approx.

Sodium polystyrene sulphonate (Resonium) 0.3–1 g/kg/dose (adult 15–30 g) 6 H NG (give lactulose) or PR.

Sodium valproate 5 mg/kg/dose (adult 200 mg) 8–12 H oral, incr if reqd to max 20 mg/kg/dose (adult 1 g) 8–12 H. Level 2 hr after dose 300–700 μmol/L (× 0.14 = mg/L).

Sorbitol 70% 0.2–0.5 mL/kg/dose (adult 20–30 mL) 8–24 H oral. With activated charcoal: 1 g/kg (1.4 mL/kg) NG, × 12.

Sorbolene cream; pure, with 10% glycerin, or with 5% or 10% olive oil or peanut oil Skin moisturiser: apply prn.

Sotalol IV: 0.5–2 mg/kg/dose (adult 25–120 mg) over 10 min 6 H. Oral: 1–4 mg/kg/dose (adult 50–160 mg) 8–12 H.

Spironolactone Oral (NOT/kg): 0–10 kg 6.25 mg/dose 12 H, 11–20 kg 12.5 mg/dose 12 H, 21–40 kg 25 mg/dose 12 H, over 40 kg 25 mg/dose 8 H. Female hirsutism 50 mg/dose 8 H. IV: see potassium canrenoate.

Streptokinase (SK) Short term (myoc infarct): 30,000 u/kg (max 1,500,000 u) IV over 60 min, repeat if occlusion recurs <5 days. Long term (DVT, pul emb, art thrombosis): 2000 u/kg (max 100,000 u) IV over 10 min, then 1000 u/kg/hr (max 100,000 u/hr); stop heparin and aspirin, if PTT <× 2 normal at 4 hr give extra 10,000 u/kg (max 500,000 u) IV over 30 min, stop SK if PTT >× 5 normal then give 1000 u/kg/hr. Local infsn: 50 u/kg/hr (continue heparin 10–15 u/kg/hr). Blocked IV cannula: 5000 u/kg in 2 mL in cannula for 2 hr then remove, may repeat × 2.

Streptomycin 20–30 mg/kg (max 1 g) IM daily.

Sucralfate 1 g tab (NOT/kg): 0–2 yr quarter tab 6 H, 3–12 yr half tab 6 H, >12 yr 1 tab 6 H oral.

Sulfadiazine 50 mg/kg/dose (max 2 g) 6 H slow IV.

Sulindac 4 mg/kg/dose (adult 200 mg) 12 H oral.

Sulphasalazine Active colitis: 20 mg/kg/dose 6–12 H (max 4 g/day) oral; remission 7.5 mg/kg/dose (max 0.5 g) 6–8 H, suppos (NOT/kg) adult 0.5–1 g 12 H. Arthritis: 5 mg/kg/dose 12 H, incr if reqd to 10 mg/kg/dose 8–12 H (max 2 g/day).

Sumatriptan Oral: 1–2 mg/kg (adult 50–100 mg) stat, may repeat twice. SC: 0.12 mg/kg (max 6 mg) stat, may repeat once after 1 hr. Nasal: 10–20 mg, may repeat × 1 after 2 hr.

Surfactant See beractant (Survanta), calfactant (Infasurf), colfosceril palmitate (Exosurf), poractant alfa (Curosurf), pumactant (ALEC).

Suxamethonium IV: neonate 3 mg/kg/dose, child 2 mg/kg/dose, adult 1 mg/kg/dose. IM: double IV dose.

Tacrolimus IV infsn: 2 mg/m^2/day. Oral: 3 mg/m^2/dose 12 H. Trough level: whole blood 10–15 ng/mL (sent to Austin daily at 1000 from RCH).

Tacrolimus ointment 2–16 yr: apply 0.03% sparingly 12 H for max 3 wk, then daily. >16 yr: apply 0.1% sparingly 12 H for max 3 wk, then 0.03% 12 H.

Tamoxifen Adult (NOT/kg): 20 mg daily, incr to 40 mg daily if no response after 1 mo.

Teicoplanin 250 mg/m^2 IV over 30 min stat, then 125 mg/m^2 IV or IM daily. Severe inftn: 250 mg/m^2 12 H × 3 doses, then 250 mg/m^2 IV or IM daily.

Temazepam 0.3 mg/kg (adult 20–40 mg) oral.

Terbinafine 62.5 mg (<20 kg), 125 mg (20–40 kg), 250 mg (adult) daily oral. 1% cream, gel: apply 12–24 H to dry skin.

Terbutaline Oral: 0.05–0.1 mg/kg/dose (adult 2.5–5 mg) 6 H. SC: 5–10 mcg/kg/dose (adult 0.25–0.5 mg). IV: child 3–6 mcg/kg/min for 1 hr, then 0.4–1 mcg/kg/min; adult 0.25 mg stat over 10 min, then 1–10 mcg/kg/hr. Inhaltn: mild resp soltn (1%, 10 mg/mL) 0.25 mL/dose diluted to 4 mL 3–6 H; moderate 0.5 mL of 1% diluted to 4 mL, or respule 5 mg/2 mL 1–2 H; severe (in ICU) undiluted continuous. Aerosol 250 mcg/puff: 1–2 puffs 4–6 H.

Terfenadine 30 mg (6–12 yr), 60 mg (adult) 12 H oral.

Testosterone Esters (NOT/kg): 100–500 mg IM every 2–4 wk. Implant: 8 mg/kg (to nearest 100 mg) every 16–24 wk. Undecanoate (NOT/kg): 40 mg daily oral, incr to 80–120 mg daily. Testosterone level: <16 yr 5–10 nmol/L, >16 yr 10–30 nmol/L.

Tetanus toxoid (Tet-Tox) 0.5 mL IM stat, 6 wk later, and 6 mo later. Boost every 10 yr, or if contaminated wound. See also diphtheria (+ pertussis) + tetanus vaccines.

Tetracycline >8 yr (NOT/kg): 250–500 mg/dose 6 H oral. Acne (NOT/kg): 500 mg/dose 12 H, reducing to 250 mg 12 H. Eye: apply 2–8 H. See also rolitetracycline.

Theophylline 80 mg theophylline = 100 mg aminophylline. Loading dose: 8 mg/kg (max 500 mg) oral. Maintenance: 1st wk life 2 mg/kg/dose 12 H; 2nd wk 3 mg/kg/dose 12 H; 3 wk–12 mo (0.1 × age in wk) + 3 mg/kg/dose 8 H; 1–9 yr 4 mg/kg/dose 4–6 H, or 10 mg/kg/dose slow rel 12 H; 10–16 yr or adult smoker 3 mg/kg/dose 4–6 H, or 7 mg/kg/dose 12 H slow rel; adult non-smoker 3 mg/kg/dose 6–8 H; elderly 2 mg/kg/dose 6–8 H. Serum level: neonate 60–80 μmol/L, asthma 60–110 (× 0.18 = mcg/mL), done as reqd at RCH.

Thiabendazole 25 mg/kg/dose (max 1.5 g) 12 H oral 3 days.

Thiopentone 2–5 mg/kg slowly stat (beware hypotension), then 1–5 mg/kg/hr IV. Level 150–200 μmol/L (× 0.24 = mcg/mL).

Thrombin glue 10,000 u thrombin in 9 mL mixed with 1 mL 10% calcium chloride in syringe 1, 10 mL cryoprecipitate in syringe 2: apply to bleeding sites together. Do not inject.

Thrombin, topical 100–2000 u/mL onto bleeding surface.

Thymidine 75 g/m^2 every 4–6 wk IV over 24 hr.

Thyroxine 50 mcg tab. 100 mcg/m^2 rounded to nearest quarter tab (adult 100–200 mcg) daily oral.

Ticarcillin 50 mg/kg/dose (adult 3 g) IV 6–8 H (1st wk life), 4–6 H or constant infsn (2+ wk). Cystic fibrosis: 100 mg/kg (max 6 g) 8 H IV.

Ticarcillin + clavulanic acid Dose as for ticarcillin.

Tilactase 200 u/drop: 5–15 drops/L added to milk 24 hr before use. 3300 u/tab: 1–3 tabs with meals oral.

Timolol 0.1 mg/kg/dose (adult 5 mg) 8–12 H, incr to max 0.3 mg/kg/dose (adult 15 mg) 8 H. Eye drops (0.25%, 0.5%): 1 drop/eye 12–24 H; see also latanoprost.

Tinidazole *Giardia*: 50 mg/kg (adult 2 g) stat, repeat after 48 hr. Amoebic dys: 50 mg/kg (adult 2 g) daily for 3 days.

Tobramycin Single daily dose IV or IM. Neonate: 5 mg/kg stat, then 2.5 mg/kg (<30 wk) 3.5 mg/kg (30–35 wk) 5 mg/kg (term <1 wk) daily. 1 wk–10 yr: 8 mg/kg day 1, then 6 mg/kg daily. >10 yr: 7 mg/kg day 1, then 5 mg/kg daily (max 240–360 mg) daily. Inhaltn: 80 mg diluted to 4 mL 12 H; or TOBI 300 mg 12 H alternate months. Eye: 1 drop or 1 cm cream 4 H. Trough level <1.0 mg/L, done daily 1000, 1600 RCH.

Tolazoline Newborn: 1–2 mg/kg slowly stat (beware hypotension), then 2–6 mcg/kg/min (0.12–0.36 mg/kg/hr) IV. Note: 1–2 mg/kg/hr too much (*Pediatrics* 1986; 77: 307).

Tolbutamide Adult (NOT/kg): initially 1 g 12 H oral, often reducing to 0.5–1 g daily.

Topiramate 1 mg/kg/dose (adult 50 mg) 12–24 H oral, incr gradually to 4–10 mg/kg/dose (adult 100–500 mg) 12 H.

Tramadol Oral: 1–2 mg/kg/dose (adult 50–100 mg) 4–6 H (max 400 mg/day). IV over 3 min, IM: 1–2 mg/kg/dose (adult 50–100 mg) 4–6 H (max 600 mg/day), or 2–8 mcg/kg/min IV.

Tranexamic acid Oral: 15–25 mg/kg/dose (adult 1–1.5 g) 8 H. IV: 10–15 mg/kg/dose (adult 0.5–1 g) 8 H.

Triamcinolone Joint, tendon (NOT/kg): 2.5–15 mg stat. IM: 0.05–0.2 mg/kg every 1–7 days. Cream or ointment 0.02%, 0.05%: apply sparingly 6–8 H. Triamcinolone has no mineralcorticoid action, 1 mg = 5 mg hydrocortisone in glucocorticoid action.

Triamcinolone 0.1% + neomycin 0.25% + gramicidin 0.025% + nystatin 100,000 u/g Kenacomb ointment: apply 8–12 H. Kenacomb otic oint, drops: apply 8–12 H (2–3 drops).

Triazolam 0.005–0.01 mg/kg (adult 0.125–0.5 mg) at night oral. 30 min preop: 0.01–0.03 mg/kg (adult 0.5 mg) oral.

Trifluoperazine 0.02–0.4 mg/kg/dose (adult 1–10 mg, occasionally 20 mg) 12 H oral. Capsule: adult 15 mg daily.

Trimethoprim 3–4 mg/kg/dose (usual max 150 mg) 12 H, or 6–8 mg/kg (usual max 300 mg) daily oral or IV. Urine prophylaxis: 1–2 mg/kg (adult 150 mg) at night oral.

Trimethoprim-sulphamethoxazole See cotrimoxazole.

Trometamol (THAM) mL of 0.3 molar (18 g/500 mL) soltn = Wt × BE (give half this) IV over 30–60 min.

Typhoid vaccine, oral (Typh-Vax) Live. 1 cap oral days 1, 3, 5 and (for better immunity) 7. Boost yearly.

Typhoid vaccine, parenteral, polysaccharide (Typherix, Typhim Vi) Inactivated. >5 yr: 0.5 mL IM once. Boost 3 yrly.

Urea 10% cream: apply 8–12 H.

Urofollitrophin See follicle stimulating hormone.

Urokinase 4000 u/kg IV over 10 min, then 4000 u/kg/hr for 12 hr (start heparin 3–4 hr later). Blocked cannula: instil 5000–25000 u (NOT/kg) in 2–3 mL saline for 2–4 hr. Empyema: 2 mL/kg of 1500 u/mL in saline, position head up/down and right side up/down 30 min each, then drain. Pericard eff: 10,000 u/mL, 1 mL/kg (max 20 mL), clamp 1 hr, drain.

Ursodeoxycholic acid 5–10 mg/kg/dose (adult 200–400 mg) 12 H oral.

Vancomycin 10 mg/kg/dose (adult 500 mg) 6 H IV over 1 hr, or 1 g/dose 12 H in adult IV over 2 hr. Newborn (any gestation): 10 mg/kg/dose 8 H IV over 1 hr. Oral: 10 mg/kg/dose to nearest 125 mg (adult 500 mg) 6 H. Intraventric (NOT/kg): 10 mg/dose 48 H. Trough 5–15 mg/L (peak 25–40 mg/L), done Mo-Fri 1000, 1600, 2200 at RCH.

Varicella vaccine (Varilix, Varivax) Live. 9 mo-12 yr: 0.5 mL SC once. >12 yr: 0.5 mL SC stat, and 4–8 wk later.

Vasopressin, aqueous IM, SC: 2.5–10 u 6–12 H. IV: put 2–5 u in 1L fluid, and replace Urine output + 10%. Brain death: 0.0003 u/kg/min (1 u/kg in 50 mL at 1 mL/hr) + adrenaline 0.1–0.2 mcg/kg/min. GI hge: 6 u/kg in 50 mL at 1–5 mL/hr IV, 1 mL/hr local IA. See desmopressin and lypressin.

Vasopressin, oily 2.5–5 u (NOT/kg) IM every 2–4 days.

Verapamil IV: 0.1–0.2 mg/kg (adult 5–10 mg) over 10 min, then 5 mcg/kg/min. Oral: 1–3 mg/kg/dose (adult 80–120 mg) 8–12 H.

Vigabatrin 40 mg/kg (adult 1 g) daily oral, incr if reqd to 80–150 mg/kg (max 4 g) daily (given in 1–2 doses).

Vitamin A High risk (NOT/kg): 100,000 IU (<8 kg), 200,000 IU (>8 kg) oral or IM every 4–6 mo. Severe measles: 400,000 IU (NOT/kg) once. Cystic fib: 1500 u daily (<3 yr) 5000 u daily (3–10 yr) 10,000 u daily (>10 yr) oral. >10,000 IU daily or >25,000 u per wk may be teratogenic.

Vitamin A, B, C, D compound (Pentavite, infant) <3 yr (NOT/kg): 0.15 mL daily, incr by 0.15 mL/day to 0.45 mL/day.

Vitamin A, B, C, D compound (Pentavite, child) <3 yr (NOT/kg): 2.5 mL daily. >3 yr (NOT/kg): 5 mL daily.

Vitamin B group Amp: IV over 30 min. Tab: 1–2/day.

Vitamin D2 (ergocalciferol) 40 u = 1 mcg = 1 mcg cholecalciferol (D3). Cystic fib, cholestasis: 10–20 mcg daily oral. Cirrhosis: adult 40–120 mcg daily oral. Deficiency: 50–100 mcg daily for 2 wk oral, then 10–625 mcg daily (more if severe malabs); or 100,000–200,000 u every 6–8 wk. Measure level after 6–8 wk. See also doxercalciferol.

Vitamin D3 (cholecalciferol) 1 mcg = 1 mcg D2. Osteodystrophy: 0.2 mcg/kg (hepatic) 15–40 mcg/kg (renal) daily oral.

Vitamin E 1 u = 1 mg. Preterm babies, Coperol E (NOT/kg): 40 u (2 drops) daily oral. CF, malabs: 50–100 u (<3 yr) 200–400 u (>3 yr) daily oral. Cholestasis: 50 u/kg daily oral, incr if reqd in 50 u/kg increments. A-beta-lipoproteinaemia: 35–70 u/kg/dose 8 H oral. HUS: 0.25 g/m^2/dose 6 H oral. See also alpha-tocopheryl.

Vitamins, parenteral MVI-12 (for adult): 5 mL in 1 litre IV fluid. MVI Paediatric, added to IV fluid: 65% of a vial (<3 kg), 1 vial (3 kg to 11 yr).

Vitaprem (RCH: Pentavite, folate, B12, C) 1 mL daily oral.

Warfarin Usually 0.2 mg/kg (adult 5 mg) stat, 0.2 mg/kg (adult 5 mg) next day providing INR <1.3, then 0.05–0.2 mg/kg (adult 2–5 mg) daily oral. INR usually 2–2.5 for prophylaxis, 2–3 for treatment. Beware drug interactions.

Whole blood 6 mL/kg raises Hb 1 g%. 1bag = 400 mL approx.

Xylometazoline <6 yr: 0.05% 1 drop or spray 8–12 H. 6–12 yr: 0.05% 2–3 drops or sprays 8–12 H. >12 yr: 0.1% 2–3 drops or sprays 6–12 H.

Yellow fever vaccine (Stamaril) Live. >12 mo: 0.5 mL SC once. Boost every 10 yr.

Zidovudine (AZT) Preterm: 1.5 mg/kg/dose 12 H to 2 wk, then 2 mg/kg/dose 8 H. Term newborn: 2 mg/kg/dose 6 H oral, 1.5 mg/kg/dose 6 H IV. Child: usually 160 mg/m^2/dose 8 H oral, 120 mg/m^2/dose 6 H IV, or 20 mg/m^2/hr IV; range 90–180 mg/m^2/dose 6–8 H. Adult (NOT/kg): usually 200 mg/dose 8 H oral, or 150 mg/dose 8 H IV.

Zinc sulphate (220 mg cap = 50 mg Zn = 765 µmol Zn). Deficiency, acroderm enteropath: initially 3 mg/kg/dose (adult 220 mg) 8–12 H oral, adjusted to achieve serum zinc 11–22 µmol/L (0.7–1.4 mg/L). Diarrhoea child (NOT/kg): 10–20 mg daily oral.

ANTIMICROBIAL GUIDELINES

Nigel Curtis, Mike Starr and Mike South

CENTRAL NERVOUS SYSTEM / EYE

Infection	*Likely organisms*	***Initial antimicrobials***[1] ***( ) = maximum dose***	***Duration of treatment***[2] ***and other comments***
Brain abscess	*S. milleri* and other streptococci Anaerobes Gram-negatives *S. aureus*	Flucloxacillin 50 mg/kg (2 g) iv 4H ***and*** Cefotaxime 50 mg/kg (2 g) iv 6H ***and*** Metronidazole 15 mg/kg (1 g) iv stat, then 7.5 mg/kg (500 mg) iv 8H	3 weeks minimum Penicillin hypersensitivity: substitute Flucloxacillin with Vancomycin 15 mg/kg (500 mg) iv 6H
. . . post neurosurgery	As above plus *S. epidermidis*	As above but substitute Flucloxacillin with Vancomycin 15 mg/kg (500 mg) iv 6H	
Encephalitis SA $(m^2) = \sqrt{\frac{ht(cm) \times wt(kg)}{3600}}$	Herpes simplex virus Enteroviruses Arboviruses *M. pneumoniae*	Aciclovir 20 mg/kg iv 8H [age < 3 months] 500 mg/m[2] iv 8H [age 3 months–12 yrs] 10 mg/kg iv 8H [age > 12 yrs]	3 weeks minimum Consider macrolide antibiotic if *M. pneumoniae* suspected
Meningitis			
. . . over 2 months of age	*S. pneumoniae*[3] *N. meningitidis* *H. influenzae* type b[4]	Cefotaxime 50 mg/kg (2 g) iv 6H	*S. pneumoniae* 10 days *N. meningitidis* 5–7 days *H. influenzae* type b 7–10 days
. . . over 2 months of age and possibility of penicillin-resistant pneumococci[3] **(www.snipurl.com/vanco)**	As above	Cefotaxime 50 mg/kg (2 g) iv 6H ***and*** Vancomycin 15 mg/kg (500 mg) iv 6H	Penicillin or cephalosporin hypersensitivity: see footnote 5

. . . under 2 months of age	As above plus Group B streptococci *E. coli* and other Gram-negative coliforms *L. monocytogenes*	Cefotaxime ***and*** Benzylpenicillin ***and*** Gentamicin[6] (for first week) [See doses in 'Septicaemia (under 2 months of age)' section]	Gram–negative 3 weeks GBS / Listeria 2–3 weeks See footnote 7 re Gentamicin dosing/monitoring Substitute Benzylpenicillin with Vancomycin if possibility of penicillin-resistant pneumococci[3]
. . . with shunt infection, post-neurosurgery, head trauma or CSF leak	As for over 2 months of age plus *S. epidermidis* *S. aureus* Gram-negative coliforms incl. *P. aeruginosa*	Vancomycin 15 mg/kg (500 mg) iv 6H ***and*** Ceftazidime 50 mg/kg (2 g) iv 8H	10 days minimum
. . . contact prophylaxis	*N. meningitidis*	Rifampicin 10 mg/kg (600 mg) po 12H	2 days (alternatives: see table 27.3)
. . . contact prophylaxis	*H. influenzae* type b[4]	Rifampicin 20 mg/kg (600 mg) po 24H	4 days (alternatives: see table 27.3)
Postseptal (orbital) cellulitis	*S. aureus* *H. influenzae* spp. *S. pneumoniae* *M. catarrhalis* Gram-negatives Anaerobes	Flucloxacillin 50 mg/kg (2 g) iv 6H ***and*** Cefotaxime 50 mg/kg (2 g) iv 6H	10 days minimum Rule out meningitis Consider adding Metronidazole if not responding

CENTRAL NERVOUS SYSTEM / EYE (continued)

Infection	*Likely organisms*	*Initial antimicrobials*[1] *( ) = maximum dose*	*Duration of treatment*[2] *and other comments*
Preseptal (periorbital) cellulitis			
. . . mild (outpatient)	Group A streptococci *S. aureus* *H. influenzae* spp.[4]	Amoxicillin/Clavulanate [400/57 mg per 5 mL] 22.5 mg/kg (875 mg) [Amoxycillin component] = 0.3 mL/kg (11 mL) po 12H	7–10 days Consider non-infective cause in trivial cases
. . . moderate (inpatient)	As above	Flucloxacillin 50 mg/kg (2 g) iv 6H	
. . . severe, or not responding, or under 5 yrs of age and non-Hib immunised	As above plus *H. influenzae* type b[4]	Flucloxacillin 50 mg/kg (2 g) iv 6H ***and*** Cefotaxime 50 mg/kg (2 g) iv 6H	

CARDIOVASCULAR

Infection	*Likely organisms*	*Initial antimicrobials*	*Duration of treatment and other comments*
Endocarditis			
... native valve or homograft	Viridans streptococci Other streptococci *Enterococcus* spp. *S. aureus*	Benzylpenicillin 60 mg/kg (2 g) iv 6H ***and*** Gentamicin 2.5 mg/kg (240 mg) iv 8H* ***and*** Flucloxacillin 50 mg/kg (2 g) iv 4–6H	4–6 weeks *Gentamicin 1 mg/kg (80 mg) iv 8H for 1–2 weeks when used only for synergy
. . . artificial valve or post surgery	As above plus *S. epidermidis*	Vancomycin 15 mg/kg (500 mg) iv 6H ***and*** Gentamicin 2.5 mg/kg (240 mg) iv 8H*	Gentamicin monitoring is generally not required when low dose is used for synergy in this setting

Endocarditis prophylaxis			
. . . low risk and dental or upper respiratory tract procedure	Viridans streptococci *S. aureus* *S. pneumoniae* Other Gram-positive cocci *Enterococcus* spp.	Amoxicillin 50 mg/kg (2 g) Local anaesthetic: give po 1 hr before procedure General anaesthetic: give iv with induction	Penicillin hypersensitivity: substitute Amoxicillin with Clindamycin 20 mg/kg (600 mg) po or iv
. . . high risk or procedure involving gastrointestinal or genitourinary tract	As above plus Gram-negative coliforms	Amoxicillin 50 mg/kg (2 g) iv or im ***and*** Gentamicin 2.5 mg/kg (240 mg) iv or im before procedure, ***followed 6 hrs later by*** Amoxicillin 25 mg/kg (500 mg) po or iv or im	Penicillin hypersensitivity: substitute Amoxicillin with Vancomycin 20 mg/kg (1 g) iv See footnote 7 re Gentamicin dosing/monitoring
GASTROINTESTINAL			
Diarrhoea			
. . . *Salmonella* spp. isolated in infant under 3 months of age or in immunocompromised	*Salmonella* spp.	Cefotaxime 50 mg/kg (2 g) iv 6H	3–5 days Antibiotic treatment is generally unnecessary for most other organisms
. . . antibiotic associated	*C. difficile*	Metronidazole 7.5 mg/kg (400 mg) po 8H	7–10 days
Giardiasis	*G. lamblia*	Metronidazole 30 mg/kg (2 g) po daily ***or*** Tinidazole 50 mg/kg (2 g) po	3 days Single dose

GASTROINTESTINAL (continued)

Infection	*Likely organisms*	*Initial antimicrobials*[1] *( ) = maximum dose*	*Duration of treatment*[2] *and other comments*
Peritonitis or ascending cholangitis	Gram-negative coliforms Anaerobes *Enterococcus* spp.	Benzylpenicillin 60 mg/kg (2 g) iv 6H ***and*** Gentamicin 7.5 mg/kg (360 mg) iv daily [< 10 yrs] 6 mg/kg (360 mg) iv daily [≥ 10 yrs] ***and*** Metronidazole 15 mg/kg (1 g) iv stat, then 7.5 mg/kg (500 mg) iv 8H	Up to 14 days See footnote 7 re Gentamicin dosing/monitoring
Threadworm (Pinworm)	*Enterobius vermicularis*	Mebendazole 50 mg po [< 10 kg] 100 mg po [≥ 10 kg]	Single dose; may need to repeat after 14 days Treat whole family

GENITOURINARY

Infection	*Likely organisms*	*Initial antimicrobials*[1] *( ) = maximum dose*	*Duration of treatment*[2] *and other comments*
Urinary tract infection			
. . . over 6 months of age and not sick	*E. coli* *P. mirabilis* *K. oxytoca* Other Gram-negatives	Trimethoprim 4 mg/kg (150 mg) po 12H ***or*** if syrup is necessary then Co-trimoxazole [Trimethoprim/Sulphamethoxazole 8/40 mg per mL] 0.5 mL/kg (20 mL) po 12H	5 days
. . . under 6 months of age or sick or acute pyelonephritis	As above plus *Enterococcus* spp.	Benzylpenicillin 60 mg/kg (2 g) iv 6H ***and*** Gentamicin 7.5 mg/kg (360 mg) iv daily [< 10 yrs] 6 mg/kg (360 mg) iv daily [≥ 10 yrs] [For infants under 1 month of age, see doses in 'Septicaemia in neonate' section]	5–7 days for UTI 10–14 days for pyelonephritis See footnote 7 re Gentamicin dosing/monitoring
. . . prophylaxis	As above	Trimethoprim 2 mg/kg (150 mg) po daily ***or*** if syrup is necessary then Co-trimoxazole [Trimethoprim/Sulphamethoxazole 8/40 mg per mL] 0.25 mL/kg (20 mL) po daily	

RESPIRATORY

Infection	*Likely organisms*	*Initial antimicrobials*[1] *( ) = maximum dose*	*Duration of treatment*[2] *and other comments*
Epiglottitis	*H. influenzae* type b[4]	Ceftriaxone 100 mg/kg (2 g) iv followed by 50 mg/kg (1 g) 24 hrs later	2 doses only
Gingivostomatitis			
. . . in immunocompromised	Herpes simplex virus	Aciclovir 500 mg/m² iv 8H [age 3 months–12 yrs] 10 mg/kg iv 8H [age > 12 yrs]	7 days Treatment is only recommended for severe primary disease in the immunocompromised
Otitis externa			
. . . acute diffuse	*S. aureus* *S. epidermidis* *P. aeruginosa* *Proteus* spp. *Klebsiella* spp.	Clean ear canal Topical steroid/antibiotic [e.g. Sofradex®] drops [± insertion of wick soaked in drops if ear canal oedematous]	7 days
. . . acute localised (furuncle) ± cellulitis	*S. aureus* Group A streptococci	Flucloxacillin 50 mg/kg (2 g) iv 6H	7–10 days
. . . failure of first line treatment, high fever or severe persistent pain	As above plus *P. aeruginosa*	Ticarcillin/Clavulanate 50 mg/kg (3 g) [Ticarcillin component] iv 6H	14 days minimum Consider fungal infection
Otitis media	Viruses *S. pneumoniae* *M. catarrhalis* *H. influenzae* spp. Group A streptococci	Consider no antibiotics for 48 hrs if over 2 yrs of age ***or*** Amoxicillin 15 mg/kg (500 mg) po 8H	5 days Consider high dose Amoxicillin 30 mg/kg (500 mg) po 8H if not responding

RESPIRATORY (continued)

Infection	*Likely organisms*	***Initial antimicrobials***[1] ***( ) = maximum dose***	***Duration of treatment***[2] ***and other comments***
Pertussis	*B. pertussis*	Clarithromycin 7.5 mg/kg (500 mg) po 12H	7 days Can be given up to 3 weeks after contact with index case
Pneumonia			
. . . mild (outpatient)	Viruses *S. pneumoniae* *H. influenzae* spp.	Amoxicillin 15 mg/kg (500 mg) po 8H	7–10 days Consider admission for all children under 1 yr of age
. . . moderate (inpatient)	As above	Benzylpenicillin 60 mg/kg (2 g) iv 6H	
. . . mild or moderate where *M. pneumoniae* is suspected (especially > 5 yrs of age)	As above plus *M. pneumoniae*	Roxithromycin 4 mg/kg (150 mg) po 12H	10 days
. . . severe systemic toxicity or pneumatocoele	As above plus *S. aureus* Group A streptococci Gram-negatives	Flucloxacillin 50 mg/kg (2 g) iv 4H ***and*** Gentamicin 7.5 mg/kg (360 mg) iv daily [< 10 yrs] 6 mg/kg (360 mg) iv daily [≥ 10 yrs] ***and*** consider Roxithromycin as above	10 days minimum
Tonsillitis	Viruses Group A streptococci *A. haemolyticum*	Consider no antibiotics [particularly if < 4 yrs] ***or*** Phenoxymethylpenicillin [Penicillin V] 250 mg po 12H [< 10 yrs] 500 mg po 12H [≥ 10 yrs]	10 days

SKIN/SOFT TISSUE/BONE

Infection	*Likely organisms*	*Initial antimicrobials*[1] *( ) = maximum dose*	*Duration of treatment*[2] *and other comments*
Adenitis	*S. aureus* Group A streptococci Oral anaerobes	Flucloxacillin 50 mg/kg (2 g) iv 6H	10–14 days
Bites (animal/human)	Viridans streptococci *S. aureus* Group A streptococci Oral anaerobes *E. corrodens* *Pasteurella* spp. (cat and dog) *C. canimorsus* (dog)	Amoxicillin/Clavulanate [400/57 mg per 5 mL] 22.5 mg/kg (875 mg) [Amoxycillin component] = 0.3 mL/kg (11 mL) po 12H	3–5 days for prophylaxis 7–14 days for treatment Check tetanus immunisation status and consider risk of hepatitis B and C, and HIV * Metronidazole should be given orally whenever possible
. . . if severe, penetrating injuries, esp. involving joints or tendons	As above	Cefotaxime 50 mg/kg (2 g) iv 6H ***and*** Metronidazole 7.5 mg/kg (400 mg) po 8H 7.5 mg/kg (500 mg) iv 8H *	
Cellulitis			
. . . mild (outpatient)	Group A streptococci *S. aureus*	Phenoxymethylpenicillin [Penicillin V] 10 mg/kg (500 mg) po 6H ***or*** if bite/injury or not responding, use Flucloxacillin 25 mg/kg (500 mg) po 6H	5–10 days Consider adding Clindamycin 10 mg/kg (600 mg) iv 6H if rapid progression suggestive of necrotising fasciitis or features of toxic shock syndrome
. . . moderate/severe (inpatient)	As above	Flucloxacillin 50 mg/kg (2 g) iv 6H	
. . . if facial cellulitis in child under 5 yrs of age and non-Hib immunised	As above plus *S. pneumoniae* *H. influenzae* spp.[4]	Flucloxacillin 50 mg/kg (2 g) iv 6H ***and*** Cefotaxime 50 mg/kg (2 g) iv 6H	

SKIN/SOFT TISSUE/BONE (continued)

Infection	*Likely organisms*	*Initial antimicrobials*[1] *( ) = maximum dose*	*Duration of treatment*[2] *and other comments*
Head lice	*Pediculus humanus* var. *capitis*	1% Permethrin liquid or cream rinse	Repeat after one week
Impetigo	Group A streptococci *S. aureus*	Mupirocin 2% ointment top 8H if localised ***or*** Flucloxacillin 15 mg/kg (500 mg) po 6H	5–10 days
Osteomyelitis	*S. aureus* Group A streptococci *S. pneumoniae*	Flucloxacillin 50 mg/kg (2 g) iv 4–6H	3 weeks for uncomplicated cases[2]
. . . if under 5 yrs of age and non-Hib immunised	As above plus *H. influenzae* type b[4]	Flucloxacillin 50 mg/kg (2 g) iv 4–6H ***and*** Cefotaxime 50 mg/kg (2 g) iv 6–8H	
. . . in patient with sickle cell anaemia	As above plus *Salmonella* spp.	Flucloxacillin 50 mg/kg (2 g) iv 4–6H ***and*** Cefotaxime 50 mg/kg (2 g) iv 6H	
. . . with penetrating foot injury	As above plus *P. aeruginosa*	Ticarcillin/Clavulanate 50 mg/kg (3 g) [Ticarcillin component] iv 6H ***and*** Gentamicin 7.5 mg/kg (360 mg) iv daily [< 10 yrs] 6 mg/kg (360 mg) iv daily [≥ 10 yrs]	Surgical intervention important See footnote 7 re Gentamicin dosing/monitoring
Scabies	*Sarcoptes scabiei*	5% Permethrin cream top	One application from neck down; may need to repeat after 14 days Treat whole family

Septic arthritis	As for osteomyelitis	As for osteomyelitis	3 weeks for uncomplicated cases[2] Always consider surgical drainage
Shingles			
. . . in immunocompromised or involving eye	Varicella zoster virus	Aciclovir 500 mg/m² iv 8H [age 3 months–12 yrs] 10 mg/kg iv 8H [age > 12 yrs] ***and*** Aciclovir ointment to eye 5 times/day	7 days Shingles in immunocompetent children does not generally require treatment
SEPTICAEMIA (UNDER 2 MONTHS OF AGE)			
Septicaemia (age < 2 months)			
. . . community-acquired infection	Group B streptococci *E. coli* and other Gram-negative coliforms *L. monocytogenes* *H. influenzae* spp.[4] plus those listed below for 'Septicaemia with unknown CSF'	Benzylpenicillin 60 mg/kg iv 12H [first week of life] 6H [1–4 weeks of age] 4H [> 4 weeks of age] ***and*** Gentamicin 2.5 mg/kg iv 12H [first week of life] 8H [> 1 week of age]	Substitute Benzylpenicillin with Flucloxacillin 50 mg/kg iv 12 H [first week of life] 8 H [1–4 weeks of age] 6 H [> 4 weeks of age] if infection with *S. aureus* suspected Duration depends on culture results
. . . if meningitis suspected	As above	Benzylpenicillin ***and*** Gentamicin[6] as above ***and*** Cefotaxime 50 mg/kg iv 12H [first week of life] 6H [> 1 week of age]	See footnote 7 re Gentamicin dosing/monitoring
. . . if abdominal source suspected	As above plus Anaerobes	Benzylpenicillin ***and*** Gentamicin as above ***and*** Metronidazole 15 mg/kg iv stat, then 7.5 mg/kg iv 12H	Premature neonates require special dosing consideration

SEPTICAEMIA (OVER 2 MONTHS OF AGE)

Infection	*Likely organisms*	***Initial antimicrobials***[1] ***( ) = maximum dose***	***Duration of treatment***[2] ***and other comments***
Septicaemia with unknown CSF **(www.snipurl.com/vanco)**	*S. pneumoniae*[3] *N. meningitidis* *S. aureus* Group A streptococci Gram-negatives	Vancomycin 15 mg/kg (500 mg) iv 6H[3] ***and*** Cefotaxime 50 mg/kg (2 g) iv 6H	See notes below
Septicaemia with normal CSF	As above	Flucloxacillin 50 mg/kg (2 g) iv 4H ***and*** Gentamicin 7.5 mg/kg (360 mg) iv daily [< 10 yrs] 6 mg/kg (360 mg) iv daily [≥ 10 yrs]	Consider adding Clindamycin 10 mg/kg (600 mg) iv 6H if suspect Gram-positive toxic shock syndrome Duration depends on culture results See footnote 7 re Gentamicin dosing/monitoring Consult local protocols and also consider anaerobic and fungal infection in neutropenic patients
. . . in non-Hib immunised	As above plus *H. influenzae* type b[4]	Flucloxacillin 50 mg/kg (2 g) iv 4H ***and*** Cefotaxime 50 mg/kg (2 g) iv 6H	
. . . in neutropenic patient	As above plus *Enterococcus* spp. *P. aeruginosa*	Ticarcillin/Clavulanate 50 mg/kg (3 g) [Ticarcillin component] iv 6H ***and*** Gentamicin 7.5 mg/kg (360 mg) iv daily [< 10 yrs] 6 mg/kg (360 mg) iv daily [≥ 10 yrs]	
. . . in neutropenic patient with potential line infection	As above plus Gram-positive cocci incl. *S. epidermidis*	Ticarcillin/Clavulanate as above ***and*** Gentamicin as above ***and*** consider Vancomycin 15 mg/kg (500 mg) iv 6H	

NOTES TO ANTIMICROBIAL GUIDELINES

These guidelines have been developed to assist doctors with their choice of initial empiric treatment. The choice of antimicrobial, dose and frequency of administration for continuing treatment may require adjustment according to the clinical situation. The recommendations are not intended to be proscriptive and alternative regimens may also be appropriate.

1 Antimicrobial choice

- Antibiotics should be changed to narrow spectrum agents once sensitivities are known.
- Dose adjustments may be necessary for neonates, and for children with renal or hepatic impairment.
- Alternative antimicrobial regimens may be more appropriate for neonates, immunocompromised patients or others with a special infection risk (e.g. cystic fibrosis, sickle cell anaemia).
- Resistance to antimicrobials is an increasing problem worldwide. Of particular concern is the increasing incidence of penicillin-resistant pneumococci (see footnote 3). It is important to take into account local resistance patterns when using these guidelines.
- Cefotaxime can usually (except in neonates) be substituted with:
  Ceftriaxone 100 mg/kg (2 g) iv daily or 50 mg/kg (1 g) iv 12H.

2 Duration of treatment

Duration of treatment is given as a guide only and may vary with the clinical situation. 'Step down' from intravenous to oral treatment is appropriate in many cases. **Durations given generally refer to the minimum total intravenous and oral treatment.**

3 Penicillin-resistant pneumococci (www.snipurl.com/vanco)

The prevalence of invasive strains that are highly resistant to penicillin or cephalosporins in Melbourne remains low. Cefotaxime remains the drug of first choice for the empiric treatment of meningitis. However, Vancomycin should be added if *S. pneumoniae* is suspected (www.snipurl.com/vanco). This should be stopped if sensitivity to Cefotaxime is shown, as will be the case with most isolates. The prevalence of resistant strains is being monitored and this recommendation may change.

Penicillin remains the drug of first choice for the empiric treatment of suspected pneumococcal pneumonia and other non-CNS infections, regardless of susceptibility. High doses of penicillin overcome resistance in this setting and should be used for confirmed non-CNS infection caused by penicillin-resistant pneumococci.

4 Invasive *H. influenzae* type b disease

Since the introduction of *H. influenzae* type b (Hib) immunisation, there has been a dramatic decline in the incidence of invasive disease. However, in children with potential invasive disease, who are not fully immunised against Hib, therapy should include cover against Hib.

5 Treatment of meningitis in patients with hypersensitivity to penicillins or cephalosporins

In patients with a history of severe (anaphylactic) penicillin hypersensitivity, avoid cephalosporins: use Chloramphenicol 25 mg/kg (1 g) iv 6H and Vancomycin 15 mg/kg (500 mg) iv 6H.

6 Empiric treatment of neonatal meningitis

Gentamicin is recommended in this setting to provide double Gram-negative cover, and for synergy with Benzylpenicillin against *Listeria monocytogenes* and group B streptococci.

7 Gentamicin dosing/monitoring

Once-daily administration of Gentamicin is safe and effective for most patients. Certain patients, such as neonates and those with cystic fibrosis, endocarditis or renal failure, may require special dosing consideration.

The regimen for monitoring Gentamicin levels is different for once-daily and 8, 12 or 18H dosing, and depends on renal function:

Once-daily dosing

- Normal renal function—if the patient is to have more than 3 doses, the trough level (pre-dose) should be checked before the third dose and then every 3 days (target level < 1 mg/L).
- Abnormal renal function—trough levels may need to be checked earlier and more frequently (target level < 1 mg/L).
- Renal failure—levels should be checked post-dose at 2, 12 and 24 hours, and adjusted accordingly. The results should be discussed with a specialist familiar with therapeutic drug monitoring.

8, 12 and 18 hourly dosing

- The trough level should be checked before the fourth dose and peak level 1 hour after the start of the fourth dose (target trough < 2 mg/L, target peak 5–10 mg/L).
- Levels should be repeated every 3 days, or more frequently if levels are inappropriate or if renal function is abnormal.

APPENDIX 4
FORMULAE

ETT tube size and position (p. 3)

Tube size (internal diameter) = (age/4) + 4 mm (for patients over 1 year of age)

Depth of insertion is approximately (age/2) + 12 cm from the lower lip

Anion gap (p. 89)

Anion gap = Na – bicarbonate – Cl

Bicarbonate administration

mmol of HCO_3 required = basic deficit (mmol/L) × weight (kg) × 0.3 (child)

mmol of HCO_3 required = basic deficit (mmol/L) × weight (kg) × 0.5 (newborn)

Dose Na replacement (p. 95)

Dose of Na^+ (mmol) = bodyweight × 0.8 × (140 – current serum Na^+)

Additives (p. 96)

Molar potassium chloride (0.75 g in 10 mL) = 1 mmol/mL of K^+ and Cl^-

Sodium chloride (20%) = 3.4 mmol/mL of Na^+ and Cl^-

Molar sodium bicarbonate (8.4%) = 1 mmol/mL of Na^+ and HCO_3^-

Calcium gluconate 10% = 0.22 mmol/mL of Ca^{2+}, which is 8.9 mg/mL of Ca^{2+}

Magnesium chloride for injection (0.48 g anhydrous in 5 mL) = 1 mmol/mL of Mg^{2+}

Conversion factors (p. 98)

Sodium chloride 1 g contains 17 mmol Na and 17 mmol Cl

Potassium chloride 1 g contains 13 mmol K and 13 mmol Cl

Sodium bicarbonate 1 g contains 12 mmol Na and 12 mmol HCO_3

Formulae (p. 98)

Anion gap = Na – (bicarbonate + Cl); normal <12

Number mmol = mEq/valence = mass (mg)/mol. wt

Sodium deficit: mL 20% NaCl = wt × 0.2 × (140 – serum Na)

Water deficit (mL) = 600 × wt (kg) × [1 – (140/Na)] (if body Na normal)

Non-catabolic anuria: urea rises of 3–5 mmol/L per day

Bicarbonate dose (mmol) = base excess × wt ÷ 3 (give 1/2 this. Note: this is different in neonates)

Osmolality serum = 2Na + glucose + urea (normal 270 – 295 mmol/L)

kcal (p. 118)

$$\text{kcal} = \frac{\text{mJ} \times 1000}{4.2}$$

BMI (p. 125)

BMI = bodyweight in kg divided by the square of height in metres (kg/m^2). Standard growth charts now include BMI centile charts.

- Overweight = BMI between 85–95th centile for age and sex.
- Obesity = BMI greater than 95th centile for age and sex.

Burns fluid resuscitation calculations. (See Fig. 17.2, p 265)

Fluid resuscitation

3 × kg × % = ...mL

See Figure 17.2.

Fluid volume

Use 3 mL/kg bodyweight per 1% burn surface area (BSA) for the first 24 h. In less severe burns 2 mL/kg bodyweight per 1% BSA may be sufficient.

Type of fluid

Use 4% normal serum albumin solution (NSAS) and Hartmann's solution, 50% of each type of solution is used concurrently.

Fluid maintenance

Type of fluid

Use 0.45% saline in 5% dextrose to provide extra sodium.

Rate of infusion (first 24 hours)

- First 8 h: one-half resuscitation fluid plus one-third maintenance fluid.
- Second 8 h: one-quarter resuscitation fluid plus one-third maintenance fluid.
- Third 8 h: one-quarter resuscitation fluid plus one-third maintenance fluid.

The 24 h period commences from the time of burning, not from the time of admission.

Rate of infusion (second 24 hours and onwards)

- Replacement fluid: approximately one-half of the volume for the first 24 h.
- Maintenance fluid as before.
- Total volume is given at an even rate over 24 h.
- The volume and type of fluid given are adjusted according to urine flow and electrolyte estimations, then decreased as the shock diminishes over the succeeding days. Diuresis occurs 2–3 days post-burn.

Osmolality (p. 328)

Calculated values

Serum osmolality = $Na^+ \times 2$ + glucose + urea

Adjusted Na^+ = plasma $Na^+ + 0.3 \times$ (plasma glucose − 5.5)

Transfusion volume (p. 413)

Packed red cells (mL) = (desired Hb − actual Hb) × weight (kg) × 4

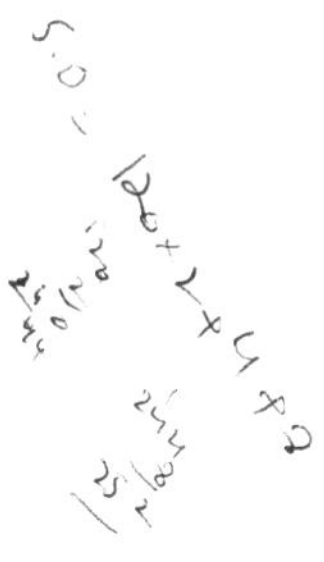

INDEX

Note: Bold page numbers refer to diagrams and tables.

PostOp manag. in children ̄c Kasai.
Any child ̄c Kasai who becomes unwell ̄c fever or hypothermia & who does not have an obvious cause sh be considered cholangitis. Other signs ↑ jaundice, ↓ stool pigment, ↑ WCC, ↑ transaminases.
— needs broad spectrum AB.

Vit. suppl ADEK.

Vacc. — usual
+ ~~pneumo~~ |

Med: Vit + proph. AB. → to prevent cholangitis.

Ongoing compl → Portal HT, → HSmegaly, hypersplenism, TCP. oesoph varices, GI bleeding, ascites.